CARDIAC EMERGENCIES

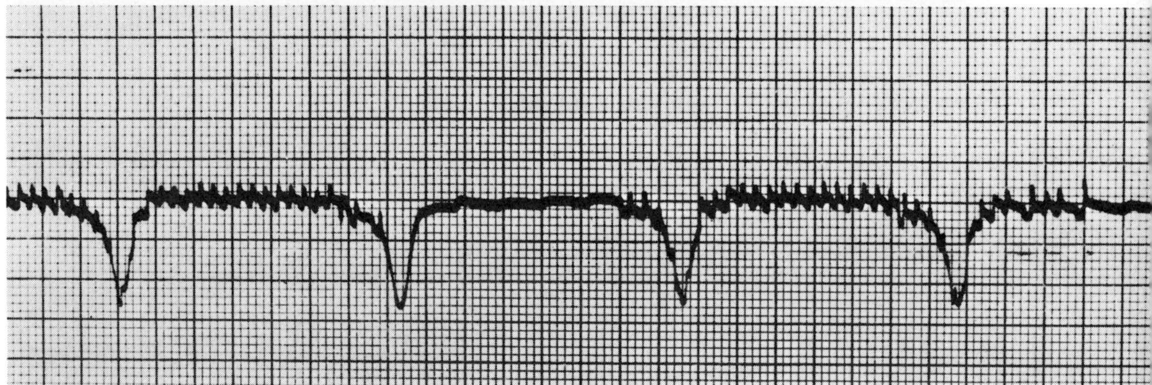

MELVIN M. SCHEINMAN, M.D.
Professor of Medicine
Division of Cardiology
University of California
San Francisco, California

1984
W.B. Saunders Company
Philadelphia • London • Toronto • Mexico City • Rio de Janeiro • Sydney • Tokyo

W. B. Saunders Company: West Washington Square
Philadelphia, PA 19105

1 St. Anne's Road
Eastbourne, East Sussex BN21 3UN, England

1 Goldthorne Avenue
Toronto, Ontario M8Z 5T9, Canada

Apartado 26370—Cedro 512
Mexico 4, D.F., Mexico

Rua Coronel Cabrita, 8
Sao Cristovao Caixa Postal 21176
Rio de Janeiro, Brazil

9 Waltham Street
Artarmon, N.S.W. 2064, Australia

Ichibancho, Central Bldg., 22-1 Ichibancho
Chiyoda-Ku, Tokyo 102, Japan

Library of Congress Cataloging in Publication Data

Scheinman, Melvin M.

Cardiac emergencies.

1. Heart—Diseases—Treatment. 2. Medical emergencies. I. Title. [DNLM: 1. Emergencies. 2. Heart diseases—Therapy. WG 205 S319c]

RC683.8.S33 1984 616.1'2025 83–4480

ISBN 0–7216–7958–7

Cardiac Emergencies ISBN 0–7216–7958–7

Last digit is the print number: 9 8 7 6 5 4 3 2 1

DEDICATION

This book is dedicated
to my parents, (Sam and Sylvia Scheinman)
my wife, and my children.
Their dedication and love is gratefully appreciated.

CONTRIBUTORS

JOSEPH A. ABBOTT, M.D.
Clinical Professor of Medicine, University of California, San Francisco

CHARLES E. BECKER, M.D.
Associate Professor of Medicine, University of California, San Francisco; Medical Director, Northern California Occupational Health Center, San Francisco General Hospital Medical Center, San Francisco, California

NEAL L. BENOWITZ, M.D.
Associate Professor of Medicine, University of California, San Francisco; Attending Physician, San Francisco General Hospital Medical Center, San Francisco, California

J. DAVID BRISTOW, M.D.
Professor of Medicine, Director, Research and Training, Cardiology Oregon Health Sciences University, Portland, Oregon

H. F. CHAMBERS, M.D.
Fellow, Division of Infectious Disease, Department of Medicine, San Francisco General Hospital, San Francisco; Clinical Instructor in Medicine, Department of Medicine, University of California, San Francisco, California

KANU CHATTERJEE, M.B., F.R.C.P.
Lucie Stern Professor of Cardiology, Professor of Medicine; Associate Chief, Cardiovascular Division; Director, Coronary Care Unit, San Francisco, California

MELVIN D. CHEITLIN, M.D.
Professor of Medicine, University of California, San Francisco; Associate Chief of Cardiology, San Francisco General Hospital, San Francisco, California

ERIC H. CONN, M.D.
Associate in Medicine; Director, Coronary Care Unit, Duke University Medical Center, Durham, North Carolina

JESSE DAVIS, M.D.
Assistant Clinical Professor of Medicine, University of California, San Francisco; Attending Cardiologist, Presbyterian Hospital of Pacific Medical Center, San Francisco, California

ROMAN W. DeSANCTIS, M.D.
Professor of Medicine, Harvard Medical School; Physician and Director of Clinical Cardiology, Massachusetts General Hospital, Boston, Massachusetts

ROBERT M. DOROGHAZI, M.D.
Cardiologist, The Boone Clinic, Columbia, Missouri

NORA GOLDSCHLAGER, M.D.
Associate Clinical Professor of Medicine, University of California, San Francisco; Director, Coronary Care Unit, and Director, Electrocardiographic Laboratory, San Francisco General Hospital, San Francisco, California

E. WILLIAM HANCOCK, M.D.
Professor of Medicine, Stanford University School of Medicine, Stanford, California

DEAN J. KEREIAKES, M.D.
Fellow in Cardiology, University of California, San Francisco; Fellow in Cardiology, University of California Hospital and Fort Miley Veterans Administration Medical Center, San Francisco, California

ROBERT M. LESTER, M.D.

Assistant Clinical Professor of Medicine, University of Pennsylvania, Philadelphia; Director, Cardiac Intensive Care, The Graduate Hospital, Philadelphia, Pennsylvania

JAY W. MASON, M.D.

Chief, Cardiology Division, University of Utah Medical Center, Salt Lake City, Utah

BARRY M. MASSIE, M.D.

Associate Professor of Medicine, University of California, San Francisco; Associate Staff, Cardiovascular Research Institute; Director, Coronary Care Unit and Hypertensive Research Unit, Veterans Administration Medical Center, San Francisco, California

MICHAEL A. MATTHAY, M.D.

Assistant Professor of Medicine and Anesthesia; Associate Director, Intensive Care Unit, University of California, San Francisco; Attending Pulmonologist and Critical Care Specialist, Moffitt Hospital, San Francisco, California

JOHN MILLS, M.D.

Associate Professor of Medicine, Microbiology, Laboratory Medicine, and Clinical Pharmacology, University of California, San Francisco; Chief, Infectious Diseases, San Francisco General Hospital, San Francisco, California

FRED MORADY, M.D.

Assistant Professor of Medicine, University of California, San Francisco; Attending Physician, Moffitt Hospital, San Francisco, California

PAUL PENTEL, M.D.

Assistant Professor of Medicine, University of Minnesota Medical School, Minneapolis; Attending Physician, Hennepin County Medical Center, Minneapolis, Minnesota

DOROTHEE PERLOFF, M.D.

Clinical Professor of Medicine, University of California, San Francisco School of Medicine; Assistant in Electrocardiography, Chief, Hypertension Clinic, and Attending Physician, University of California Hospitals, San Francisco, California

ROBERT W. PETERS, M.D.

Associate Professor of Medicine, University of Maryland School of Medicine, Baltimore; Director, Coronary Care Unit, Veterans Administration Hospital, Baltimore, Maryland

THOMAS A. PORTS, M.D.

Associate Professor of Medicine, and Director, Cardiac Catheterization Laboratories, Division of Cardiology, University of California, San Francisco, California

JON ROSENBERG, M.D.

Assistant Clinical Professor of Medicine, University of California, San Francisco; Member of Attending Staff of Medical Service, San Francisco General Hospital Medical Center, San Francisco, California

A. A. SASAHARA, M.D.

Professor of Medicine, Harvard Medical School; Chief, Medical Service, Veterans Administration Medical Center, West Roxbury, Massachusetts

MELVIN M. SCHEINMAN, M.D.

Professor of Medicine, School of Medicine, University of California, San Francisco; Chief, Electrocardiography and Clinical Cardiac Electrophysiology Section, University of California, San Francisco, California

M. SCHOOLMAN, M.D.

Instructor in Medicine, Harvard Medical School; Research Fellow in Medicine, Veterans Administration Medical Center, West Roxbury, Massachusetts

G. V. R. K. SHARMA, M.D.

Assistant Professor of Medicine, Harvard Medical School; Director, MICU-CCU, Veterans Administration Medical Center, West Roxbury, Massachusetts

PAUL SIMPSON, M.D.

Assistant Professor of Medicine, University of California, San Francisco; Chief, Hypertension Unit, Veterans Administration Hospital, San Francisco, California

EVE E. SLATER, M.D.

Assistant Professor of Medicine, Harvard Medical School; Chief, Hypertension Unit, Massachusetts General Hospital, Boston, Massachusetts

BONNIE SUDDUTH, R.N., N.P.

Supervisor, Pacemaker Surveillance Center, Veterans Administration Medical Center, San Francisco, California

RUEY J. SUNG, M.D.

Associate Professor of Medicine, University of California, San Francisco; Director, Cardiac Electrophysiology Laboratory, Moffitt Hospital, University of California, San Francisco, California

CHARLES D. SWERDLOW, M.D.

Clinical Assistant Professor of Medicine, University of Washington; Director of Cardiac Electrophysiology, Deaconess Hospital, Spokane, Washington

GALEN S. WAGNER, M.D.

Associate Professor, Duke University Medical Center, Durham; Director, Coronary Care Chairman, Department of Medicine Clinical Clerkship Grading Committee, Duke University Medical Center, Durham, North Carolina

JEANINE P. WIENER-KRONISH, M.D.

Instructor of Medicine, University of California, San Francisco; Attending Pulmonologist, University of California, Moffitt and San Francisco General Hospitals, San Francisco, California

FOREWORD

The present text attempts to pull together advances made in the management of patients with cardiovascular emergencies. The last decade has been characterized by the acquisition of new knowledge and technical advances that have been well utilized in the management of these patients. In this text, we cover the broad range of cardiac emergencies with emphasis on the practical approach to patient assessment and therapy.

The newer knowledge and techniques have been particularly fruitful for patients with acute myocardial infarction, and in this text we review newer aspects of drug therapy as well as aggressive medical and surgical approaches. Our approach in the management of patients with cardiac arrhythmias has swung from the purely empiric to that which emphasizes basic mechanisms and a more profound knowledge of antiarrhythmic drug action. Moreover, the revolution in pacemaker design and function makes it mandatory for physicians to be prepared to handle emergency malfunctions. The spectrum of cardiac trauma, aortic dissection, and acute cardiac valvular problems is fully explored.

The sections on drug effects in cardiac emergencies and adverse cardiovascular effects in drug-overdosed patients are particularly appropriate for the practitioner who is required to manage these patients. Finally, wise clinicians were taught that it is difficult to separate cardiac from pulmonary function in the critically ill cardiac patient. To this end, the text addresses the problems of management of patients with acute pulmonary embolism and those with acute respiratory emergencies.

I sincerely hope that this text will prove useful for both medical students and practitioners involved in the care of such patients. It is my profound hope that this book will in some measure result in the alleviation of pain and salvage of life.

CONTENTS

1

Acute Myocardial Infarction

ERIC H. CONN
ROBERT M. LESTER
and GALEN S. WAGNER

Ischemic heart disease is the most widespread health problem in our society. More than 600,000 people die each year from arteriosclerotic coronary disease and an additional 1.3 million sustain a nonfatal myocardial infarction.[80] Many others have congestive heart failure secondary to ischemic myocardial damage. The magnitude of this problem makes it inevitable that many physicians will become involved with the recognition and treatment of ischemic heart disease. The purpose of this chapter is to set forth clinically useful guidelines in the diagnosis and management of acute myocardial infarction derived from recently acquired data. It is recognized that there are many important areas of controversy regarding such topics as essential drug therapy and rehabilitation of the patient with acute infarction. Discussion of many of these is beyond the scope of this chapter, although reference will occasionally be made to promising areas for scientific investigation. Consideration of cardiac failure and conduction disorders has intentionally been omitted since they are discussed in other chapters.

PREHOSPITAL PLANS

The Coronary Prodrome

It is estimated that one half of the mortality associated with acute myocardial infarction occurs prior to hospital admission.[70, 96, 120, 142] Since most of these fatalities take place within the first hour of symptoms,[142] a reduction in mortality is contingent upon out-of-hospital treatment of these individuals either before or within minutes of the acute event.

The classical clinical features of acute myocardial infarction have been enumerated by Herrick.[79] Chest pain, present in most such patients, is usually described as substernal in location, often with radiation to the neck, jaw, arms, or back. It typically persists for half an hour or longer and requires opiates for relief. Associated symptoms may include diaphoresis, nausea, vomiting, breathlessness, weakness, dizziness, presyncope, and a feeling of impending doom.

Unfortunately, this clinical picture is often absent or modified, and warning symptoms other than pain may occur. The reported incidence of prodromal symptoms prior to infarction or sudden death ranges from 10 to 68 per cent,[181] thus underscoring the importance of early recognition by both patient and physician of warning symptoms when present. Solomon et al.[177] observed prodromal symptoms in 65 per cent of patients admitted to the coronary care unit with acute myocardial infarction. Chest pain was present in 91 per cent of cases and most individuals were noted to have pre-existing angina. Alonzo et al.[3] studied antecedent symptoms in a population of 169 hospitalized patients with acute myocardial infarction and compared them with symptoms in 138 individuals who died before admission. Although two thirds of those in both groups reported some warning symptoms, only 27 per cent of the hospitalized cohort and 36 per cent of the out-of-hospital group had consulted a physician before the event. The mean duration of symptoms was 29 days in those who were admitted, but only 10.5 days in those who died before hospitalization. Older and chronically ill patients were more likely to seek medical attention than were young individuals. Stowers and Short[181] analyzed the prevalence of antecedent symptoms in the two-month period prior to acute myocardial infarction in 180 patients. Of these, 68 per cent had prodromal symptoms, most commonly chest pain, but only 21 per cent with warning symptoms consulted a physician. Furthermore, one third of those who visited a physician received only reassurance, which emphasizes the point that delay in recognition of symptoms may occur at either the patient or physician level.

Although chest pain is the most common presenting feature in individuals with prodromal symptoms,[3, 177, 181] painless episodes have been observed in as many as 50 per cent of patients whose myocardial infarcts were fatal and 30 per cent of those in whom they were nonfatal.[163] Painless myocardial infarcts occur more frequently in diabetics, blacks, and persons with atrial fibrillation and hypertension.[113, 121, 163, 192] They are also more prevalent in individuals with chronic low cardiac output who may be obtunded and who therefore do not acknowledge pain. The initial clinically apparent event in the patient with an acute myocardial infarct may be syncope, pulmonary edema, shock, a tachy- or bradyarrhythmia, or a cerebrovascular accident.

The longer the interval between the occurrence of symptoms and the time of questioning, the less likely is pain to be reported. The Western Collaborative Group Study[163] found a 30 per cent prevalence of silent myocardial infarction in nonfatal cases, whereas Margolis et al.[113] documented a 17 per cent prevalence of silent myocardial infarction from the Framingham series. This latter study revealed that silent infarction was rare in persons with a previous history of angina, but not uncommon in those with hypertension or diabetes. Similar findings were confirmed by Medalie and Goldbourt,[121] who also noted age and cigarette smoking to be correlated with unrecognized infarction. Finally, Uretsky et al.[192] found that 25 per cent of patients admitted to the hospital with acute myocardial infarction mentioned no pain.

The in-hospital mortality of this group was 50 per cent compared with a similar group with antecedent pain whose mortality was 18 per cent.

For these reasons, it may be difficult for both the patient and the physician during the initial period of minutes or hours to determine whether an acute myocardial infarction is present. Many patients with typical chest pain prove not to have sustained an acute myocardial infarction since the pain is, in fact, due to acute coronary insufficiency. Thus, the pain would be identical in episodes that are reversible and termed "unstable angina" compared with episodes that are irreversible and confirmed to be acute myocardial infarction. Also, chest pain identical to that which occurs with acute coronary insufficiency may also arise in many noncardiac conditions such as esophageal spasm. Acute substernal chest pain therefore is both an insensitive and a nonspecific indicator of acute myocardial infarction. Both the patient and the physician should have a high index of suspicion that an infarction might be present when one of the other associated symptoms is present, and both should move toward rapid initiation of "coronary care" when a prolonged episode of substernal chest pain occurs.

Prehospital Coronary Care

Schroeder et al.[172] observed that the mean time between onset of symptoms and hospital arrival was over six hours in patients with chest pain suggestive of acute myocardial infarction. Pantridge et al.[142] documented that of those with premonitory symptoms, only 19 per cent sought medical attention within the first hour. Since most deaths from acute myocardial infarction occur during the first hour, attempts to reduce coronary mortality have necessarily focused on the early prehospital period.

The most extensive experience with patients in the prehospital phase of acute myocardial infarction is that of the Belfast group who during the past ten years have observed and treated more than 652 patients within the first hour of symptoms.[141, 142] Of patients who died during the first hour, ventricular fibrillation was recorded in over 90 per cent, the majority without warning dysrhythmias. Only 17 per cent of those seen in the first half-hour had normal blood pressure and heart rate. The remaining 83 per cent manifested some evidence of autonomic dysfunction. Sympathetic overactivity, with sinus tachycardia (rate > 100) or transient hypertension, was more common in patients with anterior infarction. Parasympathetic overactivity, consisting of hypotension with systolic pressure less than 80 mm Hg and bradycardia resulting from either sinus or atrioventricular nodal dysfunction, was most often seen in those with inferior infarction.

It is known from the Belfast study that the incidence of autonomic disturbances declines significantly in patients seen during the second half of the first hour after onset of symptoms. It has also been established that a high mortality rate may occur with untreated hypotension-bradycardia.[201] The incidence of hypotension and bradycardia resulting from an overbalance of parasympathetic activity is highest during the first hour of an acute infarct. Pantridge et al.[141] reported that 20 out of 23 patients with hypotension and sinus bradycardia and eight out of 12 patients with hypotension and third-degree heart block experienced a rise in both ventricular rate and blood pressure after intravenous administration of 0.3 to 0.6 mg of atropine. All three of the remaining patients with sinus bradycardia and one of the four remaining patients with complete heart block showed an increase in ventricular rate but not in blood pressure. The incidence of spontaneous resolution of these autonomic disturbances in patients presenting during the first hour of infarction is unknown. There is considerable controversy surrounding the importance and appropriate management of autonomic dysfunction complicating acute myocardial infarction.

Increased temporal dispersion of repolarization of ventricular muscle (prolonged QT interval) occurs with bradycardia and was demonstrated to promote electrical instability and predispose to ventricular fibrillation.[75, 216] Thus, it has been maintained that atropine is indicated whenever a slow heart rate is observed during acute myocardial infarction. However, Epstein et al.[45] concluded from observations in both laboratory animals and patients with acute coronary insufficiency that moderately severe bradycardia was not a harbinger of malignant ventricular tachyarrhythmias and actually had salutary effects on determinants of myocardial ischemia. These latter findings indicate that treatment of bradycardia is not required unless concomitant hypotension is present. Initiation of prompt intervention in this setting is supported by experimental studies, which have shown that a reduction in blood pressure coupled with marked bradycardia may augment the degree of myocardial ischemic injury.[114, 151] Further evidence suggests that the bradycardia-hypotension complex is a frequent occurrence in those who die suddenly before reaching a hospital.[68]

Pantridge et al.[141] have documented that in 80 per cent of cases, early intravenous administration of 0.3- to 0.6-mg aliquots of atropine abolishes the bradycardia-hypotension complex associated with inferior infarction. Warren and Lewis[201] found atropine to be a safe and effective agent in reversing hypotension and bradycardia in the early phase of myocardial infarction, with a corresponding drop in prehospital mortality. Sympathetic overactivity occasionally occurs after administration of atropine,[25, 118] which may increase myocardial ischemia. There have been several reports of ventricular fibrillation following use of atropine during acute myocardial infarction.[118, 141] Atropine should therefore be used cautiously in 0.3-mg aliquots, and only when the bradycardia is associated with hypotension.

Sympathetic overactivity is metabolically costly to the myocardium,[114] and consideration should be given to early correction of this abnormality. Preliminary investigative trials utilizing beta-blockers, such as propranolol, have shown these agents to eliminate sympathetic overactivity without causing significant hemodynamic deterioration.[114]

Several studies have now demonstrated the protective effect of chronic beta-adrenergic blockade in patients with previous myocardial infarctions.[5, 12, 85, 190] These reports all indicated that the group of patients treated with beta-blockade had a reduced mortality soon after an acute myocardial infarct, in comparison with a control group. Some of these studies[12, 85, 188] have also shown a lower incidence of recurrent acute myocardial infarcts.

The prehospital phase for acute myocardial infarction may be most benign if the patient has been on chronic beta-adrenergic blockade to protect the heart from enhanced sympathetic activity. This therapy would result in a higher incidence of enhanced parasympathetic activity, particularly in those patients who would experience a subsequent inferior myocardial infarct.

The high early incidence of malignant ventricular dysrhythmias during the early hours of acute myocardial infarction has prompted extensive clinical trials of prophylactic intramuscular lidocaine.[10, 29, 37, 142, 175, 194] Conflicting data have been presented regarding the efficacy of such a program. Pantridge et al.[142] noted no beneficial effect in the prevention of ventricular fibrillation, and that a 200-mg injection of lidocaine was not effective in terminating ventricular ectopy. Darby et al.[37] found no significant reduction in ventricular dysrhythmias after 200 mg of intramuscularly injected lidocaine coupled with a 2-mg-per-min drip. However, Bernstein et al.[10] recorded complete abolition of ventricular irritability in 75 per cent of their patients following a 300-mg intramuscular injection of lidocaine.

The therapeutic range of lidocaine is thought to be 1.2 to 5.5 μg per ml.[178] Serum levels are influenced by the site of injection, the initial dose and concentration, local fat distribution, the volume of the intravascular component, and hepatic blood flow.[30] In addition, high-velocity intramuscular injection, as occurs with the "Lidopen" autoinjector, has been shown to produce more rapid and greater tissue and capillary exposure of the drug than has use of conventional syringes.[29] The poor results observed in several studies may be secondary to subtherapeutic blood levels in patients receiving 200 mg intramuscularly. For this reason, 300 mg of a 10 per cent solution given in the deltoid muscle has been recommended as the optimal dose.[29, 175, 194] Therapeutic levels are achieved within five to ten minutes and may be maintained for as long as 120 minutes.[166] Employing this regimen, Sloman et al.[175] showed elimination of ventricular ectopic activity in 73 per cent of patients with acute myocardial infarction. Similarly, Valentine et al.,[194] using 300 mg intramuscularly in patients with suspected or proved myocardial infarction, found a statistically significant reduction in prehospital mortality between those treated with lidocaine and those given a placebo.

There is a single report[63] of a fatal complication arising from administration of lidocaine in the presence of both atrioventricular (AV) block and hypotension. The drug theoretically might exacerbate either pre-existing bradycardia or hypotension and should be used with caution in these settings. Nonetheless, since intramuscular lidocaine does yield therapeutic blood levels and experimentally lowers the fibrillatory threshold,[128, 178] it is beneficial in patients suspected of having an acute infarction. Thus, the use of intramuscular lidocaine by trained medical personnel is indicated as interim treatment prior to the insertion of an intravenous catheter.

On the basis of these considerations, the patient with symptoms suggestive of acute myocardial infarction should be managed by a regimen that includes:

1. continuous electrocardiographic monitoring.
2. an intravenous catheter.
3. lidocaine prophylaxis unless contraindicated.
4. atropine, 0.3- to 0.6-mg aliquots for bradycardia associated with hypotension.
5. availability of a synchronized defibrillator and emergency cardiac medications.
6. prompt transportation to a hospital coronary care facility.

HOSPITAL PHASE

Diagnosis

The Electrocardiogram

The electrocardiogram (ECG) is often of paramount importance in the diagnosis of acute myocardial infarction, especially when the history is atypical or unobtainable. However, in 20 to 50 per cent of cases the ECG is nondiagnostic and confirmation of the diagnosis of infarction must come from either cardiac isoenzymes or scintiscanning techniques.[54, 200] This is particularly true in the presence of left bundle branch block or left ventricular hypertrophy, which may distort the initial QRS vector and may mimic or mask the changes of infarction.[161] A normal ECG at the time of initial evaluation should never be taken to indicate that coronary care is not required.

The time course of evolutionary ST- and T-wave changes generally spans 24 to 36 hours, although new ≥0.03 Q waves may develop within two to four hours.[54] This underscores the importance of serial ECGs during the acute phase of myocardial infarction since, in some instances, ST elevation compatible with infarction may resolve without enzyme or subsequent ECG changes, thus suggesting coronary spasm or transmural ischemia without infarction. In a similar fashion, the appearance of new Q waves or loss of initial forces may sometimes be witnessed in the absence of acute infarction or ventricular volume overload. This syndrome has been described by Hassett et al.[78] in eight of 3175 patients (0.25%) who were admitted to a coronary care unit and in whom loss of forces was transient (2–6 days) and involved right precordial leads in all but one case.

As a rule, the ST-segment elevation of acute myocardial infarction persists for only one to two days, although occasionally up to two weeks are required for the ST abnormality to return to its baseline position.[54] Continued elevation beyond this time has proved to be a specific but insensitive index of advanced asynergy, with a 64 per cent incidence of ventricular aneurysm documented at autopsy or during cineangiography. Mills et al.[125] studied the natural history of ST-segment change after infarction and discovered that, in 95 per cent of inferior and 40 per cent of anterior myocardial infarctions, ST elevation resolved by two weeks. If elevation was present beyond 14 days, it was usually permanent. Moreover, persistent elevation in precordial leads was prognostically important in that these patients had a higher prevalence of left ventricular dysfunction and sudden death.

The ability of the ECG to localize the site of infarction has been evaluated by postmortem anatomic studies. Savage et al.[167] examined 24 necropsy specimens of single, well-circumscribed infarcts and correlated them with ECG alterations. They clearly refuted the assumption that infarcts must be transmural in order to produce QRS changes. Anterior infarction as evidenced by loss of initial forces in $V_{1\text{-}3}$ typically involved the anteroapical aspect of the left ventricle and spared the base. If Q waves were seen to extend to leads $V_{4\text{-}6}$, this indicated large circumferential apical involvement. This was in contrast to posterior infarcts, which predominantly spared the apex but involved the base. In a related investigation, Roark et al.[156] have shown that a 0.03-sec or greater smooth Q wave in AVF is a sensitive and specific marker for inferior myocardial necrosis. A 0.03-sec or greater Q wave in V_6 reflects posteroapical extension of the infarct process, and if the R is greater than the S wave in V_1 it indicates extension into the posterolateral free wall.

It is unusual for patients with initial myocardial infarction to reveal no alterations of the QRS complex during their hospital course. Mahoney and co-workers[110] evaluated 98 patients with enzyme-documented infarction and a previously normal QRS, and found that 89 per cent manifested QRS alterations during their hospital stay. Changes in a single area, either anterior or inferior, were observed in approximately 50 per cent of patients, whereas the remainder displayed alterations in two or more sets of leads. Only nine patients had no QRS changes.

The ECG is therefore a sensitive marker for acute myocardial infarction only in the setting of a previously normal QRS complex. Pre-existing abnormalities in the QRS complex reduce the diagnostic sensitivity of the ECG. The appearance of pathologic Q waves is almost always specific for myocardial necrosis,[78] whereas ST-segment shifts and T-wave changes are both nonspecific and insensitive indices of infarction.

Isoenzymes

In contrast with the ECG, serum enzymes are extremely sensitive indicators of myocardial necrosis. Serum glutamic oxaloacetic transaminase (SGOT), lactic dehydrogenase (LDH), and creatine kinase (CK) levels are usually elevated in the setting of acute myocardial infarction, provided that samples are obtained within 48 to 72 hours after the onset of symptoms.[161]

The diagnostic utility of total enzymes is compromised because of a lack of organ specificity, and increased levels may be observed in many noncardiac disorders.[161] For this reason, attention has been focused on the development and use of cardiac isoenzymes in the diagnosis of myocardial infarction.[13, 86, 94, 155, 157, 159, 160, 162, 174, 195, 200, 214] Each of the aforementioned enzymes exists in more than one molecular form that catalyzes the same reaction, but differs in certain physical properties that permit its identification. These forms can be demonstrated by immunologic, chromatographic, or electrophoretic techniques. For example, the electrophoretic method produces zones of enzyme activity representing different forms of the enzymes or isoenzymes. Quantitation of these isoenzymes can then be accomplished by optical means.

There are five isoenzymes of lactic dehydrogenase designated 1 to 5. Characteristically, serum levels of LDH_1 are less than those of LDH_2, but a change in this ratio such that LDH_1 is greater than LDH_2 is indicative of myocardial necrosis.[161] This reversal of the normal pattern may persist for up to six days and is therefore useful in individuals with suspected infarction who present several days after onset of symptoms when CK may have returned to normal. Wagner et al.[200] in 55 patients found the pattern of $LDH_1 > LDH_2$ to be 90 per cent sensitive and 95 per cent specific for acute myocardial infarction. False-positive results may be found with in vivo and in vitro hemolysis or renal cortical necrosis.

The most important advance in enzymology has been the use of CK isoenzymes to diagnose myocardial infarction. There are three predominant CK isoenzymes, known as MM, MB, and BB.[161] The MM form is found in skeletal and cardiac muscle and constitutes virtually all the normal serum CK activity. BB is of brain origin and absent in routine serum analysis. MB is found in significant concentrations only in heart muscle and constitutes about 20 per cent of myocardial CK content.[214] Serum CK-MB is either absent (electrophoretic method) or detected in minute amounts (chromatographic method) in normals, depending on the technique. Varat and Mercer,[195] employing ion-exchange chromatography, demonstrated that serum CK-MB levels in normal controls averaged 2 per cent. Levels above 4 per cent were diagnostic of acute myocardial infarction in 47 patients, whereas values below this effectively ruled this out as a diagnostic consideration.

Numerous observers[13, 86, 94, 155, 157, 159, 195, 200, 214] have found CK-MB to be a highly specific and sensitive marker for myocardial infarction. Irvin et al.[86] studied the relationship between onset of symptoms and appearance and disappearance of CK-MB in 27 patients with acute myocardial infarction. They noted a mean appearance time of 7.3 hours (range 2–15 hr) and elimination from the serum 17 to 85 hours (mean 48 hr) after onset of symptoms. Peak levels of the isoenzyme were found at a mean time of 19 hours from symptom onset, and correlated well with peak total CK values. It was not uncommon for the isoenzyme to be detected either before or after total CK had increased, thus emphasizing that a single normal total CK is not a reliable index of the absence of CK-MB. Moreover, these authors documented that the most productive times for sampling were 12 and 24 hours after onset of symptoms, yielding at least one positive isoenzyme value in all subjects.

A significant contribution in this regard has been made by Rivin et al.,[155] who found that 14 per cent (19 of 138) of acute myocardial infarction patients with CK-MB did not have elevated total CK values during their hospital course. An agarose electrophoretic enzyme analysis was employed. False-positive elevations were unlikely in that CK-MB values ranged from 15 to 34 per cent, the isoenzyme was present in more than one sample in 17 of 19 patients, and either QRS- or transient ST- and T-wave changes were noted in all but three individuals. These observations point out the diagnostic sensitivity of the agarose method and stress the importance of knowing which technique is being utilized for enzyme determinations.

The utility of CK-MB determinations in the community hospital setting has been analyzed by Roark et al.,[157] who ascertained that the physician had diagnosed infarction in all cases in which CK-MB was present. However, in 31 per cent of instances in which infarction was diagnosed, CK-MB was never detected. Thus, physicians tend to overdiagnose acute myocardial infarction.

Several limitations in the diagnostic value of CK-MB should be mentioned. First, it has never been established whether myocardial necrosis can occur without the isoenzyme being observed, or how much necrosis is required before detectable CK-MB is liberated into the serum. Second, the meaning of CK-MB reappearance in the serum remains to be clarified. Although it was initially thought to indicate infarct extension, Roe and Starmer[162] have suggested that secondary appearance may signify reperfusion with washout of enzyme from an ischemic zone of tissue. Third, CK-MB has reportedly been absent in several individuals with typical ECG and historical features of acute myocardial infarction.[94] This is most likely caused by inappropriate sampling times, and it underscores that the appearance of CK-MB in the plasma may be quite transient. Finally, CK-

MB is not specific for ischemic myocardial damage. It has been detected in the serum of patients with myocardial trauma, postoperatively, after DC cardioversion, in Reye's syndrome, in myositis, in Duchenne's dystrophy, and with massive skeletal muscle trauma.[157] However, these are obvious clinical conditions that should not be difficult to distinguish from myocardial infarction.

Several investigators, notably Shell et al.[174] have correlated release of CK with the extent of histologic infarction. The feasibility and accuracy of this endeavor has been questioned by Roe et al.,[160] who noted an overestimation of histologic infarction from that predicted by the Shell formula as well as an inability to differentiate large from small infarcts. Swain et al.[186] have since observed a nonlinear relationship between release of CK and the size of the infarct. Good correlation was obtained between enzyme estimates and histologic measurements for small infarctions, whereas a poor correlation was evident with large infarcts. The acceptance of mathematical models for infarct sizing must therefore await further investigative trials.

In summary, CK-MB is the most specific and sensitive enzyme marker for myocardial necrosis, and its absence, with appropriately timed serum samples, essentially excludes the diagnosis of acute myocardial infarction. It was once considered that cardiac enzyme determinations were required once daily for three days in patients with suspected myocardial infarction. However, daily sampling may not be frequent enough to detect transient appearance of CK-MB. Instead, it is recommended that in all patients who present within 24 hours from onset of symptoms, serum be obtained for total and isoenzyme CK on admission and every eight hours over the first 24 hours. This regimen should provide the greatest likelihood of enzymatic confirmation of the diagnosis of infarction. The development of techniques for detecting CK-MB has obviated the need for observation of serum levels of SGOT and total LDH and has relegated the usefulness of LDH isoenzymes to the subgroup of patients who present more than 48 hours after onset of symptoms.

Radioisotopes

To supplement the diagnostic specificity and sensitivity of the ECG and isoenzymes, there has been a proliferation of interest in the development and clinical application of radioisotope scanning techniques. A variety of "hot" (positive) and "cold" (negative) imaging agents have been evaluated, of which technetium-99m pyrophosphate (^{99m}Tc PP) and thallium-201 have been the most widely studied.

^{99m}Tc pyrophosphate is a bone-imaging agent that is believed to react with intramitochondrial calcium phosphate crystals accumulated by irreversibly damaged myocardial cells.[18] It is not taken up by necrotic cells with absent flow or normal myocardium, and is thus a "hot spot" agent that can be used to confirm the presence of acute myocardial infarction. ^{99m}Tc pyrophosphate scans become positive 12 to 24 hours after the acute episode, and positivity persists for five to six days.[205] Bruno et al.[18] noted in the dog that infarction of 1 per cent of the left ventricular mass produced a positive scan. They also observed that early localization of radioactive tracer was dependent on blood flow. In dogs with permanent occlusion, scans were negative at seven hours and invariably positive at 48 to 72 hours. With transient occlusion, scans were positive at seven hours. There was an inverse relationship between image intensity and histologic extent of infarction.

The specificity of technetium scans depends on the scintigraphic pattern observed.[112] Radionuclide uptake may produce either a diffuse or localized pattern, which is graded in intensity 1+ to 4+ based on the degree of tracer myocardial accumulation compared with bone uptake. Abnormalities less than, equal to, or greater than bone uptake are classified 2+, 3+, and 4+, respectively. Equivocal uptake is designated 1+.

Diffuse uptake scintigrams of 1+ or 2+ intensity are probably caused by blood pool imaging and are not specific indicators of myocardial necrosis. In contrast, 3+ or 4+ diffuse patterns are seen in less than 3 per cent of normal hearts and are thought to be quite specific for myocardial damage.[93, 139] Localized uptake abnormalities are almost always indicative of myocardial necrosis.[112] However, both the diffuse and localized patterns are nonspecific for acute myocardial infarction but may be observed in a variety of cardiac disorders associated with myocardial injury.[112]

In clinical practice, Bonte et al.[15] have shown a high correlation between acute myocardial infarction, confirmed by electrocardiography and serum enzymes, and the appearance of a "hot spot" three to five days after the acute episode. Willerson et al.[205] recorded a sensitivity of 96 per cent in 101 patients with acute infarction. In the 4 per cent with negative scans, imaging was performed more than seven days after onset of symptoms. In a corresponding group of 101 patients with chest pain but nondiagnostic ECG and enzymes, 92 per cent had negative scans. All nine individuals with positive images had 1+ or 2+ diffuse patterns. Klein et al.[93] found excellent concordance between the presence of CK-MB and a positive scintigram in 165 patients with suspected myocardial infarction. A positive scan was never obtained in the absence of CK-MB. Finally, Strauss and Pitt[18] in their review of radioactive tracer techniques maintain that a totally normal scan at 24 to 48 hours from the onset of symptoms is strong evidence against the diagnosis of acute infarction.

^{99m}Tc pyrophosphate scintigraphy offers several diagnostic advantages when a 3+ or 4+ localized pattern or negative scan is observed. It may be helpful in persons with pre-existing Q waves or other ECG patterns that may mimic or mask acute myocardial infarction. It is valuable in evaluating patients for acute myocardial infarction who present several days after the acute episode when CK enzymes may have disappeared. The relatively short (six-hr) half-life of ^{99m}Tc pyrophosphate enables serial determinations that may provide useful guidelines for therapy. It is safe, is relatively inexpensive, and does not adversely affect the patient's hemodynamic status.

Use of the technetium pyrophosphate scan is nonetheless limited by the ready availability of CK isoenzyme determination. This latter technique is less expensive, is less cumbersome, and does not have the problem of gray zone that is presented by the 1+ or 2+ diffusely positive scan. The diagnostic utility of ^{99m}Tc PP imaging is further compromised since it is uncertain whether the increased uptake pattern after initial infarction signifies extension or increased flow with reperfusion of an ischemic zone. Moreoever, false-positive scans with localized abnormalities may be seen in numerous conditions[205] including blunt chest trauma, ventricular aneurysm, valvular calcification, metastatic carcinoma with left ventricular involvement, and repeated high-energy cardioversion.

The predominant "cold spot" tracer is thallium-201. This radionuclide distributes in proportion to regional myocardial blood flow, with highest concentrations in areas of normal flow and diminished uptake in segments with reduced perfusion. In the setting of acute infarction, positive scintigraphic changes may be noted as early as six hours from the time of the acute episode, with progressive decline in sensitivity after 24 hours.[199] Good correlation has been obtained between thallium perfusion scintigraphy and the presence of infarction. Wackers et al.[199] documented an overall sensitivity of 82 per cent in 200 patients with acute infarction. The frequency of positive scans was significantly higher in patients studied during the first 24 hours than in those studied after 24 hours. A negative scan performed between six and 24 hours after onset of symptoms is thus strong evidence against the presence of new infarction. The major disadvantages of thallium are that it is expensive and it lacks specificity in that it cannot differentiate between new areas of infarction, reversibly ischemic myocardium, and old scars.

Perspective Regarding Diagnosis

The clinical history is the essential indicator for initiation of coronary care, but is not useful for the diagnosis or exclusion of acute myocardial infarction. The ECG is valuable in confirming acute myocardial infarction only when new pathologic Q waves are observed. Absence of new Q waves should not be used to influence clinical judgment regarding diagnosis. Appearance or persistence of ST- and T-wave alterations are not specific indications of myocardial infarction. The enzymatic hallmark of acute myocardial infarction is CK-MB, which is usually associated with a characteristic evolutionary enzyme profile. Failure to detect this isoenzyme virtually excludes the diagnosis of infarction, provided serum samples are drawn every eight hours in the first 24 hours after onset of symptoms. Total serum enzyme elevations are nonspecific markers of acute myocardial infarction and are of little value. LDH isoenzymes and radiopharmaceutical scanning with ^{99m}Tc pyrophosphate appear to be most useful clinically for detecting acute myocardial necrosis in patients admitted 48 to 72 hours after onset of symptoms.

Management

The initial treatment of most patients with chest pain who are admitted to the coronary care unit is similar. Thereafter, therapy is dictated by the manifestations of ischemic disease, regardless of whether or not an infarct is documented. These may be divided into three broad categories: (1) arrhythmic complications; (2) hemodynamic complications; (3) recurrent ischemia. In the following section, general measures for the initial hospital management of such patients are described first, followed by specific diagnostic and therapeutic considerations concerning specific complications.

General Supportive Measures

Analgesia. In a patient with suspected myocardial infarction, one of the first therapeutic goals is to relieve chest pain. This is important not only for the comfort of the patient, but because the enhanced autonomic nervous system activity may have deleterious effects. Increased sympathetic tone directly increases systemic blood pressure, heart rate, and the contractile state of the myocardium, all leading to increased myocardial work and thus increased myocardial oxygen demand. In addition, increased levels of circulating catecholamines may potentiate cardiac arrhythmias, particularly ventricular tachycardia or ventricular fibrillation.[77, 111, 206]

Several analgesic agents have been used in this setting, including meperidine and morphine, the latter being preferred. Doses of 5 to 10 mg are given intravenously every five minutes until the pain is controlled (occasional patients requiring up to 2 mg per kg total dose). Morphine has been shown to provide effective analgesia and sedation without untoward myocardial effects.[97, 187] In fact, with the reduction in the adrenergically mediated cardiovascular responses, there is a significant decrease in oxygen consumption[164] and a decrease in myocardial work. Most patients tolerate morphine well, although occasional individuals may experience nausea or vomiting requiring treatment with antiemetics. Morphine, in addition to reducing arteriolar tone, decreases venous tone, probably by central nervous system inhibition,[215] and may lead to systemic hypotension. This may be treated by volume expansion, accomplished most easily by elevation of the legs. If this proves insufficient, cautious infusion of fluids will correct filling pressures and raise the blood pressure. Respiratory depression can be a problem with administration of any narcotic agent, and is reversed with the specific opiate antagonist naloxone, in doses of 0.4 mg. intravenously as needed.

Besides narcotics, other agents that may provide beneficial physiologic effects have been used to relieve pain. At the time of initial evaluation it is difficult, if not impossible, to make a definite diagnosis of acute infarction, since the ECG is diagnostic only if new or evolving Q waves are seen. Most patients, depending on the time they are first evaluated after onset of chest pain, may have either no ECG changes or only ST- and T-wave abnormalities. Even patients with new ST-segment elevations may not evolve an infarction, as such elevations may occur in Prinzmetal's (variant) angina.[116, 147] Therefore, an initial trial of sublingual nitroglycerin may prove diagnostically and therapeutically beneficial. Patients with angina may obtain relief of symptoms immediately, along with resolution of ECG changes. Those with evolving infarction may also obtain relief, particularly if a component of spasm is involved.[152] Kim and Williams[92] have evaluated the therapeutic efficacy of large-dose sublingual nitroglycerin in patients with acute myocardial infarction, and have demonstrated a reduction or elimination of chest pain in 13 of 15 patients after 30 minutes, using a mean total dose of 24 mg. In addition, they noted a significant reduction in the evolution and size of Q waves on the ECG compared with a control group treated with morphine sulfate, suggesting a reduction in infarct size. Limitation of infarct size by nitroglycerin in both experimental and clinical studies has also been reported by Epstein and co-workers.[43]

The major common adverse effect associated with nitroglycerin administration is hypotension secondary to increased venous capacitance, and to some extent reduced arteriolar resistance. As with morphine administration, this problem can be managed by leg elevation and intravenous fluids. Interestingly, despite the hypotensive effect, the heart rate usually remains unchanged or actually decreases after nitroglycerin administration in patients with acute infarction.[92] For this reason, heart rate, as well as blood pressure, should be monitored carefully after nitroglycerin therapy.

Beta-blockers constitute another potentially useful group of drugs in the setting of a suspected myocardial infarction. In addition to possibly limiting infarct size,[114, 149] acute administration of intravenous propranolol has resulted in pain relief, both in patients with unstable angina and in those with definite myocardial infarction with pain previously unresponsive to analgesics.[133]

Finally, thrombolytic agents may have a role in acute infarction. Recent studies[38, 152] have shown that intracoronary thrombosis is involved in the pathogenesis of most acute myocardial infarctions. With lysis of intracoronary clot by fibrinolytic therapy (see Chapter 3), the pain of myocardial infarction often resolves promptly with reperfusion.[152] This would suggest that persistent chest pain represents ongoing ischemia and infarction, and that treatment with agents that can potentially increase perfusion or reduce myocardial oxygen demand may be the most appropriate treatment for the pain of myocardial infarction in the future.

Oxygen Therapy. Patients with acute myocardial infarction often demonstrate arterial hypoxemia, which is thought to be secondary to increased physiologic dead space and to ventilation-perfusion abnormalities caused by left ventricular failure.[48, 76] In an endeavor to enhance oxygen delivery to the ischemic myocardium and increase oxygen transport peripherally, thus diminishing myocardial work, supplemental oxygen is routinely administered to patients in coronary care units. Support for this comes from the experimental work of Moroko et al., who have shown a reduction in infarct size with acute coronary occlusion following oxygen inhalation.[115] Clinically, Madias and Hood[109] have demonstrated a reduction in ST-segment elevation in patients with an acute anterior wall myocardial infarction by means of oxygen therapy.

However, in evaluating the hemodynamic effects of oxygen therapy in patients with myocardial infarction, several investigators have noted possible detrimental effects. In patients with arterial desaturation ($S_AO_2 < 90\%$) administration of oxygen increased oxygen transport to the tissues by increasing both oxygen content and cardiac output. In individuals with no or only mild hypoxemia ($S_AO_2 > 90\%$), however, oxygen inhalation led to an increase in systemic vascular resistance with a rise in systolic blood pressure and a reduction in cardiac output.[184, 188]

In view of the possible adverse effects of oxygen therapy in patients without significant hypoxemia, and the cost of such therapy, it may be more prudent to restrict supplemental oxygen use for those patients with documented arterial desaturation ($S_AO_2 < 90\%$) by blood gas measurements at the time of admission to the coronary care unit. Patients with significant hypoxemia should be given oxygen delivered by nasal prongs or mask with flow rates of 2 to 4 liters per minute. Repeat blood gas determination should be made to confirm the adequacy of therapy. Patients with severe hypoxemia due to pulmonary edema or cardiogenic shock may require endotracheal intubation and high concentrations of inspired oxygen to maintain appropriate oxygen saturations.

Anticoagulation. The debate over the value of systemic anticoagulation in patients with acute myocardial infarction has continued since the work of Wright et al.[210] in 1948, which in an uncontrolled series showed a reduction in mortality in patients treated with anticoagulant drugs. Since that time, numerous studies have produced conflicting results.[165, 204] Two large randomized studies[6, 153] have failed to show any significant increase in survival of patients treated with anticoagulants, although a reduction in thromboembolic complications from 4 to 1 per cent was found. In a retrospective cumulative statistical analysis of 32 previous studies conducted from 1948 to 1975, Chalmers et al.[26] reported a 21 per cent reduction in short-term mortality (from 19.6 to 15.4%) in patients treated with anticoagulants after a myocardial infarction. Unfortunately, these studies vary drastically in patient selection, form of therapy, onset of treatment, and (in most) lack of appropriate controls. Compounding the difficulty in interpreting the results of almost 34 years of inconclusive studies is the fact that "control" therapy for a patient with acute myocardial infarction has changed. Early ambulation may counter much of the cardiac deconditioning and reduce the incidence of deep venous thrombophlebitis.[124] Likewise, "low-dose" heparin therapy is now widely used and has been shown to reduce the incidence of deep venous thrombophlebitis[209] and pulmonary embolism.[89, 171] Therefore, the potential benefit of systemic anticoagulation may have diminished. However, the risks of such therapy may be greater owing to increased use of invasive diagnostic and therapeutic modalities such as Swan-Ganz catheterization, arterial lines, intra-aortic balloon pumps, cardiac catheterization, and even emergent surgery.

In view of the unproved benefit of systemic anticoagulation in patients with acute myocardial infarction, we advocate low-dose prophylactic heparin therapy with 5000 units subcutaneously every 12 hours in all patients admitted to the coronary care unit with suspected myocardial infarction, or with evidence of an evolving infarct. This is continued until the patient begins ambulating. Systemic anticoagulation is prescribed only if there is evidence of thrombophlebitis or a thromboembolic complication.

The question of anticoagulation in the patient with unstable angina is also unresolved. Early studies by Mounsey[131] in 1951 and Wood[208] in 1961 showed a beneficial effect of anticoagulation therapy in patients with unstable angina, demonstrating a reduction in both mortality and subsequent infarction rates. However, since the advent of more precise methods for diagnosing a myocardial infarction, along with the development of numerous new drugs such as beta-blockers, long-acting nitrates, and calcium channel blockers for treatment of unstable angina, no randomized studies have been done to examine this question. The studies of DeWood et al.,[38] which demonstrated the occurrence of an intracoronary thrombosis in almost 90 per cent of patients with an acute myocardial infarction seen within four hours of onset of symptoms, suggest that some form of therapy aimed at limiting intravascular thrombosis could be potentially useful. In a preliminary report, Wolf et al.[207] offer evidence for the presence of partial coronary occlusion by intracoronary thrombosis in some patients with unstable angina.

At present, however, there is no evidence that anticoagulant therapy offers any advantage over current therapeutic modalities in the treatment of unstable angina. Data demonstrating the involvement of intracoronary thrombosis in patients with acute myocardial infarction, and perhaps in some patients with unstable angina, make some form of therapy directed at reducing clot formation attractive. Whether systemic anticoagulation, platelet inhibition, or other approaches are effective in preventing subsequent myocardial infarction or death requires further investigation.

Antifibrillatory Prophylaxis. Ventricular fibrillation is the leading out-of-hospital cause of death in patients with acute myocardial infarction.[142] Experimental studies have demonstrated that muscle necrosis is not a prerequisite for ventricular fibrillation. Rather, ischemia resulting from a coronary occlusion or reperfusion of previously ischemic muscle may precipitate electrical instability and lower the fibrillation threshold.[35, 128] Liberthson et al.[101] observed that 32 per cent of patients admitted to the coronary care unit with ventricular fibrillation had myocardial ischemia without evidence of infarction. In addition, 40 per cent of those with out-of-hospital ventricular fibrillation developed either ventricular tachycardia or fibrillation during their hospital course, the majority on the first hospital day. Thus, it is imperative that early aggressive prophylaxis against ventricular fibrillation be initiated as soon as the patient with suspected myocardial infarction comes under medical care.

Early coronary care schemes sought to identify and treat potentially lethal dysrhythmias. Lown et al.[107] advocated the use of prophylactic lidocaine for prevention of ventricular fibrillation when certain warning arrhythmias were present. It is of interest, however, that subsequent evidence from Lown's laboratory[108] indicates that warning arrhythmias might not precede ventricular fibrillation. Yasmineh et al.[214] studied 157 dogs with transient balloon occlusion of the proximal left anterior descending coronary artery; balloons were inflated and then deflated after ten minutes. Two different patterns of ventricular dysrhythmias were noted. Following initial occlusion virtually all animals developed ventricular premature beats within two to three minutes. The presence of ectopy was not a reliable predictor of the risk of fibrillation for any given animal, since in 53 per cent of dogs ventricular premature beats culminated in ventricular tachycardia and fibrillation, whereas in the remaining 47 per cent ectopy spontaneously abated within six minutes. After balloon release in those animals who survived the initial occlusion, a 40 per cent incidence of ventricular fibrillation was observed. In this setting, ventricular tachyarrhythmias developed within seconds of deflation and were not preceded by any ventricular premature beats.

It is now acknowledged that warning dysrhythmias are no longer necessary to justify antifibrillatory prophylaxis.[39, 40, 42, 102, 142] Lie et al.[102] monitored 262 consecutive patients with myocardial infarction in whom antiarrhythmic therapy was withheld. They found that warning dysrhythmias (ventricular premature beats more than five per min, runs of ventricular tachycardia, R on T phenomenon, and multifocal ventricular premature beats) were prevalent equally in those with and without subsequent primary ventricular fibrillation. Finally, these authors failed to establish any relationship between coupling interval and risk of ventricular fibrillation in that 11 of 19 patients who fibrillated had late coupled ventricular premature bests.

A similar lack of association between premonitory dysrhythmias and ventricular fibrillation was documented by Dhurandhar et al.,[39] 25 per cent of whose patients failed to manifest any warning rhythm disturbance. El-Sherif and associates[40] observed warning dysrhythmias in only 58 per cent of their patients with primary ventricular fibrillation complicating acute myocardial infarction. In addition, warning dysrhythmias were prevalent in 55 per cent of those who did not fibrillate. This underscores the physician's inability to predict the risk of ventricular fibrillation in any given patient with acute myocardial infarction.

From these data, the justification for immediate antiarrhythmic prophylaxis in all patients with acute myocardial infarction is apparent. The efficacy of this approach has also been substantiated by Lie et al.[103] in a double-blind randomized study of 212 patients with acute myocardial infarction who were admitted to the hosptial within six hours of onset of symptoms. Of these, 107 patients received a 100-mg intravenous bolus of lidocaine followed by a 3-mg-per-min infusion, while the remaining 105 received 5 per cent glucose in water. Ventricular fibrillation did not occur in those treated with lidocaine but was present in nine patients in the placebo group, four of whom had no premonitory dysrhythmias. The groups were reportedly comparable in age, infarct location, time from onset of symptoms to admission, and mortality.

In the study by Lie et al.,[103] the incidence of side effects was 15 per cent in those given lidocaine, and one third of the patients still had warning dysrhythmias despite a 3-mg-per-min infusion. This implies that further attempts to suppress all rhythm disturbances by increasing the infusion rate would undoubtedly have resulted in more toxicity, probably without demonstrable therapeutic benefit. It also serves to emphasize that the therapeutic end point during prophylaxis need not be abolition of all ventricular ectopy or warning dysrhythmias.

The goal of lidocaine prophylaxis is to achieve and sustain therapeutic serum levels as rapidly as possible without producing toxicity. The literature is unclear regarding the proper method of accomplishing this objective in patients with suspected infarction. Pharmacokinetic studies[8] have revealed that lidocaine has two half-lives, designated alpha and beta, which correspond to the distribution and the elimination phases of the drug, respectively. The alpha half-life is approximately eight minutes, and the beta decay phase is 120 to 200 minutes in persons with acute myocardial infarction. The beta half-life determines the time it takes to reach steady state levels, and is prolonged with reduced hepatic blood flow.

From these data, it is apparent that single intravenous bolus dosing is inadequate antifibrillatory prophylaxis since subtherapeutic (less than 1.2 μg per ml) blood levels may be noted owing to the rapid alpha decay phase. Similarly, in view of the long beta half-life, intravenous infusions alone are not recommended because five to seven hours may be required to attain steady state serum levels. Furthermore, the combination of a single bolus injection (1 mg per kg) and a concomitant 2-mg-per-min drip infusion has also been shown to produce a subtherapeutic hiatus. Employing this latter regimen, 25 per cent of patients were found to have subtherapeutic drug levels at five minutes, and 100 per cent had subtherapeutic levels by 15 minutes after the initial intravenous bolus.[180]

Levy et al.[100] proposed a prophylactic regimen of a 25-mg-per-min infusion for eight to 12 minutes depending on body weight, followed by a constant infusion of 20 to 30 μg per kg per min. An alternative plan is presented by Wyman et al.,[211] who administered bolus injections to 23 patients on the basis of lidocaine pharmacokinetics. An initial bolus of 75 mg was followed by a 50-mg bolus every five minutes for three subsequent doses. However, a supplemental 2-mg-per-min infusion was begun coincident with the initial bolus and increased after each additional bolus to a maximum of 4 mg per min. Serum levels were measured at one, three, five, 30, and 60 minutes and were found to be in the accepted therapeutic range in all cases. Toxic effects were relatively frequent but brief. Practical considerations such as the immediate need of a drip control apparatus and the risk of toxicity detract from the theoretical value of these approaches.

The following is our current method for lidocaine prophylaxis:[179]

1. administer 75-mg bolus over 1 min when patient is first encountered.
2. give additional 50-mg (over 1 min) bolus at 5 min.
3. give two additional 50-mg boluses at 5- to 10-min intervals.
4. begin a 2-mg-per-min drip (using a drip control apparatus) following the loading regimen.
5. do not increase lidocaine in response to warning dysrhythmias.
6. abruptly discontinue lidocaine at 36 to 48 hr if no evidence of recurrent coronary insufficiency is present.

Since the volume of distribution of lidocaine is decreased in patients with heart failure, the last one or two bolus injections should be omitted in these patients. In addition, the rate of intravenous infusion may need to be altered upward or downward depending on body weight and the degree of cardiac or hepatic failure. As with other regimens involving bolus injections of lidocaine, transient side effects (drowsiness, tinnitus) are relatively common, particularly if the bolus is given over less than the prescribed one to two minutes or if intravenous tubing containing lidocaine is flushed to the patient. An alternative method described in 1981 by Stargel et al.[179] is to administer a rapid infusion (150 mg over 18 min) following a 75-mg priming dose. With this technique, peak lidocaine levels were equivalent to the multiple injection loading method, but the incidence of side effects was reduced.

Complications of Acute Myocardial Infarction

Arrhythmic Complications

Arrhythmias complicating acute myocardial ischemia are discussed in Chapters 5, 6, and 7. However, since sinus tachycardia is so commonly present at the time of initial evaluation of a patient with chest pain, a few comments regarding management are warranted here. Sinus tachycardia occurs in about one third of patients in the early course of an acute myocardial infarction.[123] During the first 24 hours it is usually caused by enhanced sympathetic activity from anxiety, from chest pain, and possibly from direct stimulation of ventricular adrenergic receptors caused by myocardial damage.[34] Hemodynamic problems including left ventricular failure or hypovolemia (often due to previous therapy with diuretics or nitrates) may also be manifest by sinus tachycardia. Other conditions such as anemia, thyrotoxicosis, fever, pericarditis, delirium tremens or other drug withdrawal states, and hypoxemia from noncardiac causes may be responsible, but these either are rare or usually occur more than 24 hours after onset of symptoms of myocardial infarction.

One of the important variables that determine myocardial oxygen consumption is heart rate.[17] It is therefore important in the setting of a possible myocardial infarction to minimize myocardial work load by controlling heart rate. Treatment with analgesics and sedatives is often all that is necessary to modify the enhanced sympathetic drive and therefore reduce heart rate. If sinus tachycardia persists despite these measures, an aggressive approach should be made to determine whether other remediable causes are present. Hemodynamic monitoring with a Swan-Ganz catheter should be performed early in the course if tachycardia persists (see indications for Swan-Ganz catheter insertion on p. 15). Hypovolemia is not uncommon, particularly in the setting of an inferior myocardial infarction, and should be corrected by infusion with normal saline or plasma expanders. Patients with elevated pulmonary capillary wedge pressures, usually indicative of left ventricular failure, should be treated for heart failure as discussed in Chapter 2. Occasional patients, despite adequate sedation and lack of hemodynamic compromise or other known causes, may demonstrate a persistent sinus tachycardia. This occurs most commonly in patients with an anterior myocardial infarction, and may reflect a sympathetic reflex due to myocardial damage.[34] Without hemodynamic evidence of significant left ventricular dysfunction, defined as a cardiac index greater than 2.2 $l/min/m^2$, a pulmonary capillary wedge pressure less than 20 mm Hg, an AVO_2 difference less than 6.0 volumes per cent, and an adequate blood pressure, treatment with beta-blockade has been advocated.[4, 21, 52, 132] This may consist of propranolol infusion, 1 mg intravenously every five minutes to a maximum of 0.1 mg per kg, until the heart rate is reduced. Alternatively, 10 mg of propranolol may be given orally, followed by 20 mg if no effect is noted after one to two hours. After the desired effect is obtained, a dose of 20 to 40 mg orally every six hours is usually sufficient to maintain beta-blockade. The patient should be continuously monitored and therapy discontinued in the presence of heart rate less than 50, systolic blood pressure less than 95, pulmonary capillary wedge pressure greater than 22, onset of wheezing, or evidence of second- or third-degree AV block.

Hemodynamic Complications

Hemodynamic complications may occur in the setting of an acute myocardial infarction from several causes. However, regardless of the specific cause, the resultant clinical hemodynamic picture is the same and is manifest by a reduced cardiac output, an elevated left ventricular filling pressure, or both. Clinically, a reduction in the cardiac output is manifest by a lowered blood pressure and peripheral hypoperfusion with oliguria, cool extremities, and altered mentation. Nonetheless, such changes do not usually occur until the cardiac index (cardiac output/body surface area) has fallen to less than 2.2 l/min/m² (see Table 1–1).[53]

Elevations in pulmonary capillary wedge pressure to levels greater than 15 mm Hg in patients with normal lung parenchyma result in the onset of pulmonary vascular congestion. At this stage the chest radiograph demonstrates redistribution of pulmonary vascular blood flow to the upper lobes of the lung. As pulmonary capillary pressures rise to 18 to 20 mm Hg, basilar rales will be present on physical examination. The chest film will demonstrate progressive changes with increments in pulmonary venous pressure with development of perihilar haze, followed by periacinar rosette formation and interstitial edema, and finally, at pressures greater than 25 mm Hg, onset of alveolar pulmonary edema.[56, 119]

Thus, the clinical examination and x-ray are useful in evaluating the central hemodynamic status of a patient with an acute myocardial infarction. In fact, such evaluation accurately detects hemodynamic abnormalities in over 80 per cent of these patients. However, significant abnormalities may be present without clinical signs or symptoms. Twenty per cent of patients with hypoperfusion defined as a cardiac output of less than 2.2 l/min/m² and 15 per cent of those with elevated pulmonary capillary wedge pressures (> 18 mm Hg) are not recognized clinically.[53] There may be several reasons for these discrepancies. First, a "phase lag" may exist, with rales or radiologic evidence of pulmonary congestion persisting for up to 24 to 48 hours after pulmonary capillary wedge pressure has returned to normal.[119] Second, the presence of rales on a noncardiogenic basis, such as in chronic obstructive pulmonary disease, may erroneously indicate elevated pulmonary wedge pressures. Finally, compensatory mechanisms in patients with chronic left ventricular failure may alter clinical findings. Evidence of a low cardiac output may be masked by selective peripheral vasoconstriction, and elevated pulmonary venous pressures may be unsuspected owing to a thickened vascular lining in the pulmonary bed that may tolerate higher hydrostatic pressures before transudation of fluid.[52]

With the advent of the Swan-Ganz catheter in 1970, it has become possible to measure and monitor central hemodynamic parameters including cardiac output, AVO_2 difference, and pulmonary artery and pulmonary capillary wedge pressures. This modality is now widely utilized; it permits rapid and accurate assessment of a patient's status and directs appropriate therapy aimed at favora-

Table 1–1. HEMODYNAMIC SUBSETS IN ACUTE MYOCARDIAL INFARCTION

Subset	PCP > 18 mm Hg	CI < 2.2 l/min/m²	In-Hospital Mortality (%)
I	–	–	3
II	+	–	9
III	–	+	23
IV	+	+	51

PCP = pulmonary capillary pressure. CI = cardiac index.

*From Forrester et al.: Correlative classification of clinical and hemodynamic function after acute myocardial infarction. Am. J. Cardiol., 39:137, 1977. Reproduced with permission.

bly altering the hemodynamic state. The following are the generally accepted indications for insertion of a Swan-Ganz catheter in the setting of an acute myocardial infarction: (1) pulmonary venous high blood pressure or pulmonary edema; (2) hypotension or evidence of low cardiac output; (3) persistent sinus tachycardia; (4) hypoxemia; (5) recurrent chest pain; and (6) suspected ventricular septal rupture or mitral regurgitation. As with any form of cardiac catheterization, it is not without complications. Although rare, these have included: infection or bleeding at the insertion site,[24] pneumothorax, atrial and ventricular arrhythmias,[62] complete AV block,[1] intravascular knotting of the catheter,[104] pulmonary embolus or infarction,[50,69] rupture or perforation of the pulmonary artery,[144] septic and aseptic endocardial vegetations,[71,72] and pulmonary insufficiency due to pulmonary valve damage.[140] A Swan-Ganz catheter is not required for most patients with a myocardial infarction since the hemodynamic status may be accurately gauged noninvasively.

Prognostic Value of Initial Hemodynamic Data. Evaluation of central hemodynamics in a patient with an acute myocardial infarction, in addition to guiding therapy, is important from a prognostic standpoint. Since the major determinant of survival is the actual size of infarction, it is not surprising that quantitation of hemodynamic impairment, which directly reflects left ventricular dysfunction, is a potent predictor of outcome. Forrester et al.[51–53] have evaluated hospital survival in patients with acute myocardial infarction on the basis of hemodynamic status at the time of admission. Four hemodynamic subsets were defined by an elevated pulmonary capillary pressure (> 18 mm Hg) and a depressed cardiac index (2.2 l/min/m^2 or less). As shown in Table 1–1, mortality was only 3 per cent in patients in class I, whereas in Class IV it was greater than 50 per cent.[53] This strong correlation between the degree of hemodynamic abnormalities and prognosis has also been reported by Ratshin and associates.[150] In patients with a clinical diagnosis of cardiogenic shock, these authors noted a 100 per cent medical mortality in those patients with a pulmonary artery end-diastolic pressure >15 mm Hg in association with a cardiac index < 2.3 l/min/m^2, compared with a 45 per cent cumulative mortality in the other groups.

Another useful parameter to measure is the AVO_2 difference, which represents the difference in O_2 content between arterial and mixed venous blood. This is calculated by the equation:

$$AVO_2 \text{ diff. (vol. \%)} = (\text{Hemoglobin gm \%})\ (1.34\ \text{ml/gm})\ (O_2 \text{ sat. arterial} - O_2 \text{ sat. venous})$$

Provided the total body oxygen consumption remains stable, the AVO_2 difference is a simple and accurate monitor of cardiac output. Furthermore, in the absence of arteriovenous shunting or septic shock, the AVO_2 difference is a more sensitive measure of the adequacy of peripheral perfusion than is the cardiac output.[66,74] In fact, Kasnitz et al.,[91] using only the mixed venous oxygen saturation, found this to be a better predictor of hyperlactacidemia and survival than the cardiac output in patients with severe cardiopulmonary disease. Measurement of the mixed venous oxygen saturation and AVO_2 difference provides a reliable indicator of hemodynamic status and is extremely useful in monitoring therapy.

Differential Diagnosis of Hypotension. Although severe left ventricular failure is the dominant cause of hemodynamic abnormalities, several other entities may produce the same physiologic consequence. In a patient with an acute myocardial infarction and evidence of hypoperfusion or pulmonary congestion, it is important to carefully exclude the other causes, since (although these are relatively uncommon) therapy may differ markedly. The following are causes of hemodynamic impairment in the setting of an acute myocardial infarction: (1) left ventricular dysfunction; (2) hypovolemia (absolute and "relative"); (3) right ventricular infarction; (4) acute ventricular septal defect; (5) acute mitral regurgitation; (6) cardiac tamponade; and (7) arrhythmias. These are discussed in further detail below. The topic of heart failure and cardiogenic shock due to left ventricular dysfunction is presented in Chapter 2.

Hypovolemia. The most easily remedied cause of hypotension or hypoperfusion is hypovolemia. This is not an uncommon situation in patients with acute myocardial infarction, especially in the setting of an inferior infarction. Contributing factors may include vomiting, sweating, lack of fluid intake, enhanced vagal tone, and the use of drugs such as diuretics or nitrates.

If hypotension occurs in the context of vagotonia, as demonstrated by a concomitant sinus bradycardia, atropine in an initial dose of 0.6 mg should be given intravenously along with fluid administration. Patients with normal sinus rhythm or with sinus tachycardia and no evidence of pulmonary vascular congestion on physical examination or chest x-ray film may be given a fluid challenge with saline or plasma expanders. However, if there are any complicating features such as persistent chest pain, rales, an S3 gallop sound, or evidence of extensive infarction as judged by electrocardiographic criteria, hemodynamic monitoring should be performed with insertion of a Swan-Ganz catheter.

Although normal filling pressures are indicated by a pulmonary capillary wedge pressure of 6 to 10 mm Hg, optimal filling pressures during an acute myocardial infarction may be significantly higher, owing to decreased left ventricular compliance. Crexells et al.[36] have shown that pulmonary capillary wedge pressures of up to 18 mm Hg may be necessary to maximize cardiac output in the case of acute infarction. Thus, it is necessary to achieve filling pressures in this range before it may be concluded that "relative" hypovolemia is not responsible for a diminished cardiac output. This may be accomplished by intravenous fluid administration with normal saline (100 ml) or plasma expanders such as Plasmanate (50 ml) given as repeated boluses every five minutes while blood pressure, pulmonary capillary wedge pressure and cardiac output are monitored until appropriate pulmonary wedge pressures are obtained. If the patient remains hypotensive despite adequate filling pressures, other causes should be sought.

It should be appreciated that hypovolemia can cause circulatory insufficiency only through a decreased cardiac output. Therefore, one should not attempt to correct any clinically recognized abnormality in a patient with a normal cardiac index (or normal AVO_2 difference) by administering volume expansion *even* if the cardiac filling pressure is low. Volume expansion should be reserved for the patient with a low or relatively low filling pressure *and* a low cardiac index or widened AVO_2 difference.

Right Ventricular Infarction. Although it generally is not recognized clinically, right ventricular infarction assessed by hemodynamic, scintigraphic, or pathologic studies occurs in from 19 to 43 per cent of patients with inferior wall myocardial infarctions.[16, 87, 154, 198] In a series of 236 necropsy patients with acute or healed transmural myocardial infarctions, Isner and Roberts found evidence of associated right ventricular infarction in 33 (14%).[87] Right ventricular infarction occurred in none of the 97 patients with an isolated anterior wall infarction, but was present in 33 (24%) of the 139 patients with an inferior wall myocardial infarction. Right ventricular infarction was generally limited to the posterior right ventricular free wall, but in 20 per cent of cases extended to the anterolateral free wall also.

Despite the frequency of right ventricular involvement, it is often overlooked. Lorell et al.[106] reported that in 306 patients with acute inferior wall myocardial infarction, only 8 cases (2.6%) of right ventricular infarction were clinically recognized. This undoubtedly results from the relatively recent description of this entity[31] and the lack of significant hemodynamic impairment in most of these patients.[87, 182]

Clinical findings referable to right ventricular infarction range from a normal examination in patients with only minimal right ventricular involvement to the classic findings in those with marked right ventricular dysfunction, including jugular venous distention, clear lungs, and arterial hypotension. The ECG usually demonstrates an acute inferior infarction; however, there may be rare cases of isolated right ventricular infarction without evidence of left ventricular necrosis or QRS changes on the ECG.[158] Additional diagnostic information may be gained by recording the right precordial leads, particularly lead V_{4R} (a lead position analogous to the usual V_4, but recorded on the right chest wall).[22] Braat et al.[16] have reported that ST-segment elevation greater than or equal to 1 mm in this lead alone has a 92 per cent sensitivity and 100 per cent specificity for diagnosing right ventricular infarction when compared with technetium-99m pyrophosphate evidence of right ventricular involvement. ST-segment elevation may also occur in leads V_1 or V_2 (representing right ventricular infarction), but this is a less sensitive finding.[28]

A characteristic hemodynamic profile of right ventricular infarction is an elevation of right atrial and right ventricular end-diastolic pressures (to > 10 mm Hg) out of proportion to left ventricular filling pressures, which are usually normal or only minimally elevated.[31] In addition, there is often a near-equalization of the right atrial, right ventricular end-diastolic, pulmonary artery diastolic, and pulmonary capillary wedge pressures. This finding may result in a hemodynamic picture indistinguishable from that of constrictive pericarditis or cardiac tamponade.[106] Furthermore, the presence of a pulsus paradoxus, a Kussmaul sign, or an early dip and plateau configuration in the right ventricular pressure contour, which are all findings generally referable to cardiac tamponade or constrictive pericarditis, may also be noted in patients with right ventricular infarction. In the setting of an acute inferior myocardial infarction, it is important to appreciate that the likely cause of these findings is right ventricular infarction, and not cardiac tamponade due to myocardial rupture. Occasionally, the usual hemodynamic picture of right ventricular infarction may be obscured by hypovolemia. In this situation, volume loading should unmask the characteristic hemodynamic profile.[105]

The pathophysiologic mechanisms responsible for the low output state seen in patients with severe right ventricular infarction have been elucidated by Goldstein et al.[67] In experimental right ventricular infarction, these authors demonstrated that the right ventricular systolic pressure decreased by 27 per cent, with similar reductions in aortic pressure and cardiac output. In addition, they documented an increase in intrapericardial pressure, caused by massive right ventricular dilatation and encroachment on the intrapericardial volume. This produced a picture identical to that of cardiac tamponade with equalization of diastolic pressures in the right ventricle, pulmonary artery, and left ventricle. After pericardiotomy, there was prompt resolution of the equalized diastolic pressures and improved cardiac output. Thus, the basis of the hemodynamic abnormalities in patients with right ventricular infarction results from right ventricular dysfunction and increased intrapericardial pressures, both acting to reduce left ventricular preload.

The advent of noninvasive diagnostic methods for evaluating ventricular size and performance now permits a rapid means of confirming the presence of hemodynamically significant right ventricular infarction.[154, 173] Echocardiography (M-mode and two-dimensional) and radionuclide angiography have both proved valuable and demonstrate a dilated, poorly contracting right ventricle. In addition, echocardiography is useful in excluding the presence of cardiac tamponade.

Treatment of the hemodynamic complications of right ventricular infarction should consist of aggressive volume replacement, often requiring 3 to 8 liters of fluid per day. Since the right ventricle may have lost most of its pump function and serves only as a passive conduit, elevation of central venous pressure to levels of 20 mm Hg or more may be required to maintain adequate left ventricular filling pressures and systemic blood pressure. Inotropic agents including dopamine, isoproterenol, and norepinephrine have been used with variable results.[106]

Atrial pacing in selected patients may have signifcant therapeutic benefit. In one series of 12 patients with hypotension secondary to right ventricular infarction, nine required temporary pacemakers for correction of severe bradycardia or complete AV block. Loss of the functional atrial component may significantly impair right-sided cardiac output. Burks et al.[20] reported a patient with right ventricular infarction and atrial standstill who remained hypotensive despite ventricular pacing and dopamine infusion, but who responded dramatically to atrial pacing alone. Topol et al.[191] have also shown that establishment of effective synchronous atrial contractions by atrial or atrioventricular sequential pacing resulted in marked hemodynamic improvement in some patients.

Acute Ventricular Septal Defect—Mitral Regurgitation. Hemodynamic deterioration in the setting of an acute myocardial infarction, with rapid and often sudden onset of pulmonary edema and hypotension, may result from an acute ventricular septal defect or acute mitral regurgitation. Ventricular septal defect has been reported in about 1 per cent of patients dying of an acute myocardial infarction,[57] a similar incidence being noted in both inferior and anterior infarctions.[127, 170] Ventricular septal rupture occurs within 48 hours of onset of chest pain in over 50 per cent of the patients, and within the first week in over 95 per cent.[127] Acute mitral regurgitation due to myocardial infarction occurs with roughly the same frequency and timing after infarction as does ventricular septal rupture.[19] However, acute mitral regurgitation occurs more commonly after inferior infarctions (with involvement of the posterior papillary muscle) than after anterior infarctions.

Clinically, it is often very difficult to distinguish between acute ventricular septal rupture and mitral regurgitation. As discussed above, both occur in the same setting and are usually recognized by the presence of a new holosystolic murmur associated with acute hemodynamic deterioration. A thrill is often present in both instances and its location may provide some clue to the diagnosis. In ventricular septal defect, the thrill is located at the left sternal border; in mitral regurgitation, it is generally felt at the apex. However, multiple authors have stressed the frequent inability to differentiate these two conditions on physical examination.[19, 122, 203]

Right heart measurement with a Swan-Ganz catheter is valuable in differentiating these two entities.[122] Patients with ventricular septal defect demonstrate an oxygen step-up from the right atrium to the right ventricle or pulmonary artery, and inspection of the thermodilution cardiac output curve will show evidence of early recirculation indicative of a left-to-right shunt. Patients with acute mitral regurgitation may demonstrate large V waves in the pulmonary capillary wedge pressure tracing. However, there are limitations of the pulmonary wedge V waves in diagnosing mitral regurgitation.[58] Large V waves may be seen in patients with mitral obstruction (due to stenosis or mitral valve prosthesis), congestive heart failure, and ventricular septal defect in the absence of significant mitral insufficiency. On the other hand, patients with increased atrial compliance may have trivial V waves in the presence of severe regurgitation.

Noninvasive techniques are also helpful in differentiation of ventricular septal defect and mitral regurgitation. First-pass radionuclide studies have been utilized to detect the presence of a shunt (based on the premature recirculation of the radionuclide tracer activity in the lung) and thus confirm the clinical suspicion of a ventricular septal defect.[212] Two-dimensional echocardiography may demonstrate the septal defect by direct echo visualization.[46] Additionally, the injection of microcavitations (normal saline with minute air bubbles) into the right side of the heart via a peripheral arm vein may demonstrate a "negative contrast effect" produced by left ventricular blood traversing the septal defect with dilution of the contrast material in this area. Microcavitations may also traverse the septal defect and be visualized on the left side of the heart, documenting the existence of a shunt. Echocardiography is also useful in evaluating abnormalities of the mitral valve. Rupture of a papillary head or a torn chorda tendineae may be readily detected by either M-mode or two-dimensional techniques.

Definitive diagnosis requires cardiac catheterization, at which time the presence and extent of coronary artery disease should be determined along with evaluation of left ventricular performance. Medical therapy for either ventricular septal rupture or acute mitral regurgitation includes administration of vasodilator agents.[27] Although medical therapy in the past was advocated for several days to weeks until the patient had "recovered" from the myocardial injury, the early mortality is extremely high.[127] Many authors now favor urgent surgical correction once the diagnosis is established.[19, 127] Intra-aortic balloon pumping may be helpful in stabilizing a patient prior to surgical repair.[64, 203]

Recurrent Ischemia

Unstable Angina Pectoris. Unstable angina is a clinical entity that, in the spectrum of ischemic heart disease, falls in between stable angina pectoris and myocardial infarction. In fact, the propensity of this anginal pattern to presage impending myocardial infarction is reflected by previous descriptors including preinfarction angina,[55] accelerated angina,[168] intermediate coronary syndrome,[49] and acute coronary insufficiency.[95] Publication of the results of the National Cooperative Study Group's evaluation of therapy for this condition, which first appeared in 1976, has helped to establish common terms and definitions.[135] Unstable angina, as defined in this study, includes three anginal patterns: (1) the new onset of angina (within the previous month) with minimal exertion or at rest; (2) a definite change in the pain pattern of a patient with previously stable angina, including an increase in the frequency, duration, or severity of the pains; and (3) the onset of rest or nocturnal angina.

Owing to the prognostic implications of a new or changing anginal pattern and indeed often to the inability to exclude the presence of a myocardial infarction, these patients need to be admitted to a coronary care unit for further evaluation and therapy. Those with minimal or no myocardial damage when first seen are the group with the largest potential for preservation of myocardial function. A previous history of progressive, often rest angina preceding hospital admission by one week to three months is found in up to 60 per cent of patients with an acute myocardial infarction.[59] Therefore, the identification of this high-risk group is important if therapies to salvage jeopardized myocardium are to be utilized.

As noted, the history is of a changing pattern of worsening angina. The pain is similar to previous anginal pain, but typically now lasts more than 10 to 15 minutes and is less responsive to nitroglycerin. Nocturnal episodes are common. Chest pains may subside, only to return after a few minutes while the patient is still at rest. Historically, it may be impossible to distinguish a prolonged anginal episode from myocardial infarction, although with continuous pain lasting for more than 30 to 45 minutes, evidence of myocardial necrosis is usually present. It is more important to point out, however, that the distinction between a prolonged episode of angina and a small myocardial infarction may be very arbitrary. Rather than directing clinical efforts toward separation of patients into those with mycardial infarction and those without, it is important to evaluate patients for the degree of ischemia and the amount of myocardium that is jeopardized.

The ECG of patients with unstable angina usually demonstrates labile ST- and T-wave changes. Commonly, ST depression is present during an episode of pain and reverts to normal or toward the baseline tracing after pain relief.[49] Transient ST-segment elevation may also occur. Plotnick and Conti[145] noted this finding in 18 of 82 (22%) consecutive patients with unstable angina, but detected no difference in clinical presentation; in angiographic extent, location, or severity of coronary artery disease; or in resting hemodynamics as compared with patients with the more typical pattern of ST-segment depression. In the National Cooperative Study Group on unstable angina, similar findings were noted, 27 per cent of the patients demonstrating reversible ST-segment elevation with pain.[137] As in the previous study, no significant differences between patients with ST-segment elevation or depression were noted. Some patients with ST-segment elevation and pain may have focal coronary artery spasm without significant coronary artery disease, as originally described by Prinzmetal.[138, 147] These patients with unstable angina are indistinguishable on a clinical basis from those with significant coronary disease, and can be diagnosed only at the time of cardiac catheterization.

The ECG changes are thus nondiagnostic, and serial tracings should be performed, particularly comparing the ECGs obtained during and after pain. Persistent ST-segment elevation after the relief of pain generally signifies acute myocardial infarction. The evolution of Q waves is not seen in patients with unstable angina, and implies an acute infarction.

Pathophysiology. The pathophysiologic mechanism or mechanisms responsible for rest pain have been examined by several investigators. Cannom and associates[23] reported three distinctive hemodynamic subsets in patients with unstable angina and spontaneous rest pain. These subsets were defined by (1) an increase in heart rate, (2) an increase in both heart rate and brachial artery pressure, and (3) an increase in brachial artery pressure along with an increase in pulmonary artery diastolic pressure without significant heart rate changes. These authors postulated that there may be various pathogenic mechanisms responsible for rest pain. Gaasch et al.[60] noted that in four patients with Prinzmetal's angina, three had no increase in left ventricular pressure–time index before or during attacks of angina. They suggested that, since there was no increase in myocardial oxygen requirements, coronary artery spasm may play an important etiologic role. This contention was supported by Maseri and co-workers,[117] who studied 138 patients with rest pain. They also found no increase in hemodynamic determinants of myocardial O_2 demand prior to the onset of ischemia (regardless of whether the ECG showed ST-segment elevation or depression), while evidence of coronary insufficiency was demonstrated by large localized defects on thallium scintigraphy. In 37 of these authors' patients undergoing coronary angiography during pain, vasospasm was thought to be present in all. In another study of patients with rest and nocturnal angina, Figueras et al.[47] likewise found no significant alterations in the major determinants of myocardial oxygen demand at the onset of ischemia, despite the uniform presence of ischemic ECG changes, increases in pulmonary artery systolic and end-diastolic pressures, and a decrease in stroke index that always preceded the pain. Thus, a spontaneous reduction in coronary perfusion, rather than an increase in myocardial demand, would appear to be responsible for many, if not most episodes of myocardial ischemia at rest.

Angiographic Findings. Despite the relatively uniform clinical presentation, patients with unstable angina demonstrate a wide range in the severity of coronary artery disease. Alison et al.[2] prospectively evaluated 188 patients with unstable angina to determine the spectrum of anatomic coronary artery disease. They found normal coronary arteriograms in 20 patients (10.6%) and insignificant disease in 12 (6%). In the 156 patients with severe coronary artery disease defined by more than 70 per cent stenosis, 20 patients (13%) had left main coronary artery disease, and there was a 36, 38, and 26 per cent incidence of single, double, and triple vessel disease, respectively. Pugh et al.[148] reported very similar findings with a 10 per cent incidence of no angiographically significant coronary artery disease; a 16 per cent incidence of left main coronary artery disease; and a 26, 33, and 41 per cent incidence of single, double, and triple vessel disease, respectively. In the National Cooperative Study Group, patients with insignificant coronary artery disease, left main coronary artery disease, and inoperable anatomy were excluded. In their group of 288 patients, 24 per cent had single-vessel disease, 35 per cent two-vessel disease, and 39 per cent three-vessel disease.[136]

The difference in the extent of coronary artery disease noted in these studies may be related to the length of a patient's symptoms. Victor and co-workers[196] found that, in patients with unstable angina who had signs or symptoms of coronary artery disease of less than three months' duration, the incidence of single vessel disease was 52 per cent, 77 per cent of these being located in the left anterior descending artery. We have found remarkably similar results (Rosati et al., unpublished data). In 67 patients with unstable angina of new onset, 51 per cent had single-vessel coronary artery disease. Thus, the extent of disease in patients with unstable angina parallels the duration of symptoms, with a high incidence of single-vessel disease in those patients with a very short history, and a higher incidence of extensive coronary artery disease in those with a long history of symptoms.[25]

Prognosis. Patients with unstable angina as a group are at an elevated risk for subsequent myocardial infarction or death. Gazes et al.[61] studied 140 patients with unstable angina treated with only nitrates who were followed for ten years. Coronary arteriography was not performed. The incidence of subsequent myocardial infarction was 17 per cent at one month and 21 per cent at eight months. The cumulative mortality was 18 per cent at one year, 25 per cent at two years, 31 per cent at three years, and 52 per cent at ten years. In the National Cooperative Study Group study on unstable angina,[136] 288 patients were entered, but (as noted previously) patients with left main coronary artery disease, poor left ventricular function, or inoperable anatomy were excluded. Patients were treated with long-acting nitrates and beta-blockers. The rate of in-hospital myocardial infarction was 8 per cent in the medically treated group, with a mortality rate of 3 per cent. The one-year survival rate was 93 per cent. Further analysis of survival is complicated by a large cross-over of medical patients to surgical treatment (36% at 30 mo). In 1981, Mulcahy and associates[134] reported an infarction rate of 9 per cent and a mortality of 4 per cent in 101 patients with unstable angina who were treated "conservatively," this being defined as bed rest alone without the routine use of nitrates or beta-blocking agents. As exemplified in the above studies, the estimates of these risks vary depending on when the studies were done, the definitions of unstable angina used, the medical treatment prescribed, documentation of the extent of coronary artery disease, and evaluation of left ventricular function. In summary, it would seem that, despite reports in the older literature noting an incidence of subsequent myocardial infarction ranging from 22 to 80 per cent,[7, 93, 208] more recent studies generally show an 8 to 17 per cent incidence of myocardial infarction within the month following initial recognition of this syndrome. Survival statistics reported in studies over the last decade show a hospital mortality ranging from 3 to 10 per cent and a one-year mortality of 3 to 18 per cent.

Therapy. The medical management of a

patient with unstable angina should include admission to a coronary care unit for further evaluation, and treatment with bed rest, sedation, oxygen if necessary, long-acting nitrates, and beta-blocking drugs. Unfortunately, controlled trials of medical therapy for unstable angina have not been performed and such recommendations are therefore somewhat empiric. In fact, the study of Mulcahy et al.[134] implies that bed rest alone may be satisfactory in the management of many of these patients. Nonetheless, numerous studies of the use of beta-blockers in this condition[44, 49, 73, 126, 136, 143] indicate a likely beneficial role for these agents. Mizgala et al.[126] studied 15 patients who had recurrent episodes of anginal pain after a mean of 14.7 days of treatment with bed rest and nitrates. The addition of propranolol in doses of up to 400 mg a day (average 220 mg per day) resulted in pain relief for 13 patients.[32] Similarly, Fischl and colleagues[49] reported prompt relief in 17 of 22 patients with unstable angina treated with propranolol. The ability of beta-blockers to reduce heart rate, blood pressure, and myocardial contractility (all major determinants of myocardial oxygen consumption), along with the results of uncontrolled but suggestive clinical studies, have made beta-blocking drugs one of the cornerstones of therapy in the treatment of unstable angina.

For patients unresponsive to the general therapeutic strategy outlined above, other agents or modalities have recently been introduced. Intravenous nitroglycerin is now available, and may prove beneficial. A potential advantage of the parenteral route of administration is that it makes it possible to give greater amounts without untoward side effects, and to maintain steady state drug concentrations. In a preliminary report, Kaplan et al.[90] studied 27 patients with rest pain refractory to maximal medical therapy with beta-blockers and oral and topical nitrates. The addition of intravenous nitroglycerin to average maximal doses of 152 μg per min resulted in complete pain relief in 19 patients. Our experience in the last five years has also shown that many patients refractory to conventional therapy respond well to intravenous nitroglycerin, which can often be tapered and discontinued after several days without a recurrence of chest pain.

Calcium blockers, particularly nifedipine, have also been evaluated in the therapy for unstable angina.[41, 81, 82, 130, 146] Initial reports of Endo et al.[41] and Hosoda and Kimura[81] demonstrated a high degree of efficacy of nifedipine in the treatment of patients with "variant" angina who had been unresponsive to nitrates and beta-blockers. Previtali and associates[146] studied 14 patients with documented coronary artery disease and frequent ischemic episodes at rest associated with ST-segment elevation or depression. Patients were evaluated (1) during a control period on no drugs, (2) while receiving a placebo, and (3) after treatment with nifedipine. At doses of 20 mg every 4 hours, 11 of 14 patients had no further pain, and the group as a whole had a highly significant reduction in anginal attacks as compared to the placebo period. Moses et al.[130] reported similar findings in a group of 19 patients with coronary artery disease with rest pain refractory to propranolol and nitrates given to the limits of tolerance. In this group, nifedipine abolished further episodes in 14 patients, decreased its frequency in two, and was ineffective in three. Furthermore, five of seven patients maintained on long-term nifedipine (mean 6 mo) remained pain free. These agents, by blockade of inward calcium currents, have been shown to reduce or prevent coronary artery spasm and to dilate the coronary vessels.[189] Since one of the mechanisms that may be important in the pathogenesis of rest pain is coronary artery spasm, these agents, because of their unique pharmacologic action, may prove to be extremely efficacious.

Revascularization. Over the last decade, many studies have evaluated the efficacy of emergent coronary artery bypass grafting as compared with medical therapy for treatment of patients with unstable angina.[11, 14, 32, 65, 83, 136, 148, 168, 169, 213] The largest randomized, controlled study is that of the National Cooperative Study Group on unstable angina.[136] In this trial, the in-hospital mortality rate was 5 per cent in the surgical group compared with 3 per cent in the medical group—a statistically insignificant difference. The rate of myocardial infarction was greater in the surgical group (17%) than in the medical group (8%). Depending on study design, patient population selected, and other variables, very similar results have been reported in most other surgical studies examining this question. Long-term studies document no significant difference in mortality rates in patients treated with revascularization as opposed to medical therapy, but there is a marked reduction in anginal symptoms in the surgically managed group.[9, 65, 136, 148]

Current recommendations for management of patients with unstable angina are initially to employ medical therapy as outlined above. Most patients will respond with cessation of ischemic episodes. Further evaluation and treatment with cardiac catheterization and possibly coronary bypass grafting may then be performed electively, if deemed appropriate. Patients who are unresponsive to medical therapy and are thought to be surgical candidates should undergo catheterization and surgery on an urgent basis. Some groups prefer to stabilize such patients for a few days with an intra-aortic balloon pump before proceeding to surgery.[98, 99, 202]

References

1. Abernathy, W. S.: Complete heart block caused by the Swan-Ganz catheter. Chest 65:349, 1974.
2. Alison, H. W., Russell, R. O., Jr., Mantle, J. A., et al.: Coronary anatomy and arteriography in patients with unstable angina pectoris. Am. J. Cardiol. 41:204, 1978.
3. Alonzo, A., Simon, A. B., and Feinlieb, M.: Prodromata of myocardial infarction and sudden death. Circulation 52:1056, 1975.
4. Amsterdam, E. A., Hilliard, G., Williams, D. O., et al.: Hemodynamic effects of propranolol in acute myocardial infarction. Circulation 48 (Suppl. IV):138, 1973.
5. Andersen, M. P., Bechsgaard, P., Frederiksen, J., et al.: Effect of alprenolol on mortality among patients with definite or suspected acute myocardial infarction: preliminary results. Lancet 2:865, 1979.
6. Anticoagulants in acute myocardial infarction. Results of a cooperative clinical trial. J.A.M.A. 225:724, 1973.
7. Beamish, R. E., and Storrie, V. M.: Impending myocardial infarction. Recognition and management. Circulation 21:1107, 1960.
8. Benowitz, N. L.: Clinical applications of the pharmacokinetics of lidocaine. *In* Brest, A. N. (ed.): Cardiovascular Clinics. Philadelphia, F. A. Davis Co., 1976, p. 77.
9. Berndt, T. B., Miller, D. C., Silverman, J. F., et al.: Coronary bypass surgery for unstable angina pectoris. Am J. Med. 58:171, 1975.
10. Bernstein, V., Bernstein, M., Griffiths, J., et al.: Lidocaine intramuscularly in acute myocardial infarction. J.A.M.A. 219:1027, 1972.
11. Bertolasi, C. A., Tronge, J. E., Riccitelli, M. A., et al.: Natural history of unstable angina with medical or surgical therapy. Chest 70:596, 1976.
12. The beta-blocker heart attack trial. J.A.M.A. 246:2073, 1981.
13. Blomberg, D. J., Kimber, W. D., and Burke, M. D.: Creatine kinase isoenzymes: predictive value in the early diagnosis of acute myocardial infarction. Am. J. Med. 59:464, 1975.
14. Bonchek, L. I., Rahimtoola, S. H., Anderson, R. P., et al.: Late results following emergency saphenous vein bypass grafting for unstable angina. Circulation 50:972, 1974.
15. Bonte, F. J., Parkey, R. W., Graham, K. D., et al.: A new method for radionuclide imaging of myocardial infarcts. Radiology 110:473, 1974.
16. Braat, S., Brugada, P., Coenegracht, J., et al.: The value of right precordial leads in detection of right ventricular infarction: a comparison with ^{99m}Tc pyrophosphate scintigraphy. Circulation 64 (Suppl. IV):86, 1981 (abstr.).
17. Braunwald, E.: Control of myocardial oxygen consumption: physiologic and clinical considerations. Am. J. Cardiol. 27:416, 1971.
18. Bruno, F. P., Cobb, F. R., Rivas, F., et al.: Evaluation of ^{99m}technetium stannous pyrophosphate as an imaging agent in acute myocardial infarction. Circulation 54:71, 1976.
19. Buckley, M. J., Mundth, E. D., Daggett, W. H., et al.: Surgical management of ventricular septal defects and mitral regurgitation complicating acute myocardial infarction. Ann. Thorac. Surg. 16, 598, 1971.
20. Burks, J. M., Calder, J. R., and Roland, D. L.: Sinus arrest in diaphragmatic myocardial infarction: treatment of power failure with atrial pacing. Pace 2:553, 1979.
21. Cairns, J. S., and Klassen, G.: Modification of acute myocardial infarction by IV propranolol. Circulation 52 (Suppl. II): 107, 1975.
22. Candell-Riera, J., Figueras, J., Valle, V., et al.: Right ventricular infarction: relationships between ST segment elevation in V_4R and hemodynamic, scintigraphic, and echocardiographic findings in patients with acute inferior myocardial infarction. Am. Heart J. 101:281, 1981.
23. Cannom, D. S., Harrison, D. C., and Schroeder, J. S.: Hemodynamic observations in patients with unstable angina pectoris. Am. J. Cardiol. 33:17, 1974.
24. Cerra, F., Milch, R., and Lajos, T. Z.: Pulmonary artery catheterization in critically ill surgical patients. Ann. Surg. 177:37, 1973.
25. Chadda, K. D., Lichstein, E., Gupta, P. K., et al.: Effects of atropine with bradyarrhythmia complicating myocardial infarction: usefulness of an optimum dose of overdrive. Amer. J. Med. 63:503, 1977.
26. Chalmers, T. C., Matta, R. K., Smith, J., Jr., et al.: Evidence favoring the use of anticoagulants in the hospital phase of acute myocardial infarction. N. Engl. J. Med. 297:1091, 1977.
27. Chatterjee, K., Parmley, W. W., Swan, H. J. C., et al.: Beneficial effects of vasodilator agents in severe mitral regurgitation due to dysfunction of valvular apparatus. Circulation 48:684, 1973.
28. Chou, T., Van Der Bel-Kahn, J., Allen, J., et al.: Electrocardiographic diagnosis of right ventricular infarction. Am. J. Med. 70:1175, 1981.
29. Cohen, L. S., and Dunning, A. J.: Intramuscular lidocaine: practical considerations relating to its use in the pre-hospital phase of acute myocardial infarction. Publication of Survival Technology Inc., 1977.
30. Cohen, L. S., Rosenthal, J. E., Horner, D. W., et

al.: Plasma levels of lidocaine after intramuscular administration. Am. J. Cardiol. 29:520, 1972.

31. Cohn, J. N., Guiha, N. H., Broder, M. I., et al.: Right ventricular infarction: clinical and hemodynamic features. Am. J. Cardiol. 33:209, 1974.
32. Cohn, L. H., Alpert, J., Joster, J. K., et al.: Changing indications for the surgical treatment of unstable angina. Arch. Surg. 113:1312, 1978.
33. Conti, C. R., Brawley, R. K., Griffith, L. S., et al.: Unstable angina pectoris: morbidity and mortality in 57 consecutive patients evaluated angiographically. Am. J. Cardiol. 32:745, 1973.
34. Corr, P. B., and Gillis, R. A.: Autonomic neural influences on the dysrhythmias resulting from myocardial infarction. Circ. Res. 43:1, 1978.
35. Cranefield, P.: Ventricular fibrillation. N. Engl. J. Med. 298:732, 1973.
36. Crexells, C., Chatterjee, K., Forrester, J. S., et al.: Optimal level of filling pressure in the left side of the heart in acute myocardial infarction. N. Engl. J. Med. 289:1263, 1973.
37. Darby, S. Bennett, M. A., Cruickshank, J.C., et al.: Trial of combined intramuscular and intravenous lidocaine in prophylaxis of ventricular tachyarrhythmias. Lancet 2:817, 1972.
38. DeWood, M. A., Spores, J., Notske, R., et al.: Prevalence of total coronary occlusion during the early hours of transmural myocardial infarction. N. Engl. J. Med. 303:897, 1980.
39. Dhurandhar, R. W., MacMillan, R. L., and Brown, K. W. G.: Primary ventricular fibrillation complicating acute myocardial infarction. Am. J. Cardiol. 27:347, 1971.
40. El-Sherif, N., Myerburg, R. J., Scherlag, B. J., et al.: Electrocardiographic antecedents of primary ventricular fibrillation. Value of the R-on-T phenomenon in myocaridal infarction. Br. Heart J. 38:415, 1976.
41. Endo, M. Kanda, I., Hosada, S., et al.; Prinzmetal's variant form of angina pectoris. Re-evaluation of mechanisms. Circulation 36:142, 1975.
42. Engel, T. R., Meister, S. G., and Frankl, W. S.: The "R-on-T" phenomenon: an update and critical review. Ann. Intern. Med. 88:221, 1978.
43. Epstein, S. E., Borer, J. S., Kent, K. M., et al.: Protection of ischemic myocardium by nitroglycerin: experimental and clinical results. Circulation 53 (Suppl. I):191, 1976.
44. Epstein, S. E., Redwood, D. R., Goldstein, R. E., et al.: Angina pectoris: pathophysiology, evaluation and treatment. Ann. Intern. Med. 75:263, 1971.
45. Epstein, S. E., Redwood, D. R., and Smith, E. R.: Atropine and acute myocardial infarction. Circulation 45:1273, 1972.
46. Farcot, J. C., Boisante, L., Rigand, M., et al.: Two-dimensional echocardiographic visualization of ventricular septal rupture of acute anterior myocardial infarction. Am. J. Cardiol. 45:360, 1980.
47. Figueras, J., Singh, B. N., Ganz, W., et al.: Mechanisms of rest and nocturnal angina: observations during continuous hemodynamic and electrocardiographic monitoring. Circulation 59:955, 1970
48. Fillmore, S. J., Shapiro, M., and Killip, T.: Arterial oxygen tension in acute myocardial infarction. Serial analysis of clinical state and blood gas changes. Am. Heart J. 79:620, 1970.
49. Fischl, S. J., Herman, M. V., and Gorlin, R.: The intermediate coronary syndrome. Clinical, angiographic, and therapeutic aspects N. Engl. J. Med. 288:1193, 1973.
50. Foote, G. A., Sehabel, S. I., and Hodges, M.: Pulmonary complications of the flow-directed balloon catheter. N. Engl. J. Med. 290:927, 1974.
51. Forrester, J., Chatterjee, K., Parmley, W. W., et al.: Hemodynamic profiles in acute myocardial infarction and their therapeutic implications. Circulation 48 (Suppl. IV):59, 1973.
52. Forrester, J. S., Diamond, G., Chatterjee, K., et al.: Medical therapy of acute myocardial infarction by application of hemodynamic subsets. N. Engl. J. Med. 295:1356, 1404, 1976.
53. Forrester, J. S., Diamond, G. A., and Swan, H. J. C.: Correlative classification of clinical and hemodynamic function after acute myocardial infarction. Am. J. Cardiol. 39:137, 1977.
54. Fowler, N. O. (ed.): Coronary artery disease: myocardial infarction and coronary artery aneurysm. *In* Cardiac Diagnosis and Treatment, 2nd ed. New York, Harper & Row, 1976, Chapter 34.
55. Fowler, N. O.: "Preinfarctional" angina. Circulation 44:755, 1971.
56. Fraser, R. G., and Paré, J. A. P.: Diagnosis of Diseases of the Chest. Philadelphia, W. B. Saunders Co., 1977, pp. 1201–1296.
57. Friedberg, C. K.: Diseases of the Heart, 3rd ed. Philadelphia, W. B. Saunders, Co., 1966, p. 857.
58. Fuchs, R. M., Heuser, R. R., Yin, F. C., et al.: Limitations of pulmonary wedge V waves in diagnosing mitral regurgitation. Am. J. Cardiol. 49:849, 1982.
59. Fulton, M., Lutz, W., Donald, K. W., et al.: Natural history of unstable angina. Lancet 1:860, 1972.
60. Gaasch, W. H., Adyonthaya, A. V., Wang, V. H., et al.: Prinzmetal's variant angina: hemodynamic and angiographic observations during pain. Am. J. Cardiol. 35:683, 1975.
61. Gazes, P. C., Mobley, E. M., Faris, H. M., et al.: Preinfarction (unstable) angina: a prospective study: ten year follow-up. Circulation 48:331, 1973.
62. Geha, D. G., Davis, N. J., and Lappas, D. G.: Persistent atrial arrhythmias associated with placement of a Swan-Ganz catheter. Anesthesiology 39:651, 1973.
63. Gianelly, R., Vonder Groeben, J. O., Spivack, A. P., et al.: Effect of lidocaine on ventricular arrhythmias in patients with coronary heart disease. N. Engl. J. Med. 277:1215, 1967.
64. Gold, H. K., Leinbach, R. C., Sanders, C. A., et al.: Intra-aortic balloon pumping for ventricular septal defect or mitral regurgitation complicating acute myocardial infarction. Circulation 47:1191, 1973.
65. Golding, L. A., Loop, F. D., Sheldon, W. C., et al.: Emergency revascularization for unstable angina. Circulation 58:1163, 1978.
66. Goldman, R. H., Braniff, B., Harrison, D., et al.: The use of central venous oxygen saturation measurements in a coronary care unit. Ann. Intern. Med. 68:1280, 1968.
67. Goldstein, J. A., Vlahakes, G. J., Verrier, E. D., et al.: The role of right ventricular systolic dysfunction and elevated intrapericardial pressure in the genesis of low output in experimental right ventricular infarction. Circulation 65:513, 1982.
68. Goldstein, S., Moss, A. J., and Greene, W.: Sudden

death in acute myocardial infarction. Relationship to factors affecting delay in hospitalization. Arch. Intern. Med. 120:720, 1972.

69. Goodman, D. J., Rider, A. K., Billingham, M. E., et al.: Thromboembolic complications with the indwelling balloon-tipped pulmonary arterial catheter. N. Engl. J. Med. 291:777, 1974.
70. Gordon, T., and Kannel, W. B.: Premature mortality from coronary heart disease. The Framingham Study. J.A.M.A. 215:1617, 1971.
71. Greene, J. F., Jr., and Cummings, K. C.: Aseptic thrombotic endocardial vegetations: a complication of indwelling pulmonary artery catheters. J.A.M.A. 225:893, 1975.
72. Greene, J. F., Jr., Fitzwater, J. E., and Clemmer, T. P.: Septic endocarditis and indwelling pulmonary artery catheters. J.A.M.A. 218:736, 1971.
73. Guazzi, M., Fiorentini, C., Polese, A., et al.: Treatment of spontaneous angina pectoris with beta-blocking agents. A clinical, electrocardiographic and haemodynamic appraisal. Br. Heart J. 37:1235, 1975.
74. Hainsworth, R.: Mixed venous oxygen content and its meaning. Intensive Care Med. 7:153, 1981.
75. Ham, J., DeTraglia, J., Millet, D., et al.: Incidence of ectopic beats as a function of basic rate in the ventricle. Am. Heart J. 72:632, 1966.
76. Hardy, W. E., Ayres, S. M., Keyloun, V., et al.: Causes of hypoxemia and alkalosis in acute myocardial infarction. Clin. Res. 16:370, 1968.
77. Harris, A. S., Otero, H., and Bocage, A. J.: The induction of arrhythmias by sympathetic activity before and after occlusion of a coronary artery in the canine heart. J. Electrocardiol. 4:34, 1971.
78. Hassett, M. A., Williams, R. R., and Wagner, G. S.: Transient QRS changes simulating acute myocardial infarction. Circulation 62:975, 1980.
79. Herrick, J. B.: Clinical features of sudden obstruction of the coronary arteries. J.A.M.A. 59:2015, 1912.
80. Hillis, L. D., and Braunwald, E.: Myocardial ischemia. N. Engl. J. Med. 296:971, 1034, 1093, 1977.
81. Hosoda, S., and Kimura, E.: Efficacy of nifedipine in the variant form of angina pectoris. *In* Jatene, S. D., and Lichtlen, P. R. (eds.): Third International Adalat Symposium, Amsterdam, Excerpta Medica, 1976, pp. 195–199.
82. Hugenholtz, P. G., Michels, H. R., Serruys, P. W., et al.: Nifedipine in the treatment of unstable angina, coronary spasm, and myocardial ischemia. Am. J. Cardiol. 47, 163, 1981.
83. Hultgren, H. N., Pfeifer, J. F., Angell, W. W., et al.: Unstable angina: comparison of medical and surgical management. Am. J. Cardiol. 39:734, 1977.
84. Hutter, A. M., Sidel, V. W., Shine, K. I., et al.: Early hospital discharge after myocardial infarction. N. Engl. J. Med. 288:1141, 1973.
85. Improvement in prognosis of myocardial infarction by long-term beta adrenoreceptor blockade using practolol: a multicentre study. Br. Med. J. 3:735, 1975.
86. Irvin, R. G., Cobb, F. R., and Roe, C. R.: Relationship between onset of symptoms of acute myocardial infarction and appearance and disappearance of CK-MB. Arch. Intern. Med. 104:329, 1980.
87. Isner, J. M., and Roberts, W. C.: Right ventricular infarction complicating left ventricular infarction secondary to coronary heart disease. Am. J. Cardiol. 42:885, 1978.
88. Jonas, V., Hyncik, V., Chlumsky, J., et al.: Eight-year survival after perforation of ventricular septum in myocardial infarction. Acta Univer. Carol [Med] (Praha) 16:133, 1970.
89. Kakkar, U. V., Corrigan, T. P., and Fossard, D. P.: Prevention of fatal postoperative embolism by low-dose heparin: an international multicentre trial. Lancet 2:45, 1975.
90. Kaplan, K., Davison, R., Parker, M., et al.: Efficacy of intravenous nitroglycerin in the treatment of angina at rest unresponsive to standard nitrate therapy. Circulation 64 (Suppl. IV):11, 1981 (abstr.).
91. Kasnitz, P., Druger, G. L., Yorra, F., et al.: Mixed venous oxygen tension and hyperlactatemia. J.A.M.A. 236:570, 1976.
92. Kim, Y. I., and Williams, J. F.: Large-dose sublingual nitroglycerin in acute myocardial infarction: relief of chest pain and reduction of Q wave evolution. Am. J. Cardiol. 49:842, 1982.
93. Klein, M. S., Coleman, R. E., Ahmed, S. A., et al.: ^{99m}Tc (Sn) pyrophosphate scintigraphy: sensitivity, specificity and mechanisms. Circulation 52 (Suppl. II):52, 1975.
94. Konttinen, A., and Somer, H.: Specificity of serum creatine kinase isoenzymes in diagnosis of acute myocardial infarction. Br. Med. J. 1:386, 1973.
95. Krauss, K. R., Hutter, A. M., Jr., and DeSanctis, R. W.: Acute coronary insufficiency: course and follow-up. Circulation 45 (Suppl. I): 66, 1972.
96. Kuller, L., Lilienfeld, A., and Fisher, R.: Epidemiological study of sudden and unexpected deaths due to arteriosclerotic heart disease. Circulation 34:1056, 1966.
97. Lal, S., Savidge, R. S., and Chhabra, G. P.: Cardiovascular and respiratory effects of morphine and pentazocine in patients with myocardial infarction. Lancet 1:379, 1969.
98. Langou, R. A., Geha, A. S., Hammond, G. L., et al.: Surgical approach for patients with unstable angina pectoris: role of the response to initial medical therapy and intra-aortic balloon pumping in perioperative complications after aortocoronary bypass grafting. Am. J. Cardiol. 42:629, 1978.
99. Levine, F. H., Gold, H. K., Leinbach, R. C., et al.: Management of acute myocardial ischemia with intra-aortic balloon pumping and coronary bypass surgery. Circulation 58 (Suppl. I):69, 1978.
100. Levy, R. A., Charuzi, Y., and Mandell, W. J.: Lignocaine: a new technique for intravenous administration. Br. Heart J. 39:1026, 1977.
101. Liberthson, R. R., Nagel, E. L., Hirschman, J. C., et al.: Pre-hospital ventricular defibrillation: prognosis and follow-up course. N. Engl. J. Med. 291:317, 1974.
102. Lie, K. I., Wellens, H. J. J., Downar, E., et al.: Observations on patients with primary ventricular fibrillation complicating acute myocardial infarction. Circulation 52:755 1975.
103. Lie, K. I., Wellens, H. J., VanCapelle, F. J., et al.: Lidocaine in the prevention of primary ventricular fibrillation. A double-blind randomized study of 212 consecutive patients. N. Engl. J. Med. 291:1324, 1974.
104 Lipp, H., O'Donoghue, K., and Resnekow, L.: In-

tracardiac knotting of a flow-directed balloon catheter. N. Engl. J. Med. 284:220, 1971.

105. Lopez-Sendon, J., Coma-Canella, I., and Gamallo, C.: Sensitivity and specificity of hemodynamic criteria in the diagnosis of acute right ventricular infarction. Circulation 64:515, 1981.
106. Lorell, B., Leinbach, R. C., Pohort, A. M., et al.: Right ventricular infarction: clinical diagnosis and differentiation from cardiac tamponade and pericardial constriction. Am. J. Cardiol. 43:465, 1979.
107. Lown, B., Fakhro, A. M., Hood, W. B., et al.: The coronary care unit. New perspectives and directions. J.A.M.A. 199:188, 1967.
108. Lown, B., and Wolf, M.: Approaches to sudden death from coronary heart disease. Circulation 44:130, 1971.
109. Madias, J. E., and Hood, W. B., Jr.: Reduction of precordial ST-segment elevation in patients with anterior myocardial infarction by oxygen breathing. Circulation 53 (Suppl. I):198, 1976.
110. Mahoney, C., Aronin, N., and Wagner, G. S.: The excellent short and long term prognosis of patients with subendocardial infarction. Am. J. Cardiol. 41:407, 1978.
111. Maling, H. M., and Moran, N. C.: Ventricular arrhythmias induced by sympathetic amines in unanesthetized dogs following coronary artery occlusion. Circ. Res. 5:409, 1957.
112. Marcus, M. L., and Kerber, R. E.: Present status of the ^{99m}technetium pyrophosphate infarct scintigram. Circulation 56:335, 1977.
113. Margolis, J. R., Kannel, W. B., Feinlieb, M., et al.: Clinical features of unrecognized myocardial infarction—silent and symptomatic. Eighteen-year follow-up. The Framingham study. Am. J. Cardiol. 32:1, 1973.
114. Maroko, P. R., Kjekshus, J. K., Sobel, B. E., et al.: Factors influencing infarct size following experimental coronary artery occlusions. Circulation 43:67, 1971.
115. Maroko, P. R., Radvany, P., Braunwald, E., et al.: Reduction of infarct size by oxygen inhalation following acute coronary occlusion. Circulation 52:360, 1975.
116. Maseri, A., Mimmo, R., Chierchia, S., et al.: Coronary artery spasm as a cause of acute myocardial ischemia in man. Chest 68:625, 1975.
117. Maseri, A., Severi, S., DeNes, M., et al.: "Variant" angina: one aspect of a continuous spectrum of vasospastic myocardial ischemia. Am. J. Cardiol. 42:1019, 1978.
118. Massumi, R. A., Mason, D. T., Amsterdam, E. A., et al.: Ventricular fibrillation and tachycardia after intravenous atropine for treatment of bradycardias. N. Engl. J. Med. 287:336, 1972.
119. McHugh, T. J., Forrester, J. S., Adler, L., et al.: Pulmonary vascular congestion in acute myocardial infarction: hemodynamic and radiologic correlations. Ann. Intern. Med. 76:29, 1972.
120. McNeilly, R. H., and Pemberton, J.: Duration of last attack in 998 fatal cases of coronary artery disease and its relation to possible caridac resuscitation. Br. Med. J. 3:139, 1968.
121. Medalie, J. H., and Goldbourt, U.: Unrecognized myocardial infarction: five year incidence, mortality and risk factors. Ann. Intern. Med. 84:526, 1976.
122. Meister, S. G., and Helfant, R. H.: Rapid bedside differentiation of ruptured intraventricular septum from acute mitral insufficiency. N. Engl. J. Med. 287:1024, 1972.
123. Meltzer, L. E., and Kitchell, J. B.: The incidence of arrhythmias associated with acute myocardial infarction. Prog. Cardiovasc. Dis. 9:50, 1966.
124. Miller, R. R., Lies, J. E., Caretta, R. F., et al.: Prevention of lower extremity venous thrombosis by early mobilization. Confirmation in patients with acute myocardial infarction by 124 I-fibrinogen and venography. Ann. Intern. Med. 84:700, 1976.
125. Mills, R. M., Young, E., Gorlin, R., et al.: Natural history of ST segment elevation after acute myocardial infarction. Am. J. Cardiol. 35:609, 1975.
126. Mizgala, H. F., Khan, A. S., and Davies, D. O.: The effect of propranolol in acute coronary insufficiency: a preliminary report. Clin. Res. 17:637, 1969.
127. Montoya, A., McKeever, L., Scanlon, P., et al.: Early repair of ventricular septal rupture after infarction. Am. J. Cardiol. 45:345, 1980.
128. Moore, E. N., and Spear, J. F.: Ventricular fibrillation threshold: its physiological and pharmacological importance. Arch. Intern. Med. 135:446, 1975.
129. Moritz, A. R., and Zamchek, N.: Sudden and unexpected deaths of young soldiers: diseases responsible for such deaths during World War II. Arch. Pathol. 42:459, 1946.
130. Moses, J. W., Wertheimer, J. H., Bodenheimer, M. M., et al.: Efficacy of nifedipine in rest angina refractory to propranolol and nitrates in patients with obstructive coronary artery disease. Ann. Intern. Med. 94:425, 1981.
131. Mounsey, P.: Prodromal symptoms in myocardial infarction. Br. Heart J. 13:215, 1951.
132. Mueller, H. S., and Ayres, S. M.: The role of propranolol in the treatment of acute myocardial infarction. Prog. Cardiovasc. Dis. 19:405, 1977.
133. Mueller, H. S., Ayres, S. M., Religa, A., et al.: Propranolol in the treatment of acute myocardial infarction. Effect on myocardial oxygenation and hemodynamics. Circulation 49:1078, 1974.
134. Mulcahy, R., Daly, L., Graham, I., et al.: Unstable angina: natural history and determinants of prognosis. Am. J. Cardiol. 48:525, 1981.
135. National Cooperative Study Group: Unstable angina pectoris. National cooperative study group to compare medical and surgical therapy: I. Report of protocol and patient population. Am. J. Cardiol. 37:896, 1976.
136. National Cooperative Study Group: Unstable angina pectoris. National cooperative study group to compare medical and surgical therapy: II. In-hospital experience and initial follow-up results in patients with one, two, and three vessel disease. Am. J. Cardiol. 42:839, 1978.
137. National Cooperative Study Group: Unstable angina pectoris. National cooperative study group to compare medical and surgical therapy: III. Results in patients with S-T segment elevation during pain. Am. J. Cardiol. 45:819, 1980.
138. Oliva, P. B., Rotts, D. E., and Pluss, R. G.: Coronary arterial spasm in Prinzmetal angina. Documentation by coronary arteriography. N. Engl. J. Med. 288:745, 1973.
139. Olson, H. G., Lyons, K. P., and Aronow, W. S.: Follow-up technetium-99m stannous pyrophos-

phate myocardial scintigrams after acute myocardial infarction. Circulation 56:181, 1977.
140. O'Toole, J. D., Wurtzbacher, J. J., Wearner, N. E., et al.: Pulmonary valve injury and insufficiency during pulmonary artery catheterization. N. Engl. J. Med. 301:1167, 1979.
141. Pantridge, J. F., Adgey, A. A. J., Geddes, J. S., and Webb, S. W.: Acute Coronary Attack. New York, Grune & Stratton, 1975.
142. Pantridge, J. F., Webb, S. W., Adgey, A. A. J., et al.: The first hour after the onset of acute myocardial infarction. In Yu, P. N., and Goodwin, J. F. (eds.): Progress in Cardiology. New York, Lea & Febiger, 1974. Chapter 5.
143. Papazolov, N. M.: Use of propranolol in preinfarction angina. Circulation 44:303, 1971.
144. Pape, L. A., Haffajee, C. I., Markis, J. E., et al.: Fatal pulmonary hemorrhage after use of flow-directed balloon-tipped catheter. Ann. Intern. Med. 90:344, 1979.
145. Plotnick, G. D., and Conti, R.: Transient ST-segment elevation in unstable angina. Clinical and hemodynamic significance. Circulation 51:1015, 1975.
146. Previtali, M., Salerno, J. A., Tavazzi, L., et al.: Treatment of angina at rest with nifedipine: a short-term controlled study. Am. J. Cardiol. 45:825, 1980.
147. Prinzmetal, M., Kennamer, R., Merliss, R., et al.: Angina pectoris. I. A variant form of angina pectoris. Am. J. Med. 27:365, 1959.
148. Pugh, B., Platt, M. R., Mills, L. J., et al.: Unstable angina pectoris: a randomized study of patients treated medically and surgically. Am. J. Cardiol. 41:1291, 1978.
149. Rasmussen, M. M., Reimer, K. A., Klover, R. A., et al.: Infarct size reduction by propranolol before and after coronary ligation in dogs. Circulation 56:794, 1977.
150. Ratshin, R. A., Rackley, C. E., and Russell, R. O.: Hemodynamic evaluation of left ventricular function in shock complicating myocardial infarction. Circulation 45:127, 1972.
151. Redwood, D. R., Smith, E. R., and Epstein, S. E.: Coronary artery occlusion in the conscious dog. Effects of alterations in heart rate and arterial pressure on the degree of myocardial ischemia. Circulation 46:323, 1972.
152. Rentrop, P., Blanke H., Hassck, K. R., et al.: Selective intracoronary thrombolysis in acute myocardial infarction and unstable angina pectoris. Circulation 63:307, 1981.
153. Report of the Working Party to the Medical Research Council. Assessment of short-term anticoagulant administration after cardiac infarction. Br. Med. J. 1:335, 1969.
154. Rigo, P., Murray, M., Taylor, D. R., et al.: Right ventricular dysfunction detected by gated scintiphotography in patients with acute inferior myocardial infarction. Circulation 52:268, 1975.
155. Rivin, B. E., Wagner, G. S., and Calbreath, D. F.: Presence of CK-MB in the absence of abnormal total CK levels. Submitted for publication (abstr.).
156. Roark, S., Ideker, R., Wagner, G., et al.: Evaluation of the electrocardiogram in localizing and sizing inferior myocardial infarcts at necropsy. Submitted for publication (abstr.).
157. Roark, S. F., Wagner, G. S., Izlar, H. L., et al.: Diagnosis of acute myocardial infarction in a community hospital: significance of CPK-MB determination. Circulation 53:965, 1976.
158. Roberts, N., Harrison, D. G., Reimer, K. A., et al.: Right ventricular infarction, without clinical left ventricular involvement or QRS change. Submitted for publication.
159. Roberts, R., Gowda, K. S., Ludbrook, P. A., et al.: Specificity of elevated serum MB creatine phosphokinase activity in the diagnosis of acute myocardial infarction. Am. J. Cardiol. 36:433, 1976.
160. Roe, C. R., Cobb, F. E., and Starmer, C. F.: The relationship between enzymatic and histologic estimation of the extent of myocardial infarction in conscious dogs with permanent coronary occlusion. Circulation 55:438, 1977.
161. Roe, C. R., Limbird, L. E., Wagner, G. S., et al.: Combined isoenzyme analysis in the diagnosis of myocardial injury. Application of electrophoretic methods for the detection and quantitation of the creatine phosphokinase MB isoenzyme. J. Lab. Clin. Med. 80:577, 1972.
162. Roe, C. R., and Starmer, C. F.: A sensitivity analysis of enzymatic estimation of infarct size. Circulation 52:1, 1975.
163. Rosenman, R. H., Friedman, M., Jenkins, C. D., et al.: Clinically unrecognized myocardial infarction in the Western Collaborative Group Study. Am. J. Cardiol. 19:776, 1967.
164. Rouby, J. J., Eurin, B., Glaser, P., et al.: Hemodynamic and metabolic effects of morphine in the critically ill. Circulation 64:53, 1981.
165. Russek, H. I.: Anticoagulants should not be used routinely for acute myocardial infarction. Cardiovasc. Clin. 8:123, 1977.
166. Ryden, L., Wasir, H., Conradsson, T. B., et al.: Blood levels of lignocaine after intramuscular administration to patients with proven or suspected acute myocardial infarction. Br. Heart J. 34:1012 1972.
167. Savage, R. M., Wagner, G. S., Ideker, R. E., et al.: Correlation of postmortem anatomic findings with electrocardiographic changes in patients with myocardial infarction: retrospective study of patients with typical anterior and posterior infarcts. Circulation 55:279, 1977.
168. Scanlon, P. J., Nemickas, R., Moran, J. F., et al.: Accelerated angina pectoris. Clinical hemodynamic, arteriographic, and therapeutic experience in 85 patients. Circulation 47:19, 1973.
169. Selden, R., Neill, W. A., Ritzmann, L. W., et al.: Medical versus surgical therapy for acute coronary insufficiency. N. Engl. J. Med. 293:1329, 1975.
170. Selzer, A., Gerbode, F., and Keith, W. J.: Clinical, hemodynamic, and surgical considerations of rupture of the ventricular septum after myocardial infarction. Am. Heart J. 78:598, 1969.
171. Sevitt, S., and Gallagher, N. G.: Prevention of venous thrombosis and pulmonary embolism in injured patients. Lancet 2:981, 1959.
172. Schroeder, J. S., Laine, I. H., and Hu, M.: The prehospital course of patients with chest pain. Analysis of the prodromal, symptomatic, decision making, transportation and emergency room periods. Am. J. Med. 64:742, 1978.
173. Sharpe, D. N., Botvinick, E. H., Shames, D. M., et

al.: The noninvasive diagnosis of right ventricular infarction. Circulation 57:483, 1978.
174. Shell, W. E., Lovell, J. F., Covell, J. W., et al.: Early estimation of myocardial damage in conscious dogs and patients with evolving acute myocardial infarction. J. Clin. Invest. 52:2579, 1973.
175. Sloman, G., Isaac, P., Harper, R., et al.: Plasma levels of lignocaine after intramuscular injection. Heart Lung 2:669, 1973.
176. Sobel, B. E., and Braunwald, E.: The management of acute myocardial infarction. *In* Braunwald, E., (ed.): Heart Disease. Philadelphia, W. B. Saunders Co., 1980, pp. 1353–1386.
177. Solomon, H. A., Edwards, A. L. and Killip, T.: Prodromata in acute myocardial infarction. Circulation 45:463, 1969.
178. Spear, J. F., Moore, E. N., and Gerstenblith, G.: Effect of lidocaine on the ventricular fibrillation threshold in the dog during ischemia and premature ventricular contractions. Circulation 46:65, 1972
179. Stargel, W. W., Shand, D. G., Routledge, P. A., et al.: Clinical comparison of rapid infusion and multiple injection methods for lidocaine loading. Am. Heart J. 102:872, 1981.
180. Stargel, W. W., and Wagner, G. S.: Personal communication.
181. Stowers, M., and Short, D.: Warning symptoms before major myocardial infarction. Br. Heart J. 32:833, 1970.
182. Strauss, H. D., Sobel, B. E., and Roberts, R.: The influence of occult right ventricular infarction on enzymatically estimated infarct size, hemodynamics, and prognosis. Circulation 62:503, 1980.
183. Strauss, H. W., and Pitt, B.: Evaluation of cardiac function and structure with radioactive tracer techniques. Circulation 57:645, 1978.
184. Sukumalchantra, Y., Levy, S., Danzig, R., et al.: Correcting arterial hypoxemia by oxygen therapy in patients with acute myocardial infarction. Am. J. Cardiol. 24:838, 1969.
185. Surawicz, B.: Ventricular fibrillation. Am. J. Cardiol. 28:268, 1971.
186. Swain, J. L., Cobb, F. R., and Roe, C. R.: Nonlinear relationship between CK appearance and histologic infarct size. Clin. Res. 274A, 1978 (abstr.).
187. Thomas, M., Malmcrona, R., Fillmore, S., et al.: Haemodynamic effects of morphine in patients with acute myocardial infarction. Br. Heart J. 27:863, 1965.
188. Thomas, M., Malmcrona, R., Shillingford, J.: Haemodynamic effects of oxygen in patients with acute myocardial infarction. Br. Heart J. 27:401, 1965.
189. Tiefenbrunn, A. J., Sobel, B. E., Gowda, S., et al.: Nifedipine blockade of ergonovine-induced coronary arterial spasm: angiographic documentation. Am. J. Cardiol. 48:184, 1981.
190. Timolol-induced reduction in mortality and reinfarction in patients surviving acute myocardial infarction (The Norwegian Multicenter Study Group). N. Engl. J. Med. 304:801, 1981.
191. Topol, E. J., Goldschlager, N., Ports, T. A., et al.: Hemodynamic benefit of atrial pacing in right ventricular infarction. Ann. Intern. Med. 96:594, 1982.
193. Uretsky, B. F., Farquhar, D. S., Berezin, A. F., et al.: Symptomatic myocardial infarction without chest pain: prevalence and clinical course. Am. J. Cardiol. 40:498, 1977.
193. Vakil, R. J.: Intermediate coronary syndrome. Circulation 24:557, 1961.
194. Valentine, P. A., Frew, J. L., Mashford, M. L., et al.: Lidocaine in the prevention of sudden death in the pre-hospital phase of acute infarction: a double-blind study. N. Engl. J. Med. 291:1327, 1974.
195. Varat, M. A., and Mercer, D. W.: Cardiac specific creatine phosphokinase isoenzyme in the diagnosis of acute myocardial infarction. Circulation 51:855, 1975.
196. Victor, M. F., Likoff, M. J., Mintz, G. S., et al.: Unstable angina pectoris of new onset: a prospective clinical and arteriographic study of 75 patients. Am. J. Cardiol. 47:228, 1981.
197. Wackers, F. J., Becker, A. E., Samson, G., et al.: Location and size of acute transmural myocardial infarction estimated from thallium-201 scintiscans: a clinicopathologic study. Circulation 56:72, 1977.
198. Wackers, F. J., Lie, K. I., Sokole, E. B., et al.: Prevalence of right ventricular involvement in inferior wall infarction assessed with myocardial imaging with thallium-201 and technetium-99m pyrophosphate. Am. J. Cardiol. 42:358, 1978.
199. Wackers, F. J., Sokole, E. B., Samson, G., et al.: Value and limitations of thallium-201 scintigraphy in the acute phase of myocardial infarction. N. Engl. J. Med. 295:1, 1976.
200. Wagner, G. S., Roe, C. R., Limbird, L. E., et al.: The importance of identification of the myocardial-specific isoenzyme of creatine phosphokinase (MB form) in the diagnosis of acute myocardial infarction. Circulation 47:263, 1973.
201. Warren, J. V., and Lewis, R. P.: Beneficial effects of atropine in the prehospital phase of coronary care. Am. J. Cardiol. 37:68, 1976.
202. Weintraub, R. M., Aroesty, J. M., Paulin, S., et al.: Medically refractory unstable angina pectoris. I. Long-term follow-up of patients undergoing intra-aortic balloon counterpulsation and operation. Am. J. Cardiol. 43:877, 1979.
203. Wellons, H. A., Grossman, J., and Crosby, I. K.: Early operative intervention for complications of acute myocardial infarction. J. Thorac. Cardiovasc. Surg. 73:763, 1977.
204. Wessler, S.: Antithrombotic agents are indicated in the therapy of acute myocardial infarction. Cardiovasc. Clin. 9:131, 1977.
205. Willerson, J. T., Parkey, R. W., Bonte, F. J., et al.: Technetium stannous pyrophosphate myocardial scintigrams in patients with chest pain of varying etiology. Circulation 51:1046, 1975.
206. Winbury, M. M., Hausler, L. M., Prioli, N. A., et al.: Effect of epinephrine on cardiac rhythm in the miniature pig before and after coronary occlusion. J. Pharmacol. Exp. Ther. 138:287, 1962.
207. Wolf, N. M., Mandelkorn, J., Singer, S., et al.: Evidence for thrombosis in acute ischemic syndromes other than transmural infarction. Circulation 64 (Suppl. IV): 1970, 1981.
208. Wood, P.: Acute and subacute coronary insufficiency. Br. Med. J. 5242:1779, 1961.
209. Wray, R., Maurer, B., and Shillingford, J.: Prophylactic anticoagulant therapy in the prevention

of calf-vein thrombosis after myocardial infarction. N. Engl. J. Med. 288:815, 1973.
210. Wright, I. S., Marple, C. D., and Beck, D. F.: Report of committee for evaluation of anti-coagulants in treatment of coronary thrombosis with myocardial infarction. Am. Heart J. 36:801, 1948.
211. Wyman, M. G., Lalka, D., Hammersmith, L., et al.: Multiple bolus technique for lidocaine administration during the first hours of an acute myocardial infarction. Am. J. Cardiol. 41:313, 1978.
212. Wynne, J., Fishbein, M. C., Holman, B. L., et al.: Radionuclide scintigraphy in the evaluation of ventricular septal defect complicating acute myocardial infarction. Cathet. Cardiovasc. Diagn. 4:189, 1978.
213. Wysham, D. N., and Rogers, W. R.: Coronary bypass surgery for unstable angina. Arch. Surg. 114:611, 1979.
214. Yasmineh, W. G., Pyle, R. B., Cohn, J. N., et al.: Serial serum creatine phosphokinase MB isoenzyme activity after acute myocardial infarction; studies in the baboon and man. Circulation 55:733, 1977.
215. Zelis, R., Mansour, E. J., Capone, R. J., et al.: The cardiovascular effects of morphine. The peripheral capacitance and resistance vessels in human subjects. J. Clin. Invest. 54:1247, 1974.
216. Zipes, D. P.: The clinical singificance of bradycardia rhythms in acute myocardial infarction. Am. J. Cardiol. 24:814, 1969.

2

Medical Therapy for Pump Failure Complicating Acute Myocardial Infarction

BARRY M. MASSIE
and KANU CHATTERJEE

With the advent of coronary care units and the availability of effective antiarrhythmic drugs, primary electrical deaths in hospitalized patients with acute myocardial infarction have become uncommon. As a result, pump failure has become the major cause of in-hospital morbidity and mortality in acute myocardial infarction. Furthermore, survivors of pump failure often remain severely symptomatic from heart failure and continue to have a high postdischarge mortality.[81]

During the past decade, bedside hemodynamic monitoring has vastly increased our understanding of the pathophysiology of myocardial infarction. This, together with our evolving experimental knowledge of myocardial mechanics and metabolism, has led investigators to evaluate new therapeutic approaches to the patient with acute pump failure. Foremost among these are the use of vasodilating drugs and newer inotropic agents.

This chapter reviews the physiologic basis, methodology, clinical results, and limitations of therapy with these agents.

PHYSIOLOGIC BASIS FOR VASODILATOR AND INOTROPIC THERAPY

Rationale

Experimental work, in both isolated cardiac muscle and intact animals, has shown that beat-by-beat cardiac performance is modulated by three factors: the inotropic state of the myocardium, left ventricular preload, and left ventricular afterload.[16,89] The last two concepts are derived from, and best understood through, isolated cardiac muscle studies such as those illustrated in Figure 2–1. This shows the change in length (shortening) of the muscle at varying external loads. The preload is the load applied to the muscle prior to contraction, which results in a greater or lesser degree of stretch (i.e., determining the initial muscle length). Once contraction begins, an additional load (the afterload) is added. The preload and the afterload together make up the total load. For any given total load, as seen in Figure 2–1, muscle shortening is greater when the contraction is initiated at a higher preload. This is simply another way of demonstrating the Frank-Starling relationship, which shows that shortening is greater when the muscle contracts from greater initial lengths. The second point to be appreciated from Figure 2–1 is that, for any given preload, shortening increases as the total load is diminished. In other words, the less the afterload, the more the muscle is able to shorten. It is noteworthy, although not shown in Figure 2–1 that a change in the inotropic state of the muscle also results in an upward shift of these curves. Thus, as contractility increases, shortening is greater at the same total load.

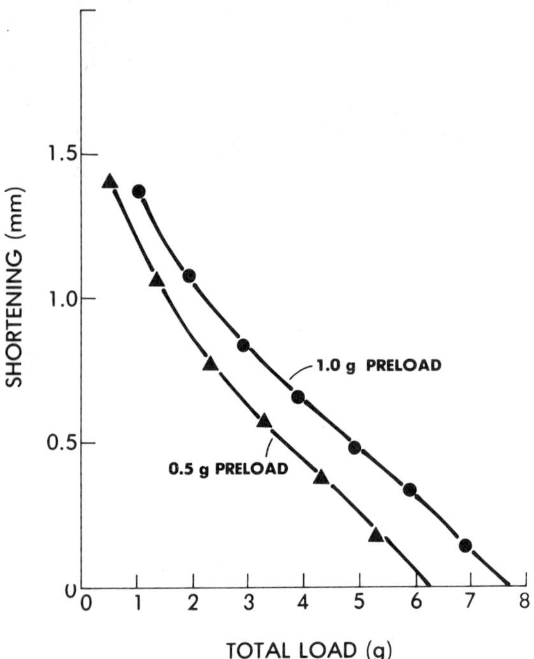

Figure 2–1. Two plots of the amount of shortening by an isolated cat papillary muscle at increasing imposed afterloads, resulting in increasing total loads. The upper line was generated at a constant initial muscle length determined by a 1.0-gm preload; the lower plot describes contractions beginning at a somewhat smaller initial length (0.5-gm preload). Note that both increasing preload and decreasing afterload result in greater shortening at any given preload.

These concepts can be extended to the clinical setting. Here, the preload would again be the length of the myocardial fibers prior to contraction, which is proportional to the left ventricular end-diastolic volume. Since ventricular volumes are difficult to measure at frequent intervals, a measurement of the left ventricular filling pressure is often used as an index of volume. As a result, the most frequently employed measure of left ventricular preload is the pulmonary capillary wedge pressure.

Afterload is a more difficult concept to apply clinically, but is best defined as the wall stress of the heart during systolic ejection. Although wall stress can be determined from measurements of intraventricular pressure, radius, and wall thickness, such calculations are difficult to make in clinical practice. Therefore, other approximations of afterload have been used, such as aortic pressure, systemic vascular resistance, and aortic impedance. The systolic blood pressure is a useful but oversimplistic measure of left ventricular afterload.[35] Thus, if other determinants of myocardial performance are kept constant, indices of systolic performance, such as ejection fraction, will decrease as blood pressure rises. However, afterload may change considerably without concomitant changes in blood pressure.[109, 110] This occurs when cardiac output rises while systemic vascular resistance decreases, yielding little change in blood pressure. As a result, systemic vascular resistance is probably a better measure of left ventricular afterload.

Some investigators believe that left ventricular afterload is best represented by a measurement of "impedance" to left ventricular outflow.[100, 109, 110] Aortic impedance is determined by a dynamic relationship between pressure and flow during phasic flow. Impedance reflects both a frequency-independent, nonpulsatile, steady state component and a frequency-dependent pulsatile component. However, measurements of impedance are difficult and generally show changes with interventions that are directionally similar changes to those in systemic vascular resistance. As a result, systemic resistance is commonly used as an approximation of left ventricular afterload or output impedance.

The inotropic state of the myocardium, although conceptually easy to understand, is the most difficult factor to measure clinically. This is so because it is not possible to keep the loading conditions of the left ventricle constant in order to assess the contractile state of the muscle. Consequently, as illustrated in Figure 2–2, hemodynamic changes produced by alterations in the inotropic state of the myocardium are similar to those produced by changes in left ventricular afterload. For example, one might see an increase in stroke volume at the same, or even at a slightly lower, left ventricular filling pressure when the patient is treated with either an inotropic agent or a peripheral vasodilator. Thus, both classes of medication are now widely used in the treatment of pump failure complicating myocardial infarction.

Pathophysiology of Pump Failure

Acute myocardial infarction results in some depression of cardiac performance in most patients.[72] The larger the infarction, the greater is the degree of hemodynamic im-

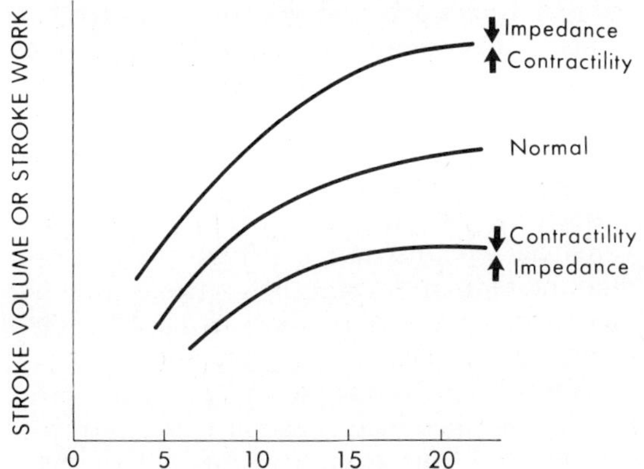

Figure 2–2. The center curve represents a normal ventricular function curve, showing an increase in stroke volume over a wide range of left ventricular filling pressures, with the maximal increment occurring between 15 and 20 mm Hg. The upper and lower curves indicate the effects of changes in myocardial contractility and afterload. Note that the hemodynamic effects of an increase in contractility are identical to those produced by a reduction in outflow impedance.

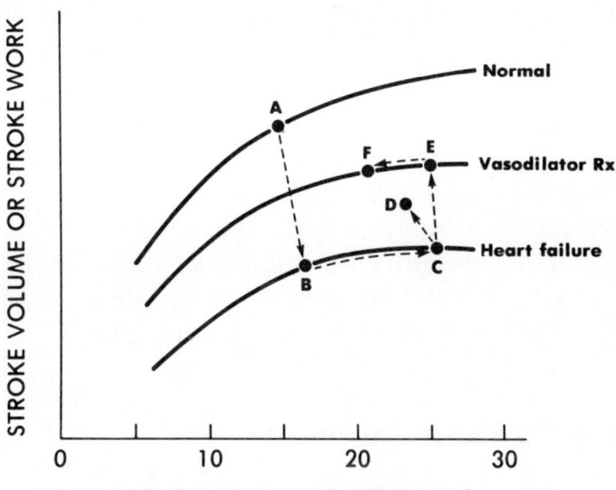

Figure 2–3. Ventricular function curve schematically indicating the effects of heart failure and vasodilator therapy. Point A indicates normal function. With heart failure, there is a downward shift to a depressed curve *(Point B).* Compensatory dilatation occurs (the Frank-Starling mechanism), causing a shift to Point C. Endogenous catecholamine stimulation may produce some improvement in function *(Point D).* Point E indicates the rise in stroke volume resulting from reduced impedance to left ventricular outflow. Point F represents the decrease in preload produced by venodilatation. Points E and F fall on a hypothetical new ventricular function curve produced by vasodilator therapy.

pairment.[81] Thus, in patients dying of cardiogenic shock, involvement of more than 40 per cent of the left ventricle is uniformly shown at postmortem examination.[4, 107] Some evidence suggests that this necrosis is an evolving process, with the hemodynamic derangements of pump failure leading to further ischemia and infarction.[71]

The cardiac performance of patients with pump failure accompanying acute myocardial infarction, then, is characterized by a shift from Point A on a normal ventricular function curve to Point B on a depressed curve (Fig. 2–3). The resulting reduction in stroke volume produces an increase in left ventricular end-diastolic volume and, therefore, filling pressure. Thus, the patient moves to the right along the depressed curve to Point C, which may result in a compensatory rise in stroke volume (the Frank-Starling mechanism) unless the patient is already on the flat portion of the curve. In addition, patients with some remaining ventricular reserve respond to endogenous catecholamine stimulation with a shift upward to a less depressed curve (Point D). When pump failure is severe, catecholamine release and reflex baroreceptor activity result in tachycardia and elevation of peripheral vascular resistance in order to maintain perfusion to vital organs, with the resultant clinical picture of vasoconstriction that characterizes the lower output state.

Each of these compensatory mechanisms paradoxically may result, either directly or indirectly, in further hemodynamic deterioration (Fig. 2–4). Tachycardia, inotropic stimulation, and the increased myocardial wall tension that results from both cardiac dilatation and elevated peripheral resistance all increase myocardial oxygen requirements,

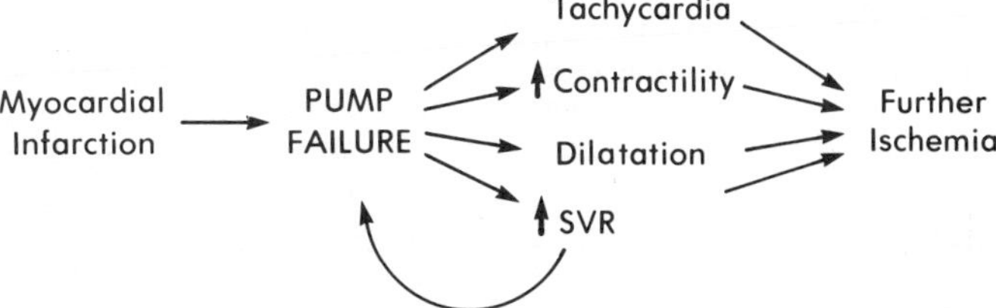

Figure 2–4. Schematic illustration of how the compensatory mechanisms for heart failure can themselves worsen ischemia and lead to further infarction and pump failure.

and may further increase the imbalance between these and the limited oxygen supply.[15] If infarct extension or ischemia result, pump failure worsens. Furthermore, the reflex increase in arterial impedance may itself further depress myocardial performance, as illustrated in Figure 2–2. Thus, the body's own compensatory mechanisms contribute to the vicious cycle of hemodynamic deterioration that characterizes cardiogenic shock.

Role of Vasodilators

Vasodilating drugs have two beneficial hemodynamic effects in patients with pump failure that may produce clinical improvement and reverse this downhill spiral.[88, 89, 98] By dilating the arterial resistance bed, they reduce afterload and produce a resultant increase in stroke volume.[90] Vasodilating drugs that reduce venous tone also decrease venous return to the heart, and thereby lower the filling pressures of both ventricles. These changes are represented hypothetically by Points E and F in Figure 2–3. Since most patients with acute pump failure have both elevated filling pressures and diminished cardiac output, the combination of these effects is usually desirable. In the setting of acute infarction, improvement of these derangements might be expected to help remedy the imbalance between myocardial oxygen supply and demand, thus reducing ischemia and potentially limiting the size of the infarction.[25] One major concern, and a frequent limitation of the use of vasodilators in severe pump failure, is that these drugs may produce excessive hypotension.[92] Hypotension may worsen ischemia both by decreasing coronary artery perfusion and by stimulating a reflex tachycardia. Thus, the hemodynamic response to vasodilators must be monitored closely in the setting of acute pump failure, in order to ensure that the beneficial effects outweigh potentially deleterious ones.

Inotropic agents may produce the same beneficial hemodynamic effects as the vasodilators. One important difference is that, by increasing contractility, these drugs necessarily increase myocardial oxygen demand. Furthermore, most inotropic agents have a propensity to produce positive chronotropic effects, and this may accentuate ischemia. Nonetheless, in selected patients, the hemodynamic improvement may outweigh these factors in causing an improvement in the myocardial oxygen supply:demand ratio. In particular, patients who develop hypotension in response to vasodilators may be better candidates for inotropic drugs.

Hemodynamic Subsets in Acute Myocardial Infarction

Since the hemodynamic status of patients with acute myocardial infarction fluctuates rapidly and is sometimes difficult to predict clinically, it is important to institute hemodynamic monitoring in patients with suspected failure. The derived information can be used to categorize patients into different subsets with different prognoses and requiring different therapeutic approaches.[30, 51] One such classification, based on measurements of stroke work index and left ventricular filling pressure, is shown in Table 2–1. The importance of classifying patients with pump failure on the basis of hemodynamic

Table 2–1. HEMODYNAMIC SUBSETS IN ACUTE MYOCARDIAL INFARCTION

Subset	Clinical Signs*	SWI g-m/m^2	LVFP mm Hg	Appropriate Therapy
I	None	≥ 40	≤ 15	None necessary
II	None or ↓ perfusion	<40	≤ 15	Volume expansion
IIIA	Pulmonary congestion	> 40	> 15	Diuretics, venodilators
IIIB	Pulmonary congestion	20–40	> 15	Diuretics, venodilators, arterial dilators
IVA	Pulmonary congestion ↓ perfusion	10–20	> 15	Combined arteriolar dilators and venodilators
IVB	Shock	≤ 10	> 15	Vasodilators, mechanical assist devices, inotropes

*Most common clinical signs, but these findings may not be present.

measurements must be emphasized, since there often are important discrepancies between the apparent status of the patient as shown by physical examination and the status as revealed by measured hemodynamics.

Patients in subset I have no hemodynamic impairment and a generally good prognosis. Patients in subset II may appear to have significant pump failure, but often are suffering only from intravascular hypovolemia resulting from a lack of oral intake, emesis, overvigorous diuresis, excessive nitrate therapy, or inappropriate reflex vasodilation. Although these latter patients are not common (making up less than 20 per cent of those with pump failure), it is particularly important that they be identified since their hemodynamic derangement can easily be rectified by volume repletion or discontinuation of unnecessary drugs. Furthermore, inotropic agents, by increasing myocardial oxygen demand, and vasodilators, by further decreasing preload and stroke volume, will aggravate these abnormalities (Fig. 2–4). Thus, patients with evidence of impaired perfusion, depressed stroke work index, and left ventricular filling pressures less than 15 to 18 mm Hg should be given a rapid infusion of 100 ml of normal saline to determine whether a rise in cardiac output results. If a beneficial response is noted, or if filling pressure does not increase into this optimal range, volume infusion should be continued until cardiac output and peripheral perfusion improve or left ventricular filling pressure rises beyond the suggested level.

Most patients with pump failure accompanying acute myocardial infarction fall into subsets III or IV. Those who clinically display normal perfusion, but have high left ventricular filling pressures together with maintained stroke work indices (subset IIIA), may be treated with diuretics or with vasodilators that predominantly reduce preload, such as the nitrates. Subset IIIB patients with moderately depressed stroke work indices may benefit from vasodilators that reduce both venous and arteriolar tone, such as sodium nitroprusside. Subset IV patients usually have obvious clinical signs of pump failure and have a very poor prognosis. In subset IVA, a trial of vasodilator therapy with sodium nitroprusside is warranted, but may result in excessive hypotension or inadequate response. In such cases, the addition or substitution of a positive inotropic agent, such as dopamine or dobutamine, may be helpful. When pump failure is very severe (subset IVB), inotropic stimulation or mechanical assist devices, such as intra-aortic balloon counterpulsation, are usually required. Subsequent addition of vasodilators may be possible and beneficial.

CLINICAL USE OF VASODILATORS IN ACUTE PUMP FAILURE

Acute pump failure generally is treated initially with parenteral medications. Three vasodilators have been studied extensively in this setting—sodium nitroprusside, phentolamine, and nitroglycerin (Table 2–2). Of these agents, sodium nitroprusside dilates both the venous capacitance vessels and the arteriolar resistance bed, whereas phentolamine has a greater effect on the arterioles and nitroglycerin has a predominant effect on the venous system.[79, 98, 99, 115] Although the explanation may be mechanistically simplistic, venodilators have been consistently noted to have a greater effect on right and left ventricular preload (decreasing right atrial and pulmonary capillary wedge pressure).[90] In contrast, arteriolar dilators have a greater effect on systemic vascular resistance, with

Table 2–2. EFFECTS OF PARENTERAL VASODILATORS IN HEART FAILURE

Medication	Dosage	Venous Tone	Arteriolar Resistance	Heart Rate	Arterial Blood Pressure	Cardiac Output	Left Ventricular Filling Pressure
Nitroprusside	8–400 μg/min	↓↓	↓↓	⟷	↓	↑↑	↓↓
Phentolamine	0.1–2 mg/min	↓	↓↓	↑	↓	↑↑	↓
Nitroglycerin	10–400 μg/min	↓↓	↓	⟷	↓	↑	↓↓

↓ or ↑ = modest change; ↓↓ or ↑↑ = marked change; ⟷ = no change.

consequent increases in cardiac output and stroke volume. Agents that act on both vascular beds produce both hemodynamic effects.

The actual clinical effects of these medications depend on the hemodynamic status of the patient. Thus, in patients with low or even normal filling pressures, venodilators such as nitroglycerin may produce a fall in stroke volume with resulting hypotension and reflex tachycardia (Fig. 2–5).[25] In patients with high filling pressures, stroke volume, arterial pressure, and heart rate are not significantly affected. Similarly, in individuals with normal or reduced preload, drugs that lower systemic vascular resistance may cause significant hypotension and reflex tachycardia, since the potential for increasing stroke volume is limited. In contrast, patients with dilated hearts rarely exhibit significant hypotension in response to arteriolar dilation. Thus, vasodilators should be avoided in persons who do not have high filling pressures, and hemodynamic measurements should be monitored closely during therapy, particularly when concomitant diuretics are employed. Some broad guidelines for the use of parenteral vasodilators in pump failure are listed in Table 2–3. The use of specific agents is discussed below.

Sodium Nitroprusside

Sodium nitroprusside has been the most widely used vasodilator in the treatment of acute pump failure.[6, 25, 55, 79] It is a potent relaxant of all vascular smooth muscle.[108] Because of its rapid onset and the short duration of its action, it is ideally suited for use in hemodynamically unstable situations. It is given as a slow intravenous infusion beginning at 8 to 16 μg per minute, increased by increments of 5 to 10 μg every five to ten minutes until the desired effect is achieved or toxicity intervenes. Arterial pressure must be continuously monitored and a diastolic pressure of at least 60 mm Hg should be maintained, in order not to compromise coronary artery perfusion. When arterial pressure cannot be maintained, concomitant use of inotropic agents or mechanical assistance devices is usually required. Doses ranging from 15 to 400 μg per minute have been used, but most patients require 50 to 150 μg per minute.

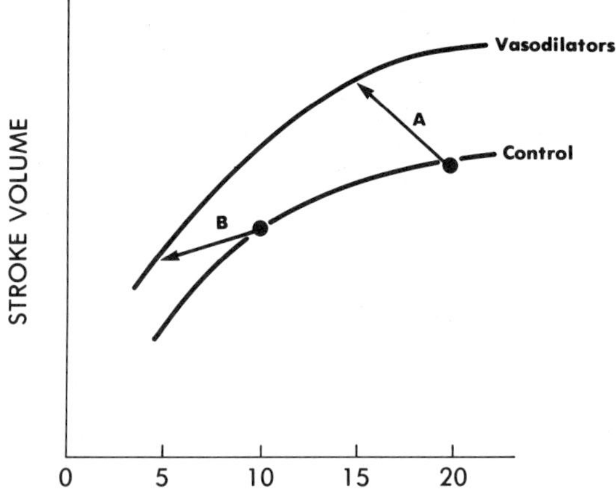

Figure 2–5. Control ventricular function curve and a curve shifted upward by vasodilator therapy. Arrow A illustrates the rise in stroke volume produced by vasodilators in patients with initially elevated filling pressures. Arrow B illustrates the potentially deleterious fall in stroke volume that may result from vasodilator therapy in patients with normal or low filling pressures.

Toxicity, aside from excessive hypotension, is uncommon and usually mild, consisting predominantly of nausea, hiccups, and transient confusion.[108] Thiocyanate may accumulate during nitroprusside infusion, with possible resultant central nervous system toxicity. Therefore, blood levels of this ion should be monitored in patients undergoing prolonged therapy. The potential complications of nitroprusside and the other com-

Table 2–3. GUIDELINES FOR INTRAVENOUS VASODILATOR THERAPY IN ACUTE PUMP FAILURE

1. Determine initial hemodynamics for selection of vasodilator.
2. Start therapy with low initial dose (nitroprusside, 15 μg/min; phentolamine, 0.1 mg/min; nitroglycerin, 10 μg/min).
3. Gradually increase infusion rate (every 5–15 min).
4. Monitor changes in blood pressure, heart rate, left ventricular filling pressure, cardiac output, systemic vascular resistance.
5. If cardiac output increases, with decrease in systemic vascular resistance and left ventricular filling pressure, and little change in blood pressure, maintain or increase infusion rate as guided by hemodynamics and clinical picture.
6. If blood pressure decreases without change in cardiac output or left ventricular filling pressure, discontinue vasodilator or add inotropic agent.
7. Substitute nonparenteral vasodilator when chronic therapy is indicated.

Table 2–4. POTENTIAL COMPLICATIONS OF PARENTERAL VASODILATOR DRUGS COMMONLY USED FOR TREATMENT OF HEART FAILURE

Nitroprusside	Phentolamine	Nitroglycerin
Hypotension	Tachycardia	Hypotension
Nausea, vomiting	Hypotension	Bradycardia
Mental confusion	Nausea, vomiting	Tachycardia
Cyanide poisoning	Diarrhea	Headache
Thiocyanate toxicity	Nasal stuffiness	Nausea
Lactic acidosis	Flushing	Hypoxemia
Hypothyroidism		
Methemoglobinemia		
Hypoxemia		

monly used parenteral vasodilators are listed in Table 2–4.

Several investigaters have reported the hemodynamic response to nitroprusside infusion in patients with acute myocardial infarction.[6, 25, 55] Table 2–5 summarizes the findings in 27 patients, who are classified into three groups on the basis of their initial left ventricular filling pressures and stroke work indices.[25] Group I patients had pulmonary capillary wedge pressures below 15 mm Hg and were largely free of evidence of impaired left ventricular performance. Group II and III patients had filling pressures above 15 mm Hg, but only Group III subjects had stroke work indices below 20 g-m/m^2. Patients in both the latter groups had clinical evidence of impaired cardiac performance, and most had pulmonary edema and/or cardiogenic shock. Nitroprusside lowered systemic vascular resistance and right atrial and left ventricular filling pressures in each group. Heart rate did not change significantly, although an increase of greater than 10 beats/min was seen in several Group I patients. Mean arterial pressure decreased modestly. As might be expected, cardiac and stroke work indices rose only in patients with elevated preload. Figure 2–6 illustrates the improvement in left ventricular performance, manifested by both reduced left ventricular filling pressure and increased stroke volume, produced by nitroprusside in Group II and III patients. In contrast, stroke volume fell in most Group I patients.

In fact, the beneficial hemodynamic effects of nitroprusside are most prominent in the patients with more severe hemodynamic impairment. Figure 2–7 illustrates the response to therapy in a larger group of patients, all of whom had elevated filling pressures and markedly reduced (≤20 g-m/m^2) stroke work indices.[31] As a result, nitroprusside is currently the vasodilator of choice for acute myocardial infarction patients in hemodynamic subset IV, and in those in subset III with evidence of both pulmonary congestion and impaired perfusion.

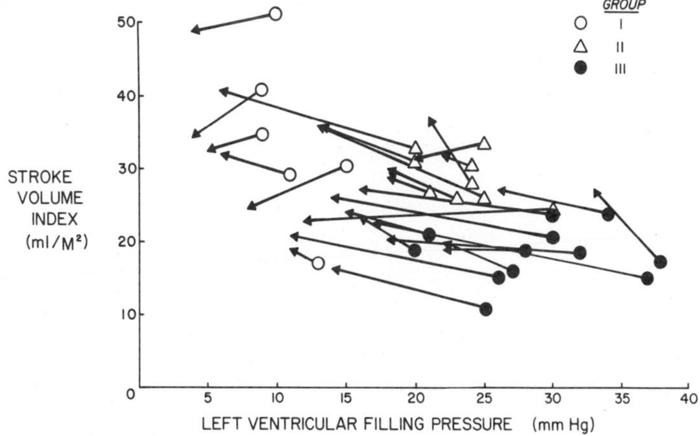

Figure 2–6. Individual changes in stroke volume (SV) and left ventricular filling pressures (LVFP) during vasodilator therapy. Each dot represents baseline measurements; the arrow head represents measurements during nitroprusside infusion. Group I patients have a baseline LVFP <15 mm Hg. Group II patients have a baseline stroke work index >20 g-m/m^2. Group III patients have a baseline LVFP >15 mm Hg and a stroke work index ≤20 g-m/m^2. (From Chatterjee, K., and Parmley, W. W.: Role of vasodilator therapy in heart failure. Prog. Cardiovasc. Dis. 19:301, 1977. Reproduced by permission.)

Table 2–5. HEMODYNAMIC EFFECTS OF NITROPRUSSIDE INFUSION IN PATIENTS WITH ACUTE MYOCARDIAL INFARCTION

	Group I (6)		Group II (9)		Group III (12)	
	C	NP	C	NP	C	NP
Heart rate (beats/min)	89.0±7.1	96.7±8.6	91.3±4.2	94.7±3.4	100.2±4.0	100.5±4.8
Mean arterial pressure (mm Hg)	91.0±2.6	85.8±3.9	100.6±4.5	87.7±4.1	82.4±2.2	76.2±2.8*
Mean pulmonary arterial pressure (mm Hg)	16.5±1.7	11.3±1.0*	31.8±1.6	23.9±2.0*	37.0±1.5	24.7±1.4
Mean right atrial pressure (mm Hg)	5.2±1.4	2.8±1.2	10.4±1.5	7.2±1.4*	12.8±1.4	8.5±1.3*
Left ventricular filling pressure (mm Hg)	11.2±4.6	6.3±1.1*	23.6±1.0	15.2±1.5*	29.0±1.6	18.7±1.8*
Cardiac index (liter/min/m^2)	2.9±.2	2.9±.2	2.6±0.1	3.1±0.2*	1.8±0.1	2.2±0.1*
Stroke work index (g-m/m^2)	38.8±7.6	34.6±2.9	33.6±2.9	34.2±1.8	13.8±1.1	17.6±1.5*
Systemic vascular resistance (dynes sec cm^{-5})	1383±148	1321±119	1577±141	1231±146	1908±260	1431±137*

Numbers in parentheses indicate number of patients.
C = control; NP = during nitroprusside therapy.
*$p<0.05$ or below (NP vs. C).
(From Chatterjee et al.: Hemodynamic and metabolic responses to vasodilator therapy in acute myocardial infarction. Circulation 48:1183, 1973. Reproduced by permission of The American Heart Association, Inc.)

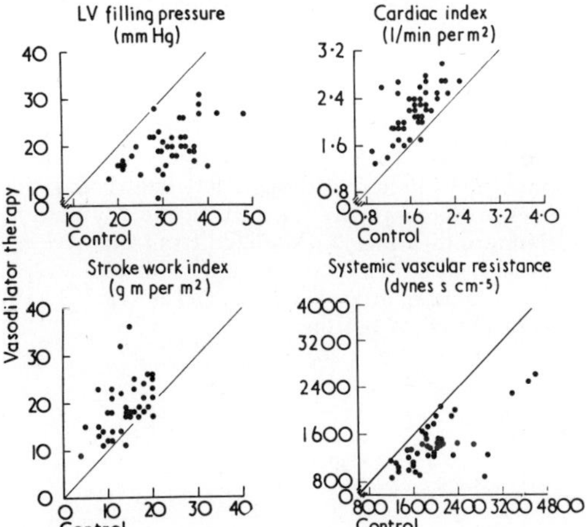

Figure 2–7. Hemodynamic effects of nitroprusside in 40 patients with acute pump failure. Note the dual hemodynamic improvement of a fall in filling pressure and rise in cardiac output. (From Chatterjee et al.: Effects of vasodilator therapy for severe pump failure in acute myocardial infarction on short-term and late prognosis. Circulation 53:797, 1976. Reproduced by permission of The American Heart Association, Inc.)

Phentolamine

Phentolamine is an alpha-adrenergic blocking agent that produces dilation of both the arterial and venous beds.[1] Some evidence suggests that phentolamine also has a direct relaxant effect on vascular smooth muscle and an indirect positive inotropic effect resulting from stimulation of norepinephrine release.[1] Therapy is usually begun at an infusion rate of 0.1 mg per minute. Only mild side effects have been reported, usually related to the gastrointestinal tract. However, some patients in each reported series have developed significant tachycardia during phentolamine therapy, irrespective of initial filling pressures.[27, 31, 66, 67, 76, 111, 123, 128] In some, this has resulted in an exacerbation of ischemia.

The hemodynamic effects of phentolamine in patients with acute myocardial infarction are otherwise quite similar to those of nitroprusside (Fig. 2–8).[66, 76, 111, 128] There are significant decreases in left ventricular filling pressure, right atrial pressure, and systemic vascular resistance, with only modest reductions of arterial pressure. In patients with elevated filling pressures, cardiac output increases significantly. However, the frequent occurrence of tachycardia and the high cost of the drug have limited the use of phentolamine in patients with acute infarction.

Intravenous Nitroglycerin and Other Nitrate Preparations

Nitroglycerin is the oldest and most widely used vasodilator. Although it is predominantly a venodilator, it has a weak effect on the arteriolar resistance vessels when administered intravenously.[87] Several preparations of intravenous nitroglycerin are now commercially available and are increasingly used for the management of acute pump failure, particularly in patients who continue to display manifestations of ischemia. The limiting side effect of intravenous nitroglycerin, just as for other nonparenteral preparations, is headache, which appears to be somewhat less common in patients with heart failure.

Figure 2–9 is a compilation of the mean findings from several studies employing nitroglycerin in patients with acute infarction.[6, 19, 48, 62, 79, 130] There is a consistent decrease in left ventricular filling pressure, with little increase in stroke volume. Nitroglycerin therefore is well suited to therapy for patients in hemodynamic subset III with dyspnea or

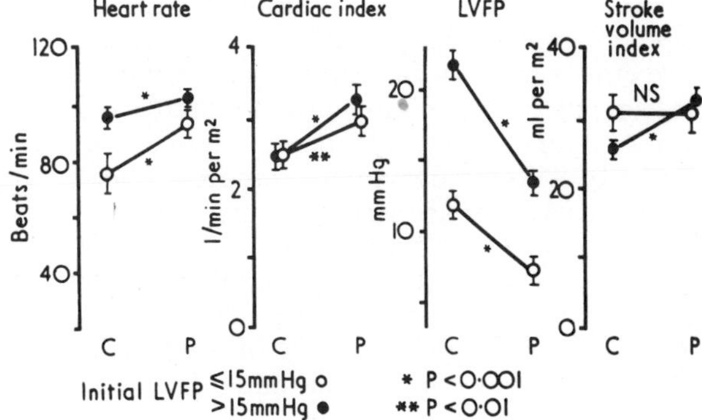

Figure 2–8. Hemodynamic effects of phentolamine in patients with acute myocardial infarction, compiled from published literature. Patients are divided according to their initial left ventricular filling pressure to emphasize the differing effect of phentolamine on stroke volume in patients with high and normal filling pressures. Note that heart rate rises significantly in both groups. (From Chatterjee, K., and Parmley, W. W.: Role of vasodilator therapy in heart failure. Prog. Cardiovasc. Dis. 19:301, 1977. Reproduced by permission.)

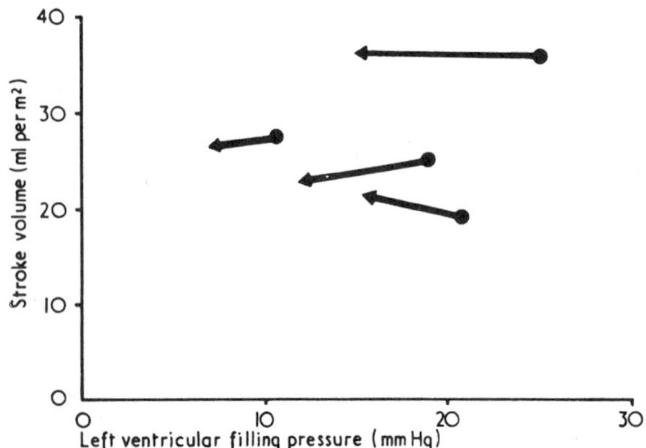

Figure 2–9. Hemodynamic effect of intravenous nitroglycerin. Lines indicate changes reported in four published studies. Although left ventricular filling pressure is markedly lowered, stroke volume is not significantly affected. (Modified from Chatterjee, K., and Parmley, W. W.: Role of vasodilator therapy in heart failure. Prog. Cardiovasc. Dis. 19:301, 1977. Reproduced by permission.)

pulmonary congestion but maintained peripheral perfusion. In patients with elevated filling pressures, there is usually no change in heart rate, arterial pressure, and cardiac output. Patients with normal or only modestly increased filling pressures may actually sustain a fall in stroke volume, with consequent tachycardia and hypotension. Rare individuals may exhibit profound bradycardia and hypotension of uncertain etiology following administration of nitroglycerin.[42]

Sublingual isosorbide dinitrate has pharmacologic effects similar to those of nitroglycerin, but its duration of action is somewhat more prolonged (up to 90 minutes) and it therefore is better suited for continuous therapy in patients with pump failure.[86] Treatment is usually started with a 2.5- or 5-mg dose every two to three hours. The dose may be increased to as much as 20 mg every one to two hours, until limited by headache or by tachycardia and hypotension (usually seen only when filling pressure is excessively reduced).

Oral isosorbide dinitrate and nitroglycerin ointment have a still longer duration of action (up to four to six hours), but individual response is more variable, especially in patients with impaired peripheral perfusion.[5, 18, 56, 124, 131] The newly available nitroglycerin patches, which produce a sustained release of nitroglycerin into the circulation for 24 hours, may also be poorly absorbed in patients with severe pump failure. These agents therefore are less well suited for the initial treatment of heart failure in the setting of acute infarction, although the use of topical nitroglycerin (1 to 4 inches every four to six hours) at night in place of sublingual medication may allow stable patients to rest more comfortably.

INOTROPIC AGENTS IN THE MANAGEMENT OF ACUTE PUMP FAILURE

The rationale for the use of positive inotropic agents is to enhance myocardial contractile function, and thereby to increase effective cardiac output. It is apparent that when contractile reserve is inadequate, the efficacy of inotropic agents is likely to be limited. With enhanced contractility, however, ventricular pump function improves with an increase in stroke volume and cardiac output.

Although all agents with positive inotropic effects have the potential to improve myocardial contractile function, their mechanisms of action are different (Table 2–6). The primary mechanism by which digitalis glycosides increase contractility is by inhibiting sodium-potassium ATPase activity, which leads to an increase in intracellular calcium content. Catecholamines such as dobutamine and dopamine increase the inotropic state by stimulating adenyl cyclase activity. The mechanisms for the inotropic action of amrinone and related compounds (MDL 17043, ARL 115) are not currently known. Although inhibition of phosphodiesterase activity has been demonstrated, this mechanism does not explain fully their inotropic effects. It appears, however, that their ability to enhance intracellular calcium content mediates increased contractility.

Digitalis

Since Herrick in early 1900 first recommended the use of digitalis after myocardial infarction,[83] its role in the treatment of acute

Table 2–6. PROPOSED MECHANISM OF ACTION OF AGENTS WITH POSITIVE INOTROPIC EFFECTS

Agent	Proposed Mechanism
Digitalis glycosides	Inhibit Na^+, K^+ ATPase activity
Glucagon	Stimulate adenyl cyclase activity
Catecholamines	Activate beta-receptors and adenyl cyclase
Methylxanthines	Inhibit phosphodiesterase
Histamine	Stimulate adenyl cyclase activity
Angiotensin	Unknown
Amrinone	Unknown
MDL 17043	Unknown
ARL 115	Unknown

myocardial infarction has been evaluated in a number of experimental and clinical studies. Although digitalis increases contractility of the nonischemic and border zones in dogs after experimental myocardial infarction, it has not been shown to have any consistent and clinically relevant beneficial effects in patients with pump failure complicating myocardial infarction.

In the absence of heart failure, digitalis does not produce any beneficial hemodynamic effects.[38, 49, 64, 75, 82, 112] Indeed, cardiac output might decrease in some patients because of increased systemic vascular resistance and arterial pressure (peripheral vascular effects of digitalis). In patients with heart failure complicating myocardial infarction, variable hemodynamic effects in response to intravenous digitalis therapy have been reported in different studies (Table 2–7). Although an increase in left ventricular stroke work index was observed in most studies, no significant increase in cardiac output or stroke volume were noted. Similarly, there was no consistent and clinically relevant decrease in pulmonary capillary wedge pressure following digitalis therapy. Most investigators observed only a slight decrease in pulmonary capillary wedge pressure following digitalis in patients with acute myocardial infarction and heart failure.

It has also been shown in patients with acute myocardial infarction that the magnitude of digitalis-induced hemodynamic improvement is inversely related to the severity of heart failure.[50] The hemodynamic effects of ouabain in 25 patients with acute myocardial infarction are illustrated in Figure 2–10. Patients were classified on the basis of clinical criteria: those in shock, those in heart failure, and those without heart failure. Ouabain produced a significant increase in cardiac output in the group without heart failure. In contrast, ouabin had no effect on either cardiac output or left ventricular filling pressure in patients with heart failure or those in shock. Furthermore, ouabain increased stroke work index only in those patients who did not have clinical heart failure. The relative ineffectiveness of digitalis in the presence of cardiogenic shock was also observed in other investigations.[59, 70]

The hemodynamic effects of digitalis have been compared with those of dobutamine, a beta-1-adrenergic receptor agonist, in patients with acute myocardial infarction. Dobutamine increased cardiac output and decreased pulmonary capillary wedge pressure consistently, but digitalis produced little or no beneficial hemodynamic effects (Table 2–8). Furthermore, the onset of hemodynamic effects of digitalis is later than that of other inotropic agents (dopamine, dobutamine, norepinephrine) that are available for clinical

Table 2–7. HEMODYNAMIC EFFECTS OF DIGITALIS IN PATIENTS WITH HEART FAILURE COMPLICATING ACUTE MYOCARDIAL INFARCTION

Study	Change in Cardiac Output (%)	Change in Stroke Work Index (%)	Change in Left Ventricular Filling Pressure (%)
Rahimtoola et al.[112]	+8	−22	−35
Cohn et al.[38]	+9	+38	−10
Hodges et al.[75]	+6	+9	−1
Forrester et al.[49]	−5	+6	−8
Lipp et al.[82]	+4	+18	−4
Goldstein et al.[64]	+9	+26	−7

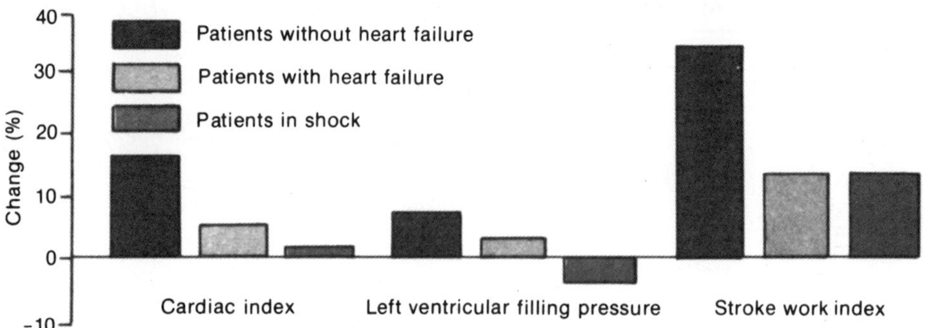

Figure 2–10. Effects of ouabain on left ventricular function in patients with acute myocardial infarction. Cardiac index and stroke work index increased in patients without heart failure; in patients with shock, there was no improvement in left ventricular function.

use. Thus, currently available information seems to indicate that digitalis is not an appropriate inotropic agent for the treatment of pump failure complicating acute myocardial infarction. When inotropic therapy is indicated, it is preferable to use more rapidly acting inotropic agents (e.g., dobutamine or dopamine) with quickly reversible hemodynamic effects. However, digitalis should be considered for the treatment of supraventricular tachyarrhythmias in patients with acute myocardial infarction, particularly for those in whom tachyarrhythmias recur following direct-current cardioversion.

Dobutamine

The beta-1-receptor agonist dobutamine is a frequently used positive inotropic agent for the management of low-output states in patients with both acute and chronic heart failure. At adequate dosages, dobutamine increases cardiac output, stroke volume, and stroke work and decreases left ventricular filling pressure without causing excessive tachycardia or changes in blood pressure (Fig. 2–11).[12] Decreased systemic vascular resistance with dobutamine appears to be primarily secondary to improved cardiac performance, although with larger dosages a direct vasodilatory effect due to partial beta-2-agonist effect can be observed. Pulmonary arterial pressure and pulmonary vascular resistance tend to decrease with dobutamine in patients with left heart failure.

Dopamine

Dopamine has both alpha- and beta-receptor stimulating effects, in addition to its effects on dopamine receptors in the mesenteric and renal vascular beds.[21] It also stimulates norepinephrine release from nerve endings. The level of circulating catecholamines, therefore, may influence the hemodynamic response to dopamine. In general, however, low doses of dopamine predominantly stimulate dopamine receptors that may be useful in improving renal function. With moderate doses of the drug, beta-stimulating effects dominate, whereas with high doses the manifestations of alpha-stimulation (increased arterial pressure and systemic vascular resistance without any significant increase in cardiac output) may be observed. In patients with severe heart failure in whom the level of circulating catecholamines is usually high, relatively smaller doses of dopamine may produce predominantly alpha-stimulating effects.

The positive inotropic effects of dopamine produce an increase in cardiac output. However, with higher doses, there may be a significant increase in arterial pressure and systemic vascular resistance, which may considerably reduce the magnitude of increase in cardiac output and stroke volume. In addition, higher doses of dopamine tend to induce tachycardia. In most patients with heart failure, dopamine does not produce a significant decrease in left ventricular filling pressure and pulmonary artery pressure.

Comparative hemodynamic studies with dobutamine and dopamine in the same patients suggest that, for a similar increase in cardiac output, dopamine produces a greater increase in arterial pressure and a smaller decrease in systemic vascular resistance.[38, 116, 121] Another difference between the two drugs is that dopamine causes no decrease, or even an increase, in left ventricular

Table 2–8. COMPARATIVE HEMODYNAMIC EFFECTS OF DOBUTAMINE AND DIGOXIN IN ACUTE MYOCARDIAL INFARCTION AND HEART FAILURE*

	Control	Dobutamine (8.5 μg/kg/min)	P	Control	Digoxin (12.5 μg/kg)	P
Heart rate (beats/min)	107.2 ± 4.4	111.0 ± 3.7	NS†	107.6 ± 5.3	102.2 ± 6.2	NS
Mean arterial pressure (mm Hg)	97.5 ± 5.7	95.5 ± 5.8	NS	97.5 ± 5.7	95.7 ± 6.4	NS
Cardiac index (l/min/m²)	2.4 ± 0.1	3.2 ± 0.2	<.005	2.2 ± 0.1	2.4 ± 0.1	<.025
Stroke work index (gm-m/m²)	24.6 ± 1.0	36.6 ± 2.8	<.02	21.9 ± 1.0	27.6 ± 2.4	<.05
Pulmonary capillary wedge pressure (mm Hg)	22.3 ± 3.1	9.8 ± 1.5	<.02	18.3 ± 3.6	17.0 ± 2	NS

*From Goldstein et al.: A comparison of digoxin and dobutamine in patients with acute infarction and cardiac failure. N. Engl. J. Med. 303:846, 1980. Reprinted, by permission, from The New England Journal of Medicine.

†NS = not significant.

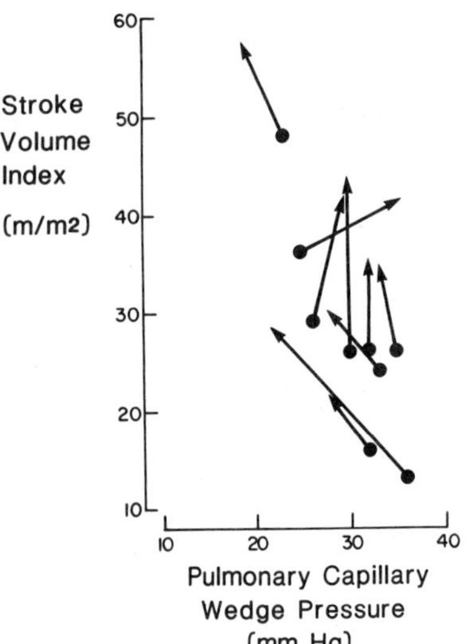

Figure 2–11. Effects of dobutamine infusion on left ventricular function in patients with chronic failure. In each patient, stroke volume index increased; pulmonary capillary wedge pressure decreased or remained unchanged in the majority. These hemodynamic effects indicated improved left ventricular function.

filling pressure, whereas dobutamine usually causes a decrease in left ventricular filling pressure. The major differences in the hemodynamic effects of dobutamine and dopamine are summarized in Table 2–9.

Norepinephrine

The hemodynamic effects of norepinephrine in patients with acute myocardial infarction appear to be related to the dose of the drug and also to the severity of heart failure.[2] In patients with severe heart failure, arterial pressure and systemic vascular resistance increase without any significant change in cardiac output or stroke volume. In patients with mild-to-moderate heart failure, cardiac output and stroke volume increase, and arterial pressure and systemic vascular resistance may not change (Table 2–10).[2] Because of its adverse effects on renal and skeletal muscle blood flow, norepinephrine should be used only in severely hypotensive patients in whom the maintenance of arterial pressure is the major objective of therapy.

Salbutamol

Salbutamol is a beta-2 agonist, but it also possesses beta-stimulating effect, particularly when larger doses are used.

The hemodynamic effects of salbutamol have been investigated both in patients with acute myocardial infarction and in those with chronic heart failure.[21] Salbutamol increases cardiac output and decreases systemic vascular resistance and left ventricular filling pressure, without any significant change in heart rate. It has also been suggested that salbutamol may improve diastolic function of the left ventricle, and thereby improve cardiac performance. Pirbuterol, an orally active beta-2-receptor agonist, produces hemodynamic effects similar to those of salbutamol, but its hemodynamic effects in patients with acute myocardial infarction have not been adequately evaluated. Furthermore, the relative advantages of salbutamol and pirbuterol compared with those of dobutamine or dopamine in the management of acute heart failure need to be evaluated.

Amrinone, MDL 17043, and ARL 115

The mechanisms of action of these newer inotropic agents differ from those of digitalis glycosides and catecholamines.[21] However, their systemic hemodynamic effects are very similar to those of dobutamine and dopamine. The hemodynamic effects of amrinone and dobutamine have been compared in patients with chronic heart failure. Both agents produced comparable increases in cardiac output and decreases in pulmonary capillary wedge pressure. Neither amrinone nor dobutamine significantly altered heart rate or blood pressure, and both agents decreased systemic vascular resistance. Thus, without further studies, the advantages of these newer inotropic agents for the management of pump failure complicating myocardial infarction remain uncertain.

Clinical Application of Inotropic Therapy

The role of inotropic agents in the management of low-output states complicating acute myocardial infarction has not been clearly defined. It appears, however, that digitalis is not indicated to improve low-output states in patients in sinus rhythm.

The choice between different intravenous inotropic agents available for clinical use should be made on the basis of the patient's hemodynamic deficits. In a patient with low

Table 2–9. COMPARATIVE HEMODYNAMIC EFFECTS OF DOBUTAMINE AND DOPAMINE IN PATIENTS WITH PUMP FAILURE*

	Cardiac Output	Arterial Pressure	Systemic Vascular Resistance	Left Ventricular Filling Pressure	Heart Rate	Peripheral Vascular Resistance	Stroke Volume	Stroke Work Index
Dobutamine	↑↑	⟷	⟷ ↓	↓ ⟷	⟷↓	⟷ ↓	↑↑	↑↑
Dopamine	↑↑	↑	⟷ ↑	↑	↑	⟷ ↓	↑↑	↑↑

↓ or ↑ = modest change; ↑ ↑ or ↓ ↓ = marked change; ⟷ = no change.

Table 2–10. HEMODYNAMIC RESPONSE TO GRADED DOSES OF NOREPINEPHRINE IN PATIENTS WITH ACUTE MYOCARDIAL INFARCTION*

	Survivors				Nonsurvivors			
	Control	*3–5 μg*	*5–8 μg*	*8–10 μg*	*Control*	*3–5 μg*	*5–8 μg*	*8–10 μg*
Mean blood pressure (mm Hg)	85.0	95.6	96.6	102.7	68.0	73.9	80.1	88.8
Heart rate (beats/min)	78.3	77.8	75.5	86.6	90.6	90.7	89.3	93.7
Cardiac output (l/min)	4.6	5.0	4.9	5.7	3.1	3.3	3.2	3.5
Stroke work (g-m/beat)	73.9	84.3	88.3	93.8	31.6	36.5	41.5	45.0
Systemic vascular resistance (dynes sec cm^{-5})	17.1	17.7	18.8	16.8	24.0	24.1	26.3	30.0

*From Abrams et al.: Variability in response to norepinephrine in acute myocardial infarction. Am. J. Cardiol. 32:919, 1973. Reproduced with permission.

Table 2–11. THE CHOICE OF AN INOTROPIC AGENT ON THE BASIS OF HEMODYNAMIC ABNORMALITIES

Cardiac Output	Arterial Pressure	Systemic Vascular Resistance	Pulmonary Capillary Wedge Pressure	Inotropic Agent
Low	Normal or slightly decreased	Normal or slightly elevated	Elevated	Dobutamine
Low	Low	Normal or low	Normal or slightly elevated	Dopamine
Low	Moderate hypotension	Elevated	Elevated	Dopamine and nitroprusside
Low	Mild hypotension	Elevated	Elevated	Dobutamine and nitroprusside
Low	Marked hypotension	Normal or elevated	Elevated	Norepinephrine + intra-aortic balloon counterpulsation + nitroprusside

cardiac output, normal or only moderately elevated left ventricular filling pressure, and low or normal systemic vascular resistance, dopamine is the drug of choice, particularly if there is coexisting hypotension. On the other hand, if the left ventricular filling pressure is elevated and systemic vascular resistance and arterial pressure are in the normal range, dobutamine can be used effectively to increase cardiac output. In the presence of severe hypotension (e.g., systolic blood pressure less than 80 mm Hg), norepinephrine can be used to maintain adequate arterial pressure until intra-aortic balloon counterpulsation therapy can be instituted to provide adequate myocardial perfusion pressure and cause systolic unloading concomitantly. The choice of an inotropic agent on the basis of hemodynamic abnormalities is suggested in Table 2–11.

COMBINED THERAPY WITH VASODILATORS AND INOTROPIC AGENTS OR INTRA-AORTIC BALLOON COUNTERPULSATION

When vasodilator agents fail to produce adequate beneficial hemodynamic effects, or when hypotension results during vasodilator therapy, the addition of inotropic agents to the vasodilators may provide optimal improvement in left ventricular function and prevent significant hypotension. In some patients with low cardiac output after acute myocardial infarction, arterial pressure is relatively normal or low and systemic vascular resistance is not elevated. In these patients, vasodilator therapy frequently produces hypotension with little or no increase in cardiac output. Inotropic agents (dobutamine or dopamine) are preferable to vasodilators in these patients. In the presence of significant hypotension, there is a potential risk of further hypotension when vasodilator therapy is initiated. Initial use of inotropic agents followed by the addition of vasodilators not infrequently prevents hypotension and causes significant hemodynamic and clinical improvement.

Several papers have demonstrated the additive effects and overall efficacy of combination therapy, employing dopamine or dobutamine together with sodium nitroprusside, in patients with chronic left ventricular failure.[13, 95, 96] This approach makes similar sense in the individual with acute heart failure complicating myocardial infarction. Figure 2–12 illustrates the effects of dobutamine and sodium nitroprusside in a patient with acute pump failure.

Unfortunately, positive inotropic agents tend to produce tachycardia and arrhythmias, and resistance often develops during chronic therapy.[101] Furthermore, the ventricular reserve of patients with severe pump failure frequently is not sufficient to maintain adequate blood pressure during vasodilator therapy. Therefore, such combined therapy is rarely efficacious in patients with true cardiogenic shock. Perhaps a more effective approach is the use of intra-aortic balloon counterpulsation in combination with vasodilators. Diastolic augmentation by balloon counterpulsation improves coronary blood flow and clinical signs of peripheral perfusion.[119] Addition of vasodilators such as nitroprusside is frequently possible after the insertion of the

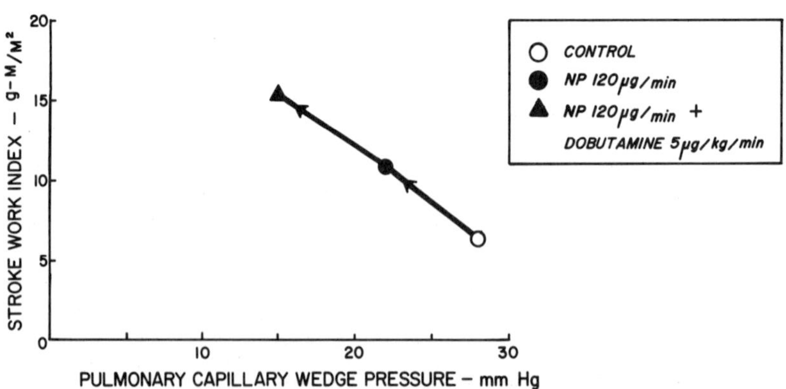

Figure 2–12. Additive improvement in left ventricular performance produced by combined infusion of a vasodilator, sodium nitroprusside, and an inotropic catecholamine, dobutamine, in a patient with acute pump failure.

balloon, even in patients in whom hypotension has previously occurred. Vasodilator therapy may further reduce left ventricular filling pressure and increase cardiac output, and thus may facilitate the weaning of these patients from mechanical assistance. Nonetheless, unless corrective surgery is feasible, the outlook for these patients is generally poor.

USE OF VASODILATORS TO TREAT MECHANICAL DEFECTS COMPLICATING MYOCARDIAL INFARCTION

In some patients with myocardial infarction, pump failure is precipitated or exacerbated by mechanical defects, such as ventricular septal rupture or mitral regurgitation caused by papillary muscle dysfunction.[103] Without surgery, which itself carries a high mortality rate in the immediate postinfarction period, these patients have previously done very poorly. In persons with these defects, the proportion of total left ventricular stroke volume entering the systemic circulation, as opposed to that returning to the left atrium or right ventricle, is determined by the relative resistance of these varying pathways to flow.[17] Therefore, vasodilators might be expected to be particularly efficacious in patients with these mechanical defects, since in addition to their beneficial effect on overall left ventricular performance, they reduce arterial impedance and thereby proportionately increase forward cardiac output.

Indeed, several studies have documented hemodynamic improvement during sodium nitroprusside therapy in patients with mitral regurgitation and ventricular septal rupture.[27, 65, 72, 122, 125] The dosage and hemodynamic guidelines for the use of nitroprusside are the same for these patients as for those in left ventricular failure. Chatterjee and colleagues administered this agent to eight patients with mitral insufficiency caused by dysfunction of the subvalvular apparatus[27] and demonstrated consistent increases in forward stroke volume and reductions in regurgitant volume, pulmonary arterial pressure, and pulmonary capillary wedge mean and "V" wave pressures. Figure 2–13 illustrates the dramatic reduction of mitral regurgitation, as demonstrated by the disappearance of the regurgitant "V" wave in a patient with acute papillary muscle dysfunction. Hydralazine, given parenterally and orally, has also been shown to decrease the amount of mitral regurgitation with similar hemodynamic and clinical improvement (Fig. 2–14).[69]

Similar improvement has been noted with sodium nitroprusside in patients with ventricular septal rupture.[122, 125] However, the actual efficacy of vasodilator therapy in these patients is determined by the relative degree to which the systemic and pulmonary resistances are lowered. Thus, hydralazine may be more effective than nitroprusside, since it acts more specifically on the peripheral arteriolar resistance vessels.

Although vasodilator agents produce beneficial hemodynamic effects in patients with mechanical defects, their clinical application in the management of this form of heart failure has not been clearly defined. In patients with severe mitral regurgitation or ventricular septal rupture complicating acute myocardial infarction, these agents can be used for immediate hemodynamic and clinical improvement. However, vasodilator therapy should be regarded as supportive rather than definitive. In most cases, surgical correction is required and should be considered as soon as the patient is stabilized.

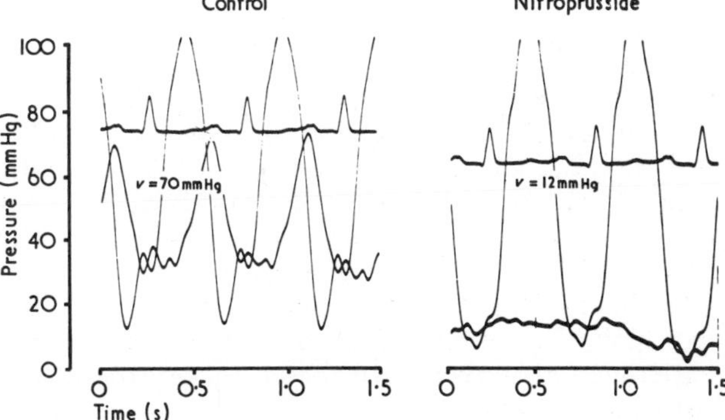

Figure 2–13. The left ventricular and pulmonary capillary wedge pressure tracings from a patient with acute papillary muscle dysfunction. Note the large "V" wave in the control tracing, which disappeared after nitroprusside was given. The mean wedge pressure and left ventricular end-diastolic pressure also fell.

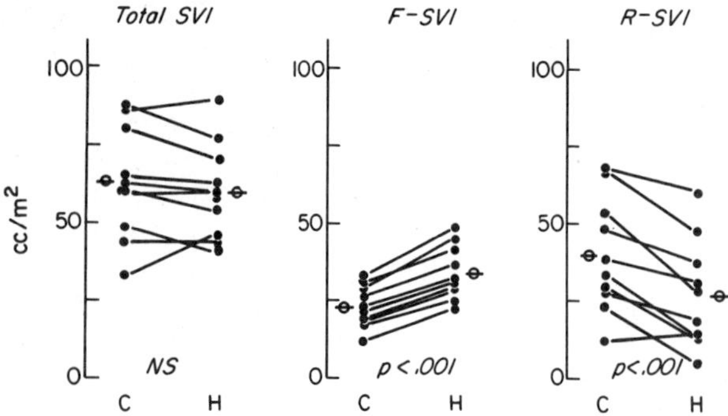

Figure 2–14. Effect of intravenous hydralazine on mitral regurgitation. Although there is no change in total left ventricular stroke volume, regurgitant volume decreases while forward stroke volume rises. Similar changes were noted during oral hydralazine therapy. (From Greenberg et al.: Beneficial effects of hydralazine in severe mitral reguritation. Circulation 58:273, 1978. Reproduced by permission of The American Heart Association, Inc.)

CLINICAL RESULTS OF VASODILATOR AND INOTROPIC THERAPY FOR ACUTE PUMP FAILURE

Effects on Myocardial Ischemia and Infarct Size

As mentioned earlier, an important goal of management of pump failure complicating acute myocardial infarction is to minimize the imbalance between myocardial oxygen supply and demand. Since both vasodilators and inotropic agents produce a variety of hemodynamic changes that may alter this balance, and since the circumstances in which they are employed are variable, their overall effect on myocardial metabolism may be difficult to predict. Thus, if arterial pressure falls excessively with the vasodilator, coronary perfusion may be impaired. If reflex tachycardia results, oxygen demand will be increased. If the inotropic state of the myocardium increases without concomitant hemodynamic improvement, overall oxygen demand will also rise. On the other hand, the decrease in both left ventricular preload and afterload with therapy should reduce oxygen requirements, and the increases in cardiac output may be associated with a rise in coronary blood flow. Another factor that must be considered is the direct effect of vasodilators on the coronary circulation, and this may vary from medication to medication.

A number of experimental studies have sought to define the effect of vasodilators on myocardial ischemia and infarct size.[10, 32, 34, 43, 44, 115, 132] Unfortunately, the results have been conflicting and difficult to extrapolate to humans. Most, but not all, experimental studies have shown that nitroprusside increases overall coronary blood flow as well as perfusion to ischemic regions. This has been associated with a shift from lactate production to extraction and functional improvement in the ischemic segment, suggesting a lessening of ischemia (Fig. 2–15).[43, 44, 77, 102, 113, 132] On the other hand, an increase in the epicardial ST-segment elevation after nitroprusside, but not nitroglycerin, has been noted.[32] These workers postulated a "coronary steal" mechanism to explain these differences. Indeed, theoretical considerations suggest that an agent with an arteriolar dilating effect would be more likely to cause a coronary steal.[11] Phentolamine, perhaps because of its direct cardiac stimulating effect, appears to be more likely to exacerbate ischemia than is nitroprusside.[113]

The results of human investigations are also conflicting. One group evaluated regional myocardial blood flow by the Xe-133 washout technique and found that nitroprusside caused a reduction in the perfusion of jeopardized regions.[85] Other studies have reported an increase in precordial ST-segment elevation and serum creatine kinase following nitroprusside administration.[32, 61, 84] In these studies, nitroglycerin has had an opposite effect to that of nitroprusside. On the other hand, another report describes a reduction in ST-segment elevation in patients given nitroprusside.[9] In prospective, randomized studies, early intervention with sodium nitroprusside was associated with a lower CPK-MB isoenzyme level compared with that of the control group.[11, 46] Chatterjee and coworkers measured coronary blood flow, myocardial oxygen consumption, and lactate metabolism in patients receiving nitroprusside for acute pump failure.[25] They found a mild reduction in coronary flow and oxygen utilization, but no change in lactate extraction, suggesting that the overall balance between

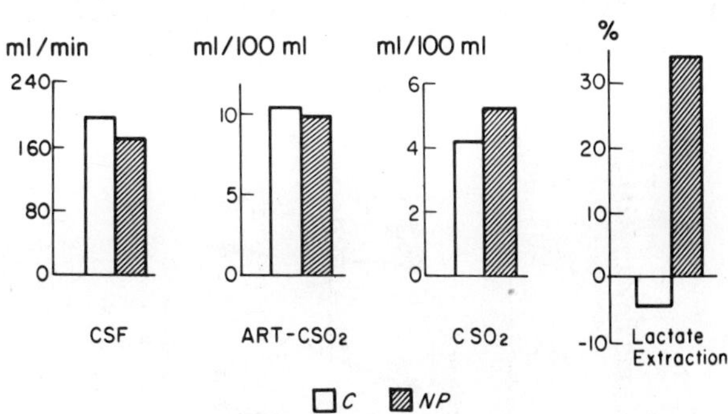

Figure 2–15. The effect of nitroprusside *(NP)* on myocardial blood flow and metabolism in a patient with pump failure complicating acute myocardial infarction is shown. Coronary sinus blood flow falls slightly from the control *(C)* value, while the arterial-coronary sinus oxygen difference (Art-CSO_2) was unchanged, resulting in a slightly lower calculated myocardial oxygen consumption. Most important, the evidence of myocardial ischemia, lactate production, disappeared. (From Chatterjee et al.: Hemodynamic and metabolic responses to vasodilator therapy in acute myocardial infarction. Circulation 48:1183, 1973. Reproduced by permission of The American Heart Association, Inc.)

oxygen supply and demand is not altered. However, the possibility of regional changes remains to be investigated.

The effect of nitroglycerin on indices of ischemia in patients with acute myocardial infarction is also somewhat controversial. The bulk of evidence suggests that if arterial pressure is maintained, the overall effect is not deleterious.[8, 14, 32, 41] At least one prospective randomized study has demonstrated a reduction in infarct size calculated by enzymatic techniques following intravenous nitroglycerin.[19] A decrease in myocardial oxygen consumption has also been demonstrated following nitroglycerin administration.[29] The particular ability of nitroglycerin to increase collateral blood flow is also potentially beneficial.

Thus, the questions of how vasodilators affect myocardial metabolism and whether they alter infarct size remain open. However, the considerable clinical experience with their use in patients with acute infarction suggests that they can be used safely, as long as patients are properly selected and careful attention is paid to the important hemodynamic parameters.

Inotropic Agents and Myocardial Ischemia

Potential also exists for the enhancement of myocardial ischemia and the deterioration of myocardial metabolic function with the use of positive inotropic agents. Augmented contractility increases myocardial oxygen demand.[15] Furthermore, if tachycardia occurs with the use of inotropic agents, not only does myocardial oxygen demand increase, but myocardial perfusion may also be compromised because of decreased diastolic perfusion time. Thus, whenever inotropic agents are used in patients with acute myocardial infarction, careful observations are needed for the occurrence of the adverse effects on myocardial ischemia and metabolic function.

The changes in coronary blood flow and myocardial oxygen consumption in a group of patients with acute myocardial infarction following intravenous digitalis are illustrated in Figure 2–16. Coronary blood flow and myocardial oxygen consumption increased in all patients. The patients who had the greatest increase in coronary blood flow and myocardial oxygen consumption also developed angina. These findings suggest that the increase in myocardial oxygen demand caused an increase in myocardial oxygen consumption, and myocardial ischemia was precipitated.

It has been demonstrated that the administration of digitalis in the acute phase of myocardial infarction can increase the extent of myocardial ischemic injury both in experimental myocardial infarction and in patients with acute myocardial infarction without heart failure.

Dopamine may enhance myocardial ischemia in patients with acute myocardial infarction and cardiogenic shock. Myocardial lactate production, the biochemical evidence of myocardial ischemia, has been observed in these patients, despite a concomitant increase in blood pressure and cardiac output. Although the effects of dobutamine on coronary hemodynamics and myocardial metabolic function have not been evaluated in patients with acute myocardial infarction, it is likely that it does increase myocardial oxygen consumption because of increased myocardial oxygen demand due to enhanced contractility. In patients with chronic ischemic heart failure, dobutamine consistently

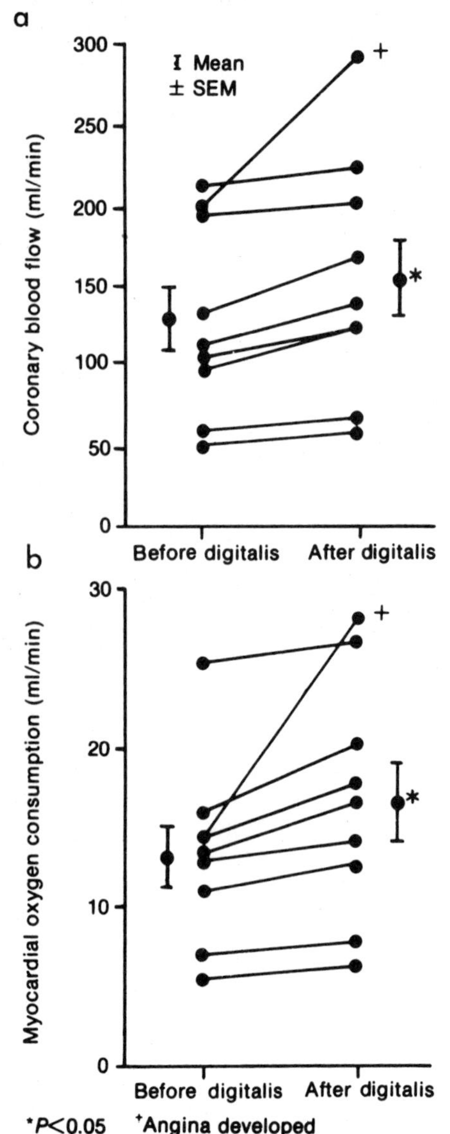

Figure 2–16. Changes in coronary blood flow *(a)* and myocardial oxygen consumption *(b)* in nine patients with acute myocardial infarction after administration of ouabain. Coronary blood flow and myocardial oxygen consumption increased in all patients, and one patient developed angina following ouabain.

increases coronary blood flow and myocardial oxygen consumption. Although in most patients no deleterious effect on myocardial metabolic function has been observed during dobutamine therapy, myocardial ischemia may be enhanced in some patients, as evidenced by the finding of myocardial lactate production during dobutamine infusion.[12] It is apparent, therefore, that irrespective of the type of inotropic agent used, myocardial metabolic function may deteriorate and the extent of myocardial ischemic injury may increase in patients with acute myocardial infarction.

Effect of Medical Therapy on Prognosis for Acute Pump Failure

It is extremely difficult to determine whether vasodilator therapy has altered the prognosis for patients with acute myocardial infarction. Recently, two controlled studies have appeared examining the effect of nitroprusside therapy in this setting. In one, a significant reduction in mortality at one week, together with a decreased incidence of clinical cardiogenic shock and left ventricular failure, was reported. Late mortality during weeks two to four was also lower in the nitroprusside-treated group.[46] In the Veterans Administration Cooperative Study, however, nitroprusside therapy was not associated with any change in either early or late mortality, but it is noteworthy that the subset of patients with persistent elevation of left ventricular filling pressure had a lower mortality rate in the group treated with nitroprusside.[37] In a study by Hockings and colleagues,[74] no reduction in hospital mortality was found following nitroprusside therapy in patients with acute myocardial infarction and elevated left ventricular filling pressure.

The reasons for the varying results from these investigations are not clear. The study with the most optimistic outcome initiated therapy sooner after the onset of symptoms.[46] This suggests that, if the prognosis for acute infarction is to be improved, early intervention is required. It is also possible that vasodilators improve prognosis only in the subset of patients with severe pump failure in cardiogenic shock, who were excluded from randomization in all of these studies.

Intravenous nitroglycerin has also been studied in a few prospective randomized investigations, but these have included only patients with mild or no left ventricular failure.[29, 33] Again, no substantial change in mortality was noted, but the number of included subjects was too small to exclude a beneficial drug effect definitively.

There are no control studies of vasodilator therapy in patients with severe pump failure or cardiogenic shock. However, it is known that the coronary care unit mortality rate for these patients is very high.[30, 81, 114, 120, 129] Before the advent of vasodilator therapy, patients with acute infarction who developed pulmonary edema had a 30 to 40 per cent mortality rate and those with cardiogenic shock had a mortality rate greater than 90 per cent. Table 2–12 catalogues some of the published mortality rates based on the initial hemodynamic measurements.[31]

The impact of vasodilator therapy on acute prognosis can be roughly assessed by comparing the survival of treated patients with these figures. Chatterjee and associates administered vasodilators to 43 patients with severe pump failure (left ventricular filling pressure > 15 mm Hg; stroke work index ≤ 20 g-m/m²).[31] Seventeen were in shock and all had pulmonary edema. Some initial hemodynamic improvement was noted in all patients. Despite continuation of intravenous vasodilators for up to 27 days, the mortality rate remained substantial (44%). However, a comparison of the mortality in comparable hemodynamic subsets from this group with the findings of other studies suggests that acute survival may be improved by vasodilators (Table 2–12). Unfortunately, only two of 11 patients with stroke work indices less than 10 g-m/m² survived, indicating that vasodilator therapy alone offers little to those with the most severe pump failure. It is in these patients that the effect of intra-aortic balloon counterpulsation and the new positive inotropic agents should be assessed.

Despite this apparent improvement in short-term prognosis by vasodilator therapy, the long-term survival of these patients is poor (Fig. 2–17).[31] After nine months, 62 per cent of the initial survivors were dead and the projected three-year survival rate was only 28 per cent. In addition, half of the chronic survivors were severely symptomatic from heart failure. In some centers, these patients undergo evaluation for surgically remediable disease such as mechanical defects, resectable aneurysm, or jeopardized myocardium that can be revascularized.

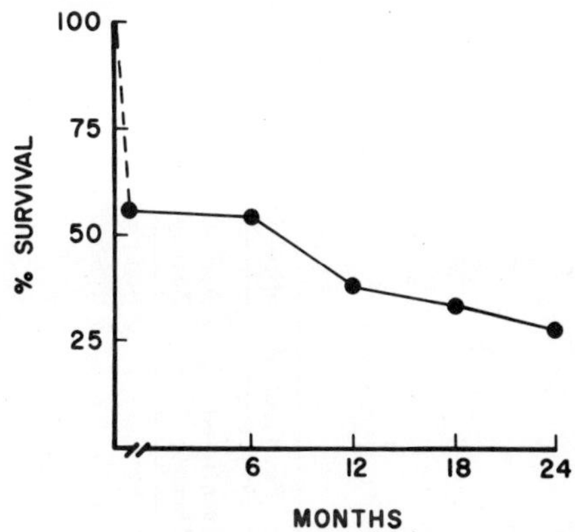

Figure 2–17. Cumulative survival rate in patients treated with vasodilators for severe pump failure accompanying acute myocardial infarction. The survival rate at 24 months was only 28 per cent. (From Chatterjee et al.: Effects of vasodilator therapy for severe pump failure in acute myocardial infarction on short-term and late prognosis. Circulation 53:797, 1976. Reproduced by permission of The American Heart Association, Inc.)

VASODILATOR THERAPY FOR CHRONIC HEART FAILURE

Most patients who survive the phase of acute pump failure complicating myocardial infarction are left with residual, usually severe, left ventricular dysfunction. In recent years, many studies have shown that hemodynamic and symptomatic improvement can be obtained in these patients with the chronic administration of vasodilators. Since this chapter is devoted primarily to the management of acute pump failure, the subject of chronic vasodilator therapy will be dealt with only briefly. Several excellent review articles devoted entirely to this subject have appeared in recent years.[23, 24, 36, 53, 89, 98, 104, 115]

As discussed above, patients with chronic heart failure generally have elevated left ventricular filling pressures and cardiac outputs that are reduced at rest or do not rise normally with activity. Dyspnea is primarily due to elevated pulmonary venous pressures, and exercise intolerance and fatigue are the major symptoms of decreased cardiac output. The objectives of vasodilator therapy are to increase cardiac output and decrease pulmonary capillary wedge pressure. Table 2–13 lists a number of currently available agents that have been shown to be hemodynamically effective in the management of chronic heart failure. To date, only captopril has been given FDA approval for this indication.

Spectrum of Nonparenteral Vasodilators

A wide variety of nitrate preparations have been studied for chronic heart failure.[5, 18, 56, 57, 62, 68, 86, 124, 130, 131] Their onset and

Table 2–12. MORTALITY FROM PUMP FAILURE IN ACUTE MYOCARDIAL INFARCTION: COMPARISON OF CONVENTIONAL THERAPY WITH VASODILATOR THERAPY*

Authors	No. of Patients	Cardiac Index 1 (liter/min/m³)	Stroke Work Index (SWI) (g-m/m³)	Left Ventricular Filling Pressure (LVFP) (mm Hg)	SWI/LVFP (g-m/m²/mm Hg)	Per Cent Mortality	
						Conventional Therapy	*Vasodilator Therapy*
Chatterjee et al.[30]	15	–	≤ 20	≥ 15	–	80	44
Ratshin et al.[114]	11	≤ 2.2	–	≥ 15	–	100	53
Scheidt et al.[120]	29	–	≤ 20	–	–	72	44
Bleifield et al.[13a]	42	–	–	–	≤ 1.2	80	44
Weber et al.[129]	84	≤ 2.0	–	≤ 15	–	95	42

*From Chatterjee and Parmley: Role of vasodilator therapy in heart failure. Prog. Cardiovasc. Dis. 19:301, 1977.

Table 2–13. DOSAGE AND HEMODYNAMIC EFFECT OF COMMONLY USED NONPARENTERAL VASODILATORS

Medication	Dosage	Venous Tone	Arteriolar Resistance	HR	BP	CO	LVFP
Nitrates	Various	↓↓	⟷↓	⟷↑	⟷↓	⟷↑	↓↓
Hydralazine	50–100 mg PO q6h	⟷	↓↓	⟷↑	⟷↓	↑↑	⟷
Minoxidil	10–80 mg PO od	⟷	↓↓	⟷↑	⟷↓	↑↑	⟷
Prazosin	3–10 mg PO q8h	↓	↓	⟷↑	⟷↓	↑	↓
Captopril	12.5–100 mg PO q8h	⟷↓	↓	↓⟷	↓↓	↑	↓↓

↓ or ↑ = modest change; ↓↓ or ↑↑ = marked change; ⟷ = no significant change. HR = heart rate; BP = arterial pressure; CO = cardiac output; LVFP = left ventricular filling pressure.

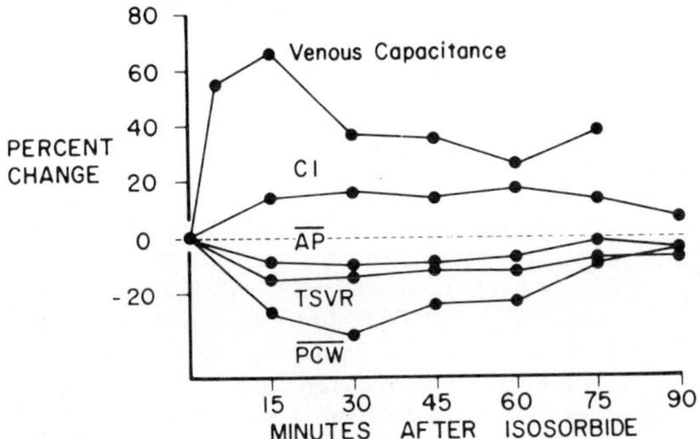

Figure 2–18. Effect of sublingual isosorbide dinitrate on hemodynamic parameters over the course of 90 min. These data indicate the mean percentage change from control values in 12 patients with chronic congestive heart failure. The most dramatic effect was an increase in venous capacitance. There was only a modest increase in cardiac index and a modest decrease in systemic vascular resistance. (From Gray et al.: Hemodynamic and metabolic effects of isosorbide dinitrate in chronic congestive heart failure. Am. Heart J. 90:346, 1975. Reproduced with permission.)

duration of action may vary, but these medications produce similar hemodynamic changes. The predominant effect is a marked increase in venous capacitance with a consequent decrease in both right atrial and pulmonary capillary wedge pressure. The hemodynamic changes following the administration of sublingual isosorbide dinitrate, in dosages ranging from 5 to 15 mg, are illustrated in Figure 2–18. By and large, the nitrates are well tolerated. The limiting side effects are generally headache and/or nausea, which may be extremely uncomfortable but tend to become less severe with chronic drug administration. Tachycardia and hypotension are uncommon in patients with elevated left ventricular filling pressures. Occasionally, these are noted when patients assume the upright position, particularly when nitrates are given in combination with other vasodilators.

Hydralazine and minoxidil are direct-acting dilators of vascular smooth muscle that have a relatively selective effect on arteriolar resistance vessels.[22, 26, 28, 54, 58, 78, 90] As a result of this afterload reduction, these drugs produce a marked rise in cardiac output in patients with heart failure. The hemodynamic effects of hydralazine in a group of such patients are illustrated in Figure 2–19. Hydralazine therapy is usually initiated with a 25-mg oral dose and increased as needed; total daily dosages in the range of 200 to 400 mg are often required. Chronic hydralazine therapy is often accompanied by side effects or drug toxicity. Most commonly seen are headaches, nausea, and other gastrointestinal symptoms, which prevent or limit therapy in nearly one third of the patients. During long-term therapy, drug-induced lupus erythematosus is sometimes seen. Fluid retention, presumably due to increased activity of the renin-angiotensin-aldosterone system, is common during long-term therapy with hydralazine or minoxidil.[106] This and other factors may lead to the development of tolerance to these drugs.[39, 104] Because of the differing but additive hemodynamic effects of nitrates and hydralazine, these agents are often used in combination to treat patients with chronic heart failure (Fig. 2–20).[90] This combination has been shown to improve exercise capacity in heart failure patients.[91]

Prazosin is a postsynaptic, alpha-adrenergic blocking agent that has been used extensively in the management of chronic heart failure.[40, 63, 97, 118] Single doses of 2 to 7 mg produce both arteriolar dilatation and venodilatation. The initial dose of prazosin may

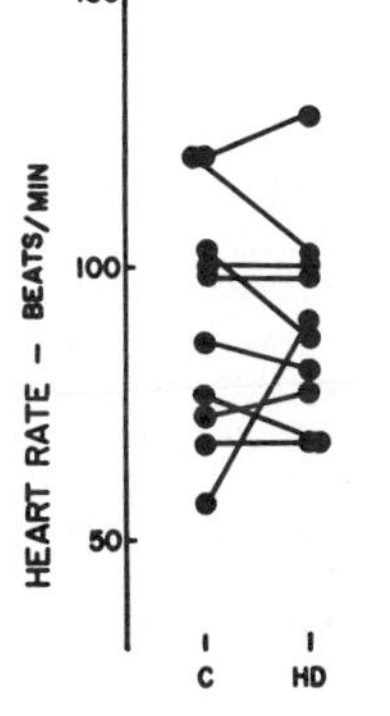

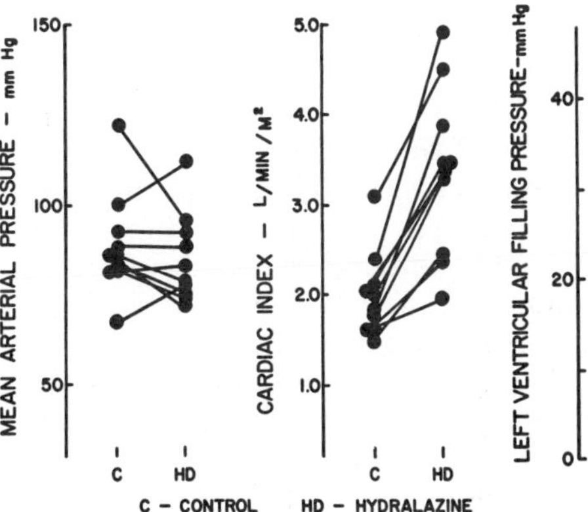

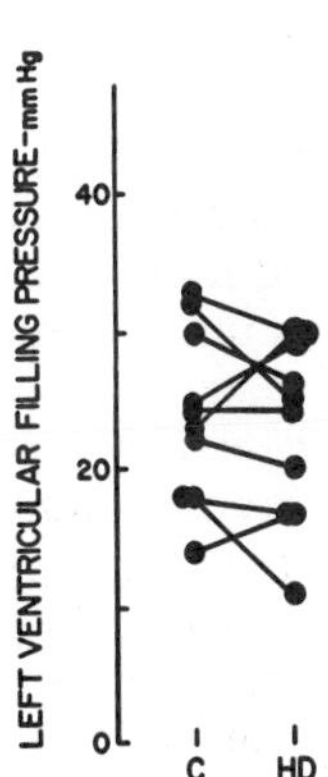

Figure 2–19. Hemodynamic effect of oral hydralazine in patients with congestive heart failure. Note the significant rise in cardiac index but relatively small changes in left ventricular filling pressure. Hydralazine did not affect heart rate or arterial pressure in these patients, in contrast to its usual effect in patients without heart failure. (From Chatterjee et al.: Oral hydralazine for chronic refractory heart failure. Circulation 54:879 1976. Reproduced by permission of The American Heart Association, Inc.)

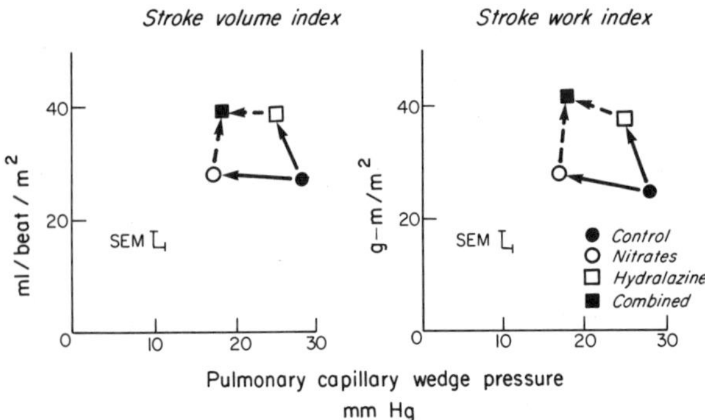

Figure 2–20. Changes in stroke volume index (SVI) and stroke work index (SWI) plotted on the vertical axis against changes in pulmonary capillary wedge (PCW) pressure on the horizontal axis during administration of nitrates, hydralazine, and combined nitrates and hydralazine in 12 patients with chronic heart failure. Nitrates significantly decreased PCW pressure without an increase in SVI or SWI. Hydralazine, on the other hand, increased SVI and SWI significantly with only a slight reduction in PCW pressure. Combined nitrates and hydralazine, however, reduced PCW pressure significantly, associated with a marked increase in SVI and SWI, indicating significant improvement in left ventricular performance. (From Massie et al.: Hemodynamic advantage of combined administration of hydralazine orally and nitrates nonparenterally in the vasodilator therapy of chronic heart failure. Am. J. Cardiol. 40:794, 1977. Reproduced with permission.)

profoundly reduce arterial pressure, so it should be started cautiously. Although hemodynamic improvement has been consistently noted following initial doses of prazosin, controversy exists regarding its continued efficacy.[7, 105] Nonetheless, some studies have documented an increase in exercise tolerance and chronic hemodynamic improvement.[40, 97]

A great deal of attention has been devoted to the use of angiotensin-converting enzyme inhibitors in the treatment of chronic heart failure.[60] Most of this work has employed captopril, which produces a dramatic decrease in pulmonary capillary wedge pressure and left ventricular volume (Fig. 2–21), usually accompanied by a modest rise in cardiac output.[3, 20, 45, 47, 52, 80, 93, 126, 127] These hemodynamic changes are not closely related to the plasma renin activity, suggesting that captopril may have other effects than those mediated by the reduction of angiotensin II. Initial doses are consistently accompanied by a reduction in blood pressure, which averages 20 to 25 per cent and can sometimes be precipitous. As a result, patients must be carefully monitored during the initiation of therapy. The severity of this hypotension can be reduced by the discontinuation of other vasodilating agents and the withholding of diuretics for 24 to 48 hours prior to captopril administration. Continuing hypotension prevents or limits chronic therapy in approximately 10 per cent of patients, but blood pressure in the remainder rises toward the pretreatment level after one to two weeks of therapy. Earlier studies employed high captopril doses (100 mg three times per day on the average), but more recent data indicate that dosages of 25 to 50 mg three times per day are often effective. Most important, captopril produces long-term improvement in exercise capacity in patients who were previously receiving optimal therapy with digoxin and diuretics (Fig. 2–22).[20, 80] Since fluid retention and drug tolerance occur rarely, if

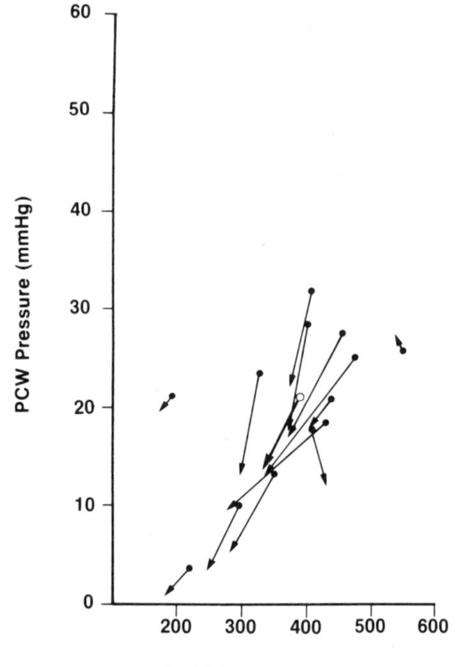

Figure 2–21. The changes produced by 25 mg oral captopril in left ventricular filling pressures (PCW pressure) and left ventricular volume, measured simultaneously. The volumes were measured by a nongeometric nuclear technique. Note that pressure and volume fell together, confirming a drug-induced reduction in preload. (From Massie et al.: Hemodynamic and radionuclide effects of acute captopril therapy for heart failure: changes in left and right ventricular volumes and function at rest and during exercise. Circulation 65:1374, 1982. Reproduced by permission of The American Heart Association, Inc.)

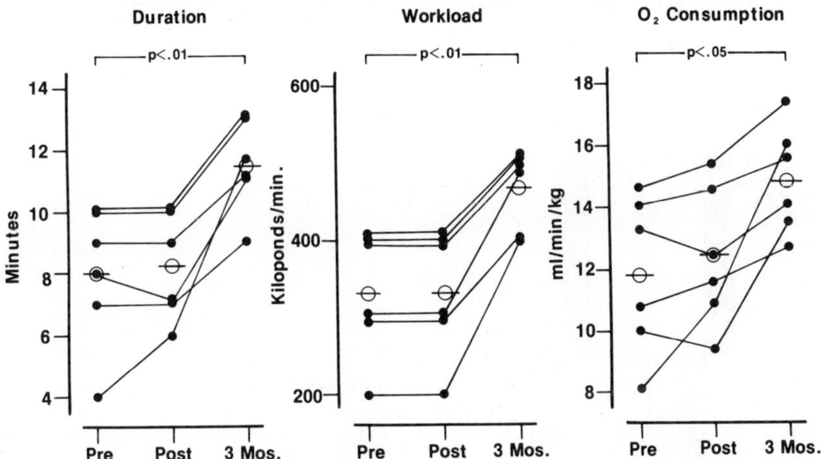

Figure 2–22. Exercise capacity on an upright ergometer was measured before treatment *(pre)*, after 24 hours of captopril *(post)* and after three months of treatment. Exercise duration, maximal workload, and maximal oxygen consumption all rose during chronic therapy. (From Topic et al.: Acute and long-term effects of captopril on exercise cardiac performance and exercise capacity in congestive heart failure. Am. Heart J. 104:1172, 1982. Reproduced with permission.)

ever, during chronic captopril therapy, this agent may become the drug of choice for chronic vasodilator therapy.

Myocardial Metabolic Effects of Vasodilators

Since patients surviving acute pump failure who go on to have chronic heart failure generally have obstructive coronary artery disease, it is important to consider the effect of drug therapy on myocardial metabolism. Figure 2–23 illustrates the relative effects of captopril, prazosin, and hydralazine on central hemodynamics and myocardial oxygen consumption in a group of patients with chronic heart failure.[117] Each of the three agents produces hemodynamic improvement, as discussed previously, but captopril appears to do so at a lower metabolic cost. This probably results from the effects of captopril on the hemodynamic determinants in myocardial oxygen consumption. Captopril lowers both blood pressure and heart rate, thus reducing double product, a frequently used index in myocardial oxygen demand. It also decreases left ventricular diastolic volume, which should result in a reduction in myocardial wall tension, another important determinant of myocardial oxygen consumption. Hydralazine and prazosin produce more variable changes in the determinants of myocardial oxygen consumption. Furthermore, they may have direct effects on the coronary vascular bed, which may redistribute coronary blood flow away from jeopardized regions.

Clinical Results of Chronic Vasodilator Therapy

A number of studies have documented short-term clinical improvement in patients treated with vasodilators, and have objectively confirmed these findings with measurements of exercise capacity.[40, 53, 57, 63, 80, 91, 126] Nonetheless, the long-term prognosis for patients with severe chronic heart failure is poor. Controlled studies evaluating the influence of vasodilator therapy on long-term prognosis are not yet available, but uncontrolled studies suggest that the mortality rate remains high. The mortality rates in a group of 56 patients treated with hydralazine and nitrates are shown in Figure 2–24.[94] The most common mode of death was sudden. Survival was significantly higher in patients who were stable before the initiation of vasodilator therapy and was worse in Class IV patients who were deteriorating when first treated. This finding suggests the need for earlier treatment if vasodilators are to have any chance of affecting prognosis.

In this group of patients, the hemodynamic changes during the initiation of vasodilator therapy did not accurately predict the re-

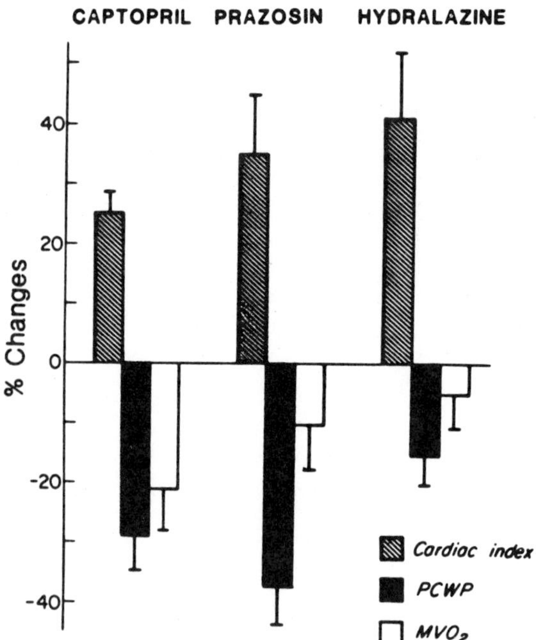

Figure 2–23. The effects of three vasodilators on central hemodynamics and myocardial oxygen consumption *(MVO_2)* are shown. Although all three increased cardiac output and lowered pulmonary capillary wedge pressure *(PCWP)*, captopril lowered MVO_2 to a significantly greater extent. (From Rouleau et al.: Alterations in left ventricular function and coronary hemodynamics with captopril, hydralazine and prazosin in chronic ischemic heart failure. A comparative study. Circulation 65:671, 1982. Reproduced by permission of The American Heart Association, Inc.)

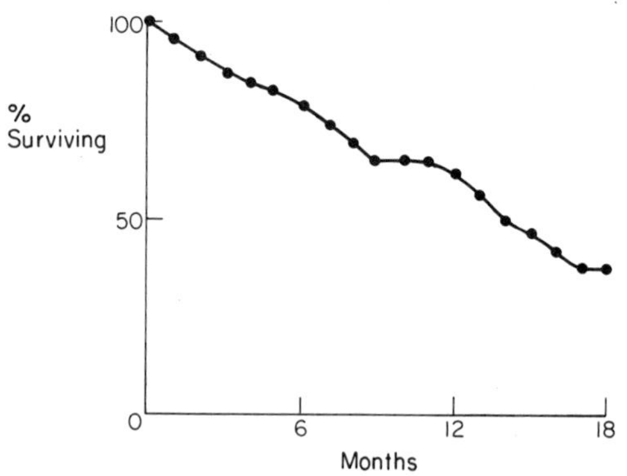

Figure 2–24. The survival curve of 56 chronic heart failure patients treated with hydralazine. Despite symptomatic improvement, the mortality rate was high: 22, 35, and 63 per cent at six, 12, and 18 months respectively. (From Massie et al.: Long-term vasodilator therapy for heart failure: clinical response and its relationship to hemodynamic measurements. Circulation 63:269, 1981. Reproduced by permission of The American Heart Association, Inc.)

sponse to therapy.[94] However, patients who showed no hemodynamic response in the first 48 hours, and those whose pulmonary capillary wedge pressure remained above 20 mm Hg and whose stroke work index was below 30 g-m/m^2 on vasodilators, had little or no response (Fig. 2–25). Retrospective studies with prazosin and captopril have also shown that patients with severe heart failure continued to have a poor prognosis despite sometimes dramatic clinical and symptomatic improvement during vasodilator therapy.[93, 117]

CONCLUSIONS

In recent years, considerable interest has been devoted to the management of acute pump failure complicating myocardial infarction. On the basis of a great deal of experience with hemodynamic measurements in

Figure 2–25. The relationship between the hemodynamic measurements obtained after initiating hydralazine and nitrates and the subsequent clinical course. Most patients with stroke work indices above 30 gm/m$_2$ and pulmonary capillary wedge pressures below 20 mm Hg were alive *(A)* and clinically improved *(I)* at latest follow-up. Conversely, those with low stroke work indices and high filling pressures usually did not improve *(NI)* and died *(D)*. (From Massie et al.: Long-term vasodilator therapy for heart failure: clinical response and its relationship to hemodynamic measurements. Circulation 63:269, 1981. Reproduced by permission of The American Heart Association, Inc.)

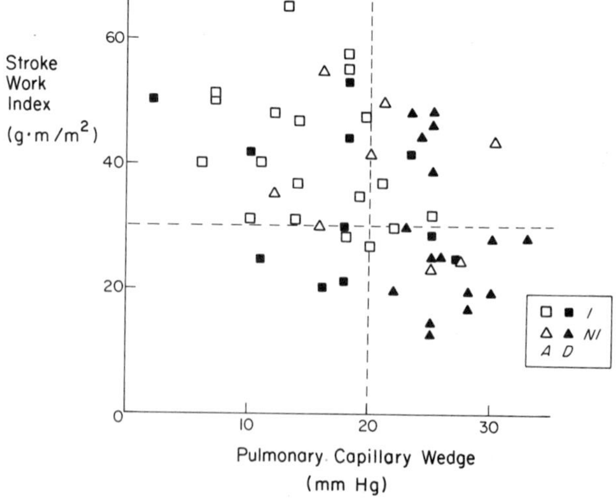

this setting, patients can be classified according to the hemodynamic findings. Both vasodilators and agents that increase myocardial contractility have proved helpful in the management of these patients. Unfortunately, despite our growing armamentarium of medications, the mortality rate remains high in patients with severe pump failure who present with cardiogenic shock. Furthermore, survivors with acute pump failure are often left with chronic cardiac dysfunction. In these patients, the chronic use of vasodilators has proved effective in reducing symptoms and improving exercise tolerance, but their effect on long-term survival remains to be studied.

References

1. Abboud, F. M., Schmid, P. G., and Eckstein, J. W.: Vascular responses after alpha-adrenergic receptor blockade. I. Responses of capacitance and resistance vessels to norepinephrine in man. J. Clin. Invest. 47:1, 1968.
2. Abrams, E., Forrester, J. S., Chatterjee, K., et al.: Variability in response to norepinephrine in acute myocardial infarction. Am. J. Cardiol. 32:919, 1973.
3. Ader, R., Chatterjee, K., Ports, T., et al.: Immediate and sustained hemodynamic and clinical improvement in chronic heart failure by an oral angiotensin converting enzyme inhibitor. Circulation 61:931, 1980.
4. Alonso, D. R., Scheidt, S., Post, M., et al.: Pathophysiology of cardiogenic shock: quantification of myocardial necrosis, clinical, pathologic and electrocardiographic correlations. Circulation 48:585, 1973.
5. Armstrong, P. W., Mathew, M. T., Boroomand, K., et al.: Nitroglycerin ointment in acute myocardial infarction. Am. J. Cardiol. 38:474, 1976.
6. Armstrong, P. W., Walker, B. C., Burton, J. R., et al.: Vasodilator therapy in acute myocardial infarction: a comparison of sodium nitroprusside and nitroglycerin. Circulation 52:1118, 1975.
7. Arnold, S., Williams, R., Ports, T. A., et al.: Attenuation of prazosin effect on cardiac output in chronic heart failure. Ann. Intern. Med. 91:345, 1979.
8. Awan, N. A., Amsterdam, E. A., Vera, Z., et al.: Reduction of ischemic injury by sublingual nitroglycerin in patients with acute myocardial infarction. Circulation 54:761, 1976.
9. Awan, N. A., Miller, R. R., Zakaruddin, V., et al.: Reduction of ST segment elevation with infusion of nitroprusside in patients with acute myocardial infarction. Am. J. Cardiol. 38:435, 1976.
10. Banka, V. S., Bodenheimer, M. M., and Helfant, R. H.: Effect of nitroprusside on local contractile performance after coronary ligation and reperfusion. Am. J. Cardiol. 37:544, 1977.
11. Becker, L. L.: Conditions for vasodilator-induced steal in experimental myocardial ischemia. Circulation 57:1103, 1978.
12. Bendersky, R., Chatterjee, K., Parmley, W. W., et al.: Dobutamine in chronic ischemic heart failure: alterations in left ventricular function and coronary hemodynamics. Am. J. Cardiol. 48:554, 1981.
13. Berkowitz, C., McKeever, L., Croke, R. P., et al.: Comparative responses to dobutamine and nitroprusside in patients with chronic low output cardiac failure. Circulation 56:918, 1977.

13a. Bleifeld, W., Hanrath, D., Mathey, D., et al.: Acute myocardial infarction. Left and right ventricular hemodynamics in cardiogenic shock. Br., Heart J., 36:822, 1974.

14. Borer, J. S., et al.: Reduction in myocardial ischemia with nitroglycerin or nitroglycerin plus phenylephrine administered during acute infarction. N. Engl. J. Med. 293:1008, 1975.
15. Braunwald, E.: Myocardial oxygen consumption: physiologic and clinical considerations. Am. J. Cardiol. 27:416, 1971.
16. Braunwald, E., Ross, J., and Sonnenblick, E. H.: Mechanisms of Contraction of the Normal and Failing Heart, 2nd ed. Boston, Little, Brown & Co., 1976.
17. Braunwald, E., Welch, C. H., and Sarnoff, S. J.: Hemodynamic effects of quantitatively varied experimental mitral regurgitation. Circ. Res. 5:539, 1957.
18. Bussmann, W., Lohner, J., and Kaltenbach, M.: Orally administered isosorbide dinitrate in patients with and without left ventricular failure due to acute myocardial infarction. Am. J. Cardiol. 39:91, 1977.
19. Bussmann, W. D., Passek, D., Seidel, W., and Kaltenbach, M.: Prospective randomized trial of intravenous nitroglycerin in acute myocardial infarction. Circulation 59 and 60:II-164, 1979.
20. Captopril Collaborative Study Group: A placebo-controlled trial of captopril in refractory chronic congestive heart failure. J. Am. Coll. Cardiol, in press.
21. Chatterjee, K.: Digitalis versus newer inotropic agents: which to use. Drug Ther. p. 83, Jan., 1982.
22. Chatterjee, K., Drew, D., Parmley, W. W., et al.: Combination vasodilator therapy for severe chronic congestive heart failure. Ann. Intern. Med. 85:467, 1976.
23. Chatterjee, K., and Parmley, W. W.: Role of vasodilator therapy in heart failure. Prog. Cardiovasc. Dis. 19:301, 1977.
24. Chatterjee, K., and Parmley, W. W.: Vasodilator therapy for acute myocardial infarction and chronic congestive heart failure. J. Am. Coll. Cardiol. 1:133, 1983.
25. Chatterjee, K., Parmley, W. W., Ganz, W., et al.: Hemodynamic and metabolic responses to vasodilator therapy in acute myocardial infarction. Circulation 48:1183, 1973.
26. Chatterjee, K., Parmley, W. W., Massie, B., et al.: Oral hydralazine for chronic refractory heart failure. Circulation 54:879, 1976.
27. Chatterjee, K., Parmley, W. W., Swan, H. J. C., et al.: Beneficial effects of vasodilator agents in severe mitral regurgitation due to subvalvular apparatus. Circulation 48:684, 1973.
28. Chatterjee, K., Ports, T. A., Brundage, B. H., et al.: Oral hydralazine in chronic heart failure: sustained beneficial hemodynamic effects. Ann. Intern. Med. 92:600, 1980.
29. Chatterjee, K., and Rouleau, J.-L.: Hemodynamic

and metabolic effects of vasodilators, nitrates, hydralazine, prazosin and captopril in chronic ischemic heart failure. Acta Med. Scand. 210 (Suppl. 651):295, 1981.

30. Chatterjee, K., and Swan, H. J. C.: Hemodynamic profile in acute myocardial infarction. *In* Corday, E., and Swan, H. J. C. (eds.): Myocardial Infraction. Baltimore, Williams & Wilkins Co., 1973, pp. 51–61.
31. Chatterjee, K., Swan, H. J., Kaushik, V. S., et al.: Effects of vasodilator therapy for severe pump failure in acute myocardial infarction on short-term and late prognosis. Circulation 53:797, 1976.
32. Chiariello, M., et al.: Comparison between the effects of nitroprusside and nitroglycerin on ischemic injury during acute myocardial infarction. Circulation 54:766, 1976.
33. Chiche, P., Baligadoo, S. J., and Derrida, J. P.: A randomized trial of prolonged nitroglycerin infusion in acute myocardial infarction. Circulation 59 and 60: II-165, 1979.
34. Cohen, M. V., Sonnenblick, E. H., and Kirk, E. S.: Comparative effects of nitroglycerin and isosorbide dinitrate on coronary collateral vessels and ischemic myocardium in dogs. Am. J. Cardiol. 37:244, 1976.
35. Cohn, J. N.: Blood pressure and cardiac performance. Am. J. Med. 55:351, 1973.
36. Cohn, J. N.: Vasodilator therapy of congestive heart failure. Adv. Intern. Med. 26:293, 1980.
37. Cohn, J. N., Franciosa, J. A., Francis, C. S., et al.: Effect of short-term infusion of sodium nitroprusside on mortality rate in acute myocardial infarction complicated by left ventricular failure. Results of Veterans Administration Cooperative Study. N. Engl. J. Med. 306:1129, 1982.
38. Cohn, J. N., Tristani, F. E., and Chatri, I. M.: Cardiac and peripheral vascular effects of digitalis in clinical cardiogenic shock. Am. Heart J. 78:318, 1969.
39. Colucci, W. S., Williams, G. H., Alexander, R. W., et al.: Mechanisms and implications of vasodilator tolerance in the treatment of congestive heart failure. Am. J. Med. 71:89, 1981.
40. Colucci, W. S., Wynne, J., Holman, B. L., and Braunwald, E.: Long-term therapy of heart failure with prazosin: a randomized double blind trial. Am. J. Cardiol. 45:337, 1980.
41. Come, P. C., Flaherty, J. T., Baird, M. G., et al.: Reversal by phenylephrine of the beneficial effects of intravenous nitroglycerin in patients with acute myocardial infarction. N. Engl. J. Med. 293:1003, 1975.
42. Come, P. C., and Pitt, B.: Nitroglycerin-induced severe hypotension and bradycardia in patients with acute myocardial infarction. Circulation 54:624, 1976.
43. da Luz, P. L., and Forrester, J. S.: Influence of vasodilators upon function and metabolism of ischemic myocardium. Am. J. Cardiol. 37:581, 1976.
44. da Luz, P. L., Forrester, J. S., Wyatt, J. L., et al.: Hemodynamic and metabolic effects of sodium nitroprusside on the performance and metabolism of regional ischemic myocardium. Circulation 52:400, 1975.
45. Davis, R., Ribner, H. S., Keung, E., et al.: Effect of captopril in heart failure. N. Engl. J. Med. 301:117, 1979.
46. Durrer, J. D., Lie, K. I., Van Capelle, F. R. J., and Durrer, D.: Effect of sodium nitroprusside on mortality in acute myocardial infarction. N. Engl. J. Med. 306:1121, 1982.
47. Faxon, D. P., Creager, M. A., Halperin, J. L., et al.: Determinants of clinical response and survival in patients with congestive heart failure treated with captopril. Am. Heart J. 104:1147, 1982.
48. Flaherty, J. T., Redd, P. R., Kelly, D. J., et al.: Intravenous nitroglycerin in acute myocardial infarction. Circulation 51:132, 1975.
49. Forrester, J., Bezdek, W., Chatterjee, K., et al.: Hemodynamic effects of digitalis in acute myocardial infarction. Ann. Intern. Med. 76:863, 1972.
50. Forrester, J. S., and Chatterjee, K.: Preservation of ischemic myocardium. *In* Vogel, J. H. K. (ed.): Advances in Cardiology. Basel, S. Karger, 1974, pp. 158–169.
51. Forrester, J. S., Diamond, G., Chatterjee, K., et al.: Medical therapy of acute myocardial infarction by application of hemodynamic subsets. N. Engl. J. Med. 295:1356 and 1404, 1976.
52. Fouad, F. M., Tarazi, R., Bravo, E. L., et al.: Long-term control of congestive heart failure with captopril. Am. J. Cardiol. 49:1489, 1982.
53. Franciosa, J. A.: Effectiveness of long-term vasodilator administration in the treatment of chronic left ventricular failure. Prog. Cardiovasc. Dis. 24:319, 1982.
54. Franciosa, J. A., and Cohn, J. N.: Effects of minoxidil on hemodynamics in patients with congestive heart failure. Circulation 63:652, 1981.
55. Franciosa, J. A., Gutha, N. M., Limas, C. J., et al.: Improved left ventricular function during nitroprusside infusion in acute myocardial infarction. Lancet 1:650, 1972.
56. Franciosa, J. A., Mikrutt, C. E., Cohn, J. N., et al.: Hemodynamic effects of orally administered isosorbide dinitrate in patients with congestive heart failure. Circulation 50:1020, 1974.
57. Franciosa, J. A., Norstrom, L. A., and Cohn, J. N.: Nitrate therapy for congestive heart failure. J.A.M.A. 240:443, 1978.
58. Franciosa, J. A., Pierpont, G., and Cohn, J.: Hemodynamic improvement after oral hydralazine in left ventricular failure. Ann. Intern. Med. 86:388, 1977.
59. Gander, M. P., Kazamias, T. M., Henry, P., et al.: Serial determinations of cardiac output and response to digitalis in patients with acute myocardial infarction. Circulation (Suppl.) 42:155, 1970.
60. Gavras, H., Faxon, D. P., Berkoberr, J., et al.: Angiotensin converting enzyme inhibition in patients with congestive heart failure. Circulation 58:770, 1979.
61. Gold, H. K., Chiariello, M., Leinbach, R. C., et al.: Deleterious effects of nitroprusside on myocardial injury during acute myocardial infarction. Herz 1:161, 1976.
62. Gold, H. K., Leinbach, R. C., and Sanders, C. A.: Use of sublingual nitroglycerin in congestive heart failure following acute myocardial infarction. Circulation 46:839, 1972.
63. Goldman, S. A., Johnson, L. L., Escala, E., et al.: Improved exercise ejection fraction with long-term prazosin therapy in patients with heart failure. Am. J. Med. 68:36, 1980.
64. Goldstein, R. A., Passamani, E. R., and Roberts,

R.: A comparison of digoxin and dobutamine in patients with acute infarction and cardiac failure. N. Engl. J. Med. 303:846, 1980.
65. Goodman, D. J., Rossen, R. M., Holloway, E. L., et al.: Effect of nitroprusside on left ventricular dynamics in mitral regurgitation. Circulation 50:1025, 1974.
66. Gould, L., Reddy, C. V. R., Kalanith, P., et al.: Use of phentolamine in acute myocardial infarction. Am. Heart J. 88:144, 1974.
67. Gould, L., Zehir, M., and Ettinger, S.: Phentolamine and cardiovascular performance. Br. Heart. J. 31:154, 1969.
68. Gray, R., Chatterjee, K., Vyden, J. K., et al.: Hemodynamic and metabolic effects of isosorbide dinitrate in chronic congestive heart failure. Am. Heart J. 90:346, 1975.
69. Greenberg, B. H., Massie, B. M., Brundage, B. H., et al.: Beneficial effects of hydralazine in severe mitral regurgitation. Circulation 58:273, 1978.
70. Gunnar, R. M., Loeb, H. S., Pietras, R. J., et al.: Hemodynamic measurements in a coronary care unit. Prog. Cardiovasc. Dis. 11:29, 1968.
71. Gutovitz, A. L., Sobel, B. E., and Roberts, R.: Progressive nature of myocardial injury in selected patients with cardiogenic shock. Am. J. Cardiol. 41:469, 1978.
72. Hamosh, P., and Cohn, J. N.: Left ventricular function in acute myocardial infarction. J. Clin. Invest. 48:523, 1970.
73. Harshaw, C. W., Grossman, W., Nunro, A. B., et al.: Reduced systemic vascular resistance as therapy for severe mitral regurgitation of valvular origin. Ann. Intern. Med. 83:312, 1975.
74. Hockings, B. E. F., Cope, G. D., Clarke, G. M., and Taylor, R. R.: Randomized controlled trial of vasodilator therapy after acute myocardial infarction. Am. J. Cardiol. 48:345, 1981.
75. Hodges, M., Friesinger, G. C., Riggins, R. C. K., et al.: Effects of intravenous administered digoxin on mild left ventricular failure in acute myocardial infarction in man. Am. J. Cardiol. 29:749, 1972.
76. Kelly, D. T., Delgado, C. E., Taylor, D. R., et al.: Use of phentolamine in acute myocardial infarction associated with hypertension and left ventricular failure. Circulation 47:729, 1973.
77. Kirk, E. S., LeJemtel, T. H., Nelson, G. R., et al.: Mechanisms of beneficial effects of vasodilators and inotropic stimulation in the experimental failing ischemic heart. Am. J. Med. 65:189, 1978.
78. Koch-Weser, J.: Hydralazine. N. Engl. J. Med. 295:320, 1976.
79. Kotter, V., Von Leitner, E. R., Wunderlich, J., and Schroder, R.: Comparison of haemodynamic effects of phentolamine, sodium nitroprusside, and glyceryl trinitrate in acute myocardial infarction. Br. Heart J. 39:1196, 1977.
80. Kramer, B., Massie, B. M., and Topic, N.: Controlled trial of captopril in chronic heart failure: a rest and exercise hemodynamic study. Circulation 67:807, 1983.
81. Kupper, W., Bleifeld, W., Hanrath, P., et al.: Left ventricular hemodynamics and function in acute myocardial infarction: studies during the acute phase, convalescence and late recovery. Am. J. Cardiol. 40:900, 1977.
82. Lipp, H., Denes, P., Gametta, M., et al.: Hemodynamic response to acute intravenous digoxin in patients with recent myocardial infarction and coronary insufficiency with and without heart failure. Chest 63:862, 1972.
83. Mackenzie, J.: Digitalis. Heart 2:273, 1911.
84. Magnusson, P., Shell, W. E., Forrester, J. S., et al.: Increased creatine phosphokinase release following blood pressure reduction in patients with acute infarction. Circulation 53:11, 1976.
85. Mann, T., Cohn, P. F., Holman, L. B., et al.: Effect of nitroprusside on regional myocardial blood flow in coronary artery disease. Circulation 57:732, 1978.
86. Mantle, J. A., Russell, R. O., Vloraski, R. E., et al.: Isosorbide dinitrate for the relief of severe heart failure after myocardial infarction. Am. J. Cardiol. 37:263, 1976.
87. Mason, D. T., and Braunwald, E.: The effects of nitroglycerin and amyl nitrate on arteriolar and venous tone in the human forearm. Circulation 32:755, 1965.
88. Massie, B. M., and Chatterjee, K.: Vasodilator therapy of pump failure complicating acute myocardial infarction. Med. Clin. North Am. 63:25, 1979.
89. Massie, B. M., Chatterjee, K., and Parmley, W. W.: Vasodilator therapy for acute and chronic heart failure. *In* Yu, P. N., and Goodwin, J. F. (eds.): Progress in Cardiology, Vol. 8. Philadelphia, Lea & Febiger, 1978, pp. 197–234.
90. Massie, B. M., Chatterjee, K., Werner, J., et al.: Hemodynamic advantage of combined administration of hydralazine orally and nitrates nonparenterally in the vasodilator therapy of chronic heart failure. Am. J. Cardiol. 40:794, 1977.
91. Massie, B. M., Kramer, B., and Haugham, F.: Acute and long-term effects of vasodilators on rest and exercise hemodynamics and exercise capacity. Circulation 64:1218, 1981.
92. Massie, B. M., Kramer, B., and Haugham, F.: Postural hypotension and tachycardia during hydralazine-isosorbide dinitrate therapy for chronic heart failure. Circulation 63:658, 1981.
93. Massie, B. M., Kramer, B. L., Topic, N., and Henderson, S. G.: Hemodynamic and radionuclide effects of acute captopril therapy for heart failure: changes in left and right ventricular volumes and function at rest and during exercise. Circulation 65:1374, 1982.
94. Massie, B. M., Ports, T., Chatterjee, K., et al.: Long-term vasodilator therapy for heart failure: clinical response and its relationship to hemodynamic measurements. Circulation 63:269, 1981.
95. Mikulic, E., Cohn, J. N., and Franciosa, J. A.: Comparative hemodynamic effects of inotropic and vasodilator drugs in severe heart failure. Circulation 56:528, 1977.
96. Miller, R. R., Awan, N. A., Joye, J. A., et al.: Combined dopamine and nitroprusside therapy in congestive heart failure: greater augmentation of cardiac performance by addition of inotropic stimulation of afterload reduction. Circulation 55:881, 1977.
97. Miller, R. R., Awan, N. A., Maxwell, K. S., and Mason, D. T.: Sustained reduction of cardiac impedance and preload in congestive heart failure with the antihypertensive vasodilator prazosin. N. Engl. J. Med. 297:303, 1977.
98. Miller, R. R., Fennell, W. H., Young, J. B., et al.:

Differential systemic arterial and venous actions and consequent cardiac effects of vasodilator drugs. Prog. Cardiovasc. Dis. 24:353, 1982.
99. Miller, R. R., Vismara, L. A., Williams, D. O., et al.: Pharmacological mechanisms for left ventricular unloading in clinical congestive heart failure. Circ. Res. 39:127, 1976.
100. Milnor, W. R.: Arterial impedance as ventricular afterload. Circ. Res. 36:565, 1975.
101. Mueller, H. S., Evans, R., and Ayres, S. M.: Effect of dopamine on hemodynamics and myocardial metabolism in shock following acute myocardial infarction in man. Circulation 57:361, 1978.
102. Mueller, H. S., Religa, A., Evans, R., et al.: Metabolic changes in ischemic myocardium by nitroprusside. Am. J. Cardiol. 33:158, 1974.
103. Mundth, E. D., et al.: Surgery for complications of acute myocardial infarction. Circulation 45:1279, 1972.
104. Packer, M., and LeJemtel, T. H.: Physiologic and pharmacologic determinants of vasodilator response: a conceptual framework for rational drug therapy for chronic heart failure. Prog. Cardiovasc. Dis. 24:275, 1981.
105. Packer, M., Meller, J., Gorlin, R., and Herman, M. V.: Hemodynamic and clinical tachyphylaxis to prazosin-mediated afterload reduction in severe chronic congestive heart failure. Circulation 59:531, 1979.
106. Packer, M., Meller, J., Medina, N., et al.: Hemodynamic characterization of tolerance to long-term hydralazine therapy in severe chronic heart failure. N. Engl. J. Med. 306:57, 1982.
107. Page, D. L., Caulfield, J. B., Kastor, J. A., et al.: Myocardial changes associated with cardiogenic shock. N. Engl. J. Med. 285:133, 1971.
108. Palmer, R. F., and Lasseter, A. Z.: Drug therapy: sodium nitroprusside. N. Engl. J. Med. 292:291, 1975.
109. Pepine, C. J., and Nichols, W. W.: Aortic input impedance in cardiovascular disease. Prog. Cardiovasc. Dis. 26:307, 1982.
110. Pepine, C. J., Nichols, W. W., Curry, R. C., et al.: Aortic input impedance during nitroprusside infusion: a reconsideration of afterload reduction and beneficial action. J. Clin. Invest. 64:643, 1979.
111. Perret, C., Cardaz, J. P., Reyneert, M., et al.: Phentolamine for vasodilator therapy in left ventricular failure complicating acute myocardial infarction. Br. Heart J. 37:640, 1975.
112. Rahimtoola, S. H., Sinno, M. Z., Chuquimia, R., et al.: Effects of ouabain on impaired left ventricular function in acute myocardial infarction. N. Engl. J. Med. 253:527, 1972.
113. Ramanathan, K. B., Bodenheimer, M. M., Banka, V. S., et al.: Contrasting effects of nitroprusside and phentolamine in experimental myocardial infarction. Am. J. Cardiol. 39:994, 1977.
114. Ratshin, R. A., Rackley, C. E., and Russell, R. O., Jr.: Hemodynamic evaluation of left ventricular function in shock complicating myocardial infarction. Circulation 45:127, 1972.
115. Ribner, H. S., Bresnahan, D., Hsieh, A. M., et al.: Acute hemodynamic responses to vasodilator therapy in congestive heart failure. Prog. Cardiovasc. Dis. 25:1, 1982.
116. Robie, N. W., and Goldberg, L. I.: Comparative systemic and regional hemodynamic effects of dopamine and dobutamine. Am. Heart J. 90:340, 1975.
117. Rouleau, J.-L., Chatterjee, K., Benge, W., et al.: Alterations in left ventricular function and coronary hemodynamics with captopril, hydralazine and prazosin in chronic ischemic heart failure. A comparative study. Circulation 65:671, 1982.
118. Rouleau, J.-L., Warnica, J. W., and Burgess, J. H.: Prazosin and congestive heart failure: short- and long-term therapy. Am. J. Med. 71:147, 1981.
119. Scheidt, S., Wilner, G., Fillmore, S., et al.: Intra-aortic balloon counterpulsation in cardiogenic shock. N. Engl. J. Med. 288:979, 1973.
120. Scheidt, S., Wilner, G., Fillmore, S., et al.: Objective haemodynamic assessment after acute myocardial infarction. Br. Heart J. 35:908, 1973.
121. Storer, J. D., Bolen, J. L., and Harrison, D. C.: Comparison of dobutamine and dopamine in treatment of severe heart failure. Br. Heart J. 39:536, 1977.
122. Synhorst, D. P., Laur, R. M., Doty, D. B., and Brody, M. J.: Hemodynamic effects of vasodilator agents in dogs with experimental ventricular septal defects. Circulation 54:472, 1976.
123. Taylor, S. H., Sutherland, G. R., MacKenzie, G. J., et al.: The circulatory effects of intravenous phentolamine in man. Circulation 31:741, 1965.
124. Taylor, W. R., Forrester, J. S., Magnusson, P., et al.: Hemodynamic effects of nitroglycerin ointment in congestive heart failure. Am. J. Cardiol. 38:469, 1976.
125. Tecklenberg, P. L., Fitzgerald, J., Allaire, B. J., et al.: Afterload reduction in the management of postinfarction ventricular septal defect. Am. J. Cardiol. 38:956, 1976.
126. Topic, N., Kramer, B., and Massie, B.: Acute and long-term effects of captopril on exercise cardiac performance and exercise capacity in congestive heart failure. Am. Heart J. 104:1172, 1982.
127. Turini, G. A., Brunner, H. R., Gribic, M., et al.: Improvement of chronic congestive heart failure by oral captopril. Lancet 1:1213, 1979.
128. Walinsky, P., Chatterjee, K., Forrester, J., et al.: Enhanced left ventricular performance with phentolamine in acute myocardial infarction. Am. J. Cardiol. 33:37, 1974.
129. Weber, K. T., Janicki, J. S., Russell, R. O., et al.: Identification of high risk subsets of acute myocardial infarction. Am. J. Cardiol. 41:197, 1978.
130. Williams, D. O., Amsterdam, E. A., and Mason, D. T.: Hemodynamic effects of nitroglycerin in acute myocardial infarction: decrease in ventricular preload at the expense of cardiac output. Circulation 51:421, 1975.
131. Williams, D. O., Bommer, W. J., Miller, R. R., et al.: Hemodynamic assessment of oral peripheral vasodilator therapy in chronic congestive heart failure: prolonged effectiveness of isosorbide dinitrate. Am. J. Cardiol. 39:84, 1977.
132. Wyatt, H. L., da Luz, P. L., Waters, D. D., et al.: Contrasting influences of alterations in ventricular preload and afterload upon systemic hemodynamics, function, and metabolism of ischemic myocardium. Circulation 55:318, 1977.

3

Thrombolytic Therapy for Acute Myocardial Infarction

THOMAS A. PORTS

The major determinant of outcome following myocardial infarction is the extent of myocardial damage.[3, 5, 9, 65] Current thinking based on animal studies is that myocardial infarction is a dynamic process evolving over several hours. During these hours early interventions may reduce the extent of myocardial necrosis, if they can alter the continuing imbalance between myocardial oxygen supply and metabolic demand caused by the acute interruption of coronary blood flow.[7, 12, 33-36, 44, 47, 63]

Most attempts to limit infarct size have attempted to do so by reduction of oxygen demand with acute interventions such as beta-blockers, nitroglycerin, calcium channel blockers, and intra-aortic balloon counterpulsation.[52] Attempts to improve oxygen supply acutely, such as emergency peri-infarction coronary bypass surgery, have been shown to be technically feasible and effective for preserving myocardial function on a long-term basis.[16, 45] However, the personnel and financial resources necessary to perform emergency coronary bypass surgery within the first few hours of myocardial infarction limit this form of therapy. Another direct approach to improvement of coronary blood flow in acute myocardial infarction is lysis of the acute intracoronary thrombus. Although the precise mechanism responsible for coronary occlusion has not been defined, it probably involves several interrelated factors, including atherosclerotic plaque ulceration and rupture, and coronary vasospasm and thrombosis.[42] The controversial nature of the relationship between myocardial infarction and coronary thrombosis has been revealed through autopsy studies for many years.[2, 6, 11, 15, 25, 51, 54] Recent clinical studies using coronary angiography and bypass surgery in the early hours of acute myocardial infarction have demonstrated a high incidence of coronary thrombotic occlusion in transmural myocardial infarction.[17] Attempts to infuse thrombolytic agents in acute myocardial infarction by the intravenous route were made by Fletcher and co-workers in 1959.[22] Infusions of a fibrinolytic agent directly into the ascending aorta during acute myocardial infarction followed in 1960, but did not employ coronary angiography to document abolition of thrombi.[8]

Intravenous infusion of streptokinase was studied in many medical centers in Europe, different protocols being used throughout the 1960s and 1970s.[1, 4, 10, 18-20, 24] The results of these studies are difficult to interpret because of varying criteria for patient selection, as well as the unknown extent of myocardial infarction and underlying coronary artery disease. The European Cooperative Study Group for Streptokinase Treatment in Acute Myocardial Infarction, which was conducted in 11 European centers, randomized patients to treatment with 24 hours of either intravenous streptokinase infusion or dextrose infusion (control).[19] The group treated with streptokinase had a significantly lower mortality both on immediate follow-up and six months after treatment.

In 1978, Rentrop and colleagues in Germany achieved mechanical reperfusion of angiographically-documented occluded coronary arteries in ten patients with acute myocardial infarction.[50] They passed a guidewire into the angiographic catheter, directly entered the thrombus, disrupted it, and restored coronary flow. The lumen of these coronary arteries increased in diameter over time, suggesting endogenous clot lysis. The following year, Rentrop and co-investigators administered streptokinase by intracoronary infusion to 29 patients within two to 15 hours from onset of chest pain,[49] and successfully re-established coronary blood flow through the occluded artery in 22 of the 29. Several subsequent studies in Germany and the United States, using different protocols but employing intracoronary infusion of streptokinase, achieved similar results.[13, 23, 38, 46] Later, other reports confirmed this early experience and demonstrated variable myocardial salvage assessed by different techniques.[28, 30, 32, 57, 58, 62] In all studies to date, total occlusion of a coronary artery corresponding approximately to one electrocardiographic site of infarction was found in 75 to 90 per cent of patients. Intracoronary nitroglycerin given to reverse possible coronary spasm failed to reopen these occluded vessels in more than 95 per cent of individuals. The infusion of intracoronary thrombolytic agents has successfully established flow through the occluded coronary artery in 75 to 85 per cent of patients.[13, 23, 28, 30, 32, 38, 46, 49, 57, 58, 62] It therefore seems probable that acute in situ coronary artery thrombus, triggered by still controversial mechanisms, is responsible for the sudden interruption of blood flow resulting in myocardial infarction.

Early in 1982 the Food and Drug Administration approved streptokinase therapy for acute myocardial infarction. The enthusiasm arising from initial studies following this sanction has resulted in the use of this technique in many catheterization laboratories. Criteria for patient selection, method of administration, dosage, and subsequent adjunctive therapy to prevent reocclusion have varied significantly among investigators employing this technique. Several reports have suggested improvement in left ventricular function following intracoronary thrombolysis, as well as improved short-term mortality.[23, 38, 39, 46, 48, 58, 62] Other studies have not demonstrated such improvement.[29, 69] Many unresolved issues remain, including quantitative assessment of the extent of myocardial salvage and short- and long-term effects of the therapy on mortality. Randomized controlled studies are in progress to help provide answers to these questions. Currently, the technique of intracoronary thrombolysis to treat acute myocardial infarction should be considered investigational. This chapter describes our approach at the University of California, San Francisco, to patient selection, technique, and adjunctive therapy, as well as complications involving intracoronary thrombolytic therapy for acute myocardial infarction.

PATIENT SELECTION

Many factors must be considered in patient selection for intracoronary thrombolytic therapy for acute myocardial infarction. Since the goal of intracoronary thrombolytic therapy is not only to re-establish blood flow through the occluded coronary artery but also to salvage significant amounts of myocardium destined to undergo necrosis, the early institution of therapy is of the utmost importance. The extent of myocardial necrosis depends on several factors, but perhaps most crucial are the completeness of occlusion, the presence and extent of functioning collateral circulation, factors affecting myocardial metabolism, and the time interval from occlusion to restoration of coronary flow. Myocardium completely deprived of blood flow (oxygen) will undergo necrosis within minutes, but ischemic cells still benefiting from blood flow, presumably from collateral channels under suitable metabolic circumstances, can resist irreversible damage for up to several hours. Therefore, candidates for thrombolytic therapy are patients presenting to the hospital within the first few hours of onset of symptoms of myocardial infarction who show electrocardiographic evidence of evolving transmural myocardial infarction and have no contraindications to thrombolysis or long-term anticoagulation. Although it is impossible to establish a rigid time limit for accepting patients for this therapy, we believe that therapy should be begun within three to four hours from onset of symptoms. Myocardial infarction usually is almost complete by six to eight hours in most patients, but some individuals with symptoms of longer duration may be appropriate candidates if there is persistence of ischemic pain and ECG evidence of continuing transmural ischemia (ST-segment elevation). The issue of time from onset of symptoms beyond which no benefit will occur from reperfusion is still unresolved. Most animal studies and preliminary investigations of this technique in man suggest that salvage is very limited beyond four to six hours. However, one study in man showed improvement of left ventricular function after thrombolysis performed within 18 hours of onset of symptoms (mean nine hours).[62]

For all candidates, the ECG should show evidence of evolving transmural infarction. If the ST elevation persists despite nitroglycerin, the presence of interrupted regional coronary blood flow, usually from thrombotic occlusion, is likely. Ideally, the ECG should not show new significant Q waves unless previous myocardial infarction has been demonstrated. Initial blood studies should not reveal CK-MB bands in the serum, as their presence implies significant necrosis of several hours' duration. These findings would indicate that the opportunity for salvage of significant amounts of myocardium had been lost.

Finally, it is very important in the selection of patients to obtain their informed consent and that of the attending physician, having regard to the potential risks and benefits of this investigational approach to the treatment of acute myocardial infarction.

CONTRAINDICATIONS TO THERAPY

There are several major and minor contraindications to thrombolytic therapy with streptokinase, in addition to late presentation to the hospital. Table 3–1 lists the contraindications to the use of streptokinase for treating acute myocardial infarction. The major potential complication of thrombolytic therapy is hemorrhage. It is important to realize that even low doses of intracoronary streptokinase can produce systemic fibrinolytic effects.[14] Since streptokinase works by way of activation of plasmin, which digests (hydrolyzes) fibrin clots indiscriminately, hemostatic clots as well as pathologic thrombi can be affected. These facts, and the realization that most patients will subsequently need to be maintained on anticoagulation to reduce the chances of rethrombosis, mean that a careful consideration of the contraindications is essential. Under certain circumstances it might be judged that the risks and potential benefits of the treatment are sufficiently great to warrant proceeding with this therapy, despite a relative contraindication to the use of streptokinase.

TECHNIQUE OF INTRACORONARY THROMBOLYSIS

Invasive procedures including needle punctures should be minimized and compression bandages applied to sites of vessel punctures. Baseline studies consisting of a 12-lead ECG; a complete blood count with platelets, prothrombin time (PT), and partial thromboplastin time (PTT); and studies of electrolytes and cardiac enzymes should be obtained before the initiation of therapy and at frequent intervals during and after intracoronary thrombolysis. We monitor the hematocrit, platelet count, PT, PTT, and cardiac enzymes during streptokinase infusion,

Table 3–1. CONTRAINDICATIONS TO THROMBOLYTIC THERAPY

Absolute
- Active internal bleeding
- Recent cerebrovascular accident or procedure
- Recent serious trauma

Relative
- Conditions with potential for serious hemorrhage, including:
  - Coagulation defects
  - Pregnancy/postpartum period
  - Uncontrolled severe hypertension
  - Diabetic retinopathy
- Conditions requiring fibrin plugs for hemostasis within preceding week:
  - Recent major surgery
  - Recent organ biopsy, thoracentesis, paracentesis, lumbar puncture
  - Cardiopulmonary resuscitation complicated by sternal or rib fracture

and every four to six hours for 24 hours after its conclusion. These parameters are then followed on a daily basis thereafter. A clot for type and crossmatch should be drawn before therapy is begun.

For intracoronary therapy, these often very unstable patients should be transported to the cardiac catheterization laboratory where complete facilities and on-call trained personnel (nurses and technicians) are available.

Intracoronary thrombolytic therapy uses the standard cardiac catheterization and coronary angiographic techniques. Femoral or brachial approaches may be made, but it is important to keep the number of venous and arterial puncture sites to a minimum; this not only decreases the chances of significant hemorrhagic complications, but also adds greatly to the convenience of obtaining hemostasis with manual compression after completion of the technique. Baseline hemodynamic measurements should be made and a temporary demand pacemaker inserted into the right ventricle; caution should be observed in patients having acute inferior wall myocardial infarction with possible right ventricular involvement, because the right ventricle is extremely irritable in these circumstances. An assessment of left ventricular function may be made either with a left ventricular angiogram, using a minimum of contrast media to lessen the risk of acute hemodynamic deterioration, or with noninvasive techniques such as two-dimensional echocardiography. To define the degree of myocardial salvage produced by intracoronary thrombolytic therapy, we perform thallium-201 perfusion studies before and after thrombolytic therapy. At the time of initiating the coronary angiograms we inject intravenous thallium-201, and proceed with the baseline nuclear imaging immediately following the coronary angiograms. The patient is scanned in the catheterization laboratory in the projections while streptokinase is being infused via the angiographic catheter positioned in the coronary ostium. Catheter position is confirmed fluoroscopically between the acquisition of each nuclear image.

By examination of the electrocardiographic site of infarction (ST-segment elevation) or regional wall motion abnormality from the left ventricular angiogram or noninvasive study, the coronary artery thought to be responsible for the acute myocardial infarction can usually be determined. We generally study first the vessel that is believed not to be responsible for the acute infarction. This choice is largely a matter of personal preference: since the entire coronary anatomy needs to be studied, it is easier to examine the nonoccluded vessel first to save catheter exchanges and to benefit from the knowledge of the entire anatomy and existing collaterals. Intracoronary thrombosis can be presumed to be present if there is an abrupt "cut-off" of the vessel. Figure 3–1 illustrates an occluded right coronary artery. Occasionally, the actual thrombus can be visualized by a contrast outline (Fig. 3–1*B*). A tapering occlusion of the coronary artery may represent thrombosis or spasm.

Regardless of the angiographic appearance of the totally occluded vessel, nitroglycerin should be administered to exclude spasm. We inject 200 to 500 μg of nitroglycerin solution into the coronary artery and repeat the angiogram one to two minutes later. If the vessel opens up following the nitroglycerin, spasm is present, and an infusion of intravenous nitroglycerin should be started and a calcium channel blocker administered. If no change in the appearance of the occluded vessel is noted, streptokinase infusion is begun. A bolus of 10,000–25,000 units is injected into the occluded artery followed by an infusion of 2000–5000 units per min of streptokinase through the angiographic catheter. The ECG should be monitored continually to note rhythm changes and decrease in ST-segment elevation, both of which accompany reperfusion. We assess the progress of clot lysis by repeating the angiogram at 15-minute intervals. If no improvement can be seen after 30 minutes, a soft-tipped 0.021- or 0.028-inch guidewire may be advanced through the site of total occlusion, in an endeavor to improve the local delivery of streptokinase by thus perforating the clot. This mechanical recanalization can be done before the start of thrombolytic therapy or during the course of the procedure if patency is not restored. The maneuver may not be necessary in most instances; it has many potential dangers and should be attempted only by individuals experienced in coronary angiography and with the intracoronary manipulation of catheters. Perforation or dissection of the coronary artery can result from improper technique. The infusion of streptokinase can be done through the standard angiographic catheters connected to a manifold and a microdrip infusion pump.

Another possible method of improving lo-

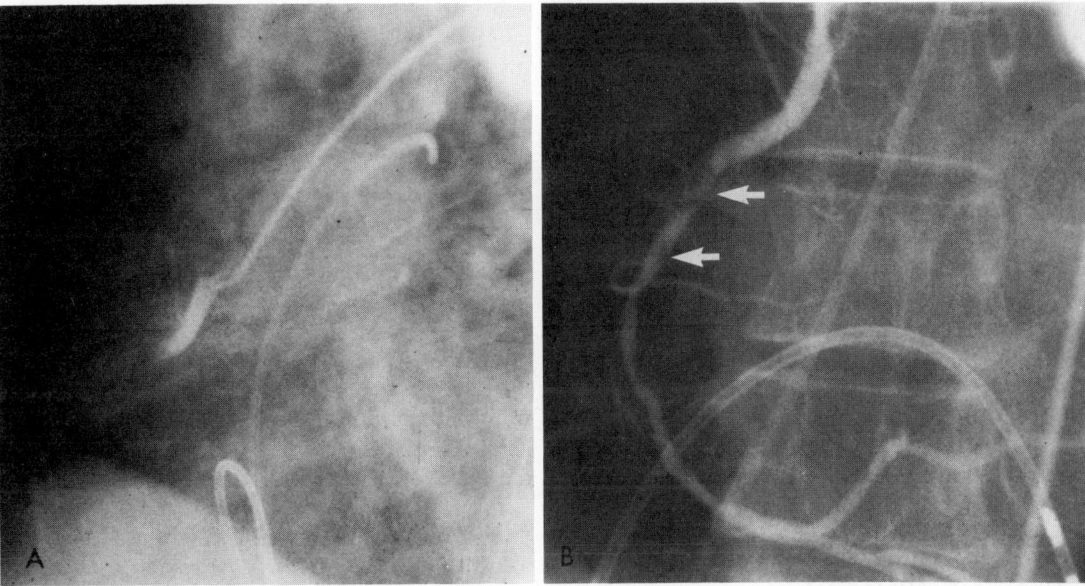

Figure 3–1. *A,* Left anterior oblique 60° projection showing completely occluded right coronary artery near its origin. *B,* Same artery after intracoronary streptokinase infusion restoring flow. Note residual thrombus within right coronary artery (*arrows*).

cal delivery of the streptokinase involves the use of various subselective intracoronary catheter delivery systems. Made by several manufacturers, these catheter systems are basically small 2–4 F flexible end-hole catheters with a radiopaque tip at one end and a manifold system at the other. Some come with guidewires to aid in their placement. These catheters are designed to be inserted through the standard angiographic catheter, which is positioned in the coronary artery ostium, advanced subselectively into the occluded arterial branch, and then positioned as close as possible to the thrombus at the site of occlusion. The necessity of using a subselective intracoronary catheter delivery system, as opposed to standard coronary ostial perfusion or even intravenous perfusion of streptokinase remains unproved. The reasoning is that more streptokinase can be delivered to the thrombus by an infusion catheter directly on or close to the thrombus and reperfusion can be established earlier by use of the subselective technique than by an infusion through the coronary ostium, where much of the streptokinase will flow through the nonoccluded coronary system. In view of the extra time that may be required to position the selective catheters, we use them only if there is evidence that the streptokinase is being diverted away from the thrombus or if the thrombus is extremely distal.

We have found that with right coronary artery occlusions and, in particular, proximal occlusions of that artery, the standard angiographic catheters are adequate for intracoronary infusion. With the left coronary system, it is often possible to advance the standard angiographic catheters into the proximal left anterior descending or circumflex coronary artery and satisfactorily deliver streptokinase directly into the occluded artery. If standard angiographic catheters are used, care should be taken to avoid pressure damping and occlusion of the other vessels. One advantage of the smaller subselective infusion catheters is that once they are positioned, the larger standard angiographic catheter can be removed from the coronary ostium and this potential compromise to coronary blood flow removed. Regardless of the system used, the intracoronary pressure should be monitored periodically to make sure that flow through the nonobstructed artery is not being impaired. Angiograms should be repeated at least every 15 minutes to assess the progress of thrombosis.

Successful thrombolysis and establishment of reperfusion are usually heralded by a relief of chest pain, a decrease in ST-segment elevation (presumably indicative of a reduction in transmural ischemia), and the appearance of frequent premature ventricular contractions or idioventricular rhythm. If the patient has had a new intraventricular conduction defect, it often resolves at this time.

The term *reperfusion arrhythmias* has been used to describe this phenomenon, which is thought to be mediated by alpha-adrenergic mechanisms. These arrhythmias are most often self-terminating and cause no hemodynamic embarrassment. Therapy is not usually required, therefore; if it should prove necessary, intravenous lidocaine is generally employed first, but this may not be successful in these circumstances. Intravenous procainamide has been used successfully, as have calcium channel blockers and even small doses of intracoronary lidocaine. Therapy, when needed, should be based on the urgency of the circumstances. We usually administer intravenous lidocaine, followed by procainamide or intracoronary lidocaine and DC cardioversion when necessary.

LENGTH OF INFUSION

The total dose and duration of infusion varies among investigators. The total dose of intracoronary streptokinase is usually in the range of 100,000 to 500,000 units. Once clot lysis has been achieved, streptokinase infusion should be continued at a reduced rate (1000 to 2000 units per minute) to digest any residual clot that might serve as a nidus for rethrombosis. Assuming no bleeding complications have arisen and the total infusion has not exceeded about 300,000 units, we continue intracoronary infusion for an additional half-hour after initial reperfusion is established. Angiograms should be repeated when the infusions are finished. With intracoronary streptokinase, reperfusion is usually established within 20 to 60 minutes, but it may take up to two hours. If clot lysis has not been partially successful after 90 to 120 minutes of intracoronary streptokinase, or if the total infusion has exceeded 300,000 units, consideration should be given to terminating the procedure, as significant myocardial salvage by this elasped time is unlikely and the potential risk of hemorrhage is magnified. Reasons for failure of intracoronary streptokinase infusion to establish coronary patency include: infusion of too low a dose; the presence of neutralizing antibodies; inadequate delivery to the thrombus owing to remote infusion; too low a concentration of plasminogen at the site of occlusion; the presence of a platelet thrombus; and the fact that, when the attempted thrombolysis is too late, the fibrin clot is no longer fresh. Before the removal of the catheter from the coronary ostium, we inject thallium-201, 0.5 mCi, directly into the coronary artery and repeat the previously obtained images. We usually leave the venous catheter in place for continued hemodynamic monitoring, and if the femoral approach is used we leave a sheath within the artery. These catheters are removed several hours to one day later when hemostasis is better and the risks of hematoma formation and bleeding are reduced.

After successful clot lysis has been achieved in the catheterization laboratory with streptokinase, the patient is transferred to the cardiac care unit for continued monitoring. Intravenous nitroglycerin, calcium channel blockers, or both are often used to reduce coronary spasm. When the PT and PTT are approximately twice control values, and if there are no significant bleeding problems, an infusion of heparin is begun without a loading dose. Patients are kept anticoagulated on heparin until warfarin, which is usually started the following day, has achieved a therapeutic effect. Anticoagulation is maintained with warfarin for three months or longer, during which time the disrupted coronary artery will re-endothelialize. Some investigators administer aspirin acutely, 500 mg to 1 gm intravenously, and maintain the patient on daily aspirin for its antiplatelet effect. Although reocclusion due to platelet thrombosis has been reported following intracoronary streptokinase reperfusion, the risks and benefits of antiplatelet therapy interaction with warfarin anticoagulation in this setting are still undefined.

Another area of controversy concerns the administration of systemic heparin in the catheterization laboratory prior to streptokinase infusion. Heparinization is standard practice during coronary angiography, but has at least theoretical disadvantages when given prior to streptokinase. Antithrombin heparin cofactor has been shown to inhibit plasmin.[27] This heparin-induced antithrombin inhibitor of plasmin may then work against the desired fibrinolytic effects induced by streptokinase. Currently, however, most investigators heparinize their patients with the introduction of the arterial catheter, and generally withhold further heparin until after streptokinase thrombolysis has been accomplished and the PTT has returned to 2 to 2.5 times control values.

Follow-up assessment of infarct size has been made by wall motion abnormalities, thallium perfusion studies, and frequent serum CK determination. The CK values are monitored every four hours. Plasma CK levels generally increase rapidly and markedly. This finding has been attributed to increased washout of enzyme from irreversibly injured cells.[61] Other explanations of this phenomenon are possible and further data need to be gathered to compare the cumulative CK release from reperfusion with cumulative CK release from infarct patients not having a thrombolysis.[64]

The resolution of ST-segment elevation that accompanies successful intracoronary thrombolysis is almost always accompanied by accelerated development of Q waves on subsequent ECGs. Figure 3–2 shows the typical ECG evolution from ST elevation to rapid normalization, with reperfusion and subsequent Q wave development.

ADJUNCT THERAPY TO PREVENT REOCCLUSION

Once patency has been restored to the thrombosed coronary artery, attention must be directed to keeping the artery patent. Anticoagulation with heparin followed by warfarin is recommended for all patients after successful thrombolysis. Warfarin is continued for from six weeks to three

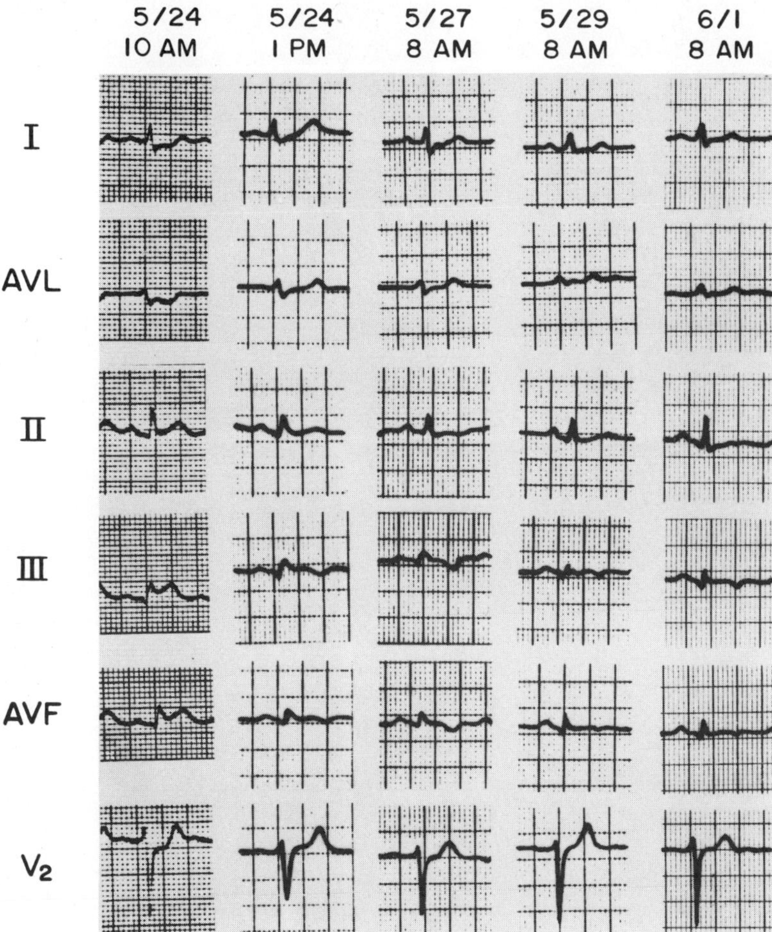

Figure 3–2. Serial ECG changes in a patient with inferior wall myocardial infarction.

months. During this period, if the patient still has continued refractory angina or ischemia and has suitable anatomy, coronary artery bypass graft surgery (CABG) can be performed without increased risk. Similarly, such patients with suitable coronary anatomy may undergo percutaneous transluminal coronary angioplasty (PTCA). We have performed PTCA on many patients without increased complications one to six weeks after thrombolysis. These individuals had refractory symptoms and demonstrable reversible thallium perfusion defects in the distribution of the coronary artery with significant residual stenosis after thrombolysis. Figure 3–3 illustrates the coronary angiograms of such a patient before and after thrombolysis, and following PTCA of the residual severe stenosis ten days later. The thallium-201 perfusion studies are shown in Figure 3–4: on the initial thallium study *(top)* there is a significant defect in the inferior and inferoseptal walls, which is significantly improved on the repeat study following thrombolysis 120 minutes later. This patient's pre-PTCA limited treadmill with thallium-201 scintigraphy showed early, reversible, exercise-induced ischemia in the same regions. The patient was asymptomatic and without exercise-induced ischemia following successful PTCA for the residual right coronary artery lesion.

Both emergency CABG surgery and PTCA

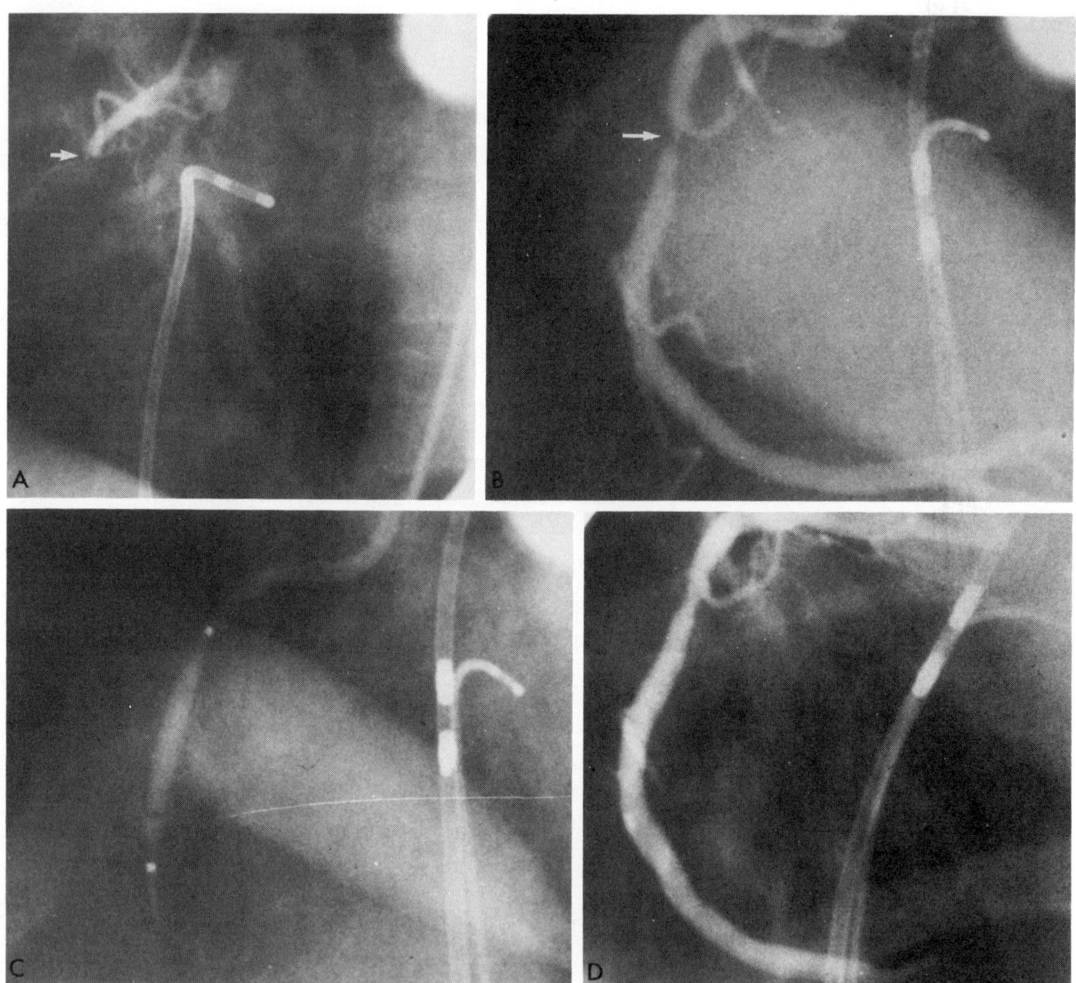

Figure 3–3. Patient with acute inferior wall myocardial infarction. *A,* 100 per cent occlusion of right coronary artery (*arrow*). Left anterior oblique (LAO) 60° projection. *B,* Flow restored through right coronary artery after streptokinase infusion. Significant residual stenosis remains in proximal right coronary artery (*arrow*). LAO 60° projection. *C,* Coronary angioplasty balloon catheter inflated within right coronary stenosis. *D,* Follow-up angiogram of right coronary artery 14 mo after thrombolysis and coronary angioplasty, showing persistent improvement in coronary lumen. LAO 60° projection.

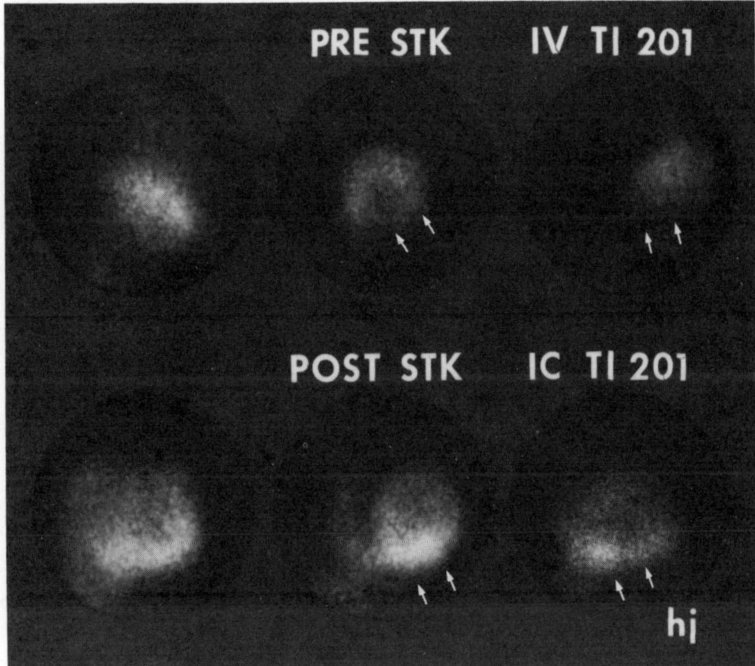

Figure 3–4. Anterior, left anterior oblique 30° and 70° projections. Anterior, Thallium-201 scintigrams pre- and poststreptokinase infusion. Note improvement in perfusion (thallium uptake) to inferior wall (*arrows*).

have been employed immediately following streptokinase thrombolysis in very unstable individuals. We have sent several patients to emergency CABG surgery from the catheterization laboratory for continued chest pain refractory to medical therapy and intra-aortic balloon counterpulsation following thrombolysis. Somewhat surprisingly, our surgeons have not encountered increased bleeding intra- or postoperatively. Emergency CABG surgery may also be indicated for abrupt reclosure following thrombolysis, assuming the coronary anatomy is suitable and salvage of significant myocardium is still feasible having regard to the time elasped. The performance of PTCA immediately after successful intracoronary thrombolysis is also feasible.[41] We have carried out PTCA immediately following streptokinase thrombolysis successfully in 19 of 21 patients who had severe residual coronary artery obstruction and were either reoccluding or threatening to do so. Figure 3–5 illustrates the use of PTCA immediately postthrombolysis in an unstable patient with significant residual left anterior descending stenosis. Figures 3–6 and 3–7 are from another patient with a right coronary artery occlusion. After intracoronary streptokinase infusion failed to restore flow, the vessel was mechanically opened with a guidewire (Fig. 3–7). The tight residual lesion was responsible for continued reocclusion and was subsequently dilated with the balloon angioplasty catheter. Successful PTCA led to resolution of the ischemia. This application of PTCA remains investigational but in selected patients offers the promise of reducing preocclusive obstructions and relieving ischemia, and the hope of diminishing the risk of reocclusion and improving the prognosis.

COMPLICATIONS

Significant hemorrhage requiring transfusion has been the most frequent complication following the use of intracoronary streptokinase, occurring in 4 to 7 per cent of patients.[53] Although gastrointestinal, retroperitoneal, and cerebrovascular bleeding have occurred, the most common locations for significant hemorrhage remain arterial and venous puncture sites. Bleeding is probably more common with the femoral approach, but should be infrequent if careful attention is paid to technique and if the vascular sheath is used and allowed to remain within the artery until systemic fibrinolysis has resolved. Some investigators consider that bleeding may be more common when the dose of streptokinase exceeds 250,000 units, or when fibrinogen levels decrease to less than 100

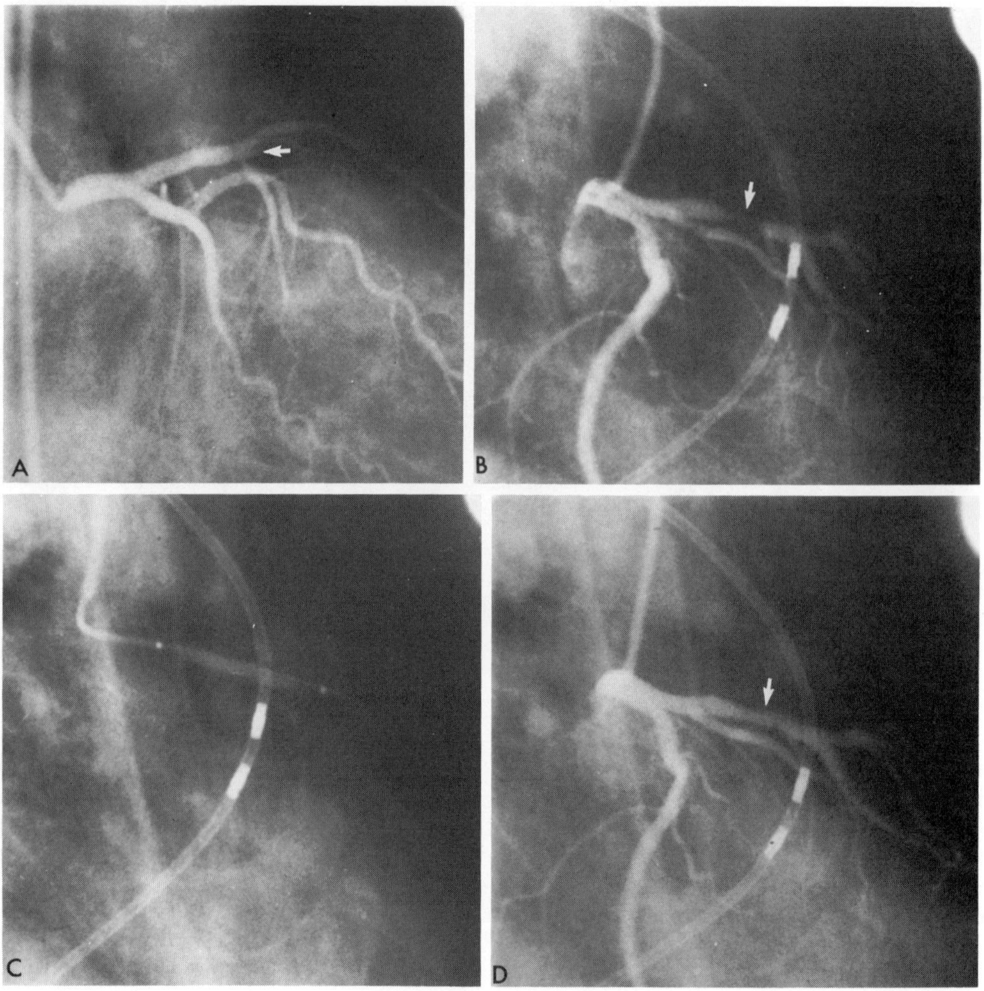

Figure 3–5. *A,* Left coronary angiogram showing complete occlusion of left anterior descending (*arrow*). Right anterior oblique (RAO) 5° projection. *B,* Left coronary angiogram RAO 45° from same patient after flow has been restored following 25 min of intracoronary streptokinase infusion. Note residual tight stenosis within left anterior descending (*arrow*). A pacing catheter is in the right ventricle. RAO 45° projection. *C,* Balloon angioplasty catheter inflated within left anterior descending stenosis. *D,* Follow-up angiogram showing improvement in left anterior descending caliber after angioplasty (*arrow*). RAO 45° projection.

mg/dl.[53] Others believe that bleeding during thrombolytic therapy is not dose dependent and reflects a previous hemostatic defect in the patient.[59] This situation is unlike anticoagulant therapy, an excessive dose of which is the most common reason for bleeding complications. We have not had serious hemorrhagic complications from streptokinase infusion, but have seen them from both the subsequent heparin and warfarin anticoagulation therapies. Treatment of hemorrhage from thrombolytic therapy depends on severity. Most bleeding that occurs at puncture sites can be controlled with local pressure. The use of a pledget soaked with aminocaproic acid (Amicar, EACA) has also been recommended to control continued minor oozing.[59] Severe bleeding, of course, calls for prompt termination of streptokinase. The lytic activity should stop within 15 minutes owing to the short half-life. Fresh whole blood is probably best for blood replacement when necessary, but packed red cells and fresh frozen plasma may be used, or cryoprecipitate.

Other complications attributed to streptokinase include fever and allergic reactions. Streptokinase is a foreign protein and therefore antigenic. Although fever occurs in about 25 per cent of patients and allergic

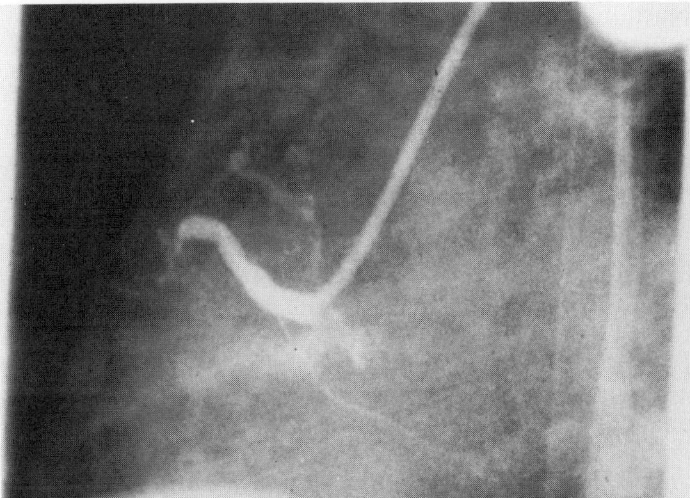

Figure 3–6. Right coronary angiogram. Left anterior oblique 60° projection. The vessel remains occluded after 30 min of streptokinase infusion.

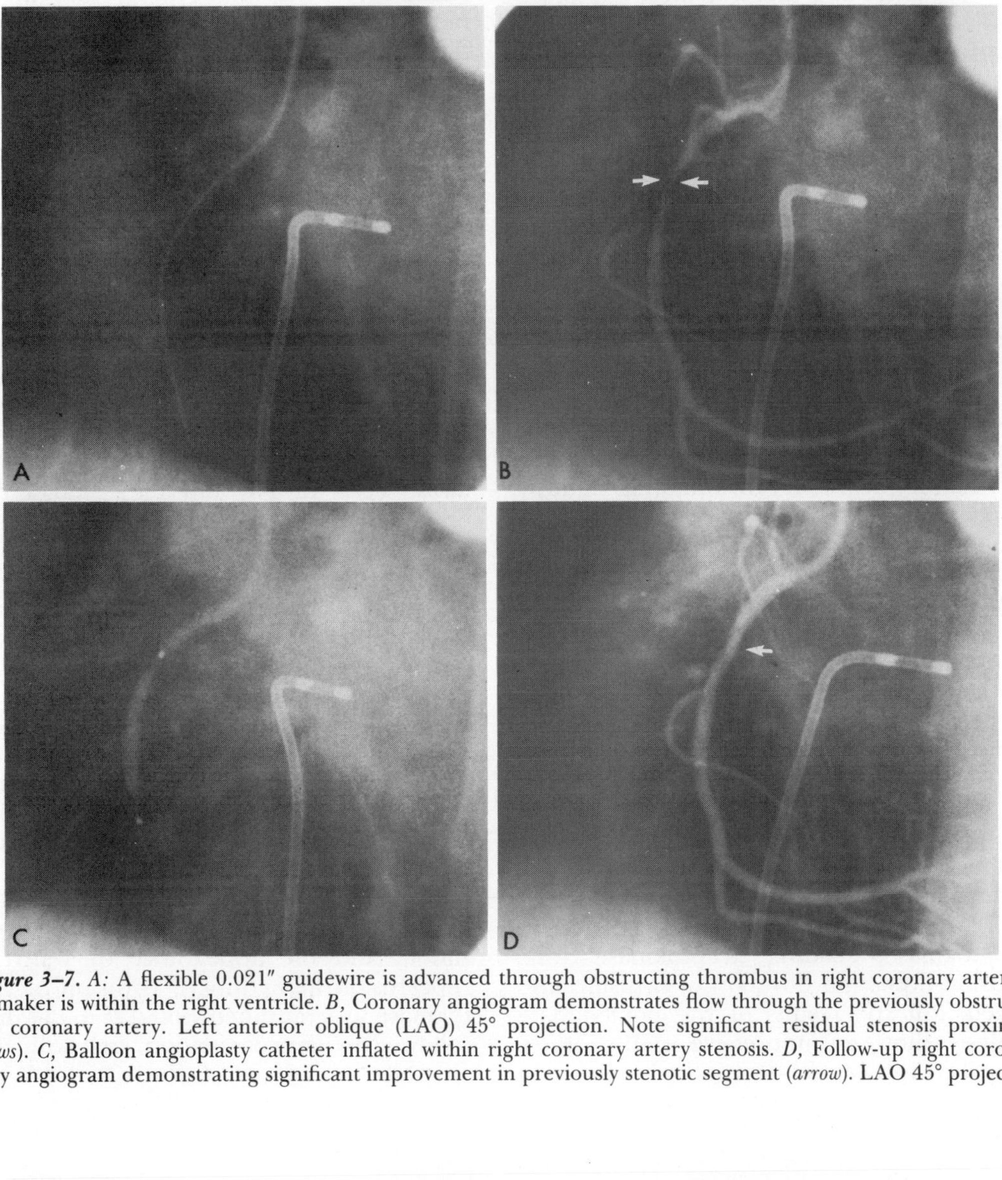

Figure 3–7. *A:* A flexible 0.021″ guidewire is advanced through obstructing thrombus in right coronary artery. A pacemaker is within the right ventricle. *B,* Coronary angiogram demonstrates flow through the previously obstructed right coronary artery. Left anterior oblique (LAO) 45° projection. Note significant residual stenosis proximally (*arrows*). *C,* Balloon angioplasty catheter inflated within right coronary artery stenosis. *D,* Follow-up right coronary artery angiogram demonstrating significant improvement in previously stenotic segment (*arrow*). LAO 45° projection.

reactions in 6 per cent, as shown in the N.I.H. systemic administration trials experience, the frequency of such reactions appears much less common in intracoronary thrombolysis studies.[59] Many investigators give 100 mg of hydrocortisone and/or Benadryl intravenously before giving streptokinase. Small streptokinase-provoked temperature rises and mild allergic reactions are usually controlled by antihistamines and acetaminophen. It is rarely necessary to discontinue therapy.

Other potential complications include the production of a transmural hemorrhagic infarction in the region of the reperfused coronary artery, and perhaps an increased incidence of cardiac rupture.[23] However, at least one animal study found that streptokinase did not augment reperfusion hemorrhage.[26] The frequency and cause of these complications in man need to be evaluated in future studies.

INTRAVENOUS SYSTEMIC THROMBOLYTIC THERAPY

Many studies have been done using systemic infusion of thrombolytic agents in acute myocardial infarction since the initial trials in 1959 by Fletcher et al.[22] These investigations employed a variety of protocols but usually did not treat patients within the first three to six hours from onset of symptoms. Because of varied protocols and late treatment, conclusions are difficult to reach and comparisons with intracoronary thrombolysis therapy are impossible to make. The 1979 European Cooperative Study for Streptokinase Treatment in Acute Myocardial Infarction did demonstrate a significantly lower mortality in the treatment group at immediate and six-month follow-ups.[19] A 1982 report of pooled results from eight European randomized studies of intravenous streptokinase treatment of acute myocardial infarction found an approximately 20 per cent reduction in mortality among patients treated with streptokinase as compared with controls.[67] The protocols varied in these randomized trials, some allowing patients with symptoms of up to 72 hours' duration to be treated with streptokinase. Loading streptokinase dose, infusion dose, and duration of infusion also varied, but the results of the pooled data analysis show an impressive reduction in mortality. Intravenous streptokinase infusion has the advantages of being easier and less costly, since the need for a catheterization laboratory and on-call trained personnel is eliminated.

There are important differences between intravenous and intracoronary streptokinase with regard to dosage, duration of infusion, and laboratory monitoring. Most of the early intravenous thrombolytic studies used a bolus of 250,000 units, followed by an infusion of 100,000 units per hour for 12 to 24 hours, and then anticoagulation therapy. Others have used larger initial doses ranging from 500,000 to 1.5 million units.[43, 56, 63] The incidence of bleeding complications was not excessive. The large loading dose of intravenous streptokinase is necessary to inhibit or neutralize the large reservoir of circulating antistreptococcal antibodies found in most individuals. With intravenous thrombolytic therapy it is necessary to obtain a systemic fibrinolytic effect. Laboratory monitoring of fibrinolytic parameters is necessary in order to determine that a degree of systemic fibrinolysis has been achieved. Once this is established, dissolution of fresh fibrin clots can be expected. Unlike anticoagulation therapy, dosage is relatively fixed and adjustments are not necessary except to ensure that a systemic lytic state has been established. The most sensitive test for fibrinolysis is thought to be the whole blood euglobulin lysis time, followed next in sensitivity by the thrombin time.[59] These tests unfortunately are often unavailable on an immediate or after-hours basis. Tests of PT and PTT and a fibrin degradation assay are acceptable substitutes. Whichever tests are employed, control values should be obtained and the tests repeated during the infusion, every four to six hours to monitor fibrinolysis and anticoagulation effects. Prolonged values of all the above-mentioned studies indicate that systemic lysis is occurring, except the euglobulin lysis time, which will be shortened. Since it is not possible to assess the progress of clot lysis angiographically with intravenous therapy taking place in the coronary care unit, it is mandatory to monitor cardiac rhythm and ST-segment changes. Reperfusion is usually marked by relief of chest pain, ST-segment normalization, and the appearance of ventricular reperfusion arrhythmias. Infusion of streptokinase is continued for 12 to 24 hours followed by anticoagulation, first with heparin and then with warfarin.

Preliminary results are available of a few intravenous streptokinase infusion studies employing coronary angiography to monitor results[43, 56, 66] In 1981, Schroeder and coworkers in Germany used an early intravenous infusion of a single dose of 500,000 units of streptokinase and were able to produce angiographic documentation of reperfusion in 10 of 22 patients (45%) within the first hour. They had 87 per cent patency at 24 hours and three weeks.[56]

Many studies are currently under way comparing early intravenous with intracoronary thrombolytic therapy. If equally beneficial results, without significant complications, are demonstrated with intravenous systemic thrombolysis, this approach may turn out to be preferable to intracoronary infusion.

OTHER THROMBOLYTIC AGENTS

The only other thrombolytic agent currently available is urokinase. This drug has F.D.A. approval for treatment of pulmonary embolism and occluded arteriovenous shunts but at this time is not approved for use in myocardial infarction. Several important differences exist between streptokinase and urokinase. Streptokinase is an enzyme produced from cultures of Group C streptococci; it is a foreign protein and therefore antigenic. Urokinase is a human enzymatic protein and is nonantigenic. Available forms are prepared by isolation of the protein from human urine or synthesized from human embryonic tissue cultures. As a result, urokinase is very expensive (about $50 per 100,000 units) in comparison with streptokinase (about $8 per 100,000 units). Both enzymes have short half-lives of about 10 to 15 minutes but differ in their activation of fibrinolysis. Streptokinase is an indirect activator, which after its infusion must combine with plasminogen to form an activator complex. This streptokinase-plasminogen complex then activates fibrinolysis by converting free plasminogen to plasmin. By contrast, urokinase is a direct activator of plasminogen and can initiate fibrinolysis without forming an activator complex. For intracoronary use urokinase is given at a rate of 6000 units per min compared with 2000 to 5000 units per min for streptokinase. For intravenous use the usual loading dose of urokinase is 4400 units per kg of body weight given over 10 minutes. The other principles of administration and laboratory monitoring are the same as outlined for streptokinase. Investigation is also currently in progress with recombinant DNA techniques to produce tissue plasminogen activator. If it becomes feasible to produce this enzyme in quantity, tissue plasminogen activator will likely become the agent of choice for thrombolysis.

CONCLUSIONS

The initial studies of intracoronary thrombolytic therapy for acute myocardial infarction have established that acute coronary thrombosis is present in about 90 per cent of patients and that successful recanalization by intracoronary streptokinase is possible in about 80 per cent of all patients treated.

Successful thrombolysis is greatest when treatment is started within the first four hours following onset of pain, after which time the success rate appears to fall.[62] Some of these initial studies have also suggested that it is possible to salvage ischemic cardiac muscle, improve impaired ventricular function, and reduce mortality.[23, 43, 49, 62] Assessment of myocardial preservation by any form of therapy to limit infarct size is currently extremely difficult because of the lack of a sensitive measure of infarct size. To assess myocardial salvage after intracoronary streptokinase, most investigators have looked at a decrease in pre- to posttreatment thallium-201 perfusion scan size or at improvement in ejection fraction. By performing thallium-201 myocardial perfusion scans prior to streptokinase infusion, a baseline differentiation between ischemic and nonischemic myocardium can be made. Immediately following thrombolysis, intracoronary thallium-201 is injected and the scan repeated. A decrease in the initial defect indicates improved perfusion to viable myocardium because thallium-201 uptake is ATP dependent, requiring viable cells. Figure 3–4 illustrates this sequence. Several investigators have noted serial improvement on pretreatment compared with immediate and late thallium-201 perfusion scans following successful thrombolysis.[23, 30, 31, 39, 55, 58] Control patients and those patients in whom thrombolysis was unsuccessful have not generally shown this improvement. Differentiation of patchy or subendocardial necrosis in this setting is difficult with this technique. The technique of simultaneous intracoronary thallium and technetium pyrophosphate imaging shows promise for the immediate assessment of reversibly ischemic and necrotic myocardium.[31, 55] Assessment of myocardial salvage with intracoronary thrombolysis has also been evaluated by comparing pre- with posttreatment ejection fractions. Many investigators have noted small but significant increases in ejection fraction for those patients having successful early intracoronary thrombolysis, but not for controls or for those patients with unsuccessful thrombolysis.[23, 38, 39, 46, 48, 58, 62] However, recent preliminary reports from randomized clinical trials have failed to show this improvement.[29, 69] Other studies have shown that, although global left ventricular ejection fraction may not improve after "successful" early thrombolysis (less than six hours), regional or segmental function improves in those segments initially impaired.[21, 60] The demonstration of changes in ventricular function is complex because of the many variables involved. The natural history of gradual improvement in ejection fraction after acute infarction must be considered[40, 68] as well as other variables, including ventricular loading condition at the time of the study, anatomic site of the infarct (anterior or inferior), degree of ventricular impairment, residual coronary stenosis, rethrombosis, and the timing of initial therapy. At this time it is difficult to establish a direct connection between successful streptokinase recanalization and the restoration of cardiac function.

MORTALITY

Some preliminary data are available from nonrandomized studies on the in-hospital and short-term mortality of patients with acute myocardial infarction treated with streptokinase. The Intracoronary Streptokinase Registry of the European Study of Cardiology of 331 patients with complete coronary occlusion found an in-hospital mortality of 7.6 per cent for those patients in whom the complete obstruction could be recanalized, compared with 21 per cent mortality for those with persistent complete obstruction. Other studies have shown similar reduced mortality among successfully treated patients.[62] Data from randomized controlled studies now in progress are not yet available.

SUMMARY

Despite many unknown factors and differences in opinion regarding patient selection, technique, and optimal therapy to prevent reocclusion, intracoronary streptokinase therapy is an exciting new technique for the treatment of acute myocardial infarction in selected patients. Its efficacy in restoring coronary blood flow early in the course of acute myocardial infarction, with relative safety in a high percentage of patients, seems to be established. It remains to be proved in carefully designed, controlled, randomized trials whether this approach will be associated with significant myocardial salvage, improved ventricular function, and reduced short- and long-term mortality.

References

1. Aber, C. P., Bass, N. M., Berry, C. L., et al.: Streptokinase in acute myocardial infarction: a controlled multicentre study in the United Kingdom. Br. Med. J. 2:1100, 1976.
2. Allison, R. B., Rodriquez, F. L., Higgins, E. A., Jr., et al.: Clinicopathologic correlations in coronary atherosclerosis. Four hundred thirty-eight patients studied with postmortem coronary angiography. Circulation 27:170, 1963.
3. Alonso, D. R., Scheidt, S., Post, M. R., and Killip, T.: Quantification of myocardial damage in cardiogenic shock. Circulation 48:588, 1973.
4. Bett, J. H. N., Biggs, J. C., Castaldi, P. A., et al.: Australian multicentre trial of streptokinase in acute myocardial infarction. Lancet 1:57, 1973.
5. Bleifeld, W., Mathey, D., Hanrath, P., et al.: Infarct size from serial serum creatinine phosphokinase in relation to left ventricular hemodynamics. Circulation 55:303, 1977.
6. Blumgart, H. L., Schlesinger, M. J., and Davis, D.: Studies on the relation of the clinical manifestations of angina pectoris, coronary thrombosis, and myocardial infarction to the pathologic findings with particular reference to the significance of the collateral circulation. Am. Heart J. 19:1, 1940.
7. Bolooki, H., Golkar, R. R., Morales, A., and Kaiser, G. A.: Effects of direct myocardial revascularization on infarct size: a clinical and experimental correlation. Surg. Forum 24:137, 1973.
8. Boucek, R. J., and Murphy, W. P., Jr.: Segmental perfusion of the coronary arteries with fibrinolysin in man following a myocardial infarction. Am. J. Cardiol. 6:525, 1960.
9. Braunwald, E.: Protection of the ischemic myocardium. Circulation 53:1, 1976.
10. Breddin, K., Ehrly, A. M., Fechler, L., et al.: Die Kurzzeitfibrinolyse beim akuten Myokardinfarkt. Dtsch. Med. Wochenschr. 98:861, 1973.
11. Chandler, A. B., Chapman, I., Erhardt, L. R., et al.: Coronary thrombosis in myocardial infarction. Report of a workshop on the role of coronary throm-

bosis in the pathogenesis of acute myocardial infarction. Am. J. Cardiol. 34:823, 1974.

12. Constantini, C., Corday, E., Lang, T. W., et al.: Revascularization after 3 hours of coronary arterial occlusion. Effects on regional cardiac metabolic function and infarct size. Am. J. Cardiol. 36:368, 1975.
13. Cowley, M. J., Hastillo, A., Vetrovec, G. W., and Hess, M. L.: Effects of intracoronary streptokinase in acute myocardial infarction. Am. Heart J. 182:1149, 1981.
14. Cowley, M. J., Hastillo, A., Vetrovec, G. W., and Hess, M. L.: Fibrinolytic effects of low dose intracoronary streptokinase administration in acute myocardial infarction. Circulation 64:10, 1981.
15. Dalen, J. D., Ockene, I. S., and Alpert, J. S.: Coronary spasm, coronary thrombosis, and myocardial infarction: a hypothesis concerning the pathophysiology of acute myocardial infarction. Am. Heart J. 104:1119, 1982.
16. DeWood, M. A., Spores, J., Notske, R. N., et al.: Medical and surgical management of myocardial infarction. Am. J. Cardiol. 44:1356, 1979.
17. DeWood, M. A., Spores, J., Notske, R. N., et al.: Prevalence of total coronary occlusion during the early hours of transmural myocardial infarction. N. Engl. J. Med. 303:897, 1980.
18. Dioguardi, N., Mannucci, P. M., Lotto, A., et al.: Controlled trial of streptokinase and heparin in acute myocardial infarction. Lancet 2:891, 1971.
19. European Cooperative Study Group for Streptokinase Treatment in Acute Myocardial Infarction: Streptokinase in acute myocardial infarction. N. Engl. J. Med. 301:797, 1979.
20. European Working Party: Streptokinase in recent myocardial infarction: a controlled multi-centre trial. Br. Med. J. 3:325, 1971.
21. Fallon, J. T., Aretz, T., and Gold, H. K.: Coronary arterial pathology following thrombolytic therapy for acute myocardial infarction. Circulation 66:II-336, 1982 (abstr.).
22. Fletcher, A. P., Sherry, S., Alkjaersig, N., et al.: The maintenance of a sustained thrombolytic state in man. II. Clinical observations on patients with myocardial infarction and other thromboembolic disorders. J. Clin. Invest. 38:1111, 1959.
23. Ganz, W., Buchbinder, N., Marcus, H., et al.: Intracoronary thrombolysis in evolving myocardial infarction. Am. Heart J. 101:4, 1981.
24. Heikinheimo, R., Ahrenberg, P., Honkapohja, H., et al.: Fibrinolytic treatment in acute myocardial infarction. Acta Med. Scand. 189:7, 1971.
25. Herrick, J. B.: Clinical features of sudden obstruction of the coronary arteries. J.A.M.A. 49:2015, 1912.
26. Higginson, L. A. J., Sheldrick, K., Temple, V., and Beanlands, D. S.: Does streptokinase augment reperfusion hemorrhage? Circulation 66:II-86, 1982 (abstr.).
27. Highsmith, R. F., and Rosenberg, R. D.: The inhibition of human plasmin by human antithrombin-hepatic cofactor. J. Biol. Chem. 249:4335, 1974.
28. Kennedy, J. W., Fritz, J. K., Ritchie, J. L., et al.: Streptokinase in acute myocardial infarction: Western Washington randomized trial—protocol and progress report. Am. Heart J. 104:899, 1982.
29. Leiboff, R. H., Katz, R. J., Wasserman, A. G., et al.: A randomized controlled trial of intracoronary streptokinase in acute MI: preliminary (cautionary) observations. Circulation 66:II-334, 1982 (abstr.).
30. Maddahi, J., Ganz, W., Ninomiya, K., et al.: Myocardial salvage by intracoronary thrombolysis in evolving acute myocardial infarction: evaluation using intracoronary injection of thallium-201. Am. Heart J. 102:664, 1981.
31. Maddahi, J., Geft, I., Hulse, S., et al.: Dual intracoronary thallium and technetium pyrophosphate imaging for immediate assessment of reversibly ischemic and necrotic myocardium following intracoronary thrombolysis. Circulation 66:II-261, 1982 (abstr.).
32. Markis, J. E., Malagold, M., Parker, J. A., et al.: Myocardial salvage after intracoronary thrombolysis with streptokinase in acute myocardial infarction: assessment by intracoronary thallium-201. N. Engl. J. Med. 305:777, 1981.
33. Maroko, P. R., Bernstein, E. F., Libby, P., et al.: The effects of intraaortic balloon counterpulsation on the severity of myocardial ischemic injury following acute coronary occlusion. Circulation 45:1150, 1972.
34. Maroko, P. R., and Braunwald, E.: Effect of metabolic and pharmacologic interventions on myocardial infarct size following coronary occlusion. Circulation 53:162, 1976.
35. Maroko, P. R., Kjekshus, J. K., Sobel, B. E., et al.: Factors influencing infarct size following experimental coronary artery occlusion. Circulation 43:67, 1971.
36. Maroko, P. R., Libby, P., Ginks, W. R., et al.: Coronary artery reperfusion. I. Early effects on local myocardial function and the extent of myocardial necrosis. J. Clin. Invest. 51:2710, 1972.
37. Mathey, D. G., Klöppel, G., Kuck, K.-H., et al.: Transmural, hemorrhagic infarction following intracoronary streptokinase: clinical, angiographic and autoptical findings. Circulation 64:IV-194, 1981 (abstr.).
38. Mathey, D. G., Kuck, K.-H., Tilsner, V., et al.: Nonsurgical coronary artery recanalization in acute transmural myocardial infarction. Circulation 63:489, 1981.
39. Mathey, D. G., Sheehan, P. H., Schofer, J., et al.: LV function following intracoronary thrombolysis in acute myocardial infarction. Circulation 66:II-335, 1982 (abstr.).
40. Meizlish, J. L., Berger, H. J., Plandey, M., et al.: Spontaneous improvement in regional wall motion in initial transmural myocardial infarction: implications for evaluating therapy. Circulation 66:II-86, 1982 (abstr.).
41. Meyer, J., Merx, W., Schmitz, H., et al.: Percutaneous transluminal coronary angioplasty immediately after intracoronary streptolysis of transmural myocardial infarction. Circulation 66:905, 1982.
42. Muller, J. E., Antman, E., Green, L. H., and Koster, J. K., Jr.: Salvage of acute ischemic myocardium by emergency coronary artery bypass grafting. Clin. Cardiol. 3:276, 1980.
43. Neuhaus, K. L., Kostering, H., Tebbe, U., et al.: High-dose intravenous streptokinase infusion in acute myocardial infarction. Z. Kardiol. 70:791, 1981.
44. O'Brien, C. M., Caroll, M., O'Rourke, P. T., et al.: The reversibility of acute ischemic injury to the myocardium by restoration of coronary flow. J. Thorac. Cardiovasc. Surg. 64:840, 1972.
45. Phillips, S. J., et al.: Emergency coronary artery revascularization: a possible therapy for acute myocardial infarction. Circulation 60:241, 1979.

46. Reduto, L. A., Smalling, R. W., Freund, G. C., and Gould, K. L.: Intracoronary infusion of streptokinase in patients with acute myocardial infarction: effects of reperfusion on left ventricular performance. Am. J. Cardiol. 48:403, 1981.
47. Reimer, K. A., Lowe, J. E., Rasmussen, M. M., and Jennings, R. B.: The wavefront phenomenon of ischemic cell death; myocardial infarction size vs. duration of coronary occlusion in dogs. Circulation 56:785, 1977.
48. Rentrop, K. P.: Mortality and functional changes after intracoronary streptokinase infusion. Circulation 66:II-335, 1982 (abstr.).
49. Rentrop, K. P., Blanke, H., Karsch, K. R., et al.: Selective intracoronary thrombolysis in acute myocardial infarction and unstable angina pectoris. Circulation 63:307, 1981.
50. Rentrop, K. P., Blanke, H., Karsch, K. R., et al.: Acute myocardial infarction: intracoronary application of nitroglycerin and streptokinase. Clin. Cardiol. 2:354, 1979.
51. Roberts, W. C.: Coronary arteries in fatal acute myocardial infarction. Circulation 45:215, 1972.
52. Rude, R. E., Muller, J. E., and Braunwald, E.: Efforts to limit the size of myocardial infarct. Ann. Intern. Med. 95:736, 1981.
53. Rutsch, W., Schartl, M., Mathey, D., et al.: Percutaneous transluminal coronary recanalization: procedure, results, and acute complications. Am. Heart J. 102:1178, 1981.
54. Saphir, O., Priest, W. S., Hamburger, W. W., et al.: Coronary atherosclerosis, coronary thrombosis, and the resulting myocardial changes. An evaluation of their respective clinical pictures including the electrocardiographic records based on their anatomical findings. Am. Heart J. 10:567, 1924.
55. Schofer, J., Stritzke, P., Kuck, K.-H., et al.: Dual intracoronary myocardial scintigraphy with thallium-201 and technetium-99m pyrophosphate predicts myocardial salvage immediately after successful intracoronary thrombolysis. Circulation 66:II-335, 1982 (abstr.).
56. Schroeder, R., Biamino, G., von Leitner, E. R., et al.: Comparisons of the effects of intracoronary and systemic streptokinase infusion in acute myocardial infarction: preliminary results. *In* Rafflenbrul, W., Lichtlen, P. R., and Balcon, R. (eds.): Unstable Angina Pectoris. Stuttgart & New York, Georg Thieme Verlag, 1981, p. 167.
57. Schuler, G., Schwarz, F., Hofmann, M., et al.: Thrombolysis in acute myocardial infarction using intracoronary streptokinase: assessment by thallium-201 scintigraphy. Circulation 66:658, 1982.
58. Schwarz, F., Schuler, G., Katus, H., et al.: Intracoronary thrombolysis in acute myocardial infarction: correlations among serum enzyme, scintigraphic and hemodynamic findings. Am. J. Cardiol. 50:32, 1982.
59. Sharma, G. V. R. K., Cella, G., Parisi, A. F., and Sasahara, A. A.: Thrombolytic therapy. N. Engl. J. Med. 306:1268, 1982.
60. Sheehan, F. H., Mathey, D., Dodge, H. T., and Kuck, K. H.: Effect of early revascularization on compensatory hyperkinesis in acute infarction. Circulation 66:II-336, 1982 (abstr.).
61. Shell, W. E., Swan, H. J. C., and Ganz, W.: Accelerated washout of creatine kinase by fibrinolytic reperfusion in man. Clin. Res. 29:241, 1981.
62. Smalling, R. W., Fuentes, F., Freund, G. C., et al.: Beneficial effects of intracoronary thrombolysis up to eighteen hours after onset of pain in evolving myocardial infarction. Am. Heart J. 104:912, 1982.
63. Smith, G. T., Soeter, J. R., Haston, H. H., and McNamara, J. J.: Coronary reperfusion in primates. Serial electrocardiographic and histologic assessment. J. Clin. Invest. 54:1420, 1974.
64. Sobel, B. E., and Bergmann, S. R.: Coronary thrombolysis: some unresolved issues. Am. J. Med. 72:1, 1982.
65. Sobel, B. E., Bresnahan, G. F., Shell, W. E., and Yoder, R. D.: Estimation of infarct size in man and its relation to prognosis. Circulation 46:640, 1972.
66. Spann, J. F., Sherry, S., Blase, A., et al.: High-dose, brief intravenous streptokinase early in acute myocardial infarction. Am. Heart J. 104:939, 1982.
67. Stampfer, M. J., Goldhaber, S. Z., Yusuf, S., et al.: Effect of intravenous streptokinase on acute myocardial infarction: pooled results from randomized trials. N. Engl. J. Med. 307:1180, 1982.
68. Wackers, F., Berger, H., and Zaret, B.: Spontaneous changes of global and regional left ventricular function during the first 24 hours of acute myocardial infarction: implications for evaluating thrombolytic therapy. Circulation 64:IV-196, 1981 (abstr.).
69. Walton, J., Jr., O'Neill, W., Colfer, H., et al.: Failure of intracoronary thrombolysis to preserve ventricular function: report of a randomized clinical trial. Circulation 66:II-334, 1982 (abstr.).

4

Intra-Aortic Balloon Counterpulsation and the Diagnosis and Management of Surgical Complications of Acute Myocardial Infarction

DEAN J. KEREIAKES
and THOMAS A. PORTS

INTRA-AORTIC BALLOON COUNTERPULSATION

Knowledge of the utility and mechanisms of action of intra-aortic balloon counterpulsation (IABP) can be of paramount importance in the management of the critically ill patient with cardiac disease. This is particularly true for the mechanical complications of acute myocardial infarction, i.e., papillary muscle dysfunction or rupture, ventricular septal rupture, and free wall rupture, in which cardiogenic shock is potentially treatable with early surgical intervention. Familiarity with the clinical presentation, appropriate diagnostic evaluation, and therapeutic approach, including proper use of IABP, can be particularly gratifying in these situations.

The intra-aortic balloon pump is the most common circulatory assist device currently in use. It uses the counterpulsation principle, as opposed to the actual pumping of blood, to achieve its beneficial hemodynamic effects. When triggered from an electrocardiographic QRS or arterial pulse tracing, the intra-aortic balloon is inflated during diastole with 20 to 40 ml of gas within the descending aorta at the level of the left subclavian artery. The balloon then deflates in systole. The diastolic filling of the balloon expands intra-aortic volume, resulting in an increase in aortic diastolic pressure, and therefore in coronary perfusion pressure.[98] With systolic deflation there is a rapid decline in aortic volume, causing pressure to fall as systole begins. The left ventricle is then ejecting blood against decreased afterload, and left ventricular performance is enhanced.[10, 60, 70] Cardiac output can increase 15 to 50 per cent,[60] forward flow improve, left ventricular end-diastolic pressure (LVEDP) decrease, and myocardial oxygen demand fall as a result of IABP.[61] Additionally, the transmyocardial coronary perfusion gradient (coronary artery pressure–LVEDP) increases.[50] As coronary blood flow occurs primarily in diastole, the increase in aortic diastolic pressure and coronary perfusion gradient may have a net effect of increasing coronary blood flow in obstructed coronary arteries.[7, 9] Coronary collateral blood flow may also be enhanced.[40, 51] A recent study did not show an increase in regional coronary blood flow in patients with coronary artery disease. The authors suggested that a reduction in myocardial oxygen consumption was the most

Table 4–1. INTRA-AORTIC BALLOON PUMP INDICATIONS

Indications
- Cardiogenic shock
  - Secondary to pump failure
  - Secondary to ventricular septal rupture
  - Secondary to acute mitral regurgitation
- Refractory ischemia
  - Unstable angina not responding to pharmacologic treatment
  - Postinfarction angina not responding to pharmacologic treatment
- Pharmacologically refractory lethal ventricular arrhythmias post myocardial infarction
- Aid to discontinuing cardiopulmonary bypass

Possible Indications
- Limitation of myocardial infarct size without shock
- Support of critically ill/high-risk patient during coronary angiography or angioplasty
- Major noncardiac surgery in a high-risk cardiac patient

likely mechanism by which IABP relieves myocardial ischemia.[96]

Considering these beneficial effects, it is not surprising that the main indications for the pump are in patients with coronary artery disease who have circulatory failure or refractory ischemia. The most common situations for using the pump are listed in Table 4–1.

The use of the pump for cardiogenic shock secondary to ventricular septal rupture and with mitral regurgitation is discussed later. For cardiogenic shock without rupture we begin IABP once the diagnosis is firmly established and other causes of low output (hypovolemia, tamponade, and right ventricular infarct) are excluded by hemodynamic measurement. Vasodilators may be added to inotropic agents once balloon support of arterial pressure is achieved.

Survival of patients with cardiogenic shock treated with inotropic agents and IABP is improved, but still poor.[2, 20, 45, 49, 69, 77, 91, 95] We usually perform emergency coronary angiography and coronary bypass surgery on those patients showing initial improvement on the pump. Some increase in survival may be expected from this approach, as indicated by several nonrandomized, noncontrolled studies.[20, 45, 49, 53, 69]

Method of Balloon Insertion

Until recently, insertion of the intra-aortic balloon was accomplished by surgical insertion in an end-to-side manner by means of a graft into the common femoral artery through which the balloon was inserted. This technique has been largely replaced by the introduction of percutaneous intra-aortic balloons; those available today have a volume of 30 to 40 ml and are designed to be inserted through an intra-arterial sheath. The 40-ml balloon is most commonly used in adult men, and the 30-ml balloon in women.

Figure 4–1 illustrates two types of percutaneous intra-aortic balloons currently available—a single-lumen and a dual-lumen model. The dual-lumen type allows the use of a movable guidewire during insertion and for direct measurement of arterial pressure. Figure 4–2 shows a dual-lumen balloon in its wrapped position with a movable "J" wire extended through the inner lumen. An inflated single-lumen balloon is shown with it. Excellent detailed descriptions of the insertion technique are available from the various manufacturers in the form of instruction manuals or instruction videotapes, and should be thoroughly reviewed by any indi-

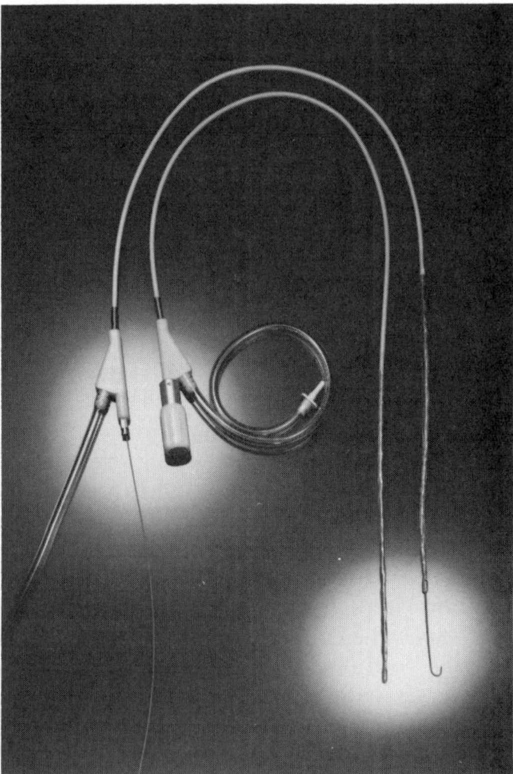

Figure 4–1. Two types of percutaneous intra-aortic balloons. Dual-lumen balloon with movable wire is on outside. Inner balloon is single-lumen type. (Courtesy of Datascope Corp., Paramus, New Jersey.)

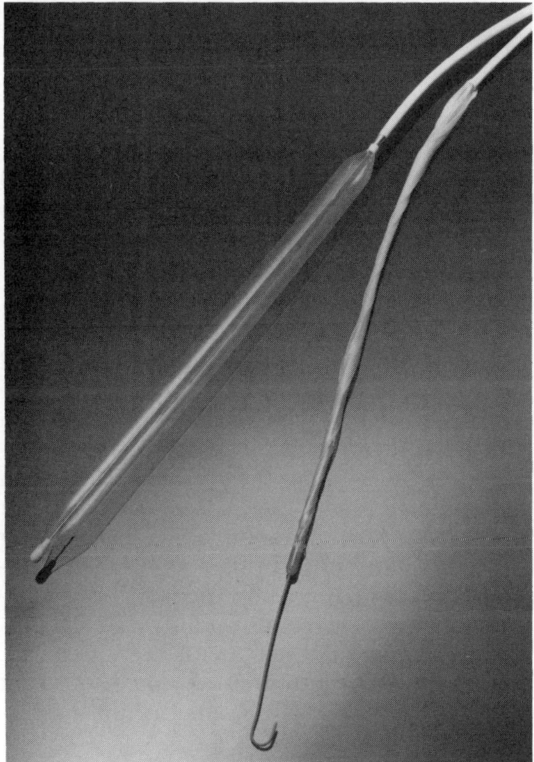

Figure 4–2. Close-up of intra-aortic balloons. A wrapped dual-lumen balloon with movable "J" wire extending from its inner lumen is seen on the right. An inflated single lumen balloon is shown to the left. (Courtesy of Datascope Corp., Paramus, New Jersey.)

vidual considering placement or use of an intra-aortic balloon. Intra-aortic balloon insertion by the percutaneous method can be safe when certain guidelines are followed.

First and foremost, it should be done only by persons experienced in both the Seldinger technique of catheter insertion and the intravascular manipulation of catheters. The patient and staff should be informed of the procedure before beginning. Necessary monitoring equipment should be available. All the intra-aortic balloon equipment should be assembled and a back-up balloon should be available. The console should be tested to make sure it is working properly, and the pressure transducers calibrated. Both groins of the patient should be widely prepped and then draped in a sterile manner; it is advantageous to drape a large, sterile working area. The balloon is prepared and tested to ensure adequate inflation and balloon competence.

After appropriate local anesthesia, the femoral artery is punctured percutaneously and a guidewire is inserted through the needle. We prefer to advance the guidewire to the level of the left subclavian artery under fluoroscopic control. If fluoroscopic monitoring is not available, the guidewire and intra-aortic balloon can be measured before insertion to approximate the level of the left subclavian artery, and this length should be marked with a sterile suture tie. We prefer to pass the guidewire to the approximate final location of the intra-aortic balloon before inserting the vascular sheath, to ensure that passage through the iliac artery and abdominal aorta is smooth and unhindered. After appropriate subcutaneous dissection, the arterial dilator and long intra-arterial sheath can be introduced. The dilator is then removed, the guidewire wiped, and the wrapped intra-aortic balloon slid over the guidewire into the intra-arterial sheath. The balloon is then advanced over the guidewire under fluoroscopic control to its proper position in the descending aorta at the level of the left subclavian artery. If fluoroscopy is not available, the balloon is advanced until the previously placed marking surgical tie reaches the sheath. We strongly favor the dual-lumen balloon as it allows the insertion over the guidewire into the aorta. This approach significantly reduces, if not eliminates, the major hazard of aortic dissection.

Once the balloon is in its proper position, the guidewire can be removed from the dual-lumen balloon and, after flushing this lumen, used as an intra-arterial pressure monitor. The retrograde passage of the intra-aortic balloon up the aorta must be done with great care in patients with iliofemoral and aortic atherosclerosis. Significant resistance should not be overcome with pressure. Because of the high incidence of significant iliofemoral and aortic atherosclerosis, we prefer the guidewire to be inserted to at least the level of the diaphragm before the vascular sheath is inserted. If the initial site proves to be unacceptable because of extensive disease, the guidewire and needle can be removed easily and hemostasis obtained quickly with manual pressure. The other femoral artery can be punctured and, it is hoped, will allow unobstructed passage of the balloon. Once the intra-aortic balloon tip is advanced to the level of the left subclavian artery and proper catheter position is confirmed by fluoroscopy, the balloon is fixed to the sheath with umbilical tape and additionally sutured to the patient's leg. A sterile pressure dressing is then applied.

Patients are anticoagulated with intravenous heparin for the duration of the balloon's use. Frequent monitoring of the perfusion of the leg through which the intra-aortic balloon is inserted is required. When the intra-aortic balloon is in its proper position, counterpulsation should be begun immediately. The proper timing of balloon inflation and deflation is absolutely essential for optimal results. Timing can be judged from the pulse contour as it appears on the intra-aortic balloon console. An electronic signal superimposed on the electrocardiogram estimates the point of balloon inflation. Adjustments are made to the point of balloon inflation and deflation within the cardiac cycle so that optimal diastolic augmentation of blood pressure is achieved.

Figure 4–3 illustrates the normal diastolic augmentation of blood pressure achieved with the intra-aortic balloon pump set on a 1:2 (every other heartbeat) timing. The end-diastolic dip in pressure caused by the deflation of the balloon should reach a minimal value just before the arterial upstroke begins. The diastolic augmentation produced by the balloon's inflation should not occur before the dicrotic notch. If inflation of the balloon is too late, the diastolic augmentation produced by the balloon may merge into the beginning of the next arterial upstroke. This situation may force the left ventricle to contract against an inflated balloon, and results in an increase in afterload rather than a decrease. Early deflation is less serious, but less than optimal reduction in afterload is achieved if too long an interval passes between balloon deflation and the beginning of left ventricular ejection. Early inflation, before the beginning of diastole, should obviously be avoided, as this forces the left ventricle to contract against the inflated balloon. Late inflation does not allow optimal diastolic augmentation to improve coronary blood flow. Figures 4–4 and 4–5 illustrate early and late inflation, respectively.

Once the patient is on the intra-aortic balloon, the hemodynamic status is constantly monitored. Therapeutic end points should be considered prior to the insertion of the intra-aortic balloon. We usually proceed with cardiac catheterization and coronary angiography supported by the intra-aortic balloon as soon as feasible. Care should be taken not to puncture the balloon while exchanging catheters, but beyond this point cardiac catheterization in patients on the intra-aortic balloon does not differ significantly from standard technique. These patients are, of course, very ill, and close attention should be directed to their hemodynamic status during the cardiac catheterization.

We usually test for balloon dependence within the first 18 to 36 hours after counterpulsation is begun. Gradual weaning from counterpulsation is done by having the balloon pump every other beat; then, if the patient is stable, inflation with every third or fourth beat is tried. The patient is closely observed and the hemodynamics are continually monitored during the period of balloon weaning. If the heart can maintain the cir-

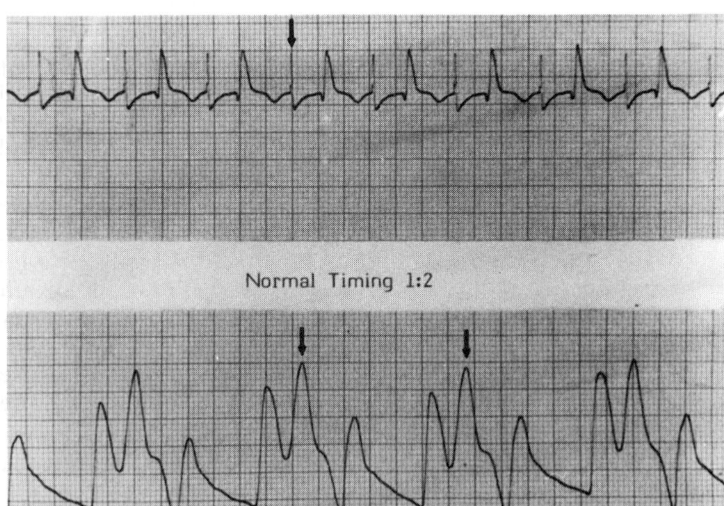

Figure 4–3. *Top,* ECG with timing marks *(arrow)* for balloon inflation. *Bottom,* Arterial pulse tracing showing diastolic augmentation *(arrows)* with every other beat (1:2) with correct timing of inflation and deflation. (Courtesy of Datascope Corp., Paramus, New Jersey.)

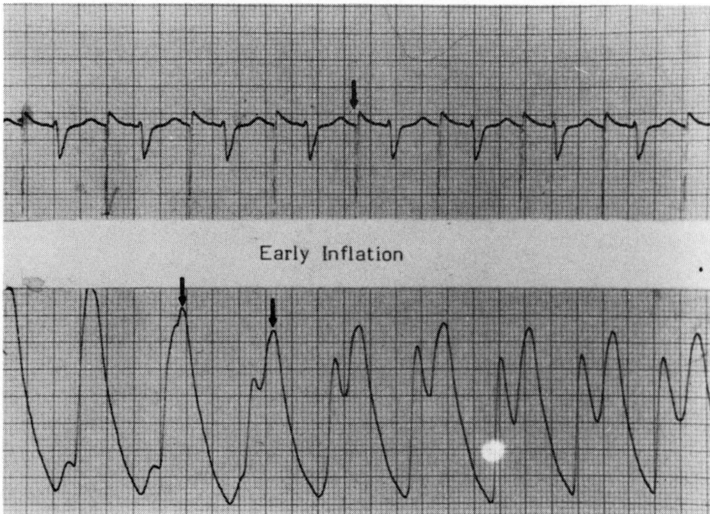

Figure 4–4. *Top,* ECG. *Bottom,* Arterial pulse tracing 1:1 diastolic augmentation *(arrows).* Inflation is occurring early before dicrotic notch during the first five cycles; onset of inflation is then corrected for the last three cycles. (Courtesy of Datascope Corp., Paramus, New Jersey.)

culation with diastolic augmentation on every fourth beat, a decision may be made for elective balloon removal. If weaning fails, further 1:1 counterpulsation is employed, and attempts can be made to wean the patient six to 12 hours later.

Removal of Percutaneous Balloon

Major complications from IABP include ischemic injuries of the leg in which the balloon is inserted. These can be due to trauma to the femoral or iliac vessels, or to obstruction caused by the balloon catheter within the vessel itself. In patients with very low cardiac output and poor perfusion pressure, particularly in association with atherosclerotic narrowing of the iliac and femoral arteries, the presence of the balloon catheter itself can significantly compromise the lumen and flow to the distal limb. Damage to the aorta and aortic dissection can also occur. Many aortic dissections have been discovered incidentally at the time of angiography or an autopsy. The incidence of aortic dissection is perhaps 5 to 10 per cent among all patients in whom an intra-aortic balloon pump is inserted. Incidence of complications in several large series utilizing the graft method of pump insertion is available.[77] Preliminary data concerning the safety of the newer percutaneous intra-aortic balloon are encouraging.[35, 85] We have not encountered any serious

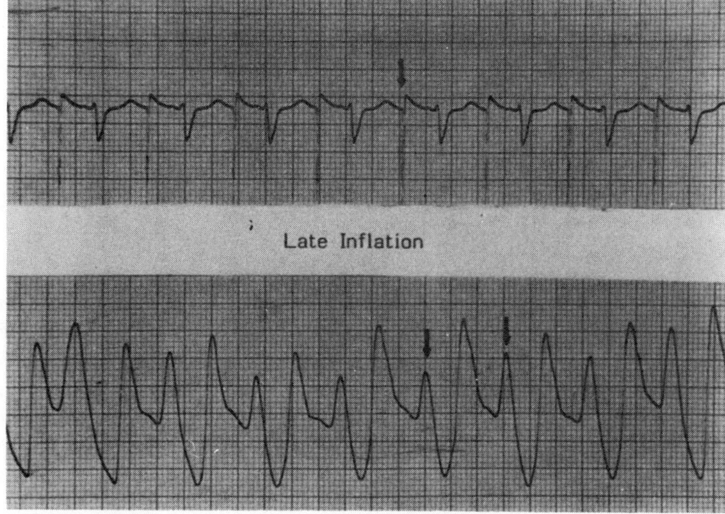

Figure 4–5. Late balloon inflation *(arrows)* is seen during cycles 2 to 8. (Courtesy of Datascope Corp., Paramus, New Jersey.)

complications from careful percutaneous intra-aortic balloon insertion in over 60 patients in whom we have used this device.

PAPILLARY MUSCLE DYSFUNCTION AND RUPTURE

Papillary muscle dysfunction (PMD) frequently accompanies myocardial ischemia and may be clinically detected in over one half of patients with infarction.[37] Ischemia may impair normal papillary muscle contraction in isovolumetric systole, or cause regional left ventricular dysfunction at the base of a papillary muscle, with consequent failure of normal systolic mitral leaflet coaptation. Dysfunction or rupture preferentially affects the posteromedial papillary muscle by virtue of its single blood supply from the posterior descending coronary artery. The anterolateral papillary muscle has a more extensive collateral circulation derived from both left circumflex and left anterior descending coronaries.[22] PMD is, therefore, more common in association with posterior or inferior infarctions.[1, 89]

The murmur of PMD is highly variable in onset, duration, and configuration. Although classically described as an ejection type (crescendo-decrescendo) murmur occurring in mid-late systole,[67, 91] the murmur is frequently pansystolic.[19] The intensity bears little relationship to the severity of regurgitation, and may be deceptively soft or absent in the presence of severe left ventricular dysfunction.[27] The murmur is heard best at the apex with radiation to the axilla and, less commonly, the base. Systolic clicks with or without murmurs may also reflect PMD.[82]

Papillary muscle rupture (PMR) may be heralded by the acute onset of an apical pansystolic murmur, dyspnea, chest pain, and hemodynamic deterioration. The murmur of PMR is frequently decrescendo in contour as rapid elevation in left atrial pressure lowers left ventricle–left atrium pressure gradient and decreases flow from the left ventricle to the left atrium in late systole. As noted above, rupture preferentially involves the posteromedial papillary muscle and occurs two to ten days following a posterior or inferior infarction. Rupture most commonly involves a solitary head of the papillary muscle, but transection of the entire trunk can occur, as illustrated in Figure 4–6. The

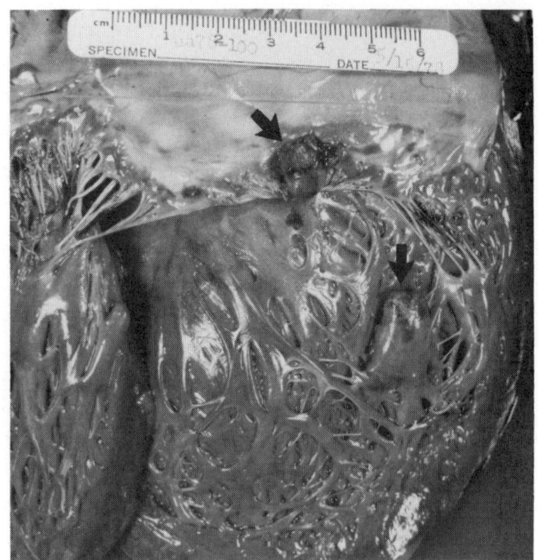

Figure 4–6. Rupture of the entire trunk of the posteromedial papillary muscle. Arrows demonstrate severed ends of muscle at the site of rupture. Specimen is from a patient who expired in florid pulmonary edema following acute inferior myocardial infarction.

course is one of rapid clinical deterioration, and mortality without surgical intervention exceeds 50 per cent by 24 hours and 90 per cent by two weeks following rupture.[41, 74] Cardiogenic shock and death are common sequelae, although the quantity of left ventricle involved with infarction is relatively small.[65, 91] Prompt diagnosis is therefore essential, as PMR is a potentially treatable form of cardiogenic shock with early surgical intervention.

The differential diagnosis of a new pansystolic murmur following myocardial infarction includes a ventricular septal rupture (VSR). The murmur of VSR is often best heard at the lower left sternal border, and is more frequently associated with a thrill than is the apical murmur of PMR. VSR may occur in the setting of either acute anterior or inferior myocardial infarction. Since the physical examination may be misleading,[24, 26] bedside cardiac catheterization with a flow-directed, balloon-tipped catheter should be performed.[54] Blood should be carefully obtained for oxygen saturation determination from the right atrium, right ventricle, and pulmonary artery by using fluoroscopic or pressure waveform guidance. The presence of an oxygen saturation step-up in excess of 5 per cent from right atrium to pulmonary artery, or a recirculation peak in the thermodilution cardiac output curve, reflects the left-to-right shunt of VSR. Large regurgitant or V waves in the pulmonary capillary wedge pressure tracing usually indicate acute mitral regurgitation. However, a large-magnitude V wave may accompany VSR.[26] The normal left atrial V wave reflects left atrial filling, and its magnitude is dependent on left atrial filling volume and compliance.[68] Augmented left atrial filling due to an acute left-to-right shunt accompanying VSR may be associated with exaggeration of normal V-wave magnitude, thus simulating acute mitral regurgitation.[5] However, the onset of this wave is normal with respect to the QRS complex of a simultaneously recorded ECG, it peaks at or beyond the apex of the ECG T wave, and it rarely exceeds peak systolic pressure in the pulmonary arterial pressure tracing. In acute mitral regurgitation, the V wave is in truth a C-V or regurgitant wave, with earlier onset obliterating the X descent of the pulmonary capillary wedge pressure tracing. This regurgitant wave not infrequently exceeds peak pulmonary arterial systolic pressure.[12]

Two-dimensional echocardiography may help establish the diagnosis of PMD or PMR.[57,66] In PMD, parasternal and apical long-axis views may demonstrate failure of one or both mitral leaflets to reach their normal systolic position in the plane of the mitral anulus, "incomplete leaflet closure."[92] The anterior leaflet is always affected irrespective of which papillary muscle is dysfunctional; the posterior leaflet is involved in a smaller percentage of cases. Segmental dysfunction of the left ventricular wall at the base of a papillary muscle may be present. In the parasternal long-axis or apical four-chamber view, PMR is suggested by the presence of a flail mitral leaflet with systolic prolapse into the left atrium. A mass of tissue representing the ruptured papillary muscle head may accompany the flail leaflet.[23] Pulsed Doppler combined with echocardiography is an excellent technique for demonstrating and helping to quantify acute mitral regurgitation.[64] Radionuclide angiography can be used to demonstrate and help to quantify and differentiate between acute mitral regurgitation and the left-to-right shunt of VSR.[36,81] First-pass radionuclide ventriculography, which can be done at the bedside, is used to confirm the presence of the shunt, and gives valuable information about global and segmental left ventricular function and the response to various interventions. If the patient can be stabilized medically, cardiac catheterization should be performed to document the severity of the defect and to evaluate associated coronary artery disease.

The treatment of severe acute mitral regurgitation complicating myocardial infarction is mitral valve replacement. Emergency medical therapy is directed at reducing impedance to forward left ventricular outflow and lowering elevated left ventricular pressure and volume. Bedside hemodynamic monitoring should be performed to exclude the diagnosis of VSR and to assess the response to therapy. We have found nitroprusside to be particularly useful because of its potent systemic impedance lowering effect and its ability to reduce left ventricular volume. Evidence suggests that mitral regurgitant orifice size is not static in disorders of the subvalve apparatus, but varies directly with left ventricular volume.[13,76,99] The importance of regurgitant orifice size is demonstrated through an adaptation of the Gorlin formula. Regurgitant flow across the mitral valve reflects the product of mitral regurgitant orifice size and the square root of the systolic pressure gradient across the valve (left ventricle to left atrium). Viewed in this context, one can appreciate the importance of even minor changes in orifice size relative to changes in the pressure gradient. Reduction of left ventricular volume will reduce regurgitant orifice size and the severity of mitral regurgitation. Experimental observations suggest that this mechanism is the predominant beneficial influence of nitroprusside in acute mitral regurgitation.[100] Hydralazine may also be given to reduce systemic vascular resistance and improve forward output.[31] Hydralazine, however, has insignificant effects on left ventricular volume and mitral regurgitant orifice size compared with nitroprusside and may result in unwanted positive chronotropic effects also. Further reduction in left ventricular outflow impedance can be obtained with IABP.[29] The augmentation of aortic diastolic pressure with balloon pumping may improve coronary blood flow and allow more aggressive use of vasodilators such as nitroprusside.

Further improvement in left ventricular function and forward output may be achieved by the addition of the inotropic agent, particularly dobutamine. By improving contractile function with subsequent reduction in left ventricular volume, mitral regurgitant orifice size and the severity of regurgitation decline. We use dobutamine instead of dopamine because of the alpha-adrenergic stimulating effect seen with dopamine, which has at least a theoretical disadvantage with respect to left ventricular outflow impedance. We do not use digoxin in the management of acute severe mitral regurgitation because of delayed onset, difficult titration, and relatively low magnitude of inotropic effect. Digoxin given by rapid intravenous infusion may increase systemic vascular resistance through direct arteriolar constriction and may exacerbate mitral regurgitation.[15] Furosemide or nitroglycerin may be useful in manipulating preload to meet the desired response.

Papillary muscle dysfunction that is transient or responds to medical therapy does not require immediate surgical intervention. Residual mitral regurgitation can be managed with an oral regimen of digitalis, diuretics, hydralazine, or other vasodilating agents as necessary. Surgery should be considered electively when symptoms of regurgitation are refractory to medical management. PMR requires early surgical intervention, the choice of procedure depending on the mechanism of mitral regurgitation and the experience of the surgeon. Most patients require mitral valve replacement, although repair may be adequate in some. Repair is accomplished through reattachment of the ruptured muscle head to the left ventricular wall or adjacent papillary muscle trunk with Teflon-reinforced mattress sutures. Surgical mortality in recent surgical series of PMR has been between 20 and 30 per cent.[33, 41, 55] Both surgical and long-term mortality are dependent on residual left ventricular function and are inversely related to preoperative ejection fraction.[41] Although concomitant coronary artery bypass grafting may not influence acute surgical mortality, improved long-term survival may accompany coronary revascularization.[55]

VENTRICULAR SEPTAL RUPTURE

Ventricular septal rupture (VSR) complicates 1 per cent or less of all myocardial infarctions and accounts for 2 to 5 per cent of all infarct deaths.[48, 89] Septal rupture usually occurs within four days of infarction and is marked by the development of a pansystolic murmur, hemodynamic deterioration, and signs of ventricular failure. VSR complicates inferior and anterior infarctions with similar frequency and often accompanies the first myocardial infarction in a patient without previous coronary symptoms.[73] Rupture most commonly involves the low muscular septum. The location of rupture correlates well with the location of infarct by ECG. The rupture may consist of multiple perforations in 40 per cent of cases.[38] As a group, patients with VSR have a paucity of septal collateral vessels, and between 30 and 40 per cent have single vessel disease.[43, 59, 71] Complete obstruction of the left anterior descending or right coronary artery is usually present. These arteries supply the anterior two thirds and posterior third of the septum, respectively. The clinical course, without surgical intervention, is usually progressive deterioration, with a mortality rate of 25 per cent in 24 hours and 65 per cent in two weeks following rupture.[1, 75]

The murmur of VSR is most frequently pansystolic, but may be descrescendo with late systolic termination, as closure of the defect accompanies contraction of the muscular septum. The murmur is best heard at the lower left sternal border and is accompanied by a palpable thrill in 50 per cent of cases.[71] Transmission of the murmur to the back between the spine and left scapula may occur.[4] When the magnitude of left-to-right shunt is large, a third heart sound, with or without accompanying mid-diastolic flow rumble, may be heard at the apex.

The differentiation between VSR and PMR by physical examination may be difficult. The location of the murmur and accompanying thrill, as discussed previously, may be helpful. Signs of right heart failure may overshadow those of left heart failure early in the course of VSR. These patients may have more marked elevation in jugular venous pressure and less pulmonary venous hypertension than patients with acute mitral regurgitation. Correspondingly, the chest radiograph shows pulmonary edema less frequently with VSR and may be read as normal in 25 per cent of cases.[71] Abnormalities of atrioventricular or intraventricular conduction may be present on the ECG in 40 per cent of patients with VSR.[42, 89]

The diagnosis of VSR can be rapidly and accurately established at the bedside following right heart catheterization with a balloon-

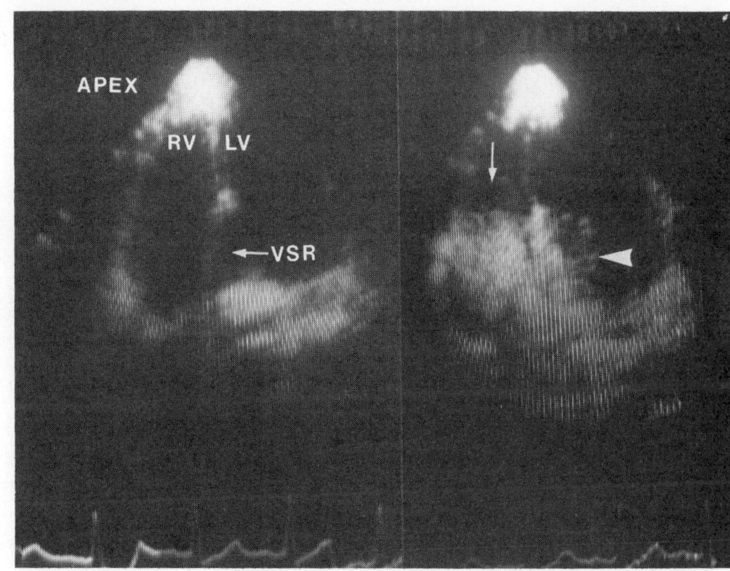

Figure 4–7. Two-dimensional echocardiogram. Apical four-chamber view with inferior angulation to demonstrate a defect in the posterobasal septum *(VSR)* in a patient with an acute inferior myocardial infarction. *Left,* prior to contrast material injection, VSR *(arrow)* is noted in the posterobasal septum. *Right,* contrast material, following intravenous injection, partially fills the right ventricle. A negative contrast effect is seen at the apex of the right ventricle *(small arrow).* Some contrast material crosses the VSR and enters the left ventricle *(arrowhead).* RV = right ventricle; LV = left ventricle.

tipped, flow-directed catheter. An increase in oxygen saturation of blood obtained from the right ventricle reflects a left-to-right shunt at this level. The intracardiac shunt also results in a recirculation peak on the thermodilution cardiac output curve. Occasionally, patients with severe acute mitral regurgitation, associated with marked left atrial hypertension and normal pulmonary vascular resistance, may have pulmonary venous to pulmonary arterial reflux of oxygenated blood, causing an oxygen saturation "step-up" in the distal pulmonary artery.[86] This may create confusion when oxygen saturations are obtained only from the right atrium and distal pulmonary artery, and may simulate intracardiac left-to-right shunt. This error can be eliminated by carefully obtaining samples from the right atrium, right ventricle, and proximal pulmonary artery with fluoroscopic or pressure waveform guidance. VSR, as noted previously, may result in an increased amplitude of the normal left atrial V wave. As discussed, this V wave can be distinguished from the regurgitant wave accompanying acute mitral insufficiency by its normal time of onset with respect to the QRS of a simultaneously recorded ECG.

The noninvasive diagnosis of VSR can be established in the coronary care unit with two-dimensional echocardiography.[21,57] Apical or subxiphoid four-chamber views, or occasionally the parasternal short-axis view, will usually demonstrate the defect. The ruptured septum often bulges paradoxically into the right ventricle during systole. Intravenous injection of saline contrast material may show the intraventricular communication by demonstrating a negative contrast effect in the right ventricle, or contrast material entering the left ventricle. These findings are illustrated in Figure 4–7. First-pass radionuclide angiography may be used to demonstrate, quantify, and help localize the left-to-right shunt of VSR.[36] Valuable information about global and segmental left ventricular function may also be obtained. Pulsed Doppler in conjunction with echocardiography offers an additional noninvasive bedside method of confirming the diagnosis of septal rupture.[83] A sample volume placed on the right side of the interventricular septum at the base is gradually directed down the septum toward the apex. Systolic turbulence is noted in the region of the VSR. Differentiation of VSR from acute mitral regurgitation is also possible with Doppler echocardiography.

Emergency medical therapy aimed at reduction of impedance to left ventricular outflow may be used to stabilize the patient with VSR for cardiac catheterization or surgery. It should be emphasized that such improvement is temporary and that deterioration, once begun, usually progresses relentlessly. Nitroprusside lowers systemic vascular resistance, reduces the severity of left-to-right shunt, and improves forward output. Further reduction in systemic resistance and shunt magnitude, with an improvement in cardiac output, can be achieved with IABP. The augmentation of diastolic blood pressure achieved with IABP may facilitate the use of vasodilator drugs. Dobutamine improves left ventricular performance without increasing systemic resistance, and is the inotropic agent of choice.

There is no unanimity of opinion regarding the role of preoperative cardiac catheterization once the diagnosis of VSR is established.[30, 32, 52] Catheterization can be used to localize the septal defect, identify an associated left ventricular aneurysm, and evaluate coronary anatomy for possible revascularization. As global and segmental left ventricular function and the location of the defect can be assessed rapidly by noninvasive techniques, we consider left ventriculography unnecessary for this purpose. If the patient is hemodynamically stable, we usually perform coronary angiography emergently to evaluate coronary anatomy. The patient with unstable hemodynamics is taken to surgery without coronary angiography. It must be noted that there are no available data proving the benefit of concomitant coronary revascularization on perioperative or long-term survival in patients with VSR.

Early reports of surgical repair in VSR showed surgical mortality to correlate inversely with time between rupture and surgery. Recommendations were made to delay surgery in the hope of lowering operative risk and allowing time for scarring and fortification of peri-infarct tissues.[17] It is now apparent that the improved survival in patients receiving late surgery for VSR reflected the greater severity of illness in those requiring early surgery and the interval attrition of patients with large defects and poor ventricular function. The single most important determinant of surgical risk is hemodynamic status. The presence of shock or multisystem failure is invariably associated with a high surgical mortality. Several series have noted a high surgical mortality in patients with diaphragmatic infarction complicated by posterior septal rupture.[32, 41, 63] This finding has been attributed to greater technical difficulty in repairing these defects and the not infrequent requirement for concomitant mitral valve replacement or replacement of the posterior left ventricular wall with a Dacron patch.

Over the past decade, great advances have been made in the surgical approach to VSR. The septum is approached through an incision made through the infarcted left ventricle. Concomitant infarctectomy or aneurysmectomy provides better septal exposure. The septal defect is closed with a Dacron or Teflon patch placed on the left ventricular side of the septum or on both sides as a "sandwich," and secured with Teflon felt-buttressed mattress sutures. In anteroapical ruptures, amputation of the cardiac apex with exclusion of the defect can be performed. Posterior ruptures are approached through the center of the infarct on the posterior surface of the heart. Posteromedial papillary muscle damage or posterior wall infarctectomy may necessitate mitral valve or posterior left ventricular wall replacement with prosthetic devices. Saphenous vein bypass of significantly stenosed coronary arteries should be performed. The overall mortality of patients operated on within four weeks of VSR approximates 40 per cent.[8, 87] Early repair can be achieved with a mortality of less than 25 per cent in patients who are hemodynamically stable.[52, 71, 87] We recommend immediate repair of VSR; postponing the operation begets hemodynamic instability and a higher surgical mortality. Most patients who survive the operation have NYHA class I or II functional capacity. Long-term prognosis is excellent and five-year survival exceeds 80 per cent.[32, 63]

CARDIAC RUPTURE

Cardiac rupture (CR) occurs in 3 per cent of patients with acute myocardial infarction and, after cardiogenic shock or arrhythmia, is the third most common cause of early death, accounting for 10 to 20 per cent of infarct-related deaths.[44, 72] CR is eight to ten times more common than rupture of a papillary muscle or the interventricular septum.[14] Over 90 per cent of ruptures involve the left ventricle and appear as a tear or hemorrhagic dissection at the lateral border of a transmural infarction.[3] This site represents the point of maximal shearing stress between normal and dysfunctional myocardium. One third of ruptures occur during the initial 24 hours of infarction, and 85 per cent within the first week.[6, 46, 72] CR is more common in older patients, women, patients with hypertension that precedes or persists after infarction, and patients without a previous history of coronary heart disease who experience their first transmural myocardial infarction.[6, 28, 46, 62, 72, 80] CR may occur in temporal relationship to a specific physical stress such as coughing or straining at stool.

The clinical diagnosis of CR frequently is not made antemortem because of the rapidity with which hemopericardium, tamponade, and death may occur. Signs and symptoms are determined by the rate and volume of hemorrhage into the pericardial space. The normal pericardium is relatively inelastic, and the rapid introduction of as little as 150 ml of blood may cause fatal tamponade. Chest pain, persisting or recurring after infarctions, and the acute onset of dyspnea may herald CR. Jugular venous pressure elevation, pulsus paradoxus, muffled heart sounds, and a pericardial friction rub may be found. New systolic, diastolic, or to-and-fro murmurs may accompany subacute rupture and the formation of false aneurysm.[25, 46] The ECG usually demonstrates a Q-wave infarction pattern, but may show only ST-segment and T-wave abnormalities in less than 10 per cent of cases. Sudden slowing of the sinus rate followed by a junctional or idioventricular rhythm with diminution in QRS amplitude is characteristic.[56, 58] Tall peaking of precordial T-waves, despite previous T-wave inversion or ST-segment depression, may suggest hemopericardium.[47]

Survival hinges on rapid diagnosis and surgical repair. With the acute onset of electromechanical dissociation, cardiopulmonary resuscitation and immediate pericardiocentesis should be attempted. Emergency sternotomy and the institution of cardiopulmonary bypass may be lifesaving in this situation.[44] With less precipitous deterioration, bedside hemodynamic monitoring may demonstrate equilization of right and left heart diastolic pressures consistent with tamponade. Two-dimensional echocardiography will show a pericardial effusion and may demonstrate septal paradoxical motion, expiratory right ventricular compression, or posterior movement of the anterior right ventricular wall in diastole.[94] The major differential diagnostic point in CR, right ventricular infarction, has no pericardial fluid and a dilated, hypocontractile right ventricle on two-dimensional echocardiography.[79] Pericardiocentesis or the insertion of an intra-aortic balloon pump may provide temporary hemodynamic improvement.[39] If pericardiocentesis is performed, a catheter draining the pericardial space should be left in place. The use of these techniques, however, must not delay emergent surgery as this represents the patient's best chance for survival. We do not recommend formal cardiac catheterization in this situation because of the risk and delay entailed.

Cardiac rupture, not causing tamponade, may result in the formation of a false aneurysm. The outer walls of these aneurysms, unlike true aneurysms, are devoid of muscular elements and are composed of pericardium and mural thrombus.[88] False aneurysms are not contained within the perimeter of the left ventricular cavity, but instead are discrete paraventricular chambers connected by a narrow orifice to the left ventricular cavity.[84] The diameter of the orifice or mouth of a false aneurysm is usually less than 40 per cent of the maximal diameter of the aneurysm. This differs from a true aneurysm, in which the orifice usually represents the point of largest diameter.[93] Cardiac catheterization may demonstrate the narrow mouth and avascular wall of a false aneurysm. Radionuclide gated blood pool imaging may also aid in differentiating false from true aneurysms.[97] Spontaneous rupture may occur unpredictably in one third of patients with false aneurysms, and prophylactic resection is advised.[18]

The authors appreciate the secretarial assistance of Pamela D. Kimball.

References

1. Barnard, P. M., and Kennedy, J. H.: Postinfarction ventricular septal defect. Circulation 32:76, 1965.
2. Baron, D. W., and O'Rourke, M. F.: Long-term results of arterial counterpulsation in acute severe cardiac failure complicating myocardial infarction. Br. Heart J. 38:285, 1976.
3. Bates, R. J., Beutler, S., Resnekov, L., and Anagnostopoulos, C. E.: Cardiac rupture—challenge in diagnosis and management. Am. J. Cardiol. 40:429, 1977.
4. Benson, R.: Paravertebral systolic murmur with septal rupture. N. Engl. J. Med. 307:1086, 1982.
5. Bethea, C. F., Peter, R. H., Behar, V. S., et al.: The hemodynamic simulation of mitral regurgitation in ventricular septal defect after myocardial infarction. Cathet. Cardiovasc. Diagn. 2:97, 1976.
6. Biorck, G., Mogensen, P. L., Nyquist, O., et al.: Studies of myocardial rupture with tamponade in acute myocardial infarction. I. Clinical features. Chest 61:4, 1972.

7. Bolooki, H.: The effects of counterpulsation with an intra-aortic balloon on cardiovascular dynamics and metabolism. *In* Bolooki, H. (ed.): Clinical Application of Intra-Aortic Balloon Pump. Mount Kisco, New York, Futura Publishing Co., 1977, p. 15.
8. Brandt, B., Wright, C. B., and Ehrenhaft, J. L.: Ventricular septal defect following myocardial infarction. Ann. Thorac. Surg. 27:580, 1978.
9. Bregman, D., Parodi, E. N., Edie, R. N., et al.: Intraoperative unidirectional intra-aortic balloon pumping in the management of left ventricular power failure. J. Thorac. Cardiovasc. Surg. 70:1010, 1975.
10. Buckley, M. J., Leinbach, R. C., Kastor, J. A., et al.: Hemodynamic evaluation of intra-aortic balloon pumping in man. Circulation 41(Suppl. 2):130, 1970.
11. Burch, G. E., DePasquale, N. P., and Phillips, J. N.: Clinical manifestations of papillary muscle dysfunction. Arch. Intern. Med. 112:112, 1963.
12. Carley, J. E., Wong, B. Y. S., Pugh, D. M., and Dunn, M.: Clinical significance of the V-wave in the main pulmonary artery. Am. J. Cardiol. 39:982, 1977.
13. Chatterjee, K., Parmley, W. W., Swan, H. J. C., et al.: Beneficial effects of vasodilator agents in severe mitral regurgitation due to dysfunction of the subvalvular apparatus. Circulation 48:684, 1973.
14. Chizner, M. A.: Bedside diagnosis of the acute myocardial infarction and its complications. Curr. Probl. Cardiol. 7:64, 1982.
15. Cohn, J. N., Tristani, F. E., and Khatri, I. M.: Cardiac and peripheral vascular effects of digitalis in clinical cardiogenic shock. Am. Heart J. 78:318, 1969.
16. Cohn, P. F.: Problems in diagnosing acute mitral regurgitation due to coronary artery disease. Chest 78:416, 1980.
17. Daggett, W. M., Guyton, R. A., Mundth, E. D., et al.: Surgery for post–myocardial infarct ventricular septal defect. Ann. Surg. 186:260, 1977.
18. Davidson, K. H., Parisi, A. F., Harrington, J. J., et al.: Pseudoaneurysm of the left ventricle: an unusual echocardiographic presentation. Review of the literature. Ann. Intern. Med. 86:430, 1978.
19. DeBusk, R. F., and Harrison, D. C.: The clinical spectrum of papillary muscle disease. N. Engl. J. Med. 281:1458, 1969.
20. DeWood, M. A., Notshe, R. N., Hensley, G. R., et al.: Intraaortic balloon counterpulsation with and without reperfusion for myocardial infarction shock. Circulation 61:1105, 1980.
21. Drobac, M., Gilbert, B., Howard, R., et al.: Ventricular septal defect after myocardial infarction: diagnosis by two-dimensional contrast echocardiography. Circulation 67:335, 1983.
22. Estes, E. H., Dalton, F. M., Entman, M. L., et al.: The anatomy and blood supply of the papillary muscles of the left ventricle. Am. Heart J. 71:356, 1966.
23. Feigenbaum, H.: Echocardiography. 3rd ed. Philadelphia, Lea & Febiger, 1981, p. 265–267.
24. Friedman, A. W., and Stein, L.: Pitfalls in the bedside diagnosis of severe acute mitral regurgitation. Chest 78:436, 1980.
25. Friedman, H. S., Kuhn, L. A., and Katz, A. M.: Clinical and electrocardiographic features of cardiac rupture following acute myocardial infarction. Am. J. Med. 50:709, 1971.
26. Fuchs, R. M., Heuser, R. R., Yin, F. C. P., and Brinker, J. A.: Limitations of pulmonary wedge V-waves in diagnosing mitral regurgitation. Am. J. Cardiol. 49:849, 1982.
27. Gahl, K., Sutton, R., Pearson, M., et al.: Mitral regurgitation in coronary heart disease. Br. Heart J. 39:13, 1977.
28. Gjol, N.: Cardiac rupture and acute myocardial infarction. Geriatrics 27:126, 1972.
29. Gold, H. K., Leinbach, R. C., Sanders, C. A., et al.: Intra-aortic balloon pumping for ventricular septal defect or mitral regurgitation complicating acute myocardial infarction. Circulation 47:1191, 1973.
30. Graham, A. F., Stinson, E. B., Daily, P. O., and Harrison, D. C.: Ventricular septal defects after myocardial infarction. Early operative treatment. J.A.M.A. 226:708, 1973.
31. Greenberg, B. H., Massie, B. M., Brundage, B. H., et al.: Beneficial effects of hydralazine in severe mitral regurgitation. Circulation 58:273, 1978.
32. Guadiani, V. A., Miller, D. C., Stinson, E. B., et al.: Postinfarction ventricular septal defect: an argument for early operation. Surgery 89:48, 1981.
33. Gula, G., and Yacouv, M. H.: Surgical correction of complete rupture of the anterior papillary muscle. Ann. Thorac. Surg. 32:88, 1981.
34. Hagemeijer, F., Laird, J. D., Hallebos, M. M. P., et al.: Effectiveness of intra-aortic balloon pumping without cardiac surgery for patients with severe heart failure secondary to a recent myocardial infarction. Am. J. Cardiol. 40:951, 1977.
35. Hauser, A. M., Gordon, S., Gangadmar, V., et al.: Percutaneous intraaortic balloon counterpulsation: clinical effectiveness and hazards. Chest 82:422, 1982.
36. Hecht, H. S., and Zibelli, L. R.: First-pass radionuclide angiography in visualization of acute myocardial infarction ventricular septal defect and assessment of ventricular function. Am. Heart J. 103:436, 1982.
37. Heikkil, A.: Mitral incompetence complicating acute myocardial infarction. Br. Heart J. 29:162, 1967.
38. Hill, J. D., Lary, D., Kerth, W. J., and Gerbode, F.: Acquired ventricular septal defects: evolution of an operation, surgical technique and results. J. Thorac. Cardiovasc. Surg. 70:440, 1975.
39. Hochreiter, C., Goldstein, J., Borer, J. S., et al.: Myocardial free wall rupture after acute infarction: survival aided by percutaneous intraaortic balloon counterpulsation. Circulation 65:1279, 1982.
40. Jacobey, J. A., Taylor, W. J., Smith, G. T., et al.: A new therapeutic approach to acute coronary occlusion: II. Opening dormant coronary collateral channels by counterpulsation. Am. J. Cardiol. 11:218, 1963.
41. Kay, J. H., Zubiate, P., Mendez, M. A., et al.: Surgical treatment of mitral insufficiency secondary to coronary artery disease. J. Thorac. Cardiovasc. Surg. 79:12, 1980.
42. Khan, M. M., Patterson, G. C., Oikane, H. O., and Adgey, A. A.: Management of ventricular septal rupture in acute myocardial infarction. Br. Heart J. 44:570, 1980.
43. Kitamura, S., Mendez, A., and Kay, J. H.: Ventric-

ular septal defect following myocardial infarction: experience with surgical repair through a left ventriculotomy and a review of the literature. J. Thorac. Cardiovasc. Surg. 61:186, 1971.
44. Kouchoukos, N. T.: Surgical treatment of acute complications of myocardial infarction. Cardiovasc. Clin. 11:141, 1981.
45. Leinbach, R. C., Gold, H. K., Dinsmore, R. E., et al.: The role of angiography in cardiogenic shock. Circulation 48 (Suppl. III):95, 1973.
46. Lewis, A. J., Burchell, H. B., and Titus, J. L.: Clinical and pathologic features of postinfarction cardiac rupture. Am. J. Cardiol. 23:43, 1969.
47. London, R. E., and London, S. B.: The electrocardiographic sign of acute hemopericardium. Circulation 25:780, 1962.
48. Longo, L. A., and Cohen, L. S.: Rupture of interventricular septum in acute myocardial infarction. Am. Heart J. 92:81, 1976.
49. Lorente, P., Gourgon, R., Beaufils, P., et al.: Multivariate statistical evaluation of intraaortic counterpulsation in pump failure complicating acute myocardial infarction. Am. J. Cardiol. 46:124, 1980.
50. Maddoux, G., Pappas, G., Henkins, M., et al.: Effect of pulsatile and nonpulsatile flow during cardiopulmonary bypass on left ventricular ejection fraction early after aortocoronary bypass surgery. Am. J. Cardiol. 37:1000, 1976.
51. Maroko, P. R., Bernstein, E. F., Libby, P., et al.: Effects of intraaortic balloon counterpulsation on the severity of myocardial ischemic injury following acute coronary occlusion. Circulation 45:1150, 1972.
52. Matsui, K., Kay, J. H., Mendez, M., et al.: Ventricular septal rupture secondary to myocardial infarction. J.A.M.A. 245:1537, 1981.
53. MeEnany, M. T., Kay, H. R., Buckley, M. J., et al.: Clinical experience with intra-aortic balloon pump support in 728 patients. Circulation 58(Suppl. 1):1, 1978.
54. Meister, S. G., and Helfant, R. H.: Rapid bedside differentiation of ruptured interventricular septum from acute mitral insufficiency. N. Engl. J. Med. 287:1024, 1972.
55. Merin, G., Giuliani, E., Pluth, J., et al.: Surgery for mitral valve incompetence after myocardial infarction. Am. J. Cardiol. 32:322, 1973.
56. Meurs, A. A. H., Vos, A. C., Verhey, J. B., and Gerbrandy, J.: Electrocardiogram during cardiac rupture by myocardial infarction. Br. Heart J. 32:232, 1970.
57. Mintz, G. S., Victor, M. F., Kotler, M. N., et al.: Two-dimensional echocardiographic identification of surgically correctable complications of acute myocardial infarction. Circulation 64:91, 1981.
58. Mogensen, L., Nyquist, O., Orinius, E., and Sjogren, A.: Studies of myocardial rupture with cardiac tamponade in acute myocardial infarction. II. Electrocardiographic changes. Chest 61:6, 1972.
59. Montoya, A., McKeever, L., Scanlon, P., et al.: Early repair of ventricular septal rupture after infarction. Am. J. Cardiol. 45:345, 1980.
60. Mueller, H., Ayres, S. M., Conklin, E. F., et al.: The effects of intraaortic counterpulsation on cardiac performance and metabolism in shock associated with acute myocardial infarction. J. Clin. Invest. 50:1885, 1971.
61. Mueller, H., Ayres, S. M., Gianelli, S., Jr., et al.: Effect of isoproterenol, l-normepinephrine and intraaortic counterpulsation on hemodynamics and myocardial metabolism in shock following acute myocardial infarction. Circulation 45:335, 1972.
62. Mundth, E.: Rupture of the heart complicating myocardial infarction. Circulation 46:427, 1972.
63. Naifeh, J., Grehl, T. M., and Hurley, E. J.: Surgical treatment of post-myocardial infarction ventricular septal defects. J. Thorac. Cardiovasc. Surg. 79:483, 1980.
64. Nichol, P. M., Boughner, D. R., and Persaud, J. A.: Noninvasive assessment of mitral insufficiency by transcutaneous Doppler ultrasound. Circulation 54:656, 1976.
65. Nishimura, R. A., Schaff, H. V., Shub, C., et al.: Papillary muscle rupture complicating acute myocardial infarction: analysis of 17 patients. Am. J. Cardiol. 51:373, 1983.
66. Nishimura, R. A., Shub, C., and Tajik, A.: Two-dimensional echocardiographic diagnosis of partial papillary muscle rupture. Br. Heart J. 47:598, 1982.
67. Phillips, J. H., Burch, G. E., and DePasquale, N. P.: The syndrome of papillary muscle dysfunction. Ann. Intern. Med. 59:508, 1963.
68. Pichard, A. D., Kay, R., Smith, H., et al.: Large V-waves in the pulmonary wedge pressure tracing in the absence of mitral regurgitation. Am. J. Cardiol. 50:1044, 1982.
69. Pierri, M. K., Zema, M., Kligfield, P., et al.: Exercise tolerance in late survivors of balloon pumping and surgery for cardiogenic shock. Circulation 62(Suppl. I):138, 1980.
70. Powell, W. J., Daggett, W. M., Magro, A. R., et al.: Effects of intra-aortic balloon counterpulsation on cardiac performance, oxygen consumption and coronary blood flow in dogs. Circ. Res. 26:753, 1970.
71. Radford, M. J., Johnson, R. A., Daggett, W. M., et al.: Ventricular septal rupture: a review of clinical and physiologic features and an analysis of survival. Circulation 64:545, 1981.
72. Rasmussen, S., Leth, A., Kjoller, E., and Pedersen, A.: Cardiac rupture in acute myocardial infarction. Acta Med. Scand. 205:11, 1979.
73. Roberts, W. C., Rowan, J. A., and Harvey, W. P.: Rupture of the left ventricular free wall or ventricular septum secondary to acute myocardial infarction: an occurrence virtually limited to the first transmural myocardial infarction in a hypertensive individual. Am. J. Cardiol. 35:166, 1975.
74. Sanders, R. F., Neuberger, K. T., and Ravin, A.: Rupture of posterior papillary muscles: occurrence of rupture of posterior muscle on posterior myocardial infarction. Dis. Chest 31:316, 1957.
75. Sanders, R. J., Kern, W. H., and Blount, S. G.: Perforation of the interventricular septum complicating myocardial infarction. Am. Heart J. 51:736, 1956.
76. Sasayama, S., Takahashi, M., Osakada, G., et al.: Dynamic geometry of the left atrium and left ventricle in acute mitral regurgitation. Circulation 60:117, 1979.
77. Scheidt, S., Collins, M., Goldstein, J., and Fisher, J.: Mechanical circulatory assistance with the intraaortic balloon pump and other counterpulsation devices. Prog. Cardiovasc. Dis. 25:55, 1982.

78. Scheidt, S., Wilner, G., Rubenfire, M., et al.: Intraaortic balloon counterpulsation in cardiogenic shock. Report of a cooperative clinical trial. N. Engl. J. Med. 288:979, 1973.
79. Sharpe, D. N., Botvinick, E. H., Shames, D. M., et al.: The noninvasive diagnosis of right ventricular infarction. Circulation 57:483, 1978.
80. Sievers, J., Blomqvist, G., and Biorck, G.: Studies on myocardial infarction in Malmö 1935–1954. VI. Some clinical data with particular reference to diabetes, menopause and heart rupture. Acta Med. Scand. 169:95, 1961.
81. Sorensen, S. G., O'Rourke, R. A., and Chadhuri, T. K.: Noninvasive quantitation of valvular regurgitation by gated equilibrium radionuclide angiography. Circulation 62:1089, 1980.
82. Steelman, R. B., White, R. S., Hill, J. C., et al.: Midsystolic clicks in arteriosclerotic heart disease: a new facet in the clinical syndrome of papillary muscle dysfunction. Circulation 44:503, 1971.
83. Stevenson, J. G., Kawabori, I., Dooley, T. K., and Guntheroth, W. G.: Diagnosis of ventricular septal defect of pulsed Doppler echocardiography—sensitivity, specificity, limitations. Circulation 58:322, 1978.
84. Stewart, S., Huddle, R., Stuard, I., et al.: False aneurysm of the left ventricle: etiology, pathology, diagnosis and operative management. Ann. Thorac. Surg. 31:259, 1981.
85. Subramanian, V., Goldstein, J., Sos, T., et al.: Preliminary clinical experience with percutaneous intraaortic balloon pumping. Circulation 62 (Suppl. 1):123, 1980.
86. Tatooles, C. J., Gault, J. H., Mason, D. T., and Ross, J., Jr.: Reflux of oxygenated blood into the pulmonary artery in severe mitral regurgitation. Am. Heart J. 75:102, 1968.
87. Thomas, C. S., Alford, W. C., Burrus, G. R., et al.: Urgent operation for acquired ventricular septal defect. Ann. Surg. 195:706, 1982.
88. Vlodaver, Z., Coe, J. I., and Edwards, J. E.: True and false left ventricular aneurysms. Circulation 51:567, 1975.
89. Vlodaver, Z., and Edwards, J. E.: Rupture of ventricular septum or papillary muscle complicating myocardial infarction. Circulation 55:815, 1977.
90. Wajszczuk, W. J., Krakauer, J., Rubenfire, M., et al.: Current indications for mechanical circulatory assistance on the basis of experience with 104 patients. Am. J. Cardiol. 33:176, 1974 (abstr.).
91. Wei, J. Y., Hutchins, G. M., and Buckley, B. H.: Papillary muscle rupture in fatal acute myocardial infarction. Ann. Intern. Med. 90:149, 1979.
92. Weyman, A. Cross-Sectional Echocardiography. Philadelphia, Lea & Febiger, 1982, pp. 176–179.
93. Weyman, A.: Cross-Sectional Echocardiography. Philadelphia, Lea & Febiger, 1982, pp. 320–322.
94. Weyman, A.: Cross-Sectional Echocardiography. Philadelphia, Lea & Febiger, 1982, pp. 484–485.
95. Willerson, J. T., Curry, G. C., Watson, J. T., et al.: Intraaortic balloon counterpulsation in patients in cardiogenic shock, medically refractory left ventricular and/or recurrent ventricular tachycardia. Am. J. Med. 58:183, 1975.
96. Williams, D., Korr, K., Gewirtz, H., and Most, A.: The effect of intraaortic balloon counterpulsation on regional blood flow and oxygen consumption in the presence of coronary artery stenosis in patients with unstable angina. Circulation 66:593, 1982.
97. Winzelberg, G. G., Miller, S. W., Okada, R. D., et al.: Scintigraphic assessment of false left ventricular aneurysms. A. J. R. 135:569, 1980.
98. Yahr, W. Z., Butner, A. N. ,Krakauer, J. S., et al.: Cardiogenic shock: dynamics of coronary blood flow with intraaortic phase shift balloon pumping. Surg. Forum 19:142, 1968.
99. Yoran, C., Yellin, E. L., Becker, R. M., et al.: Dynamic aspects of acute mitral regurgitation: effects of ventricular volume, pressure and contractility on the effective regurgitant orifice area. Circulation 60:170, 1979.
100. Yoran, C., Yellin, E. L., Becker, R. M., et al.: Mechanisms of reduction of mitral regurgitation with vasodilator therapy. Am. J. Cardiol. 43:773, 1979.

5

Emergency Treatment of Ventricular Tachycardia

CHARLES D. SWERDLOW
and JAY W. MASON

Ventricular tachycardia requires urgent evaluation and treatment because of the hemodynamic compromise and myocardial ischemia it may precipitate, the risk of degeneration to ventricular fibrillation, and the nature of the clinical events that may cause it. The therapeutic approach to a patient with ventricular tachycardia is based on correct identification of the arrhythmia and appropriate assessment of the clinical and electrophysiologic milieu in which it occurs.

CLINICAL SETTING

Ventricular tachycardia usually occurs in patients with significant, structural heart disease. In those with coronary artery disease, ventricular tachycardia commonly arises during the acute phase of myocardial infarction or weeks to years following infarction, but it may occur without antecedent infarction. Patients with previous myocardial infarction represent 60 to 75 per cent of cases in most series of those with recurrent ventricular tachycardia.[3, 44, 47, 79] Patients with cardiomyopathies and valvular heart disease account for 10 to 25 per cent of such cases.[3, 7, 44, 47, 79] Hypertrophic cardiomyopathy,[7] right ventricular dysplasia,[16, 71] idiopathic dilated cardiomyopathy,[63, 109] mitral valve prolapse,[50] acute myocarditis, sarcoidosis, and virtually any other form of structural heart disease can be associated with ventricular tachycardia. Ten to 15 per cent of patients with recurrent ventricular tachycardia have no apparent structural heart disease.[3, 44, 47, 79] Patients with idiopathic, hereditary, or drug-induced prolonged QT syndromes are included in this group.

Specific precipitating events can be identified in some patients with ventricular tachycardia. Myocardial ischemia may be the provoking factor in the setting of acute myocardial infarction, coronary artery spasm,[58] or unstable angina due to atherosclerotic coronary artery disease.[58, 92] Exercise-induced ventricular tachycardia may be due to ischemia in some patients with atherosclerotic coronary artery disease,[5, 10, 51, 143] but it also may occur in those with normal coronary arteries.[51, 90] Metabolic factors include hypoxemia, acidosis, hypokalemia, and hypomagnesemia.[64] Intracardiac catheters—including temporary or permanent transvenous pacemaker leads, central venous catheters, and pulmonary artery catheters—are the most common mechanical causes of ventricular tachycardia. Many drugs may initiate or exacerbate the condition;[4, 26, 60, 62, 64, 106, 107, 112, 120, 124, 142] the most common offenders are listed in Table 5–1.

DIAGNOSIS

The distinction between ventricular tachycardia and supraventricular tachycardia with

Table 5–1. DRUGS THAT MAY CAUSE VENTRICULAR TACHYCARDIA

Drug Class	Examples	Specific Therapy
Membrane-active antiarrhythmics	Quinidine Procainamide Disopyramide	Isoproterenol, overdrive pacing; alkali therapy for quinidine
Digitalis glycosides	Digoxin, digitoxin	Correct hypokalemia and hypomagnesemia; phenytoin, lidocaine; antidigoxin Fab antibody for digoxin
Vasoactive amines	Isoproterenol Epinephrine Dopamine	Discontinue drug; consider beta-blocking agent
Bronchodilators	Aminophylline Isoproterenol	Discontinue drug; consider beta-blocking agent
Tricyclic antidepressants	Amitryptyline Desipramine Imipramine	Hyperventilation; systemic alkalinization
Phenothiazines	Thioridazine Chlorpromazine	Isoproterenol, overdrive pacing

aberration is critical to the selection of appropriate therapy for the patient who presents with a wide-complex tachycardia. Intracardiac recording techniques have clarified the diagnostic capabilities and limitations of the surface electrocardiogram.

Using electrograms recorded from intracardiac electrode catheters, the diagnosis of a wide-complex tachycardia can be established by analyzing the temporal relationship of the His bundle electrogram to atrial and ventricular depolarization during both the arrhythmia and the patient's normal rhythm. The H-V interval, representing His-Purkinje conduction time, is measured from onset of the His bundle electrogram to the earliest onset of ventricular activation in any lead. When the His bundle is activated by antegrade impulses conducted through the atrioventricular (AV) junction, the normal H-V interval is 35 to 55 msec. In the absence of ventricular pre-excitation, the H-V interval during supraventricular tachyarrhythmias is always greater than or equal to the H-V interval recorded during sinus rhythm. During ventricular tachycardia, the His bundle usually is activated retrogradely from the ventricles. Its electrogram may be concealed in the ventricular depolarization, may precede the onset of ventricular activity with an H-V interval shorter than that measured during sinus rhythm, or may appear at random during the recording.[55] In the absence of pre-excitation, a tachyarrhythmia can be tentatively identified as ventricular tachycardia if a His bundle electrogram is no longer recorded from a catheter position in which it was recorded during sinus rhythm or atrial pacing. Only in the unusual instance of bundle branch reentry tachycardia will the H-V interval recorded during ventricular tachycardia equal or exceed the H-V interval in sinus rhythm. In such cases, ventricular tachycardia must be diagnosed by other means, such as by normalization of the QRS complex during atrial pacing rates exceeding that of the tachycardia.

His bundle electrocardiography frequently is impractical in an emergency situation. Although no surface ECG finding is pathognomonic of ventricular tachycardia, the correct diagnosis usually can be made by careful analysis of available data. The presence of AV dissociation, or varying degrees of ventriculoatrial block, allows the diagnosis of ventricular tachycardia to be made with a high degree of certainty. These findings occur in approximately two thirds of cases of ventricular tachycardia, but rarely in supraventricular tachycardia.[131, 133, 134] One-to-one AV association is uncommon in ventricular tachycardia with left bundle branch block morphology or with rates greater than 200 beats per minute (see Table 5–2). Thus, a tachycardia with left bundle branch block morphology or a rate greater than 200 beats per minute and a one-to-one AV relationship is more likely to be supraventricular in origin.[133, 134]

In the emergency situation, accurate identification of atrial electrical activity is frequently difficult. If the patient's hemodynamic status does not require immediate termination of the arrhythmia, a few minutes'

Table 5–2. CHARACTERISTICS DISTINGUISHING VENTRICULAR TACHYCARDIA FROM SUPRAVENTRICULAR TACHYCARDIA WITH ABERRANCY*

	N	VT	SVT
One to one VA conduction absent	72	72(100)	0
One to one VA conduction present	128	28(22)	100(78)
LBBB	35	4(11)	31(89)
RBBB	93	24(26)	69(74)
Rate >200/min	28	2(7)	26(93)
QRS duration > 0.14 sec	57	57(100)	0(0)
QRS axis < −30°			
LBBB	24	20(83)	4(17)
RBBB	51	48(94)	3(6)
RBBB			
Lead V_1: rsR′	53	6(11)	47(89)
R, Rs, qR, Rr′	43	42(98)	1(2)
Lead V_6: qRs	47	3(6)	44(94)
rS, QS, QR	50	46(92)	4(8)
LBBB			
Lead V_6: QR	5	5(100)	0(0)
Concordant precordial pattern	3	3(100)	0(0)

*Numbers in parentheses are percentages.
Data adapted from Wellens et. al.[31,32]

effort usually is rewarded. The presence of cannon "a" waves in the jugular venous pulse and variable intensity of the first heart sound in a patient with a regular tachycardia suggests AV dissociation. A three-channel ECG machine will facilitate identification of the regular deformations of the T wave that represent atrial activity. Vagal maneuvers may enhance diagnostic certainty by altering the rate of dissociated P waves or by inducing varying degrees of ventriculoatrial block in ventricular tachycardia with one-to-one ventriculoatrial condition.

If it is not visible on the surface ECG, atrial activity may be identified accurately using bipolar chest leads, esophageal leads, or intra-atrial leads. A recently developed bipolar esophageal "pill" electrode is easily swallowed and produces high-quality recordings.[34] Explanted permanent pacemaker leads may be passed easily into the esophagus by the nasal route. Alternatively, an adequate esophageal electrode may be created by filling a standard nasogastric tube with electrode gel, cutting off the tip, plugging the distal end with a saline-soaked cotton swab, and inserting a standard V-lead electrode into the proximal end. In patients with central venous or pulmonary arterial catheters, a unipolar atrial electrogram may be recorded from an alligator clip attached to a metal stopcock after the catheter lumen has been filled with normal or hypertonic saline.

Capture or fusion beats during tachycardia provide indirect evidence of AV dissociation. "Fusion beats" occur when the ventricle is partially activated by the ventricular impulse and partially by a premature supraventricular impulse passing through the normal conduction system. They are identified by their slight prematurity, short H-V intervals, and morphologic features intermediate between supraventricular and ventricular beats. If ventricular tachycardia is slow, supraventricular captures may produce complexes morphologically identical to sinus beats with normal H-V intervals (see Figure 5–1). Capture or fusion beats occur during approximately 10 per cent of episodes of sustained ventricular tachycardia.[131, 133, 134]

Ancillary evidence indicating the site of origin of a wide-complex tachycardia may be obtained by measurement of the QRS width and axis and assessment of the rhythm's regularity.[131, 133, 134] In patients with normal QRS duration and axis during sinus rhythm, a QRS duration greater than 0.14 seconds or left axis deviation more negative than −30° favors ventricular tachycardia (see Table 5–2). The presence of a rightward, superior axis during tachycardia (axis 180°–270°) also suggests ventricular tachycardia.[33, 133] Variations in cycle length of up to 20 msec. have been reported in 6 per cent of cases of aberrantly conducted supraventricular tachycardia and 21 per cent of cases of ventricular tachycardia.[133] When atrial fibrillation occurs in patients with Wolff-Parkinson-White syn-

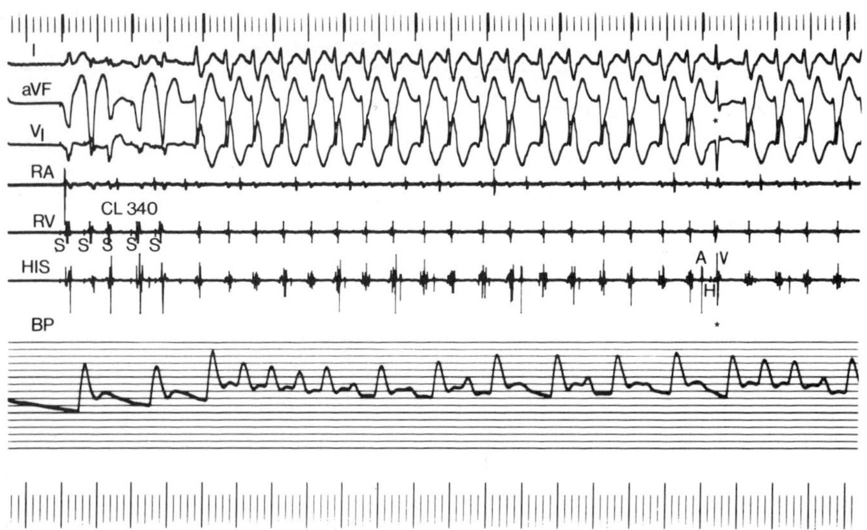

Figure 5–1. Ventricular tachycardia induced by a burst of rapid ventricular pacing at cycle length *(CL)* 340 ms. Surface leads I, aVF, and V_1 are shown together with intracardiac electrograms recorded from the right atrium *(RA)*, right ventricular apex *(RV)*, and His bundle recording position *(His)*. Blood pressure is also displayed *(BP)*. Pacing stimulus artifacts are designated by the letter *S*. During ventricular tachycardia the surface ECG shows right bundle branch block morphology with left axis deviation. A monophasic R wave is present in lead V_1. The right atrial electrogram is intermittently dissociated from the ventricular electrogram. The asterisk indicates a sinus capture beat.

drome, the irregularity of the rhythm may be difficult to identify because of extremely rapid ventricular rates. In this arrhythmia, beats with the morphologic characteristics of fusion beats end long cycles, in contrast to the slight prematurity of fusion beats during ventricular tachycardia, and considerable variation of QRS morphology usually is seen (see Figure 5–2).

The QRS morphology during tachycardia is useful in differentiating aberrant conduction from ventricular tachycardia in patients with normal resting ECGs. In patients with a right bundle branch block pattern during tachycardia, analysis of leads V_1 and V_6 is particularly helpful. A typical right bundle branch block morphology in lead V_1 (rsR′) is highly correlated with aberration, and an

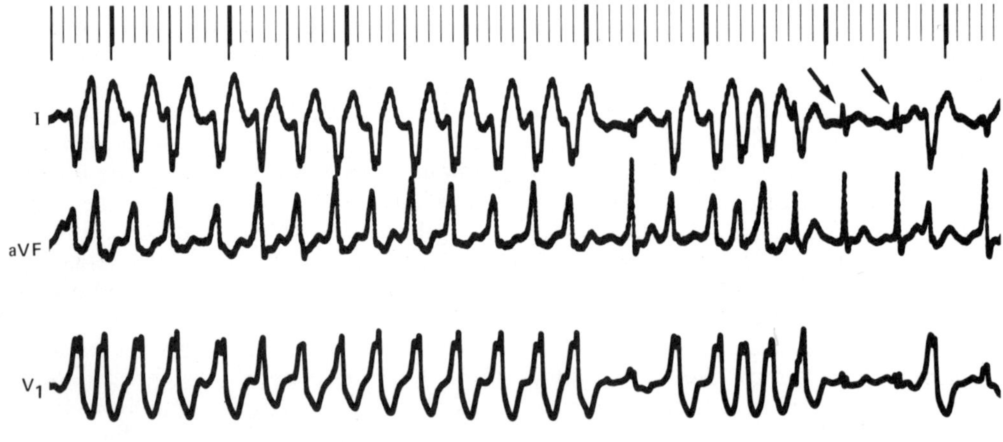

Figure 5–2. Atrial fibrillation in a patient with Wolff-Parkinson-White syndrome. Surface leads I, aVF, and V_1 are shown. In this patient, pre-excitation during sinus rhythm was intermittent. The tachycardia is irregularly irregular. There is marked beat-to-beat variation of the QRS complexes. The beats designated by the arrow are morphologically identical to normally conducted sinus beats. Note that these normally conducted beats end long RR intervals, in contrast to the capture beats seen in Figure 5–1, which end short RR intervals.

atypical pattern (R, qR, Rs, or Rr′) is highly correlated with ventricular tachycardia. A qRs configuration in lead V_6 is highly suggestive of aberration, whereas rS, QS, or QR patterns suggest a ventricular origin. The configuration of QRS complexes is less helpful in tachycardias with left bundle branch block configuration, although the uncommon finding of a QR pattern in lead V_6 suggests a ventricular origin.[131, 133, 134] Similarly, the infrequent finding of a concordant precordial QRS pattern during tachycardia is highly specific for ventricular tachycardia[105, 131] (see Table 5–2).

If inspection of the ECG does not allow definitive diagnosis of a wide-complex tachycardia, diagnostic-therapeutic interventions with rapid-acting drugs may be employed. Vagal maneuvers or edrophonium administration may produce AV block in patients with one-to-one conduction of atrial flutter or atrial tachycardia. Tachycardia termination after cholinergic intervention[128, 129] or administration of verapamil[110, 132] is more common with supraventricular arrhythmias, but can occur with ventricular tachycardia.[72, 128] Termination after lidocaine administration suggests a ventricular origin, but may occur in circus movement tachycardia utilizing an accessory AV pathway.

DRUGS

Antiarrhythmic drugs are the first line of therapy for patients with ventricular tachycardia. Although many drugs with potent electrophysiologic effects are available, the therapeutic effects required may vary from patient to patient and no single agent is uniformly safe and effective. The clinical pharmacology of antiarrhythmic drugs has been reviewed in recent years[1, 15, 37, 57, 89] and is beyond the scope of this chapter.

Lidocaine usually is the drug of choice in emergency situations because of its rapid onset and offset of action, safety, and minimal hemodynamic effects. Although often effective in the setting of acute myocardial ischemia, it is less useful in the treatment of chronic, recurrent ventricular tachycardia.[48] Lidocaine and phenytoin are effective therapy for ventricular tachycardia associated with digitalis toxicity.[42, 111] Phenytoin may occasionally be useful in patients with torsade de pointes ventricular tachycardia associated with prolonged QT syndromes.[107] Tocainide and mexiletine, two drugs chemically similar to lidocaine, are available as oral agents on an experimental basis.[2, 9, 14, 139] Dimarco et al.[14] found that ventricular tachycardias with rates greater than 175 per minute were more likely to respond to mexiletine than were slower tachycardias.

The drugs most frequently used for treatment of chronic, recurrent ventricular tachycardia are the membrane-active agents procainamide, quinidine, and disopyramide.[48, 79, 127] They decrease the rate of rapid depolarization of the cardiac action potential (phase 0) and the slope of spontaneous, diastolic depolarization (phase 4).[89] Intravenous procainamide is recommended in the emergency setting if lidocaine is ineffective. If procainamide is contraindicated because of previous toxicity or inefficacy, quinidine may be administered intravenously. Although it is used infrequently because of its possible adverse hemodynamic and electrophysiologic effects, intravenous quinidine may be given safely in an intensive care setting if adequate preload is maintained by volume administration to counteract its vasodilator properties.[117] Disopyramide is not recommended in the emergency setting because it has prominent, negative inotropic effects[94] and an intravenous preparation is not available for general use. Several other membrane-active drugs are available on an experimental basis. Two studies[121, 130] suggest that aprindine frequently may be effective in patients with mitral valve prolapse. Encainide is an experimental membrane-active agent that profoundly depresses His-Purkinje conduction.[102] Although it may prove effective when standard agents fail, it is capable of causing incessant, life-threatening ventricular tachycardia.[130]

The beta-blocking agents are effective in specific clinical settings. They are indicated in the treatment of ventricular tachycardia associated with the idiopathic long QT syndrome,[107] with catecholamine excess states (including pheochromocytoma, thyrotoxicosis, and some cases of exercise-induced ventricular tachycardia[11, 27, 118, 143]), and in rare instances when supraventricular tachycardia precipitates ventricular tachycardia. The use of these agents has been advocated in the treatment of ventricular tachycardia associated with hypertrophic cardiomyopathy[7] and mitral valve prolapse,[50] as well as for prevention of sudden death in patients with recent myocardial infarction.[119]

Bretylium tosylate acts on the heart directly to prolong the cardiac action potential, and indirectly through the initial catecholamine release and subsequent depletion it provokes.[41, 61, 140] It may also possess independent antifibrillatory properties.[103] Although it has been described as effective in refractory cases of ventricular fibrillation, reports of its use in patients with ventricular tachycardia are limited.[41] Amiodarone, a potent drug that similarly prolongs action potential duration, is effective only after two to four weeks of oral therapy,[40, 70, 93, 98] although immediate effects may be obtained with intravenous administration. Verapamil, a drug that blocks the slow, calcium-dependent plateau current, is now approved for intravenous use in patients with supraventricular tachycardias. It has been reported to be effective in some cases of ventricular tachycardia, especially those that may be provoked by exercise or atrial pacing.[63, 72, 143, 144]

Combinations of antiarrhythmic drugs often are used when individual agents prove ineffective. Some investigators have found drug combinations to be useful only infrequently when maximal doses of individual drugs have been ineffective;[48, 100] others have reported greater success with drug combinations.[20, 48, 65] In view of the potential for additive drug toxicities and the difficulty of identifying the agent responsible for an adverse reaction, we test multiple individual agents in maximally tolerated doses before considering combinations and do not combine agents that have similar electrophysiologic properties.

Emergency pharmacologic treatment of ventricular tachycardia is summarized in Table 5–3.

ASSESSMENT OF PHARMACOLOGIC THERAPY

In patients with life-threatening arrhythmias, the degree of prophylaxis against arrhythmia recurrence provided by an antiarrhythmic drug should be determined before chronic oral therapy is initiated. The limitations of empiric therapy are emphasized by the finding of Schaffer and Cobb[104] that empiric antiarrhythmic therapy had been prescribed after the initial episode of cardiac arrest and proved ineffective in 41 of 56 patients (73%) with recurrent, out-of-hospital sudden death. Furthermore, arrhythmia exacerbation occurs in up to 11 per cent of trials of antiarrhythmic drugs.[123] Two methods are used most frequently to assess antiarrhythmic efficacy. The first is noninvasive and measures suppression of spontaneous arrhythmias and arrhythmias provoked by exercise. The second is invasive and measures prophylaxis against arrhythmias induced by programmed electrical stimulation.

Noninvasive Techniques

In some patients with extremely frequent, symptomatic, spontaneous ventricular tachycardia, antiarrhythmic efficacy may be measured directly by suppression of the clinical arrhythmia.[88] In one study in which plasma concentration and continuous ECG monitoring were used to guide drug administration, effective antiarrhythmic drugs were identified for five of 11 patients with frequent, symptomatic ventricular tachycardia.[137] Similarly, in the small fraction of patients in whom clinical arrhythmias may be reliably provoked by treadmill exercise testing, limited data suggest that serial exercise tests may be used to assess antiarrhythmic efficacy.[5, 10, 51, 143] However, these approaches cannot be used in most patients with recurrent ventricular tachycardia because their clinical arrhythmias are less frequent and cannot be provoked by exercise.

Since direct assessment of clinical arrhythmia suppression often is impractical, several investigators have attempted to assess antiarrhythmic efficacy by measuring suppression of the events that may trigger ventricular tachycardia. On the basis of the observation that ventricular tachycardia may be initiated by one or more ventricular premature depolarizations (VPDs), these authors hypothesize that suppression of frequent and complex VPDs may prevent ventricular tachycardia by removing the triggering event.[68] Complex forms include multiform VPDs, early-cycle (R-on-T) VPDs, and repetitive forms (pairs of VPDs and ventricular tachycardia).

Using this approach, Lown et al. have developed the technique of trendscription to assess antiarrhythmic efficacy rapidly.[28, 67] The ECG is recorded in a compressed format

Table 5–3. EMERGENCY TREATMENT OF VENTRICULAR TACHYCARDIA: PHARMACOLOGIC THERAPY

Drug	Loading Dose	Maintenance Dose	Therapeutic Plasma Level (μg/ml)	Clinical Setting	Common Adverse Effects	Comments
Lidocaine	2–3 mg/kg over 5 min; titrate to CNS toxicity*	1–4 mg/min	2–6	Acute myocardial ischemia	CNS: tinnitus, dizziness, seizures	Initial treatment of choice for VT not associated with circulatory collapse; reduce maintenance dose in patients with liver disease and heart failure
Procainamide	10–15 mg/kg: not to exceed 0.6 mg/kg/min	1–4 mg/min	4–10 (some patients may require levels of up to 20)	Any	1. Hypotension 2. Infranodal heart block	Use if lidocaine is ineffective; stop infusion if QRS duration increases by 50%; decrease infusion rate and administer saline if hypotension occurs
Quinidine	10 mg/kg: not to exceed 0.5 mg/kg/min	NA	1.3–5.0	See comments	1. Hypotension 2. Infranodal heart block 3. Facilitation of AV nodal conduction	Use if procainamide is contraindicated or is known to be ineffective; do not combine with procainamide; follow same precautions as indicated for procainamide
Propranolol	0.075–0.15 mg/kg: not to exceed 1 mg/min	NA	Very variable	1. Catecholamine excess states 2. VT precipitated by SVT 3. Exercise-induced VT	1. Sinus bradycardia, AV block 2. Depressed myocardial contractility 3. Exacerbation of bronchospasm 4. Hypoglycemia	Contraindications: asthma, severe left ventricular dysfunction
Bretylium	5–10 mg/kg over 10 min	1–2 mg/min	0.5–1.5	VF unresponsive to defibrillation	1. Initial hypertension and exacerbation of ventricular arrhythmias 2. Late hypotension 3. Nausea and vomiting	
Phenytoin	10–15 mg/kg: not to exceed 50 mg/min	300–500 mg/day	10–20	Digitalis intoxication	1. Hypotension 2. CNS: nystagmus, ataxia	Rarely effective except in cases of digitalis intoxication

*Lidocaine should be administered at this rate only if required by the urgency of the clinical situation. For prophylaxis, 3 mg/kg should be administered over 20 min.

during a 30-minute control period and five minutes of bicycle exercise. A single oral loading dose of an antiarrhythmic agent is then administered. Trendscription is performed at selected intervals for a period of three to five hours, during which time bicycle exercise is repeated hourly. Serial plasma levels of the antiarrhythmic drug are obtained. Antiarrhythmic efficacy is defined as suppression of all repetitive forms and early-cycle VPDs. Drugs predicted effective at acute study are assessed during maintenance oral therapy after comparable plasma levels are achieved. Efficacy in this phase is defined in a similar manner using 24-hour ambulatory monitoring and exercise-treadmill testing: elimination of ventricular tachycardia and early-cycle VPDs, 90 per cent reduction in pairs, and either (1) 50 per cent reduction in number of VPDs per 24 hr or (2) 50 per cent reduction in number of hours during which 30 or more VPDs occur. In an attempt to provide a "fail-safe" system of protection against arrhythmia recurrence, chronic oral therapy is initiated with combinations of drugs that are predicted effective as single agents.

Graboys et al.[29] used this approach in 120 patients with ventricular fibrillation or ventricular tachycardia. Sudden death occurred in only five of 93 patients (5%) followed for 24.5 months in whom antiarrhythmic therapy was judged effective by this approach, compared with 18 of 27 patients (67%) for whom no therapy predicted effective could be found. However, the groups were not clinically comparable; left ventricular dysfunction was much more prevalent in the patients for whom no therapy was predicted to be effective.

Electrophysiologic Study

The study of ventricular tachycardia has been facilitated by the observation that appropriately timed premature ventricular extrastimuli can initiate and terminate ventricular tachycardia in susceptible patients (see Fig. 5–1). A stimulator is required that senses the patient's ECG and is programmed to deliver one or more stimuli at a specific time in diastole. Most pacing protocols for induction of ventricular tachycardia include the use of one and two programmed right ventricular extrastimuli in native and ventricular paced rhythms as well as bursts of rapid ventricular pacing.[12, 13, 18, 19, 78, 132] If these methods fail to initiate the arrhythmia, a third right ventricular extrastimulus,[79, 114] left ventricular stimulation,[80, 97] or stimulation during isoproterenol infusion[95, 122] may be used. In a patient with clinical, sustained ventricular tachycardia, an induced arrhythmia usually is morphologically identical to the clinical arrhythmia.[54] In some patients, additional morphologies of uncertain clinical significance may be induced.[96, 116]

For patients in whom ventricular tachycardia can be induced reliably by programmed stimulation, antiarrhythmic drug efficacy may be assessed by acute drug trials during electrophysiologic study.[12, 13, 19, 47, 48, 78, 79, 114, 122] A drug is considered acutely effective if ventricular tachycardia cannot be induced after its administration. Chronic oral therapy is instituted with an agent predicted effective, and the dose is adjusted to achieve plasma levels present during the acute study. Follow-up electrophysiologic studies for patients on oral therapy are mandatory for all drugs with active metabolites and are advisable in all cases. Mason and Winkle[79] analyzed arrhythmia recurrence in 58 trials of antiarrhythmic drugs whose efficacy had been assessed during electrophysiologic study. Patients treated with agents predicted effective had a significantly lower arrhythmia recurrence rate than those treated with agents predicted ineffective. At one year, 80 per cent of patients treated with agents predicted effective and 20 per cent of patients treated with agents predicted ineffective were free of arrhythmia recurrence by actuarial analysis. Longer follow-up of 193 patients with ventricular tachycardia who underwent acute drug trials in our laboratory demonstrated that results of pharmacologic trials during electrophysiologic study predicted arrhythmia-related mortality in medically treated patients (unpublished data) (see Fig. 5–3). However, clinical characteristics of the effective and ineffective drug groups were not comparable.

Comparison of Noninvasive Techniques and Programmed Stimulation

These individual approaches are neither universally applicable nor mutually exclusive. Except for the occasional patient with extremely frequent, spontaneous ventricular tachycardia, neither approach directly meas-

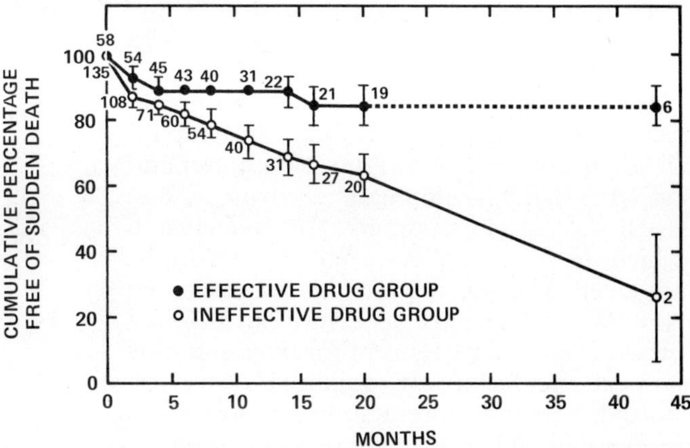

Figure 5–3. Life-table analysis of sudden death in patients with ventricular tachycardia. Sudden death–free survival is compared in 58 patients for whom an effective antiarrhythmic drug was identified at electrophysiologic study *(closed circles)* and 135 patients from whom no effective antiarrhythmic drug could be identified at electrophysiologic study *(open circles)*. Both documented arrhythmic deaths and sudden, unmonitored deaths are included in this analysis. Standard errors of the cumulative percentages are shown. The incidence of sudden death was significantly lower ($p<.04$) in the effective drug group from the eighth month throughout the rest of the follow-up period. The dashed line indicates extension of the curve beyond the last arrhythmic event to the longest duration of follow-up. The numbers above the circles represent the numbers of patients remaining in each group at various follow-up intervals.

ures the outcome variable: clinical arrhythmia recurrence. Noninvasive techniques assess suppression of presumed trigger events (VPDs). Programmed stimulation artificially provides these trigger events and, instead, measures the heart's capacity to sustain a tachycardia. There is no study that compares these techniques directly. Each has specific advantages and limitations.

Patient Eligibility. Lown et al.[68] estimate that 10 to 20 per cent of patients with recurrent, life-threatening ventricular arrhythmias have insufficient frequency or complexity of spontaneous and exercise-induced arrhythmias to allow accurate assessment of their suppression. Using programmed stimulation, ventricular tachyarrhythmias may be induced in 83 to 96 per cent of patients with recurrent, sustained ventricular tachycardia,[19, 54, 78, 80, 116] 60 to 70 per cent of those with recurrent, unsustained ventricular tachycardia,[54, 116] and 43 to 70 per cent of those with ventricular fibrillation.[56, 116] Ventricular tachycardia usually cannot be induced by programmed stimulation in patients with idiopathic, hereditary, or drug-induced prolonged QT syndromes. In one study, programmed stimulation and/or isoproterenol infusion induced ventricular tachycardia in 60 per cent of patients with exercise-induced ventricular tachycardia.[54]

Drug Efficacy Prediction. The criteria used to predict antiarrhythmic drug efficacy in both methods are arbitrary and require prospective validation. Results of acute pharmacologic testing during electrophysiologic study predict chronic oral efficacy,[79] but the degree of protection associated with various partial responses is uncertain.[13, 114] Furthermore, the incidence of acute drug efficacy depends on the pacing methods used: it is lower when drugs are assessed using three, rather than two, extrastimuli,[114] and when they are assessed by extrastimuli delivered from both ventricles rather than from the right ventricle alone.[83] In some patients, such complex stimulation techniques may be excessive and lead to rejection of potentially effective drugs.[114]

Noninvasive drug assessment also may lead to rejection of potentially effective agents. The percentage reduction in the number of VPDs required to achieve statistical significance depends on the frequency of arrhythmias in the control state and the duration of monitoring.[84, 136] In some patients, effective prophylaxis against recurrence of ventricular tachycardia may be achieved despite persistence of frequent, complex VPDs.[43, 87, 88] In others, ventricular tachycardia may recur despite suppression of virtually all VPDs. Data correlating VPD suppression with arrhythmia recurrence in patients with ventricular tachycardia are limited.

The ideal antiarrhythmic drug assessment method would detect all patients at risk for arrhythmia recurrence while recognizing clinically relevant degrees of arrhythmia prophylaxis. Such a protocol has yet to be identified.

Incidence of Successful Drug Selection. Depending on the definition of "efficacy" used, acutely effective agents are identified for 34 to 70 per cent of patients who undergo drug trials using programmed stimulation.[19, 47, 79, 114, 115] Acute efficacy rates for noninvasive assessment also are influenced by the criteria used; they have varied from 45 to 78 per cent.[66, 68, 137]

With either programmed stimulation or a noninvasive approach, efficacy rates for individual antiarrhythmic drugs may depend on the patient population, drug doses, method of drug assessment, and sequence in which the drugs are evaluated. For example, when efficacy was assessed by programmed stimulation using up to three extrastimuli, efficacy rates of 19 per cent for procainamide and 20 per cent for quinidine were reported.[115] In a different study, higher doses of procainamide prevented ventricular tachycardia induction by up to two extrastimuli in 45 per cent of trials.[48] Quinidine and procainamide have been judged effective in 61 and 71 per cent of trials, respectively, when efficacy was assessed by trendscription.[66]

Some antiarrhythmic agents may be accurately assessed by only one of these techniques. Amiodarone may prevent clinical arrhythmia recurrence much more frequently than it prohibits arrhythmia induction by programmed stimulation.[40] One study suggests that suppression of complex VPDs by amiodarone is predictive of chronic oral efficacy even though ventricular tachycardia remains inducible.[82]

No prospective, controlled comparison of the predictive accuracy of these two methods is available.

Time Required for Identification of Effective Drugs. Acute drug trials performed by trendscription or programmed stimulation may shorten the duration of the testing procedure as compared with trials performed using 24-hour continuous ECG recordings[67, 78] during chronic therapy.

Risks. Cardioversion is required in 30 to 50 per cent of patients undergoing electrophysiologic study.[78] Some patients in atrial fibrillation may be at risk for arterial embolization if they require cardioversion. We consider the presence of hypertrophic cardiomyopathy, unstable angina, and severe, global left ventricular dysfunction to be relative contraindications to programmed ventricular stimulation. Using these guidelines, we have safely performed over 1000 ventricular tachycardia induction studies without catheter-related complications or fatality.

The delays associated with drug assessment by 24-hour ECG recordings may make monitoring in an intensive care unit impractical and thereby place patients at risk for arrhythmia recurrence in a less controlled setting. Further, such delays expose patients to risks of side effects and arrhythmia exacerbation over prolonged periods.

Institutional Availability. Electrophysiologic studies require expensive equipment and extensive specialized training for physicians and ancillary personnel, and are long and labor-intensive. Noninvasive assessment of antiarrhythmic drugs uses less equipment and personnel but requires meticulous, quantitative analysis of long, continuous ECG recordings and may encroach upon a limited number of beds in the critical care unit.

Much remains to be learned about the optimal methods for antiarrhythmic drug assessment. Our current recommendations, which undoubtedly will be modified by future knowledge, are summarized in Table 5–4.

Table 5–4. GUIDELINES FOR ASSESSMENT OF ANTIARRHYTHMIC THERAPY FOR VENTRICULAR TACHYCARDIA

Electrophysiologic Study Preferred
1. Tachycardia diagnosis uncertain
2. Infrequent, life-threatening arrhythmias
3. Multiple failures of empiric drug therapy
4. Nonpharmacologic therapy considered
Noninvasive Assessment Preferred
1. Frequent, spontaneous VT
2. Electrophysiologic study contraindicated
3. Arrhythmia occurring only during exercise
Preferred Method Uncertain
1. Frequent, complex VPDs but infrequent VT
2. Unsustained VT

PACEMAKER THERAPY

Temporary or permanent pacing systems may be used to prevent or terminate ventricular tachycardia in selected patients, as shown in Table 5–5. "Overdrive" pacing of the atria or ventricles occasionally may prevent recurrent ventricular tachycardia. Suppression of late-coupled, initiating VPDs and overdrive suppression of ectopic ventricular pacemakers may account for the efficacy of overdrive pacing in some patients with ventricular tachycardia. Temporary atrial or ventricular pacing at rates of 90 to 120 per minute may prevent recurrence of ventricular tachycardia immediately after cardiac surgery[17, 113, 126, 141] or in the acute phase of myocardial infarction.[8, 59, 86] Several cases of effective chronic

Table 5–5. PACING METHODS FOR EMERGENCY TREATMENT OF VENTRICULAR TACHYCARDIA

Method	Specific Clinical Setting	Comments
Tachycardia Prevention		
Rate support	VT developing as an escape rhythm during bradycardia	
Overdrive suppression	1. Torsade de pointes VT associated with long QT interval	Atrial pacing is preferred; isoproterenol may be infused to increase sinus rate to 120/min until pacing is initiated
	2. Initiating VPDs dependent on reltive bradycardia	
Hemodynamic Improvement Without Tachycardia Termination		
Atrial overdrive	Relatively slow VT	Restoration of AV synchyrony may improve hemodynamics
Paired pacing	I VT unresponsive to cardioversion and acute drug therapy	Pulse rate is half of electrical rate; metabolic cost may provoke ischemia
Tachycardia Termination		
Diastolic scanning	Patient with implanted pacemaker	Occasionally effective if tachycardia rate is < 175/min
Burst pacing	Recurrent, sustained VT	Risk of tachycardia acceleration
Programmed extrastimuli	Recurrent, sustained VT	Required equipment usually not available in emergency setting

overdrive suppression have been reported.[6, 52, 85]

Overdrive pacing is the treatment of choice for torsade de pointes ventricular tachycardia due to antiarrhythmic drug toxicity.[108, 112] Torsade de pointes is a paroxysmal, usually unsustained, and often incessantly recurrent form of ventricular tachycardia that is characteristically initiated by a late-cycle extrasystole and occurs most commonly in the setting of marked QT or QU prolongation. In each paroxysm, the amplitude and polarity of the QRS complexes vary so that the complexes appear to twist about the isoelectric line, as shown in Figure 5–4. A rate-dependent decrease in dispersion of myocardial repolarization may be responsible for the dramatic suppression of drug-refractory paroxysms seen with pacing rates of 110 to 140 beats per minute. Atrial pacing has been advocated because it preserves the atrial transport mechanism, produces synchronous ventricular activation, and avoids catheter-induced ventricular arrhythmias. Isoproterenol may be infused to maintain sinus tachycardia at a rate of 110 to 140 beats per minute until a temporary pacing electrode is in place.[108, 112]

Pacing for tachycardia termination is more frequently effective than pacing for tachycardia prevention. As shown in Figure 5–5, many episodes of ventricular tachycardia can be terminated by appropriately timed, programmed extrastimuli or by bursts of rapid ventricular pacing.[12, 20, 55, 69, 135] Relatively slow tachycardias with rates less than 175 beats per minute are more likely to respond to single extrastimuli,[20] whereas more rapid tachycardias require more complex pacing programs for termination.[20, 69] If a patient with a permanent ventricular demand pacemaker develops ventricular tachycardia, termination may be attempted by magnet application. This converts the pacemaker to a fixed rate mode, allowing the pacing stimulus to scan diastole. Use of single, programmed ventricular extrastimuli carries minimal risk but frequently fails to terminate ventricular tachycardia.[20, 78] Similarly, rapid atrial pacing is safe but usually ineffective. Bursts of rapid ventricular pacing have been reported to terminate up to 62 per cent of tachycardias, but tachycardia acceleration occurs in 11 per cent of patients in whom this technique is used[78] (see Fig. 5–6). In one study, successful pacing rates for tachycardia termination ranged from 111 to 141 per cent of the tachycardia rate.[69] Faster burst rates are associated with greater risk of acceleration. Implantable burst generators, externally activated by patient or physician, have been successful in some cases of refractory ventricular tachycardia. Use of these devices may be considered in patients who can perceive the presence or absence of the tachycardia and who are not rapidly disabled by their arrhythmia.[21, 22, 38, 39, 49, 91, 101]

A programmable, automatic, antitachycardia pacemaker, which senses tachycardia on

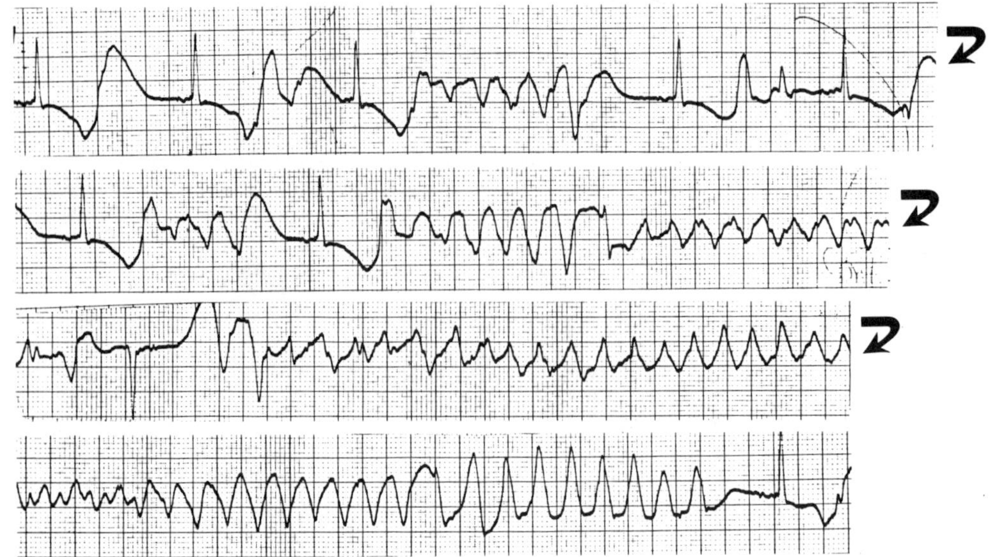

Figure 5–4. Torsade de pointes ventricular tachycardia in a patient with a long QT interval. A continuous monitor strip is shown. The first, second, and fourth beats of the top panel show sinus bradycardia with a markedly prolonged QT interval and giant, bizarre T waves. The apex of the T wave of the second QRS complex is deformed by a VPD (Ventricular premature depolarization). The apex of the T wave of the fourth QRS complex is also deformed by a VPD, which initiates a short run of ventricular tachycardia. This sequence is repeated in the subsequent strips, which demonstrate several longer runs of self-terminating ventricular tachycardia. Note that the polarity of the QRS complexes during tachycardia gradually changes from beat to beat so that the peaks of the QRS complexes appear to twist about the isoelectric line. This is best seen in the bottom panel.

the basis of rate criteria and responds with bursts of varying cycle length and duration, has been used successfully to treat supraventricular[30] and ventricular[31] tachycardia. Its use in patients with ventricular tachycardia is limited by the potentially lethal outcome if the burst pacing accelerates the tachycardia. Thorough electrophysiologic study is mandatory before implantation of an antitachycardia pacing system; reliable arrhythmia termination without acceleration must be documented, preferably over several days.

Paired ventricular pacing may improve hemodynamics during incessant ventricular tachycardias that are refractory to rapidly acting drugs, burst pacing, or repeated cardioversion. The ventricle is paced at a rate slightly faster than one half the tachycardia

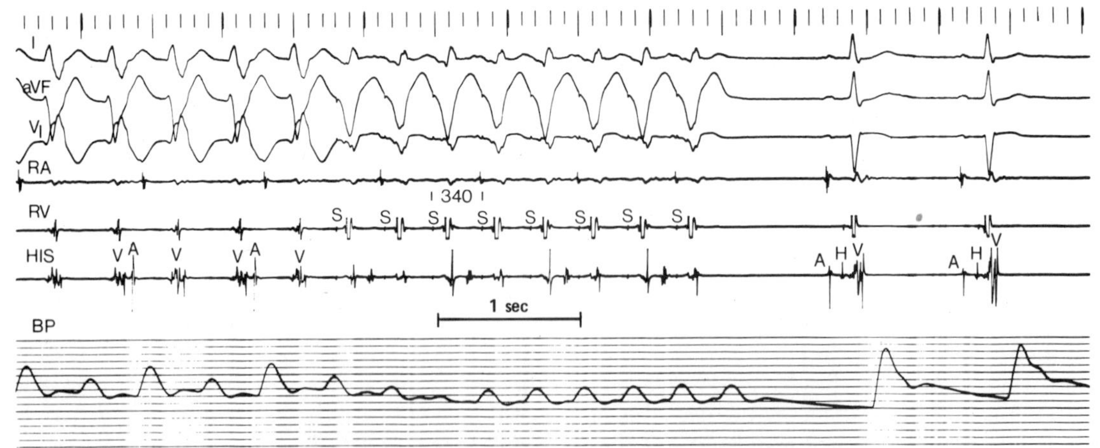

Figure 5–5. Pace termination of ventricular tachycardia. Abbreviations are as in Figure 5–1. Ventricular tachycardia is terminated by a burst of rapid ventricular pacing at cycle length 340 ms. Note the change in surface ECG morphology associated with ventricular capture by the burst of rapid ventricular pacing. Sinus rhythm resumes after termination of pacing.

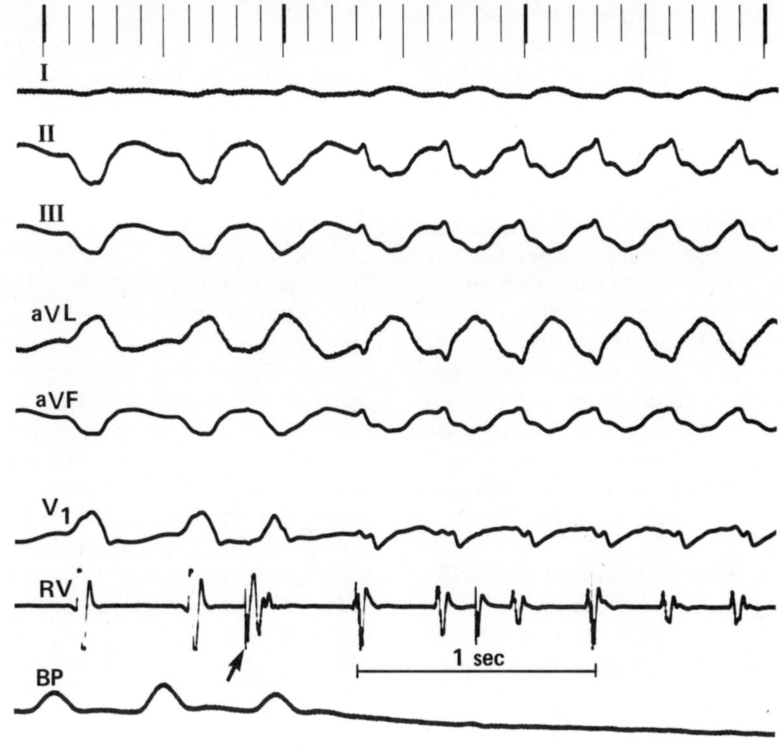

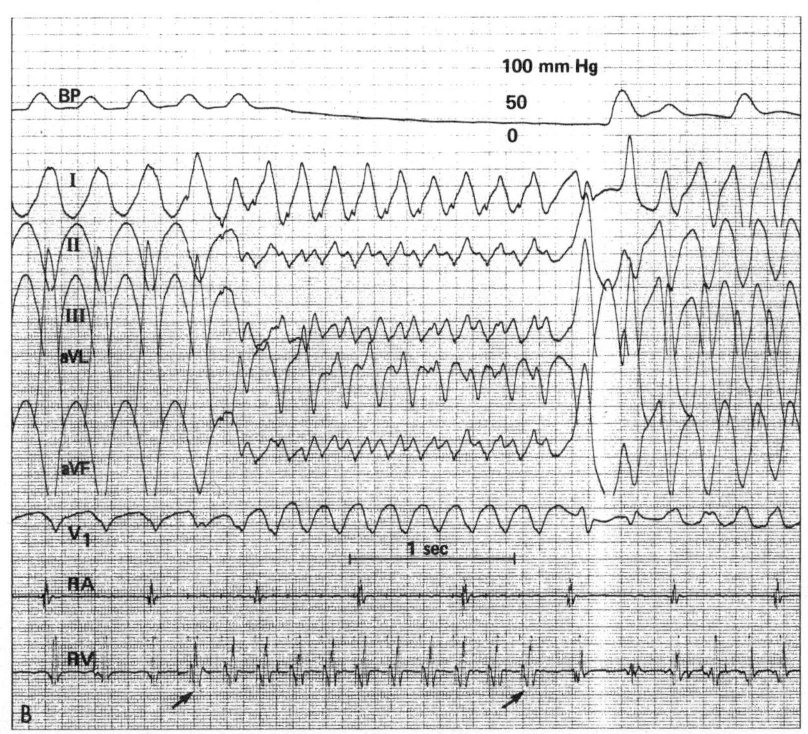

Figure 5–6. Pace acceleration of ventricular tachycardia. Surface leads I, II, III, aVL, aVF, and V_1 are displayed with the electrogram recorded from the right ventricular apex *(RV)* and the blood pressure *(BP)*. The right atrial electrogram *(RA)* also is displayed in *B*. In *A*, four pacing stimuli are delivered at a cycle length slightly longer than that of the tachycardia. Only the first pacing stimulus *(arrow)* captures the ventricle. After this capture beat, the morphology of the tachycardia changes and its rate increases. Tachycardia acceleration after a single ventricular capture is unusual. Cardioversion was required to terminate the arrhythmia. *B* shows a more typical example of tachycardia acceleration induced by a burst of rapid ventricular pacing. The first and last paced beats are designated by arrows.

rate. An extrastimulus is introduced midway between two paced beats and is brought progressively closer to the preceding QRS until it produces an electrical depolarization that is mechanically ineffective. The effective ventricular rate therefore is halved while diastolic filling is enhanced.[125] Alternatively, atrial pacing at a rate faster than that of the tachycardia may improve hemodynamics if one-to-one atrioventricular capture can be achieved.[126] This approach may be facilitated by administration of a membrane-active antiarrhythmic drug to slow the tachycardia rate. Such temporizing measures may stabilize hemodynamics until ventricular tachycardia subsides spontaneously or definitive therapy takes effect.

An automatic, fully implantable defibrillator is undergoing clinical trials. This device identifies ventricular fibrillation by the absence of isoelectric potentials and responds with a discharge of 25 to 35 joules across the heart. Preliminary experience suggests that this device may provide a satisfactory "failsafe" system for patients with life-threatening arrhythmias that are refractory to other methods of treatment.[81]

SURGERY

Although surgery is rarely indicated as an emergency measure, it is potentially curative for some patients with recurrent ventricular tachycardia. Left cervicothoracic sympathectomy is the treatment of choice for patients with idiopathic or hereditary prolonged QT syndrome associated with ventricular tachycardia that is refractory to medical therapy.[107] Some experts consider this operation preferable to attempts at drug therapy. In patients with structural heart disease, both conventional cardiac surgery techniques and new techniques designed specifically for treatment of arrhythmias have been applied.

The efficacy of coronary artery bypass grafting and/or left ventricular aneurysm resection for treatment of ventricular tachycardia in patients with coronary artery disease has been reviewed in recent years.[73] Most previous studies have reported series of only one to four patients. In 22 such reports, the extent of medical treatment was inadequate or not documented in 85 of 127 patients (79%). Reported data generally are inadequate to allow analysis of arrhythmia recurrence rates. In those studies in which sufficient data are available for analysis, arrhythmia recurrence rates are high. Mason et al.[77] reported a 50 per cent one-month recurrence rate in 32 patients undergoing standard aneurysm resection. By 94 months of follow-up, all patients at risk had suffered arrhythmia recurrence. Similarly, Harken et al.[35] reported arrhythmia recurrence in 15 of 19 patients (79%) who underwent aneurysm resection for medically refractory ventricular tachycardia. Although standard surgical techniques may be effective in some cases, they do not prevent arrhythmia recurrence in most patients with coronary disease. Currently, we employ myocardial revascularization as primary treatment for recurrent ventricular tachycardia or ventricular fibrillation only in the unusual instance in which arrhythmias are precipitated by definite episodes of myocardial ischemia without acute infarction.

Mitral valve replacement has been performed in several cases of ventricular tachycardia associated with mitral valve prolapse, with similarly mixed results.[99]

Intraoperative activation sequence mapping may be used to direct the surgical approach to ventricular tachycardia. When complete endocardial and epicardial maps are performed, sites of earliest activation, if identifiable, usually are found in the endocardium, and in some patients may represent the site of origin of the tachycardia. In other patients, electrical activity spanning diastole defines a macroscopic reentry circuit.[76] On the hypothesis that specific reentry pathways can be transected, or ectopic foci isolated, Fontaine and associates[23–25] used epicardial activation sequence mapping to direct simple transmural ventriculotomies in 19 patients with refractory ventricular tachycardia associated with primary myocardial disease. There were four postoperative deaths (21%), three due to ventricular tachycardia (16%), and one late arrhythmia recurrence (5%).[25] Guiraudon et al.[32, 33] have applied a different technique—the encircling endocardial ventriculotomy—to recurrent ventricular tachycardia in patients with previous myocardial infarction. An incision from endocardium to subepicardium is performed circumferentially around the scar and then closed. This technique is designed to electrically isolate or physically injure the tissue at the border of the infarct. Intraoperative activation sequence mapping is not required. Preliminary results have been encouraging: in a series of 23 patients, there were only two perioperative deaths (9%) and two late arrhythmia recurrences (9%).[32]

Horowitz and colleagues[36, 45, 46, 53] have used endocardial activation sequence mapping to develop an approach based on endomyocardial excision in the area of earliest electrical activation. They reported results of this technique in 39 patients with medically refractory ventricular tachycardia. There were three operative deaths (8%). Postoperatively, arrhythmia was not inducible by programmed stimulation in 31 patients (79%) and was controlled by drugs in the remaining five (13%). One late arrhythmia recurrence was noted during follow-up of two months to three years.[45]

We have reported results of surgery guided by activation sequence mapping in 50 patients with medically refractory ventricular tachycardia due to previous myocardial infarction.[75] The primary procedure was endomyocardial excision in 31 cases, cryothermal ablation in 13, and transmural or endoventriculotomy in six. There were 13 perioperative deaths (26%), eight due to left ventricular failure (16%) and three due to arrhythmia recurrence (6%). There have been two late, sudden deaths at three and six months (4%). By actuarial analysis, 69 ± 7 per cent (SEM) of patients survived at six months. Eleven patients (22%) have had documented or suspected arrhythmia recurrence. In six additional patients (12%), ventricular tachycardia was inducible by programmed stimulation postoperatively, but spontaneous arrhythmia has not recurred. Actuarial analysis shows 75 ± 7 per cent of patients at risk to be free of arrhythmia recurrence at five months.

Retrospective analysis suggests that arrhythmia recurrence is less frequent after surgery guided by activation sequence mapping than after standard surgical approaches.[35, 73, 77] Nevertheless, several difficulties limit the utility of mapping-guided surgery.[74] Ventricular tachycardia cannot be induced by programmed stimulation in all patients and may not be inducible in the cold, empty heart on cardiopulmonary bypass. The induction of multiple morphologies complicates activation sequence mapping. Very rapid tachycardias may prove unmappable owing to the absence of a discrete electrical diastole and a discernible onset of the QRS, as shown in Figure 5–7. Putative tachycardia foci may be surgically inaccessible. The significance of certain findings during mapping, such as mid-diastolic electrical activity, local block, and delayed potentials during native rhythm, remains uncertain. Similarly, the significance of induced arrhythmias immediately after resuscitation of the heart is unknown. Overall, mapping-guided surgery is plagued by our lack of understanding of the mechanisms responsible for ventricular tachycardia.

Further, mapping-guided surgery has specific risks not present in conventional cardiac surgery. Activation sequence mapping requires 20 to 60 minutes of normothermic cardiopulmonary bypass time, and the surgical technique involves destruction of some normal myocardium. Neither may be tolerated by patients with poor left ventricular function, although cryothermal ablation may be better tolerated than techniques based on ventriculotomy or endomyocardial excision.[75] Patients with inducible, sustained, unimorphic, mappable arrhythmias and ventricular dysfunction limited to discrete segments are the best candidates for surgery based on activation sequence mapping.

APPROACH TO THE PATIENT

Our approach to the patient who presents with a wide-complex tachycardia is summarized in Table 5–6. If a pulse is palpable and an ECG machine is available, there is almost always time to obtain a 12-lead ECG. If one is not available, six limb leads can be recorded on most portable defibrillator units. Arrhythmias in moderately symptomatic patients should be terminated only after the diagnosis is certain or all available diagnostic information has been extracted from the history, physical examination, and ECG.

Immediate cardioversion is indicated in patients who present with circulatory arrest due to a tachyarrhythmia. Although some ventricular tachycardias can be converted with a precordial thump or low-energy cardioversion, many require higher energies. We recommend cardioversion with at least 200 joules in cases of circulatory arrest. In moderately symptomatic patients, arrhythmia termination may be deferred if a rapidly correctable immediate cause is apparent. Therapy may help to confirm the suspected

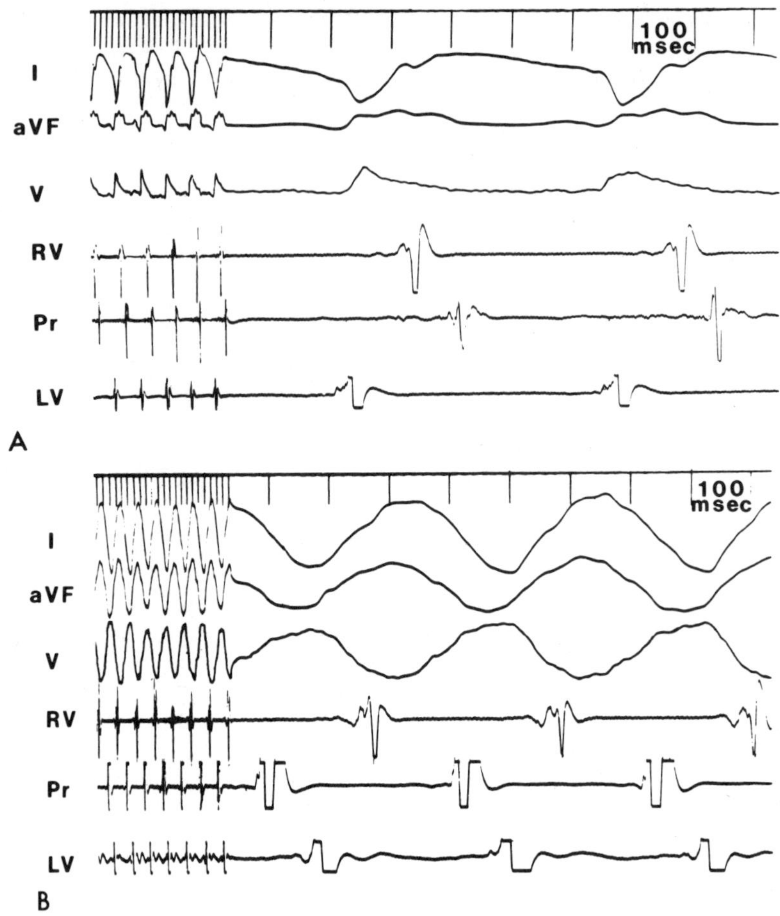

Figure 5–7. Ventricular tachycardia induced during intraoperative activation sequence mapping. Surface leads I, aVF, and a precordial lead recorded from a position on the back directly opposite the V_1 position are recorded simultaneously with right ventricular *(RV)* and left ventricular *(LV)* reference electrograms and a moving left ventricular probe electrogram *(Pr)*. Recordings are shown at 20-mm and 200-mm paper speed, respectively. The tachycardia shown in *A* is not mappable owing to the absence of discrete electrical diastole and discernible onset of the QRS complexes. *B* shows a mappable ventricular tachycardia induced in the same patient. The onset of the QRS complexes is readily identified. The probe electrogram occurs late in the QRS complex.

diagnosis. In patients with suspected ventricular tachycardia, intravenous lidocaine should be administered. If a supraventricular arrhythmia is suspected, vagal maneuvers and edrophonium should be followed by verapamil or propranolol. If these interventions fail to terminate symptomatic tachycardia and no readily correctable cause can be identified, cardioversion is indicated.

Inspect the posttachycardia ECG for evidence of pre-excitation, acute myocardial infarction, ventricular aneurysm, drug effect, electrolyte imbalance, or QT prolongation. The waste basket should be examined for valuable rhythm strips usually filed in this repository.

Define the immediate cause and correct it if possible. If acute myocardial infarction is suspected, therapy may be initiated with a lidocaine loading dose and infusion, if not contraindicated. Temporary overdrive pacing should be begun in patients with torsade de pointes ventricular tachycardia and a long QT interval.

Establish the presence and severity of structural heart disease if it is not already known. In patients with coronary artery disease, cardiac catheterization, left ventriculography, and coronary angiography usually are indicated to define the coronary anatomy, identify the presence of akinetic or dyskinetic ventricular segments, and assess the function of the remaining myocardium. In selected patients with presumed primary myocardial

Table 5–6. APPROACH TO THE PATIENT WITH A WIDE-COMPLEX TACHYCARDIA

1. Identify the rhythm.
2. Terminate the arrhythmia.
3. Inspect the posttachycardia ECG.
4. Define and correct the immediate cause. Initiate specifically indicated antiarrhythmic therapy.
5. Establish the presence and severity of structural heart disease.
6. Monitor the frequency and complexity of spontaneous arrhythmias. Perform a baseline provocative study if indicated.
7. Initiate prophylactic antiarrhythmic drug therapy.
8. Assess the efficacy of drug therapy.
9. If drug therapy is predicted to be ineffective, consider nonpharmacologic therapy.
10. Educate and provide emotional support to the patient and his family.

disease, right ventriculography to identify arrhythmogenic right ventricular dysplasia, or endomyocardial biopsy to diagnose inflammatory myocarditis or sarcoidosis, may be considered.

Assess the frequency and complexity of spontaneous arrhythmias by continuous ECG monitoring. Complex VPDs and occasional, unsustained ventricular tachycardia usually do not require immediate treatment. Specific antiarrhythmic therapy should not be initiated unil all effects of previously administered antiarrhythmic drugs have dissipated and an adequate evaluation of spontaneous arrhythmias has been made. Perform a baseline electrophysiologic study if the arrhythmia diagnosis remains uncertain, nonpharmacologic therapy is considered, or antiarrhythmic drug assessment by electrophysiologic study is selected. Perform an exercise test in patients with exercise-induced arrhythmias.

If the clinical arrhythmia recurs after all remedial causes have been corrected or if no immediate cause can be identified, initiate prophylactic pharmacologic therapy. Agents appropriate to the clinical setting should be used, taking into consideration the results of previous drug trials. In most patients, oral therapy may be initiated with quinidine or procainamide. A dosing schedule based on pharmacokinetic principles should be selected, and the plasma levels achieved documented. Meticulous records must be kept for dose and frequency of drug administration.

Assess therapeutic efficacy by programmed stimulation or noninvasive techniques. Each method is best applied when its limitations are understood: the only definite end points for therapeutic inefficacy are clinical arrhythmia recurrence on maximally tolerated doses or unacceptable drug toxicity. Arrhythmia recurrence during the loading phase of drug therapy is not an indication to discontinue the drug. If symptomatic arrhythmias recur during maintenance drug administration, it is appropriate to measure the plasma level, identify new precipitating events, and exclude the possibility of supraventricular or drug-toxic arrhythmias. Maintenance therapy should not be complicated with intravenous boluses of medication for asymptomatic arrhythmias. Doses may be increased to maximally tolerated levels before a drug is labeled ineffective. If empiric therapy is necessary, but ventricular tachycardia and ventricular premature beats are infrequent, maximum tolerated doses should be given and therapeutic plasma concentrations achieved.

One's willingness to abandon partially effective therapy should be in direct proportion to the availability of other potentially effective therapeutic modalities. Surgery should be considered earlier in patients who are good candidates by virtue of arrhythmia characteristics and cardiac anatomy. Implanted electrical devices are treatments of last resort for ventricular tachycardia.

A patient with recurrent ventricular tachycardia is subject to unpredictable, paroxysmal, disabling, and life-threatening events. The physician must assist the patient in coping with arrhythmia-associated psychologic stresses during treatment selection and during subsequent outpatient therapy. The patient should be forbidden to drive and the family must be trained to deliver effective, sustained cardiopulmonary resuscitation; a home defibrillator should be prescribed if appropriate. The patient and family must be educated so as to ensure meticulous compliance with prescribed treatment regimens.

Advances in basic and clinical electrophysiology, cardiac pharmacology, pacemaker technology, and cardiac surgery have dramatically expanded the number of therapies available for ventricular tachycardia. Nevertheless, all available therapeutic modalities have limitations. Our inability to find effective treatment for many patients is a frustrating reminder that we are profoundly ignorant of the fundamental mechanisms responsible for ventricular tachycardia.

References

1. Anderson, J. L., Harrison, D. C., Meffin, P. J., et al.: Antiarrhythmic drugs: Clinical pharmacology and therapeutic uses. Drugs 15:271, 1978.
2. Anderson, J. L., Mason, J. W., Winkle, R. A., et al.: Clinical electrophysiologic effects of tocainide. Circulation 57:685, 1978.
3. Armbrust, C. A., Jr., and Levine, S. A.: Paroxysmal ventricular tachycardia: a study of 107 cases. Circulation 1:28, 1950.
4. Brown, T. C. K., Barker, G. A., Dunlop, M. E., et al.: The use of sodium bicarbonate in the treatment of tricyclic antidepressant induced arrhythmias. Anaesth. Intens. Care 1:203, 1973.
5. Bryson, A. L., Parisi, A. F., Schechter, E., et al.: Life-threatening ventricular arrhythmias induced by exercise. Am. J. Cardiol. 32:995, 1973.
6. Burchell, H. B., and Merideth, J.: Management of cardiac tachyarrhythmias with cardiac pacemakers. Ann. N.Y. Acad. Sci. 167:546, 1969.
7. Canedo, M. I., Frank, J. J., and Abdulla, A. M.: Rhythm disturbances in hypertrophic cardiomyopathy: prevalence, relation to symptoms and management. Am. J. Cardiol. 45:848, 1980.
8. Chadda, K. D., Banka, V. S., and Helfant, R. H.: Rate-dependent ventricular ectopy following acute coronary occlusion: the concept of an optimal antiarrhythmic heart rate. Circulation 49:654, 1974.
9. Chew, C. Y. C., Collett, J., and Singh, B. N.: Mexiletine: a review of its pharmacological properties and therapeutic efficacy in arrhythmias. Drugs 17:161, 1979.
10. Codini, M. A., Sommerfeldt, L., Eybel, C. E., et al.: Efficacy of coronary bypass grafting in exercise-induced ventricular tachycardia. J. Thorac. Cardiovasc. Surg. 81:502, 1980.
11. Coumel, P., Fidelle, J., Lucet, V., et al.: Catecholamine-induced severe ventricular arrhythmias with Adams-Stokes syndrome in children. Report of four cases. Br. Heart J. (Suppl.) 40:28, 1978.
12. Denes, P., Wu, D., Wyndham, C., et al.: Chronic long-term electrophysiologic study of paroxysmal ventricular tachycardia. Chest 77:478, 1980.
13. DiMarco, J., Garan, H., and Ruskin, J. N.: Partial suppression of induced arrhythmias during serial electrophysiologic testing. Circulation 62 (Suppl. 3):III–261, 1980 (abstr.).
14. DiMarco, J. P., Garan, H., and Ruskin, J. N.: Mexiletine for refractory-ventricular arrhythmias: results using serial electrophysiologic testing. Am. J. Cardiol. 47:131, 1981.
15. Dreifus, L. S., and Morganroth, J.: Antiarrhythmic agents and their use in therapy. Pharmacol. Ther. 9:75, 1977.
16. Dungan, W. T., Garson, A., Jr., and Gillette, P. C.: Arrhythmogenic right ventricular dysplasia: a cause of ventricular tachycardia in children with apparently normal hearts. Am. Heart J. 102:745, 1981.
17. Eraklis, A. J., Green, W. T., and Watson, C. G.: Recurrent paroxysms of ventricular tachycardia following mitral valvuloplasty. Ann. Surg. 161:63, 1965.
18. Farshidi, A., Tyndall, T., and Batsford, W. P.: Inducibility of recurrent sustained ventricular tachycardia: role of stimulation mode. Circulation 61 (Suppl. 3):III–261, 1980 (abstr.).
19. Fisher, J. D.: Nonsurgical treatment of ventricular tachycardia: the value of serial provocative testing. *In* Narula, O. S. (ed.): Cardiac Arrhythmias: Electrophysiology, Diagnosis and Management. Baltimore, Williams & Wilkins Co., 1979, pp. 494–515.
20. Fisher, J. D., Cohen, H. L., Mehra, R., et al.: Cardiac pacing and pacemakers II. Serial electrophysiologic-pharmacologic testing for control of recurrent tachyarrhythmias. Am. Heart J. 93:658, 1977.
21. Fisher, J. D., Furman, S., and Kim, S. G.: Implanted automatic burst pacemakers for termination of ventricular tachycardia. Am. J. Cardiol. 45:458, 1980.
22. Fontaine, G., Frank, R., Kevorkian, M., et al.: Therapeutic use of radiofrequency pacing in the management of cardiac arrhythmias. PACE 2:A7, 25, 1979 (abstr.).
23. Fontaine, G., Guiraudon, G., and Frank, R.: Mechanism of ventricular tachycardiac with and without associated chronic myocardial ischemia: surgical management based on epicardial mapping. *In* Narula, O. S. (ed.): Cardiac Arrhythmias: Electrophysiology, Diagnosis and Management. Baltimore, Williams & Wilkins Co., 1979, pp. 529–545.
24. Fontaine, G., Guiraudon, G., Frank, R., et al.: Stimulation studies and epicardial mapping in ventricular tachycardia: study of mechanisms and selection for surgery. *In* Kulbertus, H. E. (ed.): Reentrant Arrhythmias: Mechanisms and Treatment. Baltimore, University Park Press, 1977, pp. 334–350.
25. Fontaine, G., Guiraudon, G., Frank, R., et al.: The surgical management of ventricular tachycardia. Herz 4:276, 1979.
26. Friedberg, C. K., and Donoso, E.: Arrhythmias and conduction disturbances due to digitalis. Prog. Cardiovasc. Dis. 2:408, 1959.
27. Gettes, L. S., and Surawicz, B.: Long-term prevention of paroxysmal arrhythmias with propranolol therapy. Am. J. Med. Sci. 254:257, 1967.
28. Graboys, T. B., and Lown, B.: Abbreviated electrocardiographic monitoring to expose ventricular ectopic activity. Cardiovasc. Med. 4:795, 1979.
29. Graboys, T. B., Lown, B., Podrid, P. J., et al.: Survival of patients with malignant ventricular arrhythmia treated with antiarrhythmic agents. Circulation 60 (Suppl. 2):II–155, 1980 (abstr.).
30. Griffin, J. C., Mason, J. W., and Calfee, R. V.: Clinical use of an implantable automatic tachycardia-terminating pacemaker. Am. Heart J. 100:1093, 1980.
31. Griffin, J. C., Mason, J. W., Ross, D. L., et al.: The treatment of ventricular tachycardia using an automatic tachycardia terminating pacemaker. PACE 4:582, 1981.
32. Guiraudon, G., Fontaine, G., Frank, R., et al.: Encircling endocardial ventriculotomy: a new surgical treatment following myocardial infarction. Ann. Thorac. Surg. 26:276, 1973.
33. Guiraudon, G., Fontaine, G., Frank, R., et al.: Encircling endocardial ventriculotomy: late follow-up results. Circulation 62:III–320, 1980 (abstr.).
34. Hammill, S. C., and Pritchett, E. L. C.: Simplified esophageal electrocardiography using bipolar recording leads. Ann. Intern. Med. 95:14, 1981.
35. Harken, A. H., Horowitz, L. N., and Josephson, M. E.: Comparison of standard aneurysmectomy

and aneurysmectomy with directed endocardial resection for the treatment of recurrent sustained ventricular tachycardia. J. Thorac. Cardiovasc. Surg. 80:527, 1980.
36. Harken, A. H., Josephson, M. E., and Horowitz, L. N.: Surgical endocardial resection for the treatment of malignant ventricular tachycardia. Ann. Surg. 190:456, 1979.
37. Harrison, D. C., Meffin, P. J., and Winkle, R. A.: Clinical pharmacokinetics of antiarrhythmic drugs. Prog. Cardiovasc. Dis. 20:217, 1977.
38. Hartzler, G. O.: Treatment of recurrent ventricular tachycardia by patient-activated radiofrequency ventricular stimulation. Mayo Clin. Proc. 54:75, 1979.
39. Hartzler, G. O., Osborn, M. J., and Holmes, D. R.: Termination of recurrent ventricular tachycardia by patient-activated rapid ventricular stimulation. Am. J. Cardiol. 45:457, 1980 (abstr.).
40. Heger, J. J., Prystowsky, E. N., Jackman, W. M., et al.: Amiodarone: clinical efficacy and electrophysiology during long-term therapy for recurrent ventricular tachycardia or ventricular fibrillation. N. Engl. J. Med. 305:539, 1981.
41. Heissenbuttel, R. H., and Bigger, J. T., Jr.: Bretylium tosylate: a newly available antiarrhythmic drug for ventricular arrhythmias. Ann. Intern. Med. 91:229, 1979.
42. Helfant, R. H., Scherlag, B. J., and Damato, A. N.: The electrophysiological properties of diphenylhydantoin sodium as compared to procainamide in the normal and digitalis-intoxicated heart. Circulation 36:108, 1967.
43. Herling, I. M., Horowitz, L. N., and Josephson, M. E.: Ventricular ectopic activity after medical and surgical treatment for recurrent sustained ventricular tachycardia. Am. J. Cardiol. 45:633, 1980.
44. Hermann, G. R., Park, H. M., and Hejtmancik, M. R.: Paroxysmal ventricular tachycardia: a clinical and electrocardiographic study. Am. Heart J. 57:166, 1959.
45. Horowitz, L. N., Harken, A. H., and Josephson, M. E.: Electrophysiologically-directed ventricular resection for recurrent sustained ventricular tachycardia. *In* Harrison, D. C., Winkle, R. A., and Mason, J. W. (eds.): Cardiac Arrhythmias—A Decade of Progress. Boston, G. K. Hall & Co., 1981, pp. 457–473.
46. Horowitz, L. N., Harken, A. H., Kastor, J. A., et al.: Ventricular resection guided by epicardial and endocardial mapping for treatment of recurrent ventricular tachycardia. N. Engl. J. Med. 302:589, 1980.
47. Horowitz, L. N., Josephson, M. E., Farshidi, A., et al.: Recurrent sustained ventricular tachycardia. 3. Role of the electrophysiologic study in selection of antiarrhythmic regimens. Circulation 58:986, 1978.
48. Horowitz, L. N., Josephson, M. E., and Kastor, J. A.: Intracardiac electrophysiologic studies as a method for the optimization of drug therapy in chronic ventricular arrhythmia. Prog. Cardiovasc. Dis. 23:81, 1980.
49. Hyman, A. L.: Permanent programmable pacemakers in the management of recurrent tachycardias. PACE 2:28, 1979.
50. Jeresaty, R. M.: Mitral valve prolapse–click syndrome. Prog. Cardiovasc. Dis. 15:623, 1973.
51. Jetlinek, M. V., and Lown, B.: Exercise stress testing for exposure of cardiac arrhythmias. Prog. Cardiovasc. Dis. 16:497, 1974.
52. Johnson, R. A., Hutter, A. M., Jr., DeSanctis, R. W., et al.: Chronic overdrive pacing in the control of refractory ventricular arrhythmias. Ann. Intern. Med. 80:380, 1974.
53. Josephson, M. E., Harken, A. H., and Horowitz, L. N.: Endocardial excision: a new surgical technique for the treatment of recurrent ventricular tachycardia. Circulation 60:1430, 1979.
54. Josephson, M. E., and Horowitz, L. N.: Electrophysiologic approach to therapy of recurrent sustained ventricular tachycardia. Am. J. Cardiol. 43:631, 1979.
55. Josephson, M. E., Horowitz, L. N., Farshidi, A., et al.: Recurrent sustained ventricular tachycardia. I. Mechanisms. Circulation 57:431, 1978.
56. Josephson, M. E., Horowitz, L. N., Spielman, S. R., et al.: Electrophysiologic and hemodynamic studies in patients resuscitated from cardiac arrest. Am. J. Cardiol. 46:948, 1980.
57. Keefe, D. L., Kates, R. E., and Harrison, D. C.: New antiarrhythmic drugs: their place in therapy. Drugs 22:363, 1981.
58. Kerin, N. Z., Rubenfire, M., Mansoor, N., et al.: Arrhythmias in variant angina pectoris. Circulation 60:1343, 1979.
59. Kimball, J. T., and Killip, T.: Aggressive treatment of arrhythmias in acute myocardial infarction (procedures and results). Prog. Cardiovasc. Dis. 10:483, 1968.
60. Kingston, M. E.: Hyperventilation in tricyclic antidepressant poisoning. Crit. Care Med. 7:550, 1979.
61. Koch-Weser, J.: Medical intelligence. N. Engl. J. Med. 300:473, 1979.
62. Kounis, N. G.: Iatrogenic "torsade de pointes" ventricular tachycardia. Postgrad. Med. J. 55:832, 1979.
63. Krikler, D. M.: Ventricular tachycardia as part of unusual clinical syndromes: a review. *In* Sandoe, E., and Julia, D. G. (eds.): Management of Ventricular Tachycardia—Role of Mexiletine. Amsterdam, Excerpta Medica, 1978, pp. 401–408.
64. Krikler, D. M., and Curry, P. V. L.: Torsade de pointes, an atypical ventricular tachycardia. Br. Heart J. 38:117, 1976.
65. Lown, B., and Graboys, T. B.: Management of patients with malignant ventricular arrhythmias. Am. J. Cardiol. 39:910, 1977.
66. Lown, B., and Graboys, T. B.: Ventricular premature beats and sudden cardiac death. Baylor Cardiology Series 3, No. 1:6, 1980.
67. Lown, B., Matta, R. J., and Besser, H. W.: Programmed trendscription. A new approach to electrocardiographic monitoring. J.A.M.A. 232:39, 1975.
68. Lown, B., Podrid, P. J., DeSilva, R. A., et al.: Sudden cardiac death—management of the patient at risk. Curr. Probl. Cardiol. 4:1, 1980.
69. MacLean, W. A. H., Plumb, V. J., and Waldo, A. L.: Transient entrainment and interruption of ventricular tachycardia. PACE 4:358, 1981.
70. Marcus, F. I., Fontaine, G. H., Frank, R., et al.: Clinical pharmacology and therapeutic applications of the antiarrhythmic agent, amiodarone. Am. Heart J. 101:480, 1981.

71. Marcus, F. I., Fontaine, G. H., Guiraudon, G., et al.: Right ventricular dysplasia: a report of 24 adult cases. Circulation 65:384, 1982.
72. Mason, J. W.: Efficacy of verapamil in recurrent ventricular tachycardia (VT). Am. J. Cardiol. 49:1015, 1982 (abstr.).
73. Mason, J. W., Buda, J., Stinson, E. B., et al.: Surgical therapy of ventricular tachyarrhythmias in ischemic heart disease using conventional techniques. *In* Bircks, W., Loogen, F., Schulte, H. D., and Seipel, L. (eds.): Medical and Surgical Management of Tachyarrhythmias. Berlin. Heidelberg, Springer-Verlag, 1980, pp. 177–182.
74. Mason, J. W., Stinson, E. B., Derby, G., et al.: Advantages of intraoperative activation sequence mapping for recurrent ventricular tachycardia. *In* Harrison, D. C., Winkle, R. A., and Mason, J. W. (eds.): Cardiac Arrhythmias—A Decade of Progress. Boston, G. K. Hall & Co., 1981, pp. 533–543.
75. Mason, J. W., Stinson, E. B., Oyer, P. E., et al.: Mapping-guided surgical therapy of refractory ventricular tachycardia (VT) due to coronary artery disease. Am. J. Cardiol. 49:947, 1982 (abstr.).
76. Mason, J. W., Stinson, E. B., Winkle, R. A., et al.: Mechanisms of ventricular tachycardia: wide, complex ignorance. Am. Heart J. 102:1083, 1981.
77. Mason, J. W., Stinson, E. B., Winkle, R. A., et al.: Surgery for ventricular tachyarrhythmia: efficacy of left ventricular aneurysm resection compared to operation guided by electrical activation mapping. Circulation 65:1148, 1982.
78. Mason, J. W., and Winkle, R. A.: Electrode-catheter arrhythmia induction in the selection and assessment of antiarrhythmic drug therapy for recurrent ventricular tachycardia. Circulation 58:971, 1978.
79. Mason, J. W., and Winkle, R. A.: Accuracy of the ventricular tachycardia–induction study for predicting long-term efficacy and inefficacy of antiarrhythmic drugs. N. Engl. J. Med. 303:1073, 1980.
80. Michelson, E. L., Speilman, S. R., Greenspan, A. M., et al.: Electrophysiologic study of the left ventricle: indications and safety. Chest 75:592, 1979.
81. Mirowski, M., Reid, P. R., Mower, M. M., et al.: Termination of malignant ventricular arrhythmias with an implanted automatic defibrillator in human beings. N. Engl. J. Med. 303:322, 1980.
82. Morady, F., Scheinman, M., and Hess, D.: Amiodarone in the management of patients with malignant ventricular arrhythmias. Circulation 64 (Suppl. 4):35, 1981 (abstr.).
83. Morady, F., Scheinman, M., and Hess, D.: The importance of left ventricular programmed stimulation during drug-testing in patients with ventricular tachycardia. Circulation 64 (Suppl. 4):IV–87, 1981 (abstr.).
84. Morganroth, J., Michelson, E. L., Horowitz, L. N., et al.: Limitations of routine long-term electrocardiographic monitoring to assess ventricular ectopic frequency. Circulation 58:408, 1978.
85. Moss, A. J., and Rivers, R. J., Jr.: Termination and inhibition of recurrent tachycardias by implanted pervenous pacemakers. Circulation 50:942, 1974.
86. Mounsey, P.: Intensive coronary care: arrhythmias after acute myocardial infarction. Am. J. Cardiol. 20:475, 1967.
87. Myerburg, R. J., Conde, C., Sheps, D. S., et al.: Antiarrhythmic drug therapy in survivors of prehospital cardiac arrest: comparison of effects on chronic ventricular arrhythmias and recurrent cardiac arrest. Circulation 59:855, 1979.
88. Myerburg, R. J., Kessler, K. M., Kiem, I., et al.: Relationship between plasma levels of procainamide, suppression of premature ventricular complexes and prevention of recurrent ventricular tachycardia. Circulation 64:280, 1981.
89 Opie, L. H.: Drugs and the heart: IV antiarrhythmic agents. Lancet 1:861, 1980.
90. Palileo, E., Ashley, W., Lam, W., et al.: Exercise-provocable right ventricular outflow tract tachycardia. Circulation 62 (Suppl. 3):III–276, 1980 (abstr.).
91. Peters, R. W., Shafton, E., Thomas, F. S., et al.: Radio-frequency-triggered pacemakers: uses and limitations—a long-term study. Ann. Intern. Med. 88:17, 1978.
92. Plotnick, G. D., Carliner, N. M., Fisher, M. L., et al.: Rest angina with transient S–T segment elevation. Correlation of clinical features with coronary anatomy. Am. J. Med. 65:257, 1978.
93. Podrid, P. J., and Lown, B.: Amiodarone therapy in symptomatic, sustained refractory atrial and ventricular tachyarrhythmias. Am. Heart J. 101:374, 1981.
94. Podrid, P. J., Schoeneberger, A., and Lown, B.: Disopyramide-induced congestive heart failure. N. Engl. J. Med. 302:614, 1980.
95. Reddy, C. P., and Gettes, L. S.: Use of isoproterenol as an aid to electric induction of chronic recurrent ventricular tachycardia. Am. J. Cardiol. 44:707, 1979.
96. Reddy, C. P., and Sartini, J. C.: Nonclinical polymorphic ventricular tachycardia induced by programmed cardiac stimulation: incidence, mechanisms and clinical significance. Circulation 62:988, 1980.
97. Robertson, J. F., Caine, M. E., Horowitz, L. H., et al.: Anatomic and electrophysiologic correlates of ventricular tachycardia requiring left ventricular stimulation. Am. J. Cardiol. 48:263, 1981.
98. Rosenbaum, M. B., Chiale, P. A., Halpern, M. S., et al.: Clinical efficacy of amiodarone as an antiarrhythmic agent. Am. J. Cardiol. 38:934, 1978.
99. Ross, A., DeWeese, J. A., and Yu, P. N.: Refractory ventricular arrhythmias in a patient with mitral valve prolapse. Successful control with mitral valve replacement. J. Electrocardiol. 11:289, 1978.
100. Ross, D. L., Keefe, D. L., Swerdlow, C. D., et al.: Efficacy of drug combinations in preventing induction of refractory ventricular tachycardia at electrophysiologic study. Circulation, 66:1205, 1982.
101. Ruskin, J. N., Garan, H., Poulin, F., et al.: Permanent radiofrequency ventricular pacing for management of drug-resistant ventricular tachycardia. Am. J. Cardiol. 46:317, 1980.
102. Sami, M., Mason, J. W., Peters, F., et al.: Clinical electrophysiologic effects of encainide, a newly developed antiarrhythmic agent. Am. J. Cardiol. 44:526, 1979.
103. Sanna, G., and Arcidiancon, R.: Chemical ventricular defibrillation of the human heart with bretylium tosylate. Am. J. Cardiol. 32:982, 1973.

104. Schaffer, W. A., and Cobb, L. A.: Recurrent ventricular fibrillation and modes of death in survivors of out-of-hospital ventricular fibrillation. N. Engl. J. Med. 293:259, 1975.
105. Schamroth, L.: Ventricular extrasystoles, ventricular tachycardia, and ventricular fibrillation: clinical-electrocardiographic considerations. Prog. Cardiovasc. Dis. 23:13, 1980.
106. Scherf, D., and Schott, A.: Extrasystoles and Allied Arrhythmias. 2nd ed. London, Heinemann, 1973, pp. 561–807.
107. Schwartz, P. J., Periti, M., and Malliani, A.: The long QT syndrome. Am. Heart J. 89:378, 1975.
108. Sclarovsky, S., Strasberg, B., Lewin, P. F., et al.: Polymorphous ventricular tachycardia: clinical features and treatment. Am. J. Cardiol. 44:339, 1979.
109. Segal, J. P., Stapleton, J. F., McClellan, J. R., et al.: Idiopathic cardiomyopathy: clinical features, prognosis and therapy. *In* Harvey, W. P. (ed.): Current Problems in Cardiology. Chicago-London, Year Book Medical Publishers, 1978, 3, No. 6, pp. 1–49.
110. Singh, B. N., Ellrodt, G., and Peter, C. T.: Verapamil: a review of its pharmacological properties and therapeutic use. Drugs 15:169, 1978.
111. Smith, T. W., Haber, E., Yeatman, L., et al.: Reversal of advanced digoxin intoxication with Fab fragments of digoxin–specific antibodies. N. Engl. J. Med. 294:797, 1976.
112. Smith, W. M., and Gallagher, J. J.: "Les torsades de pointes": an unusual ventricular arrhythmia. Ann. Intern. Med. 93:578, 1980.
113. Swedberg, J., and Malm, A.: Pacemaker stimulation in ventricular paroxysmal tachycardia. Acta Chir. Scand. 128:610, 1964.
114. Swerdlow, C. D., Blum, J., Winkle, R. A., et al.: Decreased incidence of antiarrhythmic drug efficacy at electrophysiologic study associated with use of a third extrastimulus. Am. Heart J., 104:1004, 1982.
115. Swerdlow, C. D., Echt, D. S., Winkle, R. A., et al.: Incidence of acute antiarrhythmic drug efficacy at electrophysiologic study. Circulation 82:IV–137, 1981.
116. Swerdlow, C. D., Echt, D. S., Winkle, R. A., et al.: Incidence of induction and drug prophylaxis of ventricular tachyarrhythmias: dependence on arrhythmia type. Clin. Res. 30:21A, 1982 (abstr.).
117. Swerdlow, C. D., Yu, E. O., Jacobson, E., et al.: Safety and efficacy of intravenous quinidine. Am. J. Cardiol. 49:1043, 1982 (abstr.).
118. Taylor, R. R., and Halliday, E. J.: Beta-adrenergic blockade in the treatment of exercise-induced paroxysmal ventricular tachycardia. Circulation 32:778, 1965.
119. The Norwegian Multicenter Study Group: Timolol-induced reduction in mortality and reinfarction in patients surviving acute myocardial infarction. N. Engl. J. Med. 304:801, 1981.
120. Tobis, J., and Das, B. N.: Cardiac complications in amitryptyline poisoning. Successful treatment with physostigmine. J.A.M.A. 235:1474, 1976.
121. Troup, P. J., and Zipes, D. P.: Aprindine treatment of recurrent ventricular tachycardia in patients with mitral valve prolapse. Am. Heart J. 97:322, 1979.
122. Vandepol, C. J., Farshidi, A., Spielman, S. R., et al.: Incidence and clinical significance of induced ventricular tachycardia. Am. J. Cardiol. 45:725, 1980.
123. Velebit, V., Podrid, P., Lown, B., et al.: Aggravation and provocation of ventricular arrhythmias by antiarrhythmic drugs. Circulation 65:886, 1981.
124. Von Cappeler, D., Copeland, G. D., Stern, T. N., et al.: Digitalis intoxication. A clinical report of 148 cases. Ann. Intern. Med. 50:869, 1959.
125. Waldo, A. L., Krongrad, E., Kupersmith, J., et al.: Ventricular paired-pacing to control rapid ventricular heart rate following open heart surgery. Circulation 53:176, 1976.
126. Waldo, A. L., and MacLean, W. A. H.: The Diagnosis and Treatment of Arrhythmias Following Open Heart Surgery—Emphasis on the Use of Epicardial Wire Electrodes. Mt. Kisco, N.Y., Futura, 1980.
127. Warnowicz, M. A., and Denes, P.: Chronic ventricular arrhythmias: comparative drug effectiveness and toxicity. Prog. Cardiovasc. Dis. 23:225, 1980.
128. Waxman, M. B., and Wald, R. W.: Termination of ventricular tachycardia by an increase in cardiac vagal drive. Circulation 56:385, 1977.
129. Waxman, M. B., Wald, R. W., Finley, J. P., et al.: Valsalva termination of ventricular tachycardia. Circulation 62:843, 1980.
130. Wei, J. Y., Bulkley, B. H., Schaeffer, A. H., et al.: Mitral-valve prolapse syndrome and recurrent ventricular tachyarrhythmias. Ann. Intern. Med. 89:6, 1978.
131. Wellens, H. J. J., Bär, F. W. H. M., and Lie, K. I.: The value of the electrocardiogram in the differential diagnosis of tachycardia with a widened QRS complex. Am. J. Med. 6:27, 1978.
132. Wellens, H. J. J., Bär, F. W. H. M., Lie, K. I., et al.: Effect of procainamide, propranolol and verapamil on mechanism of tachycardia in patients with chronic recurrent ventricular tachycardia. Am. J. Cardiol. 40:579, 1977.
133. Wellens, H. J. J., Bär, F. W. H. M., Vanagt, E. J. D. M., et al.: The differentiation between ventricular tachycardia and supraventricular tachycardia with aberrant conduction: the value of the 12–lead electrocardiogram. *In* Wellens, H. J. J., and Kulbertus, H. E. (eds.): What's New in Electrocardiography. The Hague, Martinus Nijhoff, 1981, pp. 184–199.
134. Wellens, H. J. J., Bär, F. W. H. M., Vanagt, E. J. D. M., et al.: Medical treatment of ventricular tachycardia: considerations in the selection of patients for surgical treatment. Am. J. Cardiol. 49:186, 1982.
135. Wellens, H. J. J., Schuilenburg, R. M., and Durrer, D.: Electrical stimulation of the heart in patients with ventricular tachycardia. Circulation 46:216, 1972.
136. Winkle, R. A.: Antiarrhythmic drug effect mimicked by spontaneous variability of ventricular ectopy. Circulation 57:1116, 1978.
137. Winkle, R. A., Alderman, E. L., Fitzgerald, J. W., et al.: Treatment of recurrent symptomatic ventricular tachycardia. Ann. Intern. Med. 85:1, 1976.
138. Winkle, R. A., Mason, J. W., Griffin, J. C., et al.: Malignant ventricular tachyarrhythmias associated with the use of encainide. Am. Heart J. 102:857, 1981.

139. Winkle, R. A., Meffin, P. J., and Harrison, D. C.: Long-term tocainide therapy for ventricular arrhythmia. Circulation 57:1088, 1978.
140. Wit, A., Steiner, C., and Damato, A.: Electrophysiologic effects of bretylium tosylate on single fibers of the canine specialized conducting system and ventricle. J. Pharmacol. Exp. Ther. 173:344, 1970.
141. Woodson, R. D., Friesen, W. G., and Ames, A. L.: Use of atrial pacing in cardiac surgical patients. Circulation 36 (Suppl. 2):275, 1967 (abstr.).
142. Worthley, L. I. G.: Lithium toxicity and refractory cardiac arrhythmia treated with intravenous magnesium. Anaesth. Intensive Care 2:357, 1974.
143. Wu, D., Lou, H. C., and Hung, J. S.: Exercise-triggered paroxysmal ventricular tachycardia. Ann. Intern. Med. 95:410, 1981.
144. Zipes, D. P., Foster, P. R., Troup, P. J., et al.: Atrial induction of ventricular tachycardia: Reentry versus triggered automaticity. Am. J. Cardiol. 44:1, 1979.

6

Emergency Treatment of Supraventricular Tachyarrhythmias

JESSE DAVIS
and RUEY J. SUNG

Supraventricular tachyarrhythmias are abnormally rapid rhythms originating above the bifurcation of the bundle of His. In many clinical settings, supraventricular tachyarrhythmias do not cause symptoms or hemodynamic instability and do not constitute clinical emergencies. However, prompt restoration to a hemodynamically stable rhythm is imperative in patients with symptomatic hypotension or critical compromise of blood flow to vital organs. Hemodynamic tolerance of supraventricular tachyarrhythmias depends primarily on the ventricular rate, the duration of each attack, and the presence of associated cardiovascular disease. Adverse interaction among these factors can produce dizziness, confusion, syncope, angina pectoris, and dyspnea. Rarely, supraventricular tachyarrhythmia can degenerate to ventricular flutter-fibrillation.

This chapter emphasizes the clinical presentation and electrocardiographic features of patients with supraventricular tachyarrhythmias requiring emergency treatment. This review will update current understanding of the mechanisms of these tachyarrhythmias, stress ECG features facilitating prompt diagnosis, and recommend treatment based on underlying mechanisms and the associated clinical setting.

The supraventricular tachyarrhythmias considered are sinus tachycardia; the paroxysmal supraventricular tachycardias; atrial fibrillation; atrial flutter; and atrial tachycardia including automatic or ectopic atrial tachycardia, atrial tachycardia with atrioventricular block, and multifocal atrial tachycardia.

MECHANISMS

At least three basic mechanisms may account for the occurrence of supraventricular tachyarrhythmias: reentry, enhanced automaticity, and triggered activity.

Reentry. Reentry requires the presence of two pathways differing in conduction velocity and refractoriness.[87, 104] A premature beat that is blocked in one pathway can conduct slowly through the other pathway. If slow conduction in the latter pathway is sufficient to allow recovery of excitability in the previously blocked area, the impulse may reenter this area. Perpetuation of this reentry phenomenon produces circus movement and a reentrant tachycardia.

Enhanced Automaticity. Enhanced automaticity may occur in normal or diseased cardiac fibers, through different mechanisms. In specialized atrial and ventricular fibers, acceleration of spontaneous diastolic (phase 4) depolarization normally occurs during adrenergic stimulation.[60] In contrast, abnormal automaticity develops differently. Diseased fibers have depressed or abnormally low resting transmembrane voltages. Membrane instability or extraneous current can depolarize these diseased fibers the shortened distance to threshold, producing spontaneous action potentials.[92]

Triggered Activity. Triggered activity has been described as a third mechanism for tachyarrythmias.[106] This form of automaticity never arises spontaneously but can be triggered in susceptible fibers. Immediately after full repolarization, these fibers partially depolarize, an event recorded as delayed after-depolarization.[78, 79] If the after-depolarization reaches threshold voltage, a new action potential is triggered. Repetition of these events can lead to sustained tachycardia. To date, the clinical behavior of triggered arrhythmias has been incompletely characterized. Full confirmation of a triggered mechanism for clinical arrhythmias still awaits future study.

HEMODYNAMIC CONSEQUENCES OF SUPRAVENTRICULAR TACHYARRHYTHMIA

If loss of coordinated atrial contraction occurs during supraventricular tachyarrhythmias, resting cardiac output may fall by 5 to 15 per cent in patients with normal hearts[6] and by as much as 20 to 40 per cent in those with heart disease.[4, 6, 63] Rapid ventricular rates shorten diastole and compromise ventricular filling, thereby decreasing cardiac output and blood pressure (Fig. 6–1).

Blood pressure usually falls dramatically with onset of supraventricular tachycardia.[18] After 20 to 30 seconds, blood pressure is partially restored by baroreceptor mechanisms that increase systemic arterial resistance and slow the tachycardia rate.[18, 34] If reflex mechanisms fail to rescue blood pressure, the patient may develop symptoms. The severity of hemodynamic instability usually depends on the ventricular rate, the duration of tachycardia, and the functional competence of the left ventricle.

Patients with normal hearts may experience no initial symptoms during supraventricular tachyarrhythmias other than an awareness of rapid heart action.[4] As the tachyarrhythmia continues for hours to days, cardiac output and blood pressure may decline, even in individuals with normal hearts.[4] Pulmonary vascular congestion and dyspnea may develop or polyuria can occur in patients who do not have congestive heart failure.[51, 107] Angina can also arise during supraventricular tachycardia in the absence of fixed coronary obstruction, but the mechanism of angina in this setting is unknown.[34]

Heart disease will lower hemodynamic tolerance of rapid heart rates if the lesion interferes with left ventricular filling, ventricular contraction, or outflow of ventricular blood.[22, 37, 81] Inflow obstruction by atrial thrombus, tumor, or mitral valvular stenosis acts to limit ventricular filling during tachycardia, resulting in pulmonary venous congestion and dyspnea as well as reduced cardiac output. Ventricular hypertrophy may also compromise diastolic filling. Concentric or asymmetric hypertrophy is accompanied by sluggish relaxation and poor diastolic compliance,[81] which may impede ventricular filling, reduce the cardiac index, and lead to dyspnea, hypotension, or syncope during tachycardia. Loss of atrioventricular (AV) coordination during AV nodal reentrant tachycardia or atrial fibrillation would further aggravate these hemodynamic derangements.[6] Increased resistance to coronary flow has been demonstrated in hypertrophied ventricles and could limit subendocardial coronary flow during the stress of tachycardia,[72] although any relation to clinical angina is as yet unproved. In patients with congestive cardiomyopathy, depressed ventricular ejection and shortened diastole may severely compromise cardiac output during tachycardia.[62] Obstruction to ventricular emptying by severe aortic stenosis[37] or midventricular hypertrophy[22] may also compromise cardiac output, decrease aortic diastolic pressure, and reduce coronary perfusion during tachycardia, leading to angina, hypotension, or syncope.

Regional blood flow may also be compromised during tachycardia in patients with vascular disease. Disease in coronary, cerebral, renovascular, or peripheral vascular circulations may be unmasked or vascular symptoms worsened during supraventricular tachyarrhythmias.[35] Although angina pectoris may develop during tachycardia in the absence of coronary obstruction,[34] chest pain has also occurred in middle-aged patients with subclinical coronary disease who become pain-free after conversion to sinus rhythm.[98]

DIAGNOSIS AND MANAGEMENT

Sinus Tachycardia

Sinus tachycardia is due to acceleration of sinus rhythm to a rate between 100 and 150 beats per minute or higher.[3] The P-wave morphology and P-R interval are identical to

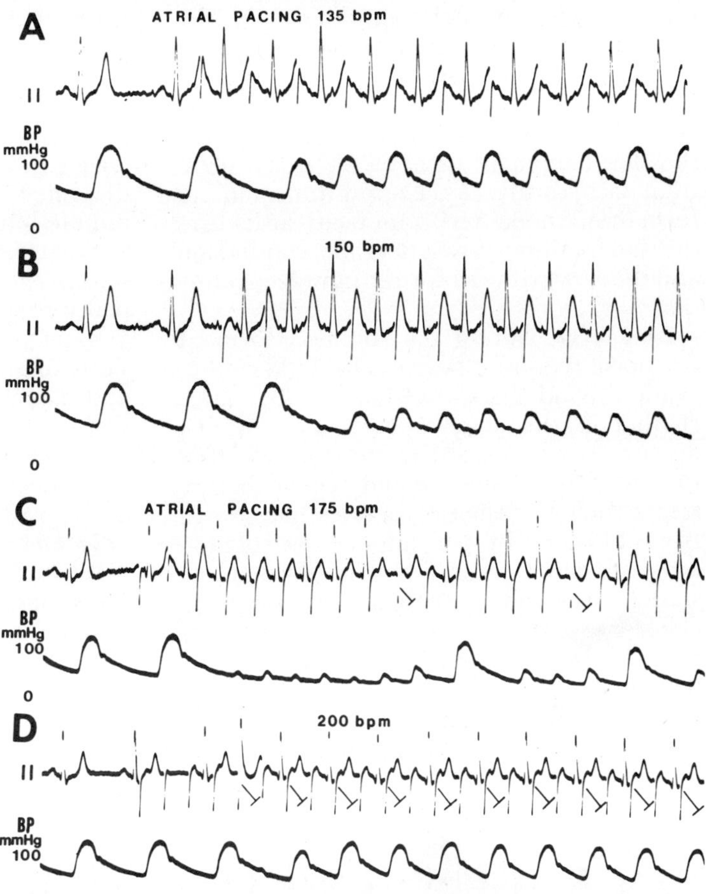

Figure 6–1. Effects of heart rate on blood pressure. ECG lead II and femoral arterial pressure are simultaneously recorded. *A,* During atrial pacing at a rate of 135 beats per min (bpm), systolic pressure falls from 130 to 115 mm Hg. *B,* An increase in atrial pacing rate to 150 bpm drops systolic pressure to 100 mm Hg. *C,* A further increase in atrial pacing rate to 175 bpm drops systolic pressure to 70 mm Hg. It is of note that development of AV Wenckebach intermittently restores the blood pressure response. *D,* During atrial pacing at 200 bpm, 2:1 AV block (ventricular response of 100 per min) prevents a fall in blood pressure.

those during sinus rhythm at comparable heart rates. Carotid sinus massage may slow the tachycardia rate transiently during application but does not terminate sinus tachycardia. The electrophysiologic mechanism is presumed to be enhancement of normal sinus node automaticity, possibly related to autonomic dysfunction in some patients.[3] Sinus tachycardia is usually a physiologic response to such conditions as fever, hypovolemia, congestive heart failure, infection, high cardiac output states, or endocrinopathy, and seldom requires specific treatment. Correction of the underlying disease process usually slows the rate of sinus tachycardia. Propranolol or other beta-adrenergic blocking agents may be required in symptomatic patients in whom no underlying illness can be identified.

The Paroxysmal Supraventricular Tachycardias (PSVT)

Of patients admitted to major referral centers for electrophysiologic study of clinical PSVT, 60 to 70 per cent demonstrate reentry over dual AV nodal pathways, 10 to 30 per cent have reentry utilizing an extranodal pathway, 4 per cent demonstrate sinoatrial node reentry, 4 per cent have intra-atrial reentry, and 4 per cent have automatic atrial tachycardia.[48, 109]

PSVT Due to Reentry Within Atrioventricular Node

This form of PSVT results from reentry over two functionally distinct pathways, probably within the AV node.[46, 108] In the most common form of PSVT, a faster conducting pathway has a relatively long refractory period and a more slowly conducting pathway has a shorter refractory period. During sinus rhythm, an atrial impulse enters both pathways but reaches the His-Purkinje system over the fast pathway. A premature impulse may block in the fast pathway and conduct slowly over the slow pathway, prolonging the P-R interval of the surface ECG. After completing slow antegrade conduction, the impulse could travel retrograde over a recovered fast pathway, generate an atrial echo complex,[46] and reenter the slow pathway to establish circus movement tachycardia (Fig. 6–2). This is sometimes referred to as the slow-fast (common) form of AV nodal reentrant tachycardia. A fast-slow (uncommon) form of AV nodal reentrant tachycardia uses the fast pathway for antegrade conduction and the slow pathway for retrograde conduction.[106, 108]

Diagnosis. During the common form of AV nodal reentrant tachycardia, QRS configuration is identical to that during sinus rhythm in the absence of bundle branch disease. The tachycardia rate is usually 150 to 180 beats per minute and regular before treatment, but tachycardia rates may range from 115 to 214 per minute. Retrograde atrial activation occurs over the fast pathway so that atrial and ventricular activation coincide in two thirds of patients, or P waves closely follow QRS in about one third of these patients[49, 109] (Fig. 6–2*A*).

By contrast, retrograde atrial activation occurs over the slow pathway in the uncommon form of AV nodal reentrant tachycardia, so that retrograde P waves are inscribed far after the QRS complex (Fig. 6–2*B*). This "uncommon" pattern is seen in only 4 to 12 per cent of patients with AV nodal reentrant tachycardia.[49, 108] In these patients, tachycardia rates vary from 133 to 187 beats per minute but average 150 per minute.[108]

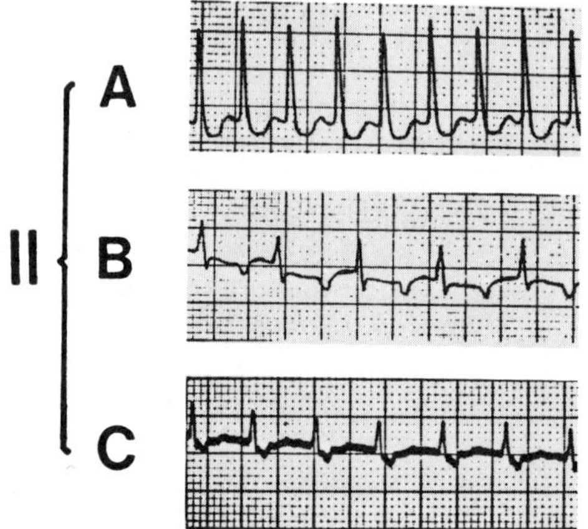

Figure 6–2. Three different forms of PSVT. *A,* The common (slow-fast) form of AV nodal reentrant tachycardia uses a slow AV nodal pathway for antegrade conduction and a fast AV nodal pathway for retrograde conduction. During the tachycardia, the retrograde P wave is inscribed within the QRS complex, hardly discernible on the ECG. *B,* The uncommon (fast-slow) form of AV nodal reentrant tachycardia uses a fast AV nodal pathway for antegrade conduction and a slow AV nodal pathway for retrograde conduction. During the tachycardia, the retrograde P wave is inscribed far behind the QRS complex. *C,* AV reciprocating tachycardia uses the AV node–His-Purkinje system for antegrade conduction and an accessory bypass tract for retrograde conduction. During the tachycardia, the retrograde P wave is inscribed immediately behind the QRS complex.

Treatment. Dual AV nodal pathways are sensitive to autonomic influence with the slow pathway showing greatest vulnerability to vagotonia.[46] Reflex vagotonia during carotid sinus massage slows conduction in the slow pathway and usually decelerates tachycardia slightly, before termination. Termination occurs with an atrial echo complex in the common form of AV nodal reentrant tachycardia, or without an atrial echo complex in the uncommon form.[46, 47, 99]

When tachycardia is unaltered by carotid sinus massage alone, the Valsalva maneuver may be helpful (Fig. 6–3). Breath-holding during facial immersion in cold water may also be effective in nonanxious patients. If these vagal maneuvers fail to convert tachycardia in asymptomatic patients, pharmacologic agents can often be used to supplement vagotonia.[99] Edrophonium (Tensilon), a reversible inhibitor of acetylcholine esterase, may enhance the effect of concurrent carotid sinus massage (Fig. 6–4). Metaraminol (Aramine) or phenylephrine (Neo-Synephrine) can be used to elevate blood pressure in young, mildly hypotensive patients without cardiac or cerebrovascular disease. The resultant baroceptor stimulation may augment vagotonia of carotid sinus massage, to terminate PSVT.

Vagal maneuvers fail to terminate AV nodal reentrant tachycardia in less than 10 per cent of clinically stable patients,[99] necessitating the use of antiarrhythmic agents in emergency management. Verapamil has impressive credentials for successfully terminating PSVT after intravenous infusion[83, 91] and decreasing its prevalence during chronic oral administration;[40] it is probably the drug of choice for PSVT due to AV nodal reentry.[88] Digitalis and propranolol may also be used. Verapamil, digitalis, and beta-adrenergic blocking agents act to prolong refractoriness and slow conduction within the AV node.[102] The predominant effect involves the slow pathway,[47] producing antegrade conduction block in the common form of AV nodal reentrant tachycardia.

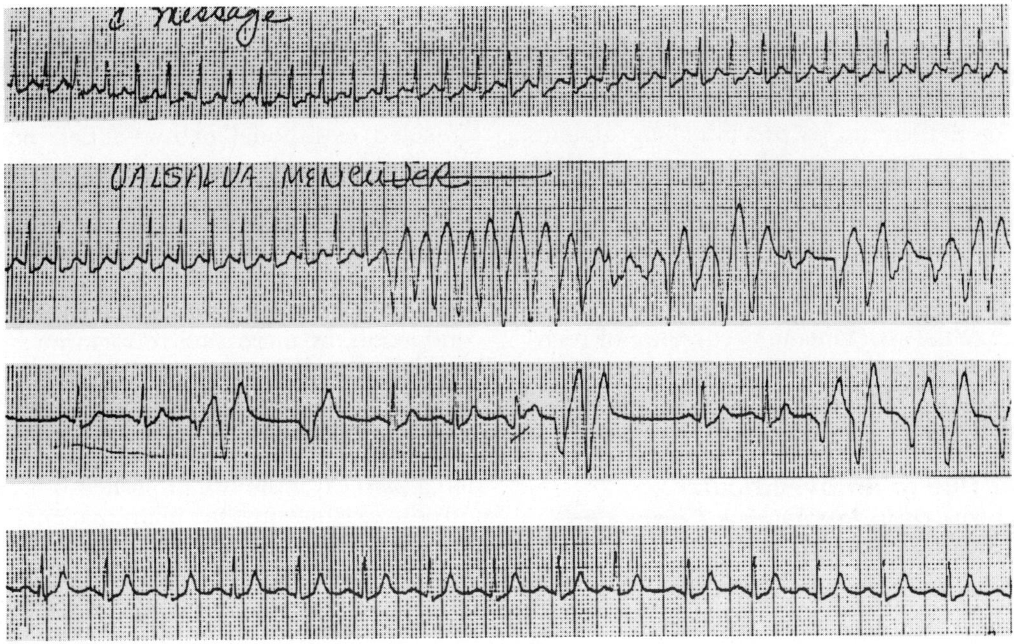

Figure 6–3. Termination of PSVT with vagal maneuvers. The tracings are continuous. Carotid sinus massage fails to terminate the supraventricular tachycardia at a rate of 215 beats per min (top tracing). Valsalva maneuver induces transient ventricular irritability and converts the tachycardia to sinus rhythm.

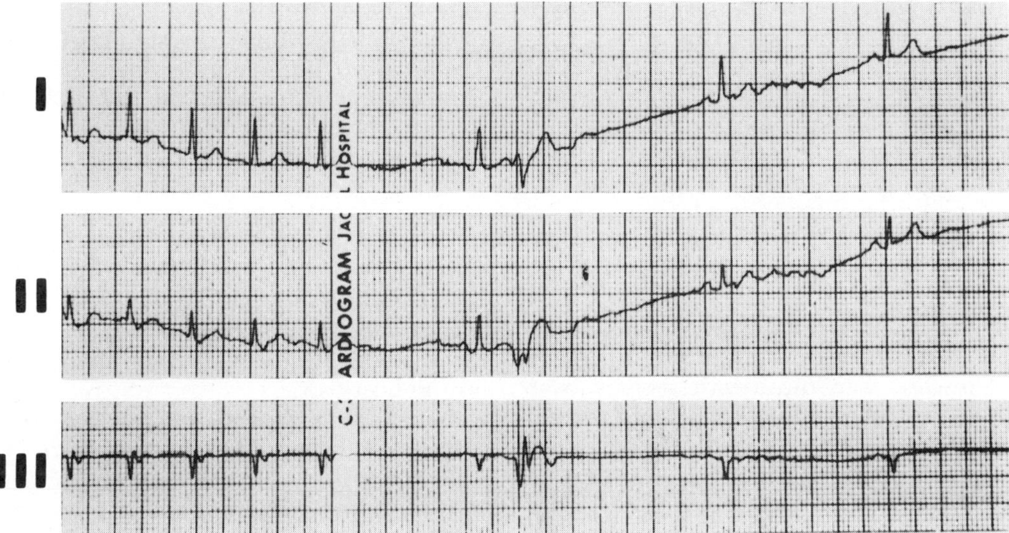

Figure 6–4. Termination of PSVT with intravenous edrophonium (Tensilon). After a bolus injection of 10 mg edrophonium, the supraventricular tachycardia at a rate of 137 beats per min is converted to a normal sinus rhythm. Note postedrophonium effects—sinus bradycardia and one ventricular premature beat.

Procainamide, a quinidine-like (type I) agent has been used intravenously for acute control of AV nodal reentrant tachycardia.[73, 111] It is not the agent of first choice, but can be used when verapamil, digitalis, or beta-adrenergic blocking agents fail to prevent symptomatic supraventricular tachycardia or if their use is precluded by digitalis excess, bronchospasm, allergy, or risk of adverse drug interaction. Procainamide disrupts reentry by prolonging refractoriness in fast AV nodal pathways.[111] Type I agents also suppress premature atrial and ventricular depolarizations and therefore serve to discourage the spontaneous occurrence of reentrant tachycardia. Finally, intravenous amiodarone may terminate PSVT in unusually resistant cases.[88, 97]

PSVT Due to Atrioventricular Reciprocation Involving a Concealed Extranodal Pathway

In approximately 15 to 20 per cent of patients with PSVT, tachycardia occurs by way of a "macro-reentry" pathway. This route incorporates the AV node and Purkinje system for antegrade conduction to the ventricle. The impulse returns to the atrium via an extranodal pathway.[48] These patients do not demonstrate ventricular pre-excitation during sinus rhythm since the extranodal pathway conducts only in a retrograde direction, i.e., the accessory pathway is "concealed." Tachycardia starts when a premature atrial impulse conducts antegrade via the AV node and bundle branches, and then proceeds retrograde over the extranodal pathway to the atrium and reenters the AV node to continue the circus movement. A retrograde P wave is inscribed immediately after the QRS complex in the ECG (Fig. 6–2*C*).

Diagnosis. As a group, these patients are slightly younger with a lower prevalence of heart disease than those with reentry over dual AV nodal pathways. The tachycardia rate is slightly faster at 156 to 230 beats per minute, averaging 178 per minute, despite the larger anatomic reentry pathway.[85] The ECG shows P waves closely following the QRS complex. Most patients have left-sided concealed pathways and this should be suspected if the P wave in lead I is inverted. The development of left bundle branch block slows the tachycardia rate, presumably because the circulating impulse must proceed from the right bundle branch through ventricular muscle mass to reach the concealed extranodal pathway. For this reason, abrupt slowing of the tachycardia rate with the development of left bundle branch block strongly suggests AV reentry via a concealed left-sided extranodal pathway. Left bundle branch block during AV nodal reentrant tachycardia is unusual.[46, 48]

Treatment. Carotid sinus massage and the Valsalva maneuver may terminate reciprocating supraventricular tachycardia, which uses an extranodal pathway for retrograde conduction, by increasing refractoriness and blocking antegrade conduction within the AV node

Drug response of PSVT is less predictable when reentry occurs via a concealed extranodal pathway although published trials may introduce a bias in that many patients may have proved refractory to digoxin before referral for study.[29, 48, 91] Verapamil is usually effective in blocking antegrade conduction in the AV node and in terminating tachycardia.[91] Propranolol alone or in combination with digoxin will slow conduction and increase antegrade refractoriness within the AV node, preventing tachycardia in 30 to 70 per cent of patients.[29, 91] Procainamide and amiodarone prolong refractoriness at multiple sites including the atrium, bundle branches, ventricular muscle, and extranodal pathway, but are not consistently effective in controlling this reciprocating tachycardia. Amiodarone also effects the AV node.

PSVT Due to Sinoatrial Reentry

Reentry can also occur at the sinoatrial node or intra-atrial sites. Despite similar mechanisms, the clinical behavior of sinoatrial and intra-atrial reentrant tachycardia appears to differ, probably reflecting differences in the electrophysiologic characteristics of the host tissue.

Sinoatrial reentrant tachycardia (SART) is present in 4 per cent of patients with PSVT referred for cardiac electrophysiologic study.[29] This arrhythmia can be initiated and terminated by extrastimuli, suggesting a reentrant mechanism. As fibers in the sinoatrial node and perinodal region are functionally similar to AV node fibers,[70] a premature impulse can conduct slowly through the sinoatrial node and exit to re-excite sur-

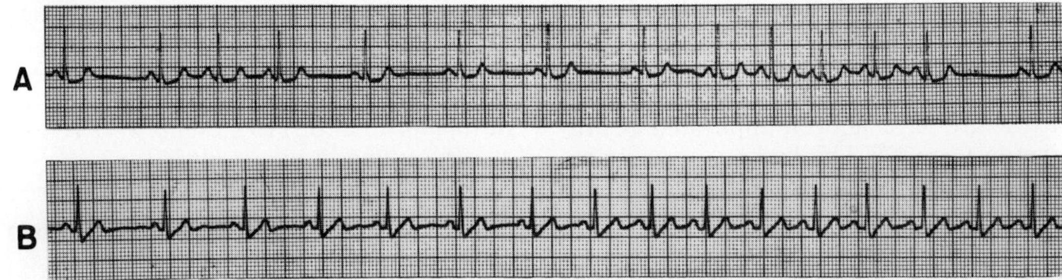

Figure 6–5. Sinoatrial reentrant tachycardia. *A*, Bursts of sinoatrial reentrant rhythm. *B*, Spontaneous initiation of sustained SART at a rate of 105 beats per min. Note that the P-wave morphology during the tachycardia is similar to that of sinus rhythm, and that the initiation of tachycardia does not require prolongation of the P-R interval.

rounding atrial tissue. Tachycardia initiation does not require P-R interval prolongation as in AV nodal reentrant tachycardia (Fig. 6–5).

Diagnosis. The existence of SART has been well documented.[19, 70] ECGs taken during this tachycardia show P waves similar to those pressnt during normal sinus rhythm. P waves always precede the QRS complex, and the P-R interval is similar to that during sinus rhythm at comparable rates. Heart rates during SART tend to be slower than rates typical for AV node reentry, ranging from 80 to 200 per minute but usually below 150 per minute. Typically, SART is sustained for only brief periods or single sinoatrial echo complexes.[55] An abrupt change in sinus rate could suggest paroxysmal sinoatrial reentry.

Treatment. Asymptomatic episodes of SART may not require treatment. The sinoatrial node has extensive vagal innervation and carotid massage has been reported to terminate SART successfully.[19, 69, 70] P-R interval prolongation may occur during carotid sinus massage, but careful review of ECG recordings should confirm that P-R prolongation and sinus slowing are not consistently coincident in patients with SART. Propranolol and verapamil may also be effective, but caution is required in patients with known sinus node dysfunction.

PSVT Due to Intra-Atrial Reentry

Intra-atrial reentrant tachycardia (IART) has been described but the number of carefully studied patients is small.[69, 110] The clinical setting and ECG presentation of IART may be similar to those of SART. However, P-wave morphology does not resemble sinus P waves in all 12 ECG leads, and the P-R interval may be short. Owing to the dearth of reported experience with IART as documented by clinical electrophysiologic study, its response to antiarrhythmic drug intervention is not well characterized. As a practical matter, the ECG appearance of IART may be indistinguishable from that of atrial tachycardia due to enhanced automaticity, so that emergency management of tachycardia by these two mechanisms is identical in many cases. Intravenous procainamide may abolish intra-atrial reentry. Digoxin or verapamil may increase AV nodal refractoriness to slow the ventricular rate.

Atrial Fibrillation

The bulk of evidence favors multiple reentrant pathways, usually in the presence of atrial disease.[49] Atrial fibrillation can be induced by atrial pacing at 400 to 600 beats per minute but self-terminates within seconds in normal atria. Induced atrial fibrillation may persist in patients who develop sustained atrial fibrillation clinically.

Diagnosis. Atrial fibrillation can occur at any age but tends to appear in patients with heart disease, so most cases arise in those over 40 years of age.[25] Both paroxysmal and sustained forms exist, and the paroxysmal pattern may evolve to established atrial fibrillation in patients with diseased atria.[2, 25] Paroxysmal atrial fibrillation often develops during clinical illness. Apathetic hyperthyroidism, alcoholic cardiomyopathy with or without heavy ("binge") drinking, febrile illness such as pneumonia or sepsis, pulmonary embolus, and acute myocardial infarction are common examples. Less commonly, myocarditis, chest trauma, subarachnoid hemorrhage, surgical procedures, or electrolyte disturbances provide the clinical setting.

Atrial fibrillation develops in 10 per cent of patients during acute myocardial infarction. Pericarditis, atrial ischemia or infarction, and atrial distention during congestive heart failure have all been implicated as precipitating factors.[37] The higher mortality associated with atrial fibrillation in this setting has been attributed to a subset of patients with more extensive myocardial damage.[17, 39]

Electrocardiographic hallmarks of atrial fibrillation include irregular baseline oscillations at 400 to 700 per minute and irregular ventricular response. The "f" waves are most visible in lead VI or the inferior frontal leads II, III, and aVF.

Occasionally, the ventricular rate is slow and regular during atrial fibrillation owing to advanced AV block with junctional or idioventricular escape rhythm. This presentation results from abnormally prolonged refractoriness in the AV node caused by disease or excessive digitalis intake.

Six to 15 per cent of patients with atrial fibrillation have no demonstrable heart disease.[66] These individuals tend to be asymptomatic, have moderate ventricular rates, and rarely constitute cardiac emergencies, but their arrhythmia resists conversion to sinus mechanism.[25, 66]

Treatment. The approach to treatment of atrial fibrillation depends on hemodynamic tolerance and symptoms. DC cardioversion is required for severe hypotension or hypoperfusion of vital organs. Propranolol may reduce the risk of ventricular arrhythmias during emergency cardioversion after excessive digoxin loading.

Drug therapy may be attempted in less urgent settings to increase AV node refractoriness and slow ventricular response. Digoxin is still the agent of choice in patients with atrial fibrillation and congestive heart failure, but it is also well tolerated in those with normal hearts. The objective of digitalis therapy is to reduce the ventricular rate. Digitalis administration can be performed rapidly using ventricular rate reduction as a guide.[108] Large intravenous doses of rapid-acting digitalis preparations are sometimes required but the safety of large doses in this setting is controversial.[58, 66] Ventricular deceleration may be resistant to digitalis in ill patients with increased sympathetic tone.[58] Low-dose propranolol is an effective adjunct to digoxin, to control the ventricular rate if active bronchospasm or severely compromised ventricular function do not preclude its use.

Intravenous verapamil is also effective in controlling the ventricular rate during atrial fibrillation: 111 of 115 patients were reported as responding in one study.[83]

Atrial Fibrillation in the Pre-Excitation Syndromes

Patients with pre-excitation syndromes may be at unique risk if they develop atrial fibrillation or flutter. Ordinarily, AV node refractoriness limits the ventricular rate to less than 180 beats per minute during atrial fibrillation, but very rapid ventricular rates may develop in patients with accessory pathways that bypass the AV node.[27] These extranodal or partial AV nodal bypass tracts do not share the same rate-related refractoriness characteristics of the normal AV node, so that ventricular rates may exceed 250 per minute during atrial fibrillation in up to 25 per cent of these patients.[52] At very rapid rates, early ventricular activation can lead to fibrillation.[52]

During sinus rhythm, extranodal AV pathways may shorten the P-R interval and distort the initial QRS vector (delta wave) owing to ventricular pre-excitation in Wolff-Parkinson-White syndrome. Partial AV nodal bypass tract or rapid AV node conduction may shorten the P-R interval without a delta wave in Lown-Ganong-Levine syndrome. Atrial fibrillation is the second most common supraventricular arrhythmia in Wolff-Parkinson-White syndrome (20–30%) after reciprocating tachycardia; atrial flutter is rare.[49] Ventricular fibrillation developed in 11 per cent of 163 patients with pre-excitation evaluated at one large referral center[27] and was related to atrial fibrillation in most cases.[52]

Diagnosis. During atrial fibrillation, the ECG demonstrates an irregular, wide-complex tachyarrhythmia due to antegrade impulse movement over the extranodal connection. In patients with partial AV node bypass tracts or short AV node refractoriness, an irregular, narrow-complex tachyarrhythmia develops at rapid ventricular rates.

Treatment. External DC cardioversion is required during atrial fibrillation or flutter with hemodynamic compromise.[27, 52] Pre-excitation may be observed after cardioversion to sinus rhythm. At that time, procainamide should be administered to prolong refractoriness in the bypass tract and to discourage atrial ectopy or recurrent atrial fibrillation.

If the ventricular rate is hemodynamically tolerated, intravenous procainamide can be used to prolong refractoriness in the extranodal pathways and to slow ventricular response. If this is successful, the QRS complex will narrow as the ventricular rate slows, indicating that all antegrade conduction is occurring over the AV node and bundle branches. Lidocaine has inconsistent effects on ventricular response over extranodal pathways, especially for those patients with pathways having short refractory periods[1] (Fig. 6–6). Digitalis will speed the ventricular rate in up to 30 per cent of adults with atrial fibrillation and extranodal pathways,[27] and should be avoided both during emergency treatment and for prophylaxis.

After rate stabilization, careful cardiac electrophysiologic study is required to select an appropriate antiarrhythmic regimen. This procedure allows prospective evaluation of drug effect on bypass tract refractoriness and ventricular rate after elective reinduction of atrial fibrillation. Surgical and transvenous ablation techniques to destroy the AV node and His bundle have been used successfully in a few patients who were completely refractory to medical management.[65] The transvenous technique is not effective for atrial fibrillation with antegrade conduction over a bypass tract.

Occasionally, atrial fibrillation in adults presents as a narrow-complex arrhythmia with very rapid ventricular rates. In these patients, ventricular rates may exceed 220 beats per minute owing to shortened refractoriness and enhanced conduction through the AV node or over an atrionodal or atriohisian bypass tract.[8] Syncopal or presyncopal patients should receive DC cardioversion. In hemodynamically stable individuals, vagal maneuvers with propranolol and/or digoxin may slow the ventricular rate.

Atrial Flutter

Current evidence favors either reentry or triggered automaticity as the mechanism for atrial flutter.[15, 49, 78] Most significantly, atrial flutter can be induced and terminated by extrastimulation or rapid pacing.[15, 99] On the other hand, substrates for reentry, enhanced automaticity, and triggered activity may coexist in diseased cardiac tissue.[87] Thus, an automatic ectopic depolarization falling in the atrial vulnerable period could precipitate a reentrant arrhythmia.

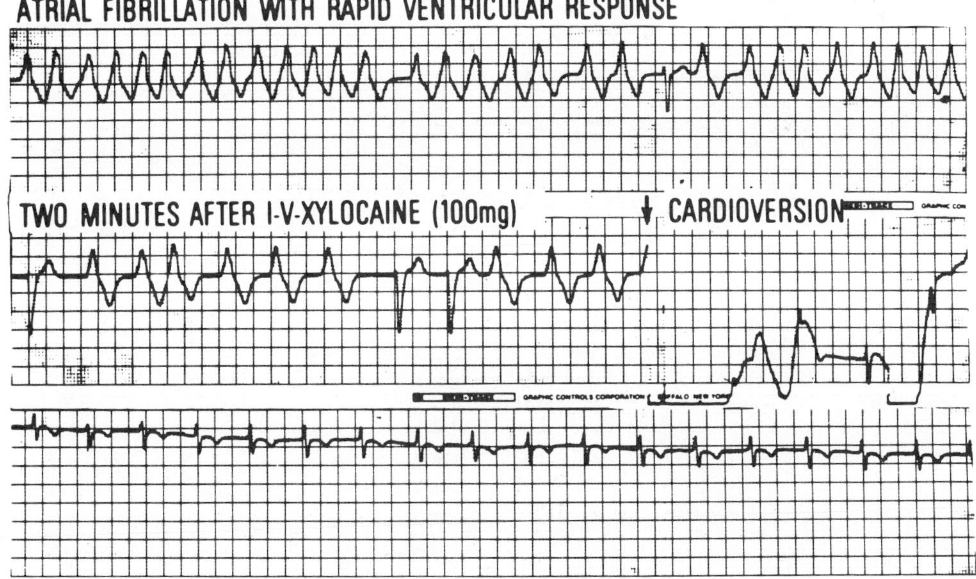

Figure 6–6. Rapid ventricular response during atrial fibrillation associated with Wolff-Parkinson-White syndrome. The tracings are not continuous. The ventricular rate averages 190 beats per min during atrial fibrillation. Antegrade conduction over an accessory bypass tract is evident. Lidocaine (Xylocaine) slows the ventricular rate to approximately 110 bpm by its action on the accessory bypass tract. DC countershock subsequently converts atrial fibrillation to sinus rhythm.

Diagnosis. The atrial flutter rate is typically 300 per minute (range 260–360) in the absence of antiarrhythmic drugs; physiologic block at the AV node usually limits ventricular rates to 140 to 180 per minute. Carotid massage helps differentiate atrial flutter from supraventricular tachycardia by transiently increasing AV block to expose the flutter waves.

Treatment. Angina, pre-syncope, or symptoms of hemodynamic instability necessitate prompt DC cardioversion of atrial flutter. Hemodynamic instability may manifest as myocardial ischemia, severe hypotension, congestive heart failure, myocardial infarction, cerebrovascular insufficiency, bowel ischemia, or rapidly worsening azotemia. Correction of acidosis and electrolyte imbalance will enhance rhythm stability after cardioversion.

Once conversion to sinus rhythm occurs, the patient may still be at risk for recurrent atrial flutter. Pharmacologic block at the AV node with beta-adrenergic blocking drugs, digitalis, or verapamil tends to control the ventricular rate during recurrence while a search is made for factors predisposing to atrial flutter. Such factors include congestive heart failure, acute myocardial infarction or active ischemia, pulmonary embolism, thyrotoxicosis at any age, acid-base or electrolyte imbalance, acute exacerbation of chronic lung disease, intra- or extracardiac infection, and severe anemia.

Patients with atrial flutter often require large doses of digitalis for rate control. The reason for this relative resistance to AV block by digoxin is unknown. In some patients, pulmonary embolus, unstable angina, or thyrotoxicosis can increase sympathetic tone. Digitalis has reflex vagotonic and antiadrenergic effects,[31] but enhanced sympathetic tone or circulating catecholamines may overwhelm the digitalis effect during atrial flutter in unstable patients. Low-dose propranolol, timolol, or other beta-adrenergic blocking agents may help to slow the ventricular rate in these patients. Verapamil may also assist in controlling the ventricular rate in atrial flutter (Fig. 6–7). However, caution is required in patients with severely depressed ventricular function, since verapamil or propranolol may worsen ventricular performance.[88]

Intravenous propranolol or verapamil also prove effective in increasing AV block to expose flutter waves. Rarely, verapamil converts atrial flutter to sinus rhythm.[88] Verapamil should be used with caution in patients receiving beta-adrenergic blocking agents. The beta-blockers and verapamil may show additive effects and markedly increase AV block or depress sinus node function after termination of atrial flutter.

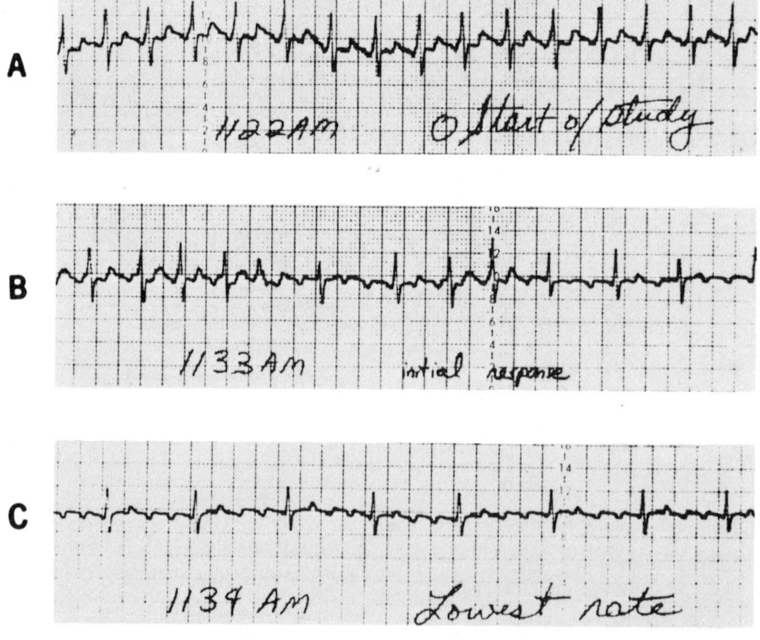

Figure 6–7. Effects of verapamil on the ventricular rate during atrial flutter. *A,* Control, atrial flutter with 2:1 AV block (ventricular rate 150 beats per min). Following 10 mg intravenous verapamil, 2:1 AV block progresses to 3:1 AV block (ventricular rate 100 bpm) and then 4:1 AV block (ventricular rate 75 bpm).

Procainamide, a quinidine-like agent, may be effective in terminating atrial flutter. It slows atrial and ventricular rates by slowing intra-atrial conduction and prolonging AV nodal refractoriness. Rarely, prolonged AV node refractoriness may be opposed by indirect autonomic actions of procainamide, resulting in 1:1 AV conductance at the reduced atrial rate.[46] Pretreatment with digoxin or propranolol may prevent this complication. Verapamil may also control the ventricular rate during atrial flutter and may convert atrial flutter to atrial fibrillation, a rhythm more easily controlled with pharmacologic agents.

When vagal maneuvers and pharmacologic agents fail to control the ventricular rate, termination of atrial flutter by transvenous right atrial pacing may be considered in hospitalized patients. Pacing is particularly useful when atrial flutter waves are distinct and the atrial rate is 250 to 340 beats per minute, as in type I or classic atrial flutter.[94, 96] Right atrial pacing is less effective when the flutter waves are less distinct and the atrial rate is 340 to 430 per minute, i.e., type II flutter. Attempts at entrainment of classic atrial flutter before termination may enhance the likelihood of success in some cases.[96]

After conversion to sinus rhythm, quinidine may reduce atrial ectopy and the risk of recurrent atrial flutter. Verapamil or propranolol are also effective in prolonging AV node refractoriness and may be used in lieu of digitalis in patients with good ventricular function.

Atrial Flutter in the Pre-Excitation Syndromes

Atrial flutter with 1:1 conduction over an accessory pathway presents as a wide-complex, regular tachycardia. Precise differentiation from ventricular tachycardia may be difficult but emergency treatment decisions are based primarily on the patient's hemodynamic tolerance of this dysrhythmia. DC cardioversion is required for syncope, angina, severe congestive heart failure, or other evidence of hemodynamic instability related to the tachyarrhythmia. In hemodynamically stable patients, intravenous procainamide may block extranodal conduction, thereby shifting antegrade conduction to the AV node and slowing the ventricular rate.

Atrial Ectopic Tachycardia

Reports characterizing the electrophysiologic behavior of atrial ectopic tachycardia are sparse.[30, 33, 82] However, isolated atrial tissue from enlarged atria obtained at open-heart surgery develops phase 4 automaticity and delayed after-depolarizations.[43] This behavior is not seen in tissue from normal atria[59] unless it is exposed to excess digitalis.[44]

Diagnosis. In a few reported cases, clinical behavior of atrial tachycardia suggests an enhanced automaticity mechanism.[30, 33, 82] These tachycardias arise spontaneously without requiring P-R interval prolongation and are not terminated by overdrive pacing or DC cardioversion.[30, 33] At the onset of tachycardia, its rate may accelerate gradually or "warm up" over the initial four to six beats.[33] Atrial ectopic tachycardia may persist for days, may be refractory to treatment,[82] or may be transient during underlying illness, metabolic derangement, or drug toxicity. Typical clinical settings for atrial ectopic tachycardia include acute exacerbation of chronic obstructive pulmonary disease, acidosis, acute infection, hypoxia, atrial dilatation, and excess administration of drugs, especially digitialis. Atrial ectopic tachycardia is perhaps more prevalent in children.[46, 50]

Treatment. Treatment for transient atrial tachycardia is targeted to the precipitating factors. Although digitalis is not consistently effective in suppressing atrial ectopy, it may slow the ventricular rate and improve ventricular function.[50] Excessive digitalis loading should be avoided. In symptomatic patients, procainamide can be given intravenously. The response of atrial ectopic tachycardia to verapamil and amiodarone has been disappointing.[54, 80] Surgical resection or transvenous catheter ablation of the AV node and His bundle may be required when medical management fails.

Atrial Tachycardia With Atrioventricular Block

Atrial tachycardia with AV block develops in less than 10 per cent of individuals with digitalis excess,[11] but most patients with this arrhythmia prove to have digitalis toxicity[57] (Fig. 6–8). Hypokalemia and underlying heart disease have caused atrial tachycardia with AV block in patients not receiving digi-

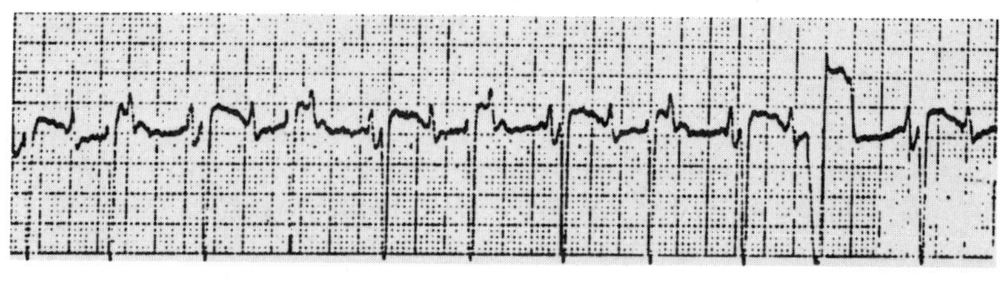

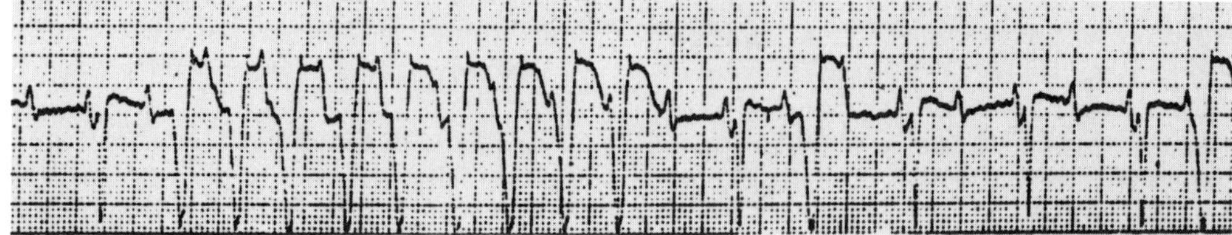

Figure 6–8. Atrial tachycardia with AV block. 3:2 AV Wenckebach in the upper tracing and 2:1 AV block in the lower tracing due to digitalis overdosage (serum digoxin level 4.6 ng/ml). A short burst of ventricular tachycardia (9 beats) is also noted in the lower tracing.

talis.[11] Phase 4 automaticity and delayed after-depolarizations have been observed in human atrial tissue exposed to digitalis,[77] and may interact to produce the clinically observed tachyarrhythmias.

Diagnosis. The atrial rate is usually 150 to 190 beats per minute.[57] P–P cycles may be irregular and ectopic activity often precedes the development of AV block. First-degree AV block or Wenckebach periodicity (Mobitz I) are typical (Fig. 6–8); Mobitz II AV block is unusual in digitalis intoxication.[57]

Treatment. The initial treatment is discontinuation of digitalis. Patients with mild AV block, hemodynamic stability, and rare ventricular ectopy often return to pre-digitialis rhythm in a few days. Improvement in AV block usually precedes the reduction in atrial ectopic activity. Restriction from physical and emotional activity has also been suggested during digitalis clearance.[11] Hypokalemia should be corrected cautiously since rapid intravenous potassium infusion can worsen P-R interval prolongation.[23] Frequently, ventricular ectopia after excess digitalis can be suppressed by intravenous lidocaine or propranolol.[11] Fab fragments of digoxin-specific antibodies were used successfully to reverse AV block after a patient had ingested massive digoxin doses in a suicide gesture.[90]

Multifocal Atrial Tachycardia

Published experience in cardiac electrophysiologic evaluation of multifocal atrial tachycardia has been meager, but the few available reports suggest that it is similar in origin to automatic atrial tachycardia but arises from several foci.[13, 86] The arrhythmia is not terminated by overdrive pacing or DC cardioversion.

Diagnosis. Multifocal atrial tachycardia is an arrhythmia of elderly men. The male:female ratio is 6:1 and the average age approximately 70 years.[74, 86] Chronic pulmonary disease or arteriosclerotic disease is found in up to 80 per cent of the patients.[86] Tachycardia rates may vary from 100 to 250 beats per minute but are slightly faster in chronic pulmonary disease.[86]

The ECG characteristics of multifocal atrial tachycardia include (1) the presence of discrete P waves with at least three different morphologies; (2) irregular variation in P-P, P-R, and R-R intervals; and (3) an isoelectric line between P waves.[86] Alteration of P-wave morphology and rate by respiratory excursion should be excluded.[86] Blocked premature P waves and QRS aberrancy may confound ECG interpretation.

Differentiation of multifocal atrial tachycardia from other atrial arrhythmias requires careful scrutiny of the ECGs. Absence of a dominant P-wave morphology distinguishes multifocal atrial tachycardia from sinus tachycardia with frequent atrial premature depolarizations. Differentiation of atrial flutter with varying AV block from multifocal atrial tachycardia is done by identifying the characteristic atrial flutter rate of 260 to 340 per minute and the sawtooth appearance of the baseline. In patients with paroxysmal atrial tachycardia and varying AV block, the P-morphology and P-P interval are constant. The exclusion of atrial fibrillation may be difficult but the rapid atrial rate, indistinct "f " waves, and absence of isoelectric baseline are key diagnostic observations favoring atrial fibrillation.

Treatment. Multifocal atrial tachycardia tends to develop during intercurrent illness, and effective treatment should be directed toward the precipitating illness. In elderly patients with obstructive lung disease, the arrhythmia often wanes after improved oxygenation, correction of metabolic or serum electrolyte abnormalities, control of infection, and reversal of bronchospasm. Digitalis is not consistently helpful, but in combination with quinidine it has been used empirically to help control multifocal atrial tachycardia.[74,86] Excess serum digoxin may elicit dangerous ventricular arrhythmias or advanced AV block. The arrhythmia often remains refractory to drug administration unless the underlying precipitating factors (usually severe pulmonary disease) are controlled.

TREATMENT MODALITIES FOR SUPRAVENTRICULAR TACHYARRTHYTHIAS

Vagal Maneuvers

Sinus and AV nodal tissue have generous autonomic innervation. Arrhythmias that depend on abnormal conduction at these sites may respond to manuevers that increase vagal tone.[99] Recommended vagal maneuvers include carotid massage, the Valsalva maneuver, facial immersion in cold water, and the pharmacologic interventions: edrophonium chloride (Tensilon), phenylephrine (Neo-Synephrine), and metaraminol tartrate (Aramine). These manipulations or drugs are most effective in patients with normal reflex autonomic sensitivity.[99] Baroreceptor sensitivity is diminished by congestive heart failure,[21] hypertension,[9] and age.[21,36] Pressor infusion may be dangerous in patients with hypertension or markedly depressed ventricular function.

Carotid Sinus Massage

Correct application of carotid sinus massage avoids unnecessary prolongation of tachycardia and can obviate any need for drugs.[99] The patient should be in the Trendelenburg position with the head turned away from the massaged artery. The carotid pulse is palpated just below the angle of the jaw, and the carotid sinus is trapped between the fingers and the transverse processes of the cervical vertebrae. Firm movement of the fingertips is performed in a cephalad-caudad direction under direct ECG observation. The carotid arteries are never massaged simultaneously; first the right, then the left carotid artery should be massaged in sequence, and the procedure should not last longer than five seconds.[40] Massage is immediately discontinued on termination of tachycardia or with the appearance of ventricular ectopy, in order to avoid ventricular fibrillation or post-conversion bradyarrhythmias, especially in digitalized patients.[112] Ipsilateral cerebral infarction with contralateral hemiplegia has occurred following carotid massage.[10] Auscultation for bruit and avoidance of carotid massage in patients with known cerebrovascular disease or carotid hypersensitivity may reduce the risk of this complication.

Valsalva Maneuver

The Valsalva maneuver requires forced expiration against a closed glottis or calibrated manometer. Ideally, 40 mm Hg positive intrathoracic pressure is maintained for 10 to 20 seconds. When the maneuver is properly performed, venous return to the thorax is diminished. In patients with normal baroreceptor sensitivity[9,20,21] and without congestive heart failure,[35] up to four phases of arterial pressure change may be seen: (1) an initial rise in blood pressure as intrathoracic pressure is reflected to the arterial tree; (2) a gradual fall in systolic, diastolic, and pulse pressures as the heart rate accelerates as a result of reduced ventricular filling, with attendant fall in cardiac output; (3) on Valsalva release, the sudden drop in intrathoracic pressure reflected to the arteries as a fall in blood pressure; followed by (4) restored ventricular filling and cardiac output, which cause an "overshoot" elevation in blood pressure. Only the fourth phase is useful in terminating tachycardia. The "overshoot" blood pressure elevation leads to baroreceptor stimulation and hypervagotonia, which slow the heart before terminating tachycardia.

Breath-Holding During Facial Immersion in Cold Water

Voluntary apnea during facial immersion in cold water is a potent stimulus for cardiac hypervagotonia.[103] This maneuver elicits bradycardia and peripheral vasoconstriction through a postulated "vestigial diving reflex" in man. Apnea and cold stimulation of nerve endings in the nose and face elicit reflex sympathetic stimulation to the peripheral vasculature (except brain and heart) and vagal stimulation with sympathetic withdrawal in cardiac nerves.[103] In man, heart rate slows by 10 to 40 per cent, blood pressure rises slightly, and cerebral blood flow is not compromised.[64, 103]

Apnea and facial cold stimulation has successfully terminated PSVT in over 50 per cent of patients not converted by carotid sinus massage.[103] During therapeutic application, the patient sits before an open pan of water cooled to 2° to 10° C. Room temperature should be approximately 25° C.[64] After the patient has taken a deep breath without exhaling, his face is submerge for up to 40 seconds. Continuous ECG monitoring is required. Tachycardia conversion occurs within 5 to 35 seconds, so that prolonging the maneuver beyond 40 seconds is not useful. A second trial, if needed, may be successful. The procedure may be uncomfortable to the novice patient, so careful explanation and reassurance from the physician are important. The intensity of elicited vagotonia is greatest when water is less than 10° C and room temperature is at least 25° C, but water temperature should be titrated to patient tolerance.[64, 103] Apnea and cold facial immersion has been effective in patients unresponsive to carotid massage and in those with ischemic heart disease.[103] The procedure should probably be avoided in patients with acute myocardial infarction since abrupt elevation in systemic vascular resistance could worsen ischemia. Severe bradycardia after conversion from PSVT could increase the risk of ventricular ectopy and fibrillation. Patients with known sick sinus syndrome or underlying AV block may develop prolonged asystole during apnea and cold facial immersion.

Edrophonium Chloride (Tensilon)

Edrophonium competitively inhibits the enzyme acetylcholinesterase to delay destruction of the neurotransmitter acetylcholine. Edrophonium is approved for use in the diagnosis of myasthenia gravis, but enjoys widespread use in the treatment of supraventricular tachycardia despite lack of F.D.A. approval. Sinus deceleration and depression of AV nodal conduction are the primary responses to edrophonium. This drug terminates PSVT in 50 to 75 per cent of patients (Fig. 6–4). In patients with atrial flutter or fibrillation, edrophonium slows the ventricular rate to facilitate the evaluation of atrial activity.[26, 67] Peak edrophonium effect begins within 30 to 60 seconds after infusion and persists for approximately 10 minutes.[26]

During edrophonium administration, the patient should be supine and kept informed of potential adverse symptoms. A syringe containing 1 mg atropine should be available at the bedside. Edrophonium is given as a 5-mg intravenous bolus over 20 to 30 seconds, during constant ECG monitoring. The 5-mg bolus may be repeated after five minutes if conversion to sinus rhythm has not occurred. Concurrent carotid sinus massage may augment the effect of edrophonium.

Adverse responses are common if edrophonium is infused too quickly or if the dose exceeds 10 mg.[26] Retching, diaphoresis, dizziness, blurred vision, increased salivation, bronchorrhea, nausea, crampy abdominal pain, and loose stools may occur. Transient fasciculations in skeletal and ocular muscle result from motor end-plate stimulation by acetylcholine. If present, these adverse symptoms begin one or two minutes after intravenous injection and subside within five to ten minutes. Informed patient consent and reassurance by the physician may improve tolerance of these adverse responses, should they occur.

Phenylephrine (Neo-Synephrine)

Phenylephrine is a synthetic amine that is structurally similar to epinephrine and causes peripheral vasoconstriction in both resistance and capacitance vessels. When infused during sinus rhythm, phenylephrine increases blood pressure and reflexly slows the heart rate. During tachycardia, increased AV node refractoriness and slowed AV node conduction are the desired reflex responses to phenylephrine.

In treating PSVT, 0.5 mg phenylephrine is diluted with 1 to 10 ml isotonic saline and injected over 20 seconds. The ECG is continuously observed, and blood pressure is monitored via intra-arterial cannula or sphygmomanometric cuff every 30 seconds. Maximal diastolic pressure should be 90 to 100 mm Hg, and systolic pressure should not exceed 180 mm Hg.

In an alternative method used by Waxman et al.,[99] phenylephrine is administered in escalating intravenous doses, starting at 0.1 mg and increasing by 0.1- to 0.2-mg increments depending on blood pressure response. Blood pressure is measured every 15 seconds. The maximal phenylephrine dose should not increase systolic pressure above 180 mm Hg, and blood pressure must be allowed to return to control values before each subsequent dose.

In a third method, phenylephrine is administered by continuous intravenous infusion.[32] Ten mg phenylephrine is diluted in 100 ml 5 per cent dextrose in water (100 μg/ml). Starting at 25 μg per min, the phenylephrine infusion rate is gradually increased to achieve systolic blood pressure approaching 160 mm Hg; 160/100 is an acceptable peak blood pressure. Blood pressure is recorded every 30 seconds and infusion is stopped when PSVT terminates, peak blood pressure is reached, or adverse symptoms such as headache or nausea develop.

Adverse reactions are minimized by careful monitoring of blood pressure and the ECG.[99] Postconversion pauses exceeding 3.5 seconds may occur but recovery time is usually less than 2 seconds, especially in young patients.[99] Anxiety, tremor, palpitations, and headache are reversible reactions that resolve promptly when phenylephrine infusion is stopped. More ominous reactions include intracranial hemorrhage, ventricular fibrillation, and acute pulmonary edema, but these are rare. Phenylephrine should not be used in the elective treatment of PSVT if patients have symptomatic coronary artery disease or intolerance to afterload elevation.

Metaraminol Bitartrate (Aramine)

Metaraminol is a sympathomimetic amine that, during rapid infusion, causes vasoconstriction and blood pressure elevation by displacing norepinephrine from sympathetic nerve terminals. It also acts as a false neurotransmitter but has less than 5 per cent of the potency of norepinephrine. As a result, tachyphylaxis develops after prolonged metaraminol infusion.[113] Metaraminol resembles norepinephrine in initial hemodynamic response but has less potency, slower onset, and longer duration of action. Metaraminol does not cross the blood-brain barrier and has no direct stimulant effect on the central nervous system.

When infused during PSVT, metaraminol causes a rise in systolic and diastolic arterial pressures, followed by reflex vagotonia and increased AV node refractoriness. In patients who are mildly hypotensive during PSVT, metaraminol is particularly effective in restoring blood pressure and augmenting vagotonia. Tachyphylaxis is not observed during these brief infusions.

Patients with symptomatic hypotension during PSVT should receive prompt DC cardioversion. Asymptomatic patients not converted by "noninvasive" vagal maneuvers may be candidates for metaraminol infusion. Metaraminol is primarily suited for young patients with PSVT and no underlying cardiovascular disease. Typically, 100 mg metaraminol is dissolved in 500 ml sterile isotonic saline or 5 per cent dextrose in water (0.2 mg/ml). The infusion rate is titrated to the patient's blood pressure response. Diastolic blood pressure should be increased to 90 to 100 mm Hg, with systolic pressure not exceeding 180 mm Hg. This may require 0.05 mg to 1.0 mg per min of intravenous metaraminol.[32] Incremental adjustments in metaraminol infusion rate should be separated by at least 10 minutes, since blood pressure gradually rises over 10 to 15 minutes after changes in steady state infusion rate. Metaraminol should be infused into a fully patent vein to avoid extravasation and local tissue sloughing.

Metaraminol is best avoided in patients with symptomatic coronary artery disease, and is less likely to be effective in those with elevated blood pressure or long-standing hypertension. Reductions in renal and cerebral blood flow occur during metaraminol infusion, so caution is suggested in patients with renal and cerebrovascular disease.

Pharmacologic Antiarrhythmic Agents

Propranolol

Beta-adrenergic blocking agents compete with neurotransmitter norepinephrine or circulating catecholamines for beta-adrenergic receptors and are most effective when the level of beta-adrenergic stimulation is high. Propranolol is the only member in this group currently approved for use in the United States to control supraventricular tachyarrhythmias. Hemodynamic response to propranolol includes a reduction in force and velocity of myocardial contraction; in an occasional patient, a mild elevation of arterial pressure may occur after intravenous infusion. ECG responses include sinus slowing, P-R interval prolongation, and QTc shortening in patients with prolonged QT syndromes.

Propranolol effectively slows the ventricular rate in sinoatrial tachycardia, PSVT, atrial fibrillation, and atrial flutter, and it is effective in digitalis-related supraventricular tachyarrhythmias with or without AV block in either terminating the arrhythmia or slowing the heart rate.

An intravenous infusion of 0.1 to 0.15 mg per kg provides propranolol concentrations of 100 to 200 ng per ml and adequate beta-adrenergic blockade.[105] Distribution to tissues causes an early fall in plasma propranolol levels consistent with its distribution half-life of ten minutes. Later, metabolism accounts for a slower fall in plasma concentration consistent with an elimination half-life of two to three hours.

After arrhythmia control with intravenous propranolol, therapeutic serum propranolol levels can be maintained with oral propranolol. First-pass hepatic metabolism limits bioavailability of oral propranolol, but 10 to 20 mg orally every six hours usually achieves adequate plasma levels.[105]

In the emergency management of supraventricular tachyarrhythmias, an initial dose of 1 to 3 mg propranolol can be infused at 1 mg per min during careful monitoring of the ECG and blood pressure. Additional propranolol of up to 0.1 to 0.15 mg per kg can be safely infused at 1 mg per min in patients without severe myocardial dysfunction.[45] Ventricular slowing begins within three minutes, peaks in 10 to 15 minutes, and lasts from one to six hours after intravenous propranolol.[45]

The most common adverse effect after propranolol is transient hypotension. Severe hypotension and congestive heart failure develop in patients with chronically failed ventricles that depend on sympathetic drive.[12] Symptomatic AV block may follow intravenous propranolol in patients with pre-existent AV node disease, but propranolol does not worsen infranodal conduction.[12] Asthmatic bronchospasm and congestive heart failure not due to the rapid tachycardia rate are contraindications to intravenous propranolol.

Verapamil

Verapamil is a papaverine derivative with coronary vasodilator and antiarrhythmic properties. It inhibits the movement of calcium and sodium ions through slow transmembrane channels in cardiac fibers; this action is thought to account for its depressant effects on automaticity and conduction velocity as well as the prolongation of refractoriness of the sinoatrial and AV nodes.[88] Intravenous verapamil converts AV nodal reentrant tachycardia to sinus rhythm with success rates approaching 90 to 100 per cent and represents a major breakthrough in the management of patients with this arrhythmia.[83, 88] Tachycardia is also slowed or converted when reentry occurs over a concealed extranodal pathway, through the action of verapamil on the AV node. When infused during atrial fibrillation or flutter, verapamil slows the ventricular rate (Fig. 6–7) and occasionally converts the tachyarrhythmia to sinus rhythm.[88] Regularization of ventricular response occurs in 25 to 60 per cent of patients receiving verapamil for atrial fibrillation, but this does not indicate drug excess as with ventricular regularization during digitalis treatment. Intravenous verapamil is contraindicated for patients with atrial fibrillation or flutter and Wolff-Parkinson-White syndrome since antegrade refractoriness of the extranodal pathways may decrease, resulting in an increased heart rate.[91]

During emergency administration, up to 10 mg (0.075–0.15 mg/kg) of intravenous verapamil can be given over one to two minutes. This results in serum verapamil concentrations ranging from 72 to 195 mg per ml (average 123 ± 40) and termination of PSVT often within two to ten minutes.[91] After 30 to 45 minutes, serum verapamil concentrations are 50 per cent of peak levels and the antiarrhythmic effect may wane.[91] A repeat dose of 5 to 10 mg may be administered after 30 minutes, or a favorable verapamil response may be maintained by an intravenous verapamil infusion of 0.005 mg per kg per min (5 μg/kg/min) after the initial bolus.[88]

The most common adverse response to verapamil is transient mild hypotension. Blood pressure usually falls within five minutes of an intravenous verapamil bolus and is recovered after ten minutes.[88] The rare patient who develops severe hypotension or congestive heart failure has often received verapamil as a rapid bolus exceeding 10 mg or concomitantly with beta-adrenergic blocking agents. Verapamil is contraindicated in patients with the sick sinus syndrome or impaired AV node conduction unless a transvenous demand pacemaker is in place. Digitalis, procainamide, and quinidine are compatible with verapamil in emergency settings, but the manufacturer recommends caution when verapamil is combined with these drugs.[20] Verapamil may elevate serum digoxin concentration during chronic treatment.

Diltiazem

Diltiazem is a benzothiazepine derivative with calcium channel blocking actions and cardiac electrophysiologic properties similar to but less potent than those of verapamil.[63A, 68A] Diltiazem slows sinus rate, slows AV node conduction, and prolongs refractoriness within the AV node. Predictably, the antiarrhythmic efficacy of diltiazem is most evident in dysrhythmias that involve the AV node. Intravenous diltiazem abolished supraventricular tachycardia due to AV node reentry in four of five patients in one study.[80A] Diltiazem promptly slows ventricular rate during atrial fibrillation and has caused ventricular regularization.[80A] It does not measurably alter conduction or refractoriness over concealed bypass tracts, but verapamil prolongs AV node refractoriness and may block antegrade reentry of atrial echos into the AV node and thereby prevent reciprocating tachycardia.

The optimal intravenous diltiazem dose is not established, but 0.25 mg per kg infused over 60 seconds is clinically effective.[80A] Oral diltiazem has recently been marketed in the United States for angina pectoris. The initial oral dose is typically 30 mg four times daily. Sixty mg four times daily is the maximal recommended dose; the safety of higher diltiazem doses is under investigation. Dizziness, headache, fatigue, blurred vision, flushing, and minor degrees of AV block are potential adverse reactions.[87A] Diltiazem is relatively contraindicated in patients with sinus node dysfunction or second-degree AV block.

Digitalis

The major clinical electrophysiologic effects of digitalis are indirect, through its effects on autonomic tone. Therapeutic doses of digoxin and ouabain increase vagal tone, inhibit sympathetic tone, and sensitize carotid baroreceptors.[31] This results in decreased automaticity in the sinus node, hyperpolarization and shortened refractoriness in atrial muscle, and prolonged AV node refractoriness.

The ECG manifestations of digitalis effect include sinus slowing, QTc shortening, scooping deformity of ST segments, and lowered T-wave amplitude. Reduced atrial irritability and acceleration of atrial flutter rate may result from hyperpolarization and shortened atrial refractoriness, respectively. In toxic doses, digitalis may increase sympathetic nerve activity, leading to ectopic rhythms that are suppressed by beta-adrenergic blocking drugs.[31]

Digoxin and ouabain are effective in the semiemergent treatment of atrial fibrillation, atrial flutter, and ectopic atrial rhythms unrelated to digitalis excess. The most clinically useful action of these agents is to increase the duration of AV node refractoriness, thereby slowing ventricular response during rapid atrial arrhythmias.[102] In atrial flutter, digitalis slows ventricular response less effectively at "therapeutic" serum concentrations but may result in conversion to atrial fibrillation, a dysrhythmia more easily slowed by digitalis.[66] In PSVT, digitalis preparations are used prophylactically to discourage recurrent attacks.

Oral ouabain is poorly absorbed from the gastrointestinal tract but intravenous ouabain is quite useful. Clinical effects appear after three to ten minutes, are maximal after 30 minutes to two hours, and wane over eight to 12 hours after infusion. Plasma half-life of ouabain is 21 hours in normal patients.[84] The digitalizing dose for ouabain is 1 mg; typically, 0.25 mg to 0.5 mg is given intravenously, followed by an additional 0.1-mg dose each hour until the desired level of ventricular slowing is achieved, or until 1 mg has been given.[32] Oral digoxin may be started six to 12 hours after the final ouabain dose, to maintain digitalis effect. Ouabain should be avoided in patients who have received digoxin or digitoxin within the previous two weeks.

Digoxin is effective both orally and intravenously. Onset of clinical response is most easily observed in patients with atrial fibrillation. Ventricular slowing begins after 15 to 30 minutes, is maximal in one to two hours, and wanes eight to ten hours after digoxin infusion.[89] The serum half-life of orally administered digoxin is 33 to 46 hours in normal patients. The digitalizing dose is 8 to 12 μg per kg but up to 15 μg per kg may be required in patients with atrial fibrillation (up to 1 mg in a 70-kg patient). Maintenance doses should be reduced in patients with renal failure or those receiving quinidine, verapamil, or amiodarone. During semiemergent administration, 0.25 to 0.50 mg digoxin is given intravenously, followed by an additional 0.1 to 0.3 mg after four to eight hours, until the desired ventricular rate or full loading doses are achieved.[32] The loading dose should be lower in patients who have taken digoxin within the previous two weeks. Hypokalemia, hypocalcemia, and hyponatremia may reduce the safety of digitalis administration.

Potential adverse responses to acute digitalization include worsening AV block and dysrhythmias. Digitalis-toxic dysrhythmias include atrial tachycardia, AV junctional tachycardia, bidirectional tachycardia, ventricular depolarizations, ventricular tachycardia, and ventricular fibrillation. Lidocaine, phenytoin, or propranolol may be effective in suppressing ventricular irritability induced by digitalis. Gastrointestinal symptoms (nausea, vomiting, salivation, and diarrhea) and neurologic effects (blurred vision, scotomata, and diplopia) respond to excretion of excess digitalis.

Procainamide

Procainamide is a local anesthetic with antiarrhythmic effects similar to those of quinidine. Procainamide decreases excitability in cardiac fibers. Both depolarization and repolarization are altered, resulting in slowed conduction, prolonged refractoriness, and depressed excitability.[41, 42] ECG effects include slight P-R interval prolongation, widened QRS duration, prolonged QTc interval, and nonspecific changes in T-wave amplitude.

Dose-related reductions in myocardial contractility and systemic vascular resistance account for elevated ventricular end-diastolic pressures and hypotension after intravenous procainamide. The distribution of intravenous procainamide is rapid (half-life 4–9 min) and the elimination half-life is three hours.[53] The *N*-acetyl procainamide metabolite has antiarrhythmic activity but is less potent than procainamide.

Procainamide is effective in atrial flutter, atrial fibrillation, and paroxysmal atrial tachycardia through actions that suppress atrial activity and slow ventricular response. Emergency administration of intravenous procainamide is quite effective in atrial fibrillation or flutter with antegrade conduction over extranodal pathways. Suppression of atrial premature depolarizations may help prevent recurrences during chronic treatment.

Intravenous procainamide can be administered as a 100-mg bolus every five minutes until 1 gm has been given, systolic blood pressure falls 15 mm Hg, or the desired antiarrhythmic effect is achieved. Alternatively, procainamide can be infused at 25 to 50 mg per min. Serum procainamide levels of 4 to 10 μg/ml are safely achieved with both schedules. QRS widening by more than 35 per cent, QTc QRS widening by more than 35 per cent, QTc block usually require discontinuation of procainamide infusion.

Common adverse responses to intravenous procainamide include hypotension, nausea, bradycardia, and advanced AV block.

Amiodarone

Amiodarone is a benzofuran derivative with potent relaxant effects on peripheral and coronary vessels. It is a powerful antiarrhythmic agent with clinical effectiveness in a variety of supraventricular and ventricular arrhythmias.[5, 16, 80] Undesirable effects from prolonged use make amiodarone a second- or third-choice agent in treating supraventricular tachyarrhythmias, reserved for patients unresponsive to or intolerant of other drugs.[16]

Intravenous amiodarone promptly terminates tachycardia in patients with PSVT due to AV nodal reentry, concealed extranodal pathway reentry, and intra-atrial reentry.[14] It slows conduction and prolongs refractoriness in extranodal pathways and should be effective in controlling the ventricular rate of atrial flutter or fibrillation with Wolff-Parkinson-White syndrome.[14] Unfortunately, amiodarone may be least effective in patients with atrial fibrillation or flutter if antegrade conduction occurs over extranodal pathways with short refractory characteristics.[101] Amiodarone also slows the ventricular rate during atrial flutter in the absence of antegrade extranodal conduction.[5] It is not particularly effective for atrial ectopic tachyarrhythmias.[80]

The recommended intravenous dose is 5 to 10 mg per kg infused over three minutes.[14, 88] A clinical antiarrhythmic response occurs in five to ten minutes. This dose has little adverse effect on ventricular function, and its action in decreasing systemic vascular resistance may improve cardiac output. As a result, amiodarone does not worsen congestive heart failure, and its negative chronotropic and coronary vasodilating effects may be favorable in patients with ischemic heart disease.

Oral amiodarone is effective in the chronic suppression of a variety of supraventricular tachyarrhythmias, particularly when used in conjunction with digoxin.[14, 16, 80, 88] Amiodarone increases serum digoxin concentration, so adjustment of maintenance digoxin dose is required when adding amiodarone.[68]

Cardiac Pacing

Atrial pacing techniques are rapid, safe, and effective means of terminating reentrant tachycardias or slowing the ventricular rate in ectopic (automatic) atrial tachyarrhythmia.[94] This approach is particularly useful when hemodynamically unstable dysrhythmias resist pharmacologic suppression.[93-96]

Atrial pacing is useful in terminating atrial flutter and PSVT (Fig. 6–9). The hemodynamic response to ectopic atrial tachycardia may be improved by atrial pacing in selected patients.[94, 95]

Atrial Flutter

Atrial flutter is best managed by DC cardioversion or pharmacologic slowing of the ventricular rate. When these objectives are frustrated by arrhythmia recurrence or drug intolerance, atrial pacing by means of transvenous electrodes may be considered.

Only type I atrial flutter responds to atrial pacing; rates may range from 230 to 350 per minute but are usually 290 to 310 per minute. Atrial rate is regular and the ventricular rate is usually a multiple of the atrial rate, typically 2:1 in those with normal AV nodal function, although irregular ventricular response may occur. The type II atrial flutter rate is usually faster than that of type I atrial flutter, being greater than 350 per minute. Type II flutter does not usually respond to overdrive pacing.

When it is proposed to attempt overdrive pacing to terminate type I atrial flutter, transvenous bipolar electrodes are first introduced percutaneously into an antecubital, subclavian, or internal jugular vein and advanced under fluoroscopy to the high right atrium. Fluoroscopic guidance is important in order to avoid rapid ventricular pacing.

After proper electrode placement in the high right atrium, overdrive pacing is attempted. Successful termination of atrial flutter requires atrial capture by atrial pacing at 110 to 140 per cent of the spontaneous atrial flutter rate for approximately 10 seconds (successful range 2–22 sec) at current strength 10 to 20 mA.[94] Either ramp pacing, constant-rate pacing, or burst pacing techniques can be used.

In the ramp technique, bipolar atrial pacing is begun at 10 beats per minute faster than the atrial flutter rate. The pacing rate is gradually escalated until the morphology

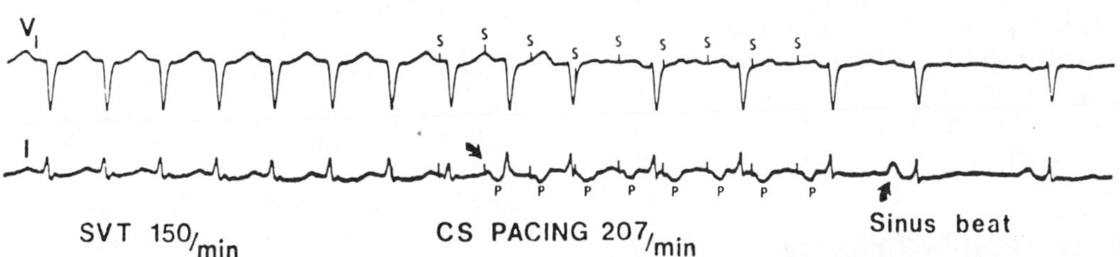

Figure 6–9. Termination of PSVT with overdrive atrial pacing. The rate of supraventricular tachycardia is 150 beats per min. Overdrive atrial pacing at 207 bpm converts the tachycardia to sinus rhythm.

of atrial flutter waves changes. Typically, "negative" atrial complexes in lead II become positive with high right atrial pacing. Rapid atrial pacing is continued for 10 to 20 seconds after the atrial morphology changes. Pacing is then abruptly terminated and the ECG examined for normal sinus rhythm. In patients at risk for postconversion bradyarrhythmias, atrial pacing may be progressively slowed to 100 per minute (ramp down-pacing) or changed in one step to 110 per minute before discontinuation.[94]

In the constant-rate technique, pacing is begun at 10 beats per minute faster than the atrial flutter rate and continued for 30 seconds before discontinuation. During successive trials of repeat stimulation, the atrial pacing rate is increased by 10-per-min increments until flutter is terminated. In the burst technique, a rapid pacing rate that is 120 to 130 per cent of spontaneous flutter rate is arbitrarily selected as "usually effective."

Failure to achieve atrial capture may result from technical problems, including insufficiently rapid pacing rate, inadequate duration of pacing, low stimulus current strength, or incorrect diagnosis (e.g., type II atrial flutter).[94] Fractured electrode wire, a weak battery, poor catheter electrode contact with the endocardium, or poor catheter connection with the pulse generator should be excluded.[94]

Paroxysmal Supraventricular Tachycardia

Failure to control PSVT with vagal techniques or drugs is rare,[99] but bipolar pacing is effective in terminating these reentrant dysrhythmias[94, 95] (Fig. 6–9). The simplest approach involves high right atrial pacing via transvenous electrodes at 5 to 20 beats per minute faster than the tachycardia rate. After atrial capture and tachycardia termination, the ventricular rate may slow to a ratio of the atrial pacing rate, usually 2:1 or higher AV ratio. Pacing is then abruptly discontinued. If the last paced atrial impulse blocks at the AV node, sinus rhythm usually ensues. If pacing is stopped with an atrial impulse that conducts through the AV node, tachycardia reinduction can occur, necessitating repeat stimulation.

Ectopic Atrial Tachycardia

Although overdrive pacing does not terminate ectopic (automatic) atrial tachycardia, atrial stimulation helps to improve hemodynamic tolerance of this atrial tachycardia, when it is refractory to medical management. Overdrive acceleration of the atrial rate increases impulse bombardment and concealment at the AV node, converting 1:1 to 2:1 AV conduction, and thereby slowing the ventricular rate. This can yield a beneficial hemodynamic result in patients with hypotension or ischemia during drug-resistant tachycardia.[94, 95]

Cardioversion

Direct current cardioversion is the treatment of choice for patients with severe hypotension or inadequate perfusion to vital organs during supraventricular tachyarrhythmia. These patients may develop stupor or syncope, anuria, dyspnea, or hypotension as clinical signs of hemodynamic instability. Patients with regional vascular disease and blood flow compromise to vital organs may develop angina, anuria, focal neurologic deficits, or extremity pain.

The objective of DC cardioversion is to drive 1.5 to 2.0 amperes of current across the heart. This should cause simultaneous depolarization of the entire heart, and consequent restoration of sinus rhythm. In clinical practice, cardioversion paddles act as capacitors to which 10 to 400 joules of energy are stored by applying up to 7000 volts during paddle charging.[75, 76] During semiemergent or emergency application of transthoracic shock, an anesthesiologist or anesthetist should be in attendance to maintain an adequate airway, administer the anesthetic, make possible the undivided attention of the person performing cardioversion, and assist if inadvertent ventricular fibrillation develops. Thiopental, a short-acting barbiturate, is the anesthetic of choice, but the hypnotic agent diazepam (Valium) also provides adequate relaxation and amnesia to the procedure.

Direct current cardioversion is applied under continuous ECG monitoring. The discharge should be synchronized to the QRS to avoid current delivery during ventricular repolarization (T-wave inscription), especially when small-to-moderate levels of energy are used.[38, 75] Adult paddles ideally should be 9 cm in diameter, with adequate electrode paste or gel. Either anteroposterior or precordial paddle placement may be used.[75] Once the patient is anesthetized and electrically isolated, R wave–synchronized energy adequate to terminate the specific arrhythmia is applied. If required, a second shock should be administered at 150 to 200 joules. A third shock should have maximal energy, usually 300 to 400 joules. Failure to terminate tachyarrhythmia requires expeditious evaluation of technique; replacement equipment; and review of the acid-base, pharmacologic, and general clinical status of the patient. Alternative methods for tachyarrhythmia termination may be considered, including pharmacologic suppression or atrial pacing techniques. The ultimate approach depends on an appraisal of the patient's specific clinical setting.

Role of the Clinical Electrophysiology Laboratory

In most cases, supraventricular tachyarrhythmias can be correctly diagnosed and successfully treated without invasive electrophysiologic study. This procedure is generally reserved for the more difficult clinical cases:[24]

1. When symptomatic PSVT is resistant to empiric pharmacologic control, precise characterization of the reentry pathway may allow rational selection of antiarrhythmic drugs targeted to specific components of the pathway.

2. Severely symptomatic PSVT may require prospective documentation of drug effectiveness before patients are discharged from a hospital setting. In these individuals, PSVT is associated with syncope, angina, congestive heart failure, or evidence of critical compromise to regional flow in obstructive vascular disease. The effectiveness of drugs in preventing tachycardia induction can be determined acutely in the Electrophysiology Laboratory. In this way, effective drug regimens can be tailored to the patient.

3. In patients with Wolff-Parkinson-White syndrome, atrial flutter or fibrillation may lead to very rapid ventricular rates, syncope, or sudden death. The effectiveness of drugs in slowing the ventricular rate can be confirmed by elective induction of atrial flutter or fibrillation in the Electrophysiology Laboratory.

4. When symptomatic supraventricular tachycardia is resistant to pharmacologic control, precise diagnosis and characterization of the arrhythmia is required before pacemaker therapy or surgical intervention are undertaken. The pacing site and rate most effective in terminating tachycardia is determined, and the reliability of the pacing technique in terminating tachycardia can be repeatedly tested.

References

1. Akhtar, M., Gilbert, C. J., and Shenasa, M.: The effects of lidocaine on atrioventricular response via the accessory pathway in patients with Wolff-Parkinson-White syndrome. Am. J. Cardiol. 38:189, 1981.
2. Bailey, G. W. H., Braniff, B. A., Hancock, E. W., and Cohn, K. E.: Relation of left atrial pathology to atrial fibrillation in mitral valvular disease. Ann. Intern. Med. 69:13, 1968.
3. Bauernfeind, R. A., Fernando, A., Dhingra, R. C., et al.: Chronic nonparoxysmal sinus tachycardia in otherwise healthy persons. Ann. Intern. Med. 91:702, 1979.
4. Bellet, S. (ed.): Hemodynamics. *In* Clinical Disorders of the Heartbeat. Philadelphia, Lea & Febiger, 1971, pp. 105–114.
5. Benaim, R., Denizeau, J., Melon, J., et al.: Les effets antiarrhythmiques de l'amiodarone injectable. Arch. Mal. Coeur 69:513, 1976.
6. Benchimol, A.: Significance of the contribution of atrial systole to cardiac function in man. Am. J. Cardol. 23:568, 1969.
7. Benditt, D., Pritchett, E. L. C., and Gallagher, J. J.: Spectrum of regular tachycardia with wide QRS complexes in patients with accessory atrioventricular pathways. Am. J. Cardiol. 42:828, 1978.
8. Bissett, J. K., deSoyza, N., Kane, J., and Murphy, M. L.: Altered refractory periods in patients with short PR intervals and normal QRS complex. Am. J. Cardiol. 35:487, 1975.
9. Bristow, D. J., Honour, A. J., Pickering, G. W., et al.: Diminished baroreflex sensitivity in high blood pressure. Circulation 39:48, 1969.
10. Calverley, J. R., and Millikan, C. H.: Complications of carotid manipulation. Neurology 11:185, 1961.
11. Chung, E. K. (ed.): Digitalis-induced cardiac arrhythmias. *In*, Principles of Cardiac Arrhythmias; 2nd ed. Baltimore, Williams & Wilkins Co., 1977, pp. 616–649.
12. Conolly, M. E., Kershing, F., and Dollery, C. T.: The clinical pharmacology of beta-adrenergic blocking drugs. Prog. Cardiovasc. Dis. 19:203, 1976.
13. Cotoi, S., and Dragulescu, S. I.: Complex atrial arrhythmias studied by suction electrode technique. Am. Heart J. 90:241, 1975.
14. Coumel; P., and Fiddle, J.: Amiodarone in the treatment of cardiac arrhythmias in children: 135 cases. *In* Harrison, D. C. (ed.): Cardiac Arrhythmias: A Decade of Progress. Boston, G. K. Hall & Co., 1981, pp. 347–357.
15. Coumel, P., LeClercq, J. F., Attuel, P., et al.: Autonomic influences in the genesis of atrial arrhythmias: atrial flutter and fibrillation of vagal origin. *In* Narula, O. S. (ed.): Cardiac Arrhythmias: Electrophysiology, Diagnosis and Management. Baltimore, Williams & Wilkins Co., 1979, pp. 243–255.

16. Coumel, P., Rosengarten, M. D., Leclerq, J., and Attuel, P.: Efficacy of new antiarrhythmic drugs. *In* Harrison, D. C. (ed.): Cardiac Arrhythmias: A Decade of Progress. Boston, G. K. Hall & Co., 1981, pp. 147–167.
17. Cristal, N., Peterburg, I., and Szwarcberg, J.: Atrial fibrillation developing in the acute phase of acute myocardial infarction. Chest 70:8, 1976.
18. Curry, P. V. L.: The hemodynamic and electrophysiological effects of paroxysmal tachycardia. *In* Narula, O. S. (ed.): Cardiac Arrhythmias: Electrophysiology, Diagnosis and Management. Baltimore, Williams & Wilkins Co., 1979, pp. 364–381.
19. Curry, P. V. L., Evans, T. R., and Krikler, D. M.: Paroxysmal reciprocating sinus tachycardia. Eur. J. Cardiol. 6:199, 1977.
20. Davis, J. C., Glassman, R., and Wit, A. L.: Method of evaluating the effects of antiarrhythmic drugs on ventricular tachycardias with different electrophysiologic characteristics and different mechanism in the infarcted canine heart. Am. J. Cardiol. 49:1176, 1982.
21. Eckberg, D. L., Drabinsky, M., and Braunwald, E.: Defective cardiac sympathetic control in patients with heart disease. N. Engl. J. Med. 285:872, 1971.
22. Falicov, R. E., and Resnekov, L.: Midventricular obstruction in hypertrophic obstructive cardiomyopathy. Br. Heart J. 39:701, 1977.
23. Fisch, C.: Effect of potassium on AV conduction. Circulation 41:575, 1970.
24. Fisher, J. D.: Role of electrophysiologic testing in the diagnosis and treatment of patients with known and suspected bradycardias and tachycardia. Prog. Cardiovasc. Dis. 24:25, 1981.
25. Friedberg, C. K.: Diseases of the Heart, 3rd ed. Philadelphia, W. B. Saunders Co., 1966, pp. 534–562.
26. Frieden, J., Cooper, J. A., and Grossman, J. I.: Continuous infusion of edrophonium (Tensilon) in treating supraventricular arrhythmias. Am. J. Cardiol. 27:294, 1971.
27. Gallagher, J. J., Pritchett, E. L. C., Sealy, W. C., et al.: The preexcitation syndromes. Prog. Cardiovasc. Dis. 20:285, 1978.
28. Giardina, E. G. V., Heissenbuttel, R. H., and Bigger, J. T., Jr.: Intravenous procainamide to treat ventricular arrhythmias. Ann. Intern. Med. 78:183, 1973.
29. Gillette, P.: Concealed anomalous cardiac conduction pathways: a frequent cause of supraventricular tachycardia. Am. J. Cardiol. 40:848, 1977.
30. Gillette, P., and Garson, A., Jr.: Electrophysiologic and pharmacologic characteristics of automatic ectopic atrial tachycardia. Circulation 56:571, 1977.
31. Gillis, R. A., Pearle, D.L., and Levitt, B.: Digitalis: a neuroexcitatory drug. Circulation 52:739, 1975.
32. Goldberger, E.: Treatment of Cardiac Emergencies. St. Louis, C. V. Mosby Co., 1982.
33. Goldreyer, B. N., Gallagher, J. J., and Damato, A. N.: The electrophysiologic demonstration of atrial ectopic tachycardia in man. Am. Heart J. 85:205, 1973.
34. Goldreyer, B. N., Kastor, J. A., and Kershbaum, K. L.: The hemodynamic effects of induced supraventricular tachycardia in man. Circulation 54:783, 1976.
35. Gorlin, R., Knowles, J. H., and Story, C.: The Valsalva maneuver as a test of cardiac function: pathologic physiology and clinical significance. Am. J. Med. 22:197, 1957.
36. Gribbein, B., Pickering, T. G., Sleight, P., and Peto, R.: Effect of age and high blood pressure on baroreflex sensitivity in man. Circ. Res. 29:424, 1971.
37. Gunther, S., and Grossman, W.: Determinants of ventricular function in pressure-overload hypertrophy in man. Circulation 59:679, 1979.
38. Han, J.: Ventricular vulnerability to fibrillation. *In* Dreifus, L. S., and Likoff, W. (eds.): Cardiac Arrhythmias: The 25th Hahnemann Symposium. New York, Grune & Stratton, 1973, pp. 87–95.
39. Harrison, D. C.: Atiral fibrillation in acute myocardial infarction. Chest 70:3, 1976.
40. Hilal, H., and Massumi, R.: Fatal ventricular fibrillation after carotid sinus stimulation. N. Engl. J. Med. 275:157, 1966.
41. Hoffman, B. F., Rosen, M. R., and Wit, A. L.: Electrophysiology and pharmacology of cardiac arrhythmias. VII. Cardiac effects of quinidine and procainamide. A. Am. Heart. J. 89:804, 1975.
42. Hoffman, B. F., Rosen, M. R., and Wit, A. L.: Electrophysiology and pharmacology of cardiac arrhythmias. VII. Cardiac effects of quinidine and procainamide. B. Am. Heart J. 90:117, 1975.
43. Hordof, A. J., Edie, R., Malm, J. R., et al.: Electrophysiologic properties and response to pharmacologic agents of fibers from diseased human atria. Circulation 54:774, 1976.
44. Hordof, A. J., Spotnitz, A., Mary-Rabine, L., et al.: The cellular electrophysiologic effect of digitalis on human atrial fibers. Circulation 57:223, 1978.
45. Iron, G. V., Ginn, W. N., and Orgain, E. S.: Use of beta-adrenergic receptor blocking agent (propranolol) in the treatment of cardiac arrhythmias. Am. J. Med. 43:161, 1967.
46. Josephson, M. E., and Kastor, J. A.: Supraventricular tachycardia: mechanisms and management. Ann. Intern. Med. 87:346, 1977.
47. Josephson, M. E., Seides, S. F., Batsford, W. B., et al.: The effects of carotid sinus massage in reentrant paroxysmal supraventricular tachycardia. Am. Heart J. 88:694, 1974.
48. Josephson, M. E., and Seides, S. F.: Clinical Cardiac Electrophysiology: Techniques and Interpretations. Philadelphia, Lea & Febiger, 1979; pp. 147–190.
49. Josephson, M. E., and Seides, S. F.: Clinical Cardiac Electrophysiology: Techniques and Interpretations. Philadelphia, Lea & Febiger, 1979, pp. 191–194.
50. Keane, J. F., Plauth, W. H., and Nadas, A. S.: Chronic ectopic tachycardia of infancy and childhood. Am. Heart J. 84:748, 1972.
51. Kinney, M. J., Stein, R. M., and DiScala, V. A.: The polyuria of paroxysmal atrial tachycardia. Circulation 50:429, 1974.
52. Klien, G. J., Bashone, J. M., Sellars, T. D., et al.: Ventricular fibrillation in the Wolff-Parkinson-White syndrome. N. Engl. J. Med. 301:1080, 1979.
53. Koch-Weser, J., and Klein, S. W.: Procainamide dosage schedules, J.A.M.A. 215:1454, 1971.
54. Krikler, D. M., and Spurrell, R. A.: Verapamil in the treatment of paroxysmal supraventricular tachycardia. Postgrad. Med. J. 50:447, 1974.
55. Lipson, M. J., and Naimi, S.: Multifocal atrial tachycardia (chaotic atrial mechanism). Circulation 42:397, 1970.

56. Lown, B., and Levine, S.: The carotid sinus: clinical value of its stimulation. Circulation 23:766, 1961.
57. Lown, B., Wyatt, N. F., and Levine, H. D.: Paroxysmal atrial tachycardia with block. Circulation 21:129, 1960.
58. Marcus, F. I.: Current concepts of digoxin therapy. Mod. Concepts Cardiovasc. Dis. 45:77, 1976.
59. Mary-Rabine, L., Hordof, A. J., Danilo, P., et al.: Mechanisms for impulse initiation in isolated human atrial fibers. Circ. Res. 47:267, 1980.
60. Mary-Rabine, L., Hordof, A. J., Bowman, F. O., et al.: Alpha and beta adrenergic effects on human atrial specialized conducting fibers. Circulation 57:84, 1978.
61. Mauritson, D., Winniford, M. D., Walker, W. S., et al.: Oral verapamil for paroxysmal supraventricular tachycardia: a long term, double blind randomized trial. Ann. Intern. Med. 96:409, 1982.
62. McIntosh, H. D., and Morris, J. J.: The hemodynamic consequences of arrhythmias. Prog. Cardiovasc. Dis. 8:330, 1966.
63. Mitchell, J. H., and Shapiro, W.: Atrial function and the hemodynamic consequences of atrial fibrillation in man. Am. J. Cardiol. 23:556, 1969.
63A. Mitchell, L. B., Schroeder, J. S., and Mason, J. W.: Comparative clinical and electrophysiologic effects of diltiazem, verapamil and nifedipine: a review. Am. J. Cardiol. 49:629, 1982.
64. Moore, T. O., Lin, Y. C., Lally, D. A., and Hong, S. K.: Effects of temperature, immersion and ambient pressure on human apneic bradycardia. J. Appl. Physiol. 33:36, 1972.
65. Morady, F., Scheinman, M. M. and Hess, D. S.: Mechanisms and management of paroxysmal supraventricular tachycardia. Cardiovasc. Rev. Rep. 2:1014, 1981.
66. Morris, D. C., and Hurst, J. W.: Atrial fibrillation. Curr. Probl. Cardiol. 5:5, 1980.
67. Moss, A. J., and Aldort, C. M.: Use of edrophonium (Tensilon) in the evaluation of supraventricular tachycardias. Am. J. Cardiol. 17:58, 1966.
68. Moysey, J. O., Jaggarao, N. S. V., Grundy, E. N., and Chamberlain, D. A.: Amiodarone increases plasma digoxin concentrations. Br. J. Med. 282:272, 1981.
68A. Nakaya, H., Schwartz, A., and Milliard, R. W.: Reflex chronotrophic and inotrophic effects of calcium channel blocking agents in conscious dogs: diltiazem, verapamil and nifedipine compared. Circ. Res. 52:302, 1983.
69. Narula, O. S. (ed.): Paroxysmal supraventricular tachycardia due to sinus and intraatrial reentry. *In* Cardiac Arrhythmias: Electrophysiology, Diagnosis and Management. Baltimore, Williams & Wilkins Co., 1979, pp. 272–293.
70. Narula, O. S.: Sinus node reentry: a mechanism for supraventricular reentry. Circulation 50:1114, 1982.
71. Nayler, W. G., and Drikler, D.: Verapamil and the myocardium. Postgrad. Med. J. 50:441, 1974.
72. O'Keefe, D. D., Hoffman, J. I. E., Cheitlin, R., et al.: Coronary blood flow in experimental canine left ventricular hypertrophy. Circ. Res. 43:43, 1978.
73. Peters, R. W., and Scheinman, M. M.: Emergency treatment of supraventricular tachycardia. Med. Clin. North Am. 63:73, 1979.
74. Phillips, J., Spano, J., and Burch, G.: Chaotic atrial mechanism. Am. Heart J. 78:171, 1969.
75. Resnekov, L.: High-energy electrical current in the management of cardiac dysrhythmias. *In* Mandel, W. J.: Cardiac Arrhythmias: Their Mechanism, Diagnosis and Management. Philadelphia, J. B. Lippincott Co., 1980, pp. 589–604.
76. Resnekov, L.: Present status of electroversion in the management of cardiac dysrhythmias. Circulation 47:1356, 1973.
77. Rosen, M., and Danilo, P.: Effects of tetrodotoxin, lidocaine, verapamil and AHR-2666 on ouabain-induced delayed afterdepolarizations in canine Purkinje fibers. Circ. Res. 46:117, 1980.
78. Rosen, M., and Reder, R.: Does triggered activity have a role in the genesis of cardiac arrhythmias? Ann. Intern. Med. 94:794, 1981.
79. Rosen, M. R., Fisch, C., Hoffman, B. F., et al.: Can accelerated atrioventricular junctional escape rhythms be explained by delayed after depolarizations? Am. J. Cardiol. 45:1272, 1980.
80. Rosenbaum, M. B., Chiale, P. A., Halpern, M. S., et al.: Clinical efficacy of amiodarone as an antiarrhythmic agent. Am. J. Cardiol. 38:934, 1976.
80A. Rozanski, J. J., Zaman, L., and Castellanos, A.: Electrophysiologic effects of diltiazem on supraventricular tachycardia. Am. J. Cardiol. 49:621, 1982.
81. Saunderson, J. E., Gibson, D. G., Brown, D. J., and Goodwin, J. F.: Left ventricular filling in hypertrophic cardiomyopathy— an angiographic study. Br. Heart J. 39:661, 1977.
82. Scheinman, M. M., Basu, D., and Hollenberg, M.: Electrophysiologic studies in patients with persistent atrial tachycardia. Circulation 50:266, 1974.
83. Schramroth, L., Krikler, D. M., and Garrett, C.: Immediate effects of intravenous verapamil in cardiac arrhythmias. Br. Med. J. 1:660, 1972.
84. Selden, R., and Smith, T. W.: Ouabain pharmacokinetics in dog and man. Circulation 45:1176, 1972.
85. Sellers, T. D., Bashore, T. M., and Gallagher, J. J.: Digitalis in the preexcitation syndrome: analysis during atrial fibrillation. Circulation 52:552, 1975.
86. Shine, K. I., Kastor, J., and Yurchak, P. M.: Multifocal atrial tachycardia. N. Engl. J. Med. 279:344, 1968.
87. Singer, D. H., Baumgarten, C. M., and Ten-Eick, R. E.: Cellular electrophysiology of ventricular and other dysrhythmias: studies on diseased and ischemic hearts. Prog. Cardiovasc. Dis. 24:97, 1981.
87A. Singh, B.: The role of calcium antagonist in arrhythmias. Drug Ther. 13:121, 1983.
88. Singh, B. N., Collett, J. T., and Chew, C. Y. C.: New perspectives in the pharmacologic control of cardiac arrhythmias. Prog. Cardiovasc. Dis. 22:243, 1980.
89. Smith, T. W.: Digitalis. *In* Levine, H. J. (ed.): Clinical Cardiovascular Physiology. New York, Grune & Stratton, 1976, pp. 333–365.
90. Smith, T. W., Haber, E., Yeatman, C., and Butler, V. P., Jr.: Reversal of advanced digoxin intoxication with Fab fragments of digoxin-specific antibodies. N. Engl. J. Med. 294:797, 1976.
91. Sung, R. J., Elsef, B., and McAllister, R. G., Jr.: Intravenous verapamil for termination of reentrant supraventricular tachycardias: intracardiac studies correlated with plasma verapamil concentration. Ann. Intern. Med. 93:682, 1980.
92. Ten-Eick, R. E., Baumgarten, C. M., and Singer, D. H.: Ventricular dysrhythmia: membrane basis

or of currents, channels, gates and cables. Prog. Cardiovasc. Dis. 24:157, 1981.

93. Waldo, A. L., and MacLean, W. A. H.: Diagnosis and Treatment of Cardiac Arrhythmias Following Open Heart Surgery. Mt. Kisco, Futura Publishing Co., 1980, pp. 115–159.
94. Waldo, A. L., and MacLean, W. A. H.: Diagnosis and Treatment of Cardiac Arrhythmias Following Open Heart Surgery. Mt. Kisco, Futura Publishing Co., 1980, pp. 187–200.
95. Waldo, A. L., MacLean, W. A. H., Karp, R. B., et al.: Continuous rapid atrial pacing to control recurrent or sustained supraventricular tachycardias following open heart surgery. Circulation 54:245, 1976.
96. Waldo, A. L., MacLean, W. A. H., Karp, R. B., et al.: Entrainment and interruption of atrial flutter with atrial pacing. Studies in man following open heart surgery. Circulation 56:737, 1977.
97. Waleffe, A., Brunibx, P., and Kulbertus, H. E.: Effects of amiodarone studied by programmed electrical stimulation of the heart in patients with paroxysmal reentrant supraventricular tachycardia. J. Electrocardiol. 11:253, 1978.
98. Walston, A., and Behar, V. S.: Spectrum of coronary artery disease in idiopathic hypertrophic subaortic stenosis. Am. J. Cardiol. 38:12, 1976.
99. Waxman, M. B., Wald, R. W., Sharma, A. D., et al.: Vagal techniques for termination of supraventricular tachycardia. Am. J. Cardiol. 46:655, 1980.
100. Weisfogel, G. M., Batsford, W. P., Paulay, K. L., et al.: Sinus node reentrant tachycardia in man. Am. Heart J. 90:295, 1975.
101. Wellens, H. J. J., Bär, F. W., Bassen, W. R., et al.: Effects of drugs in the Wolff-Parkinson-White syndrome. Am. J. Cardiol. 46:665, 1980.
102. Wellens, H. J. J., Düren, D. R., Liem, K. L., and Lie, K. I.: Effects of digitalis in patients with paroxysmal atrioventricular nodal tachycardia. Circulation 52:779, 1975.
103. Wildenthal, K., and Atkins, J. M.: Use of the "diving reflex" for the treatment of paroxysmal supraventricular tachycardia. Am. Heart J. 98:536, 1979.
104. Wit, A. L., and Cranefield, P. F.: Reentrant excitation as a cause of cardiac arrhythmias. Am. J. Physiol. 235:H1, 1978.
105. Wit, A. L., Hoffman, B. F., and Rosen, M. R.: Electrophysiology and pharmacology of cardiac arrhythmias. IX. Cardiac electrophysiologic effects of beta-adrenergic receptor stimulation and blockade. Am. Heart J. 90:665, 1975.
106. Wolff, G. S., Sung, R. J., Pickoff, A., et al.: The fast-slow form of atrioventricular nodal reentrant tachycardia in children. Am. J. Cardiol. 43:1181, 1979.
107. Wood, P.: Polyuria in paroxysmal tachycardia and paroxysmal atrial flutter and fibrillation. Br. Heart J. 25:273, 1968.
108. Wu, D.: Dual atrioventricular nodal pathways: a reappraisal. PACE 5:72, 1982.
109. Wu, D., and Amat-y-Leon, F.: Clinical, electrocardiographic and electrophysiologic observations in patients with paroxysmal supraventricular tachycardia. Am. J. Cardiol. 41:1045, 1978.
110. Wu, D., Amat-y-Leon, F., Denes, P., et al.: Demonstration of sustained sinus and atrial reentry as a mechanism of paroxysmal supraventricular tachycardia. Circulation 51:234, 1975.
111. Wu, D., Denes, P., Bauerfeind, R., et al.: Effects of procainamide on atrioventricular nodal reentrant paroxysmal tachycardia. Circulation 57:1171, 1978.
112. Yurchak, P. M.: Supraventricular arrhythmias. *In* Johnson, R. A., Haber, E., and Austen, W. G. (eds.): The Practice of Cardiology. Boston, Little, Brown & Co., 1980, pp. 96–131.
113. Zaimes, E.: Vasopressor drugs and catecholamines. Anesthesiology 29:732, 1968.

7

Bradyarrhythmias and Bundle Branch Block

FRED MORADY,
ROBERT W. PETERS,
and MELVIN M. SCHEINMAN

Rational treatment for patients with bradyarrhythmias depends on an understanding of the anatomy, blood supply, and electrophysiology of the specialized conduction system. The sinus node is an ovoid structure located on the epicardial surface between the right atrium and superior vena cava. It consists of four cell types: large, pale-staining P cells; ovoid nodal cells; transitional cells; and ordinary atrial muscle cells. The sinus node is heavily innervated by both sympathetic and parasympathetic fibers and receives its blood supply from the sinoatrial nodal artery, which arises as a branch from either the right or left circumflex artery.

The automatic cells in the sinus node have characteristics of calcium-dependent slow-response cells. These cells have a low resting membrane potential, relatively slow rate of rise of the action potential, and a short action potential duration. The impulse formed within the sinus node travels through a transitional zone to activate the atrial myocardium. The presence of preferential atrial pathways linking the sinus and atrioventricular (AV) nodes is still a matter of controversy.

The AV node is a small, ovoid structure embedded in the subendocardium of the right atrium near the ostium of the coronary sinus. It is richly endowed with both sympathetic and parasympathetic fibers and receives its major blood supply from the large AV nodal artery, a branch of the right coronary artery in 90 per cent of individuals (Fig. 7–1). The common bundle (or His bundle) arises from fibers in the anterior and inferior positions of the AV node, passes through the AV ring near the central fibrous body, and courses down the interventricular septum until it divides in the area of membranous septum. The right bundle branch is a slender band of fibers that often appears as a direct anatomic continuation of the common bundle. The left bundle branch is generally much broader and splits into several parts 20 to 30 mm from its origin. The thickest portion extends down the posterior aspect of the septum toward the posterior papillary muscle, while the thinner anterior division advances toward the anterior papillary muscle. In addition, there is often a third group of fibers that spreads out over the septum. Unlike the AV node, there is relatively little autonomic innervation of the bundle of His and bundle branches. The blood supply to these areas is predominantly from septal perforating branches of the left anterior descending coronary artery and also from branches of the AV nodal artery. There is marked variation in the anatomic configuration and blood supply of the ventricular con-

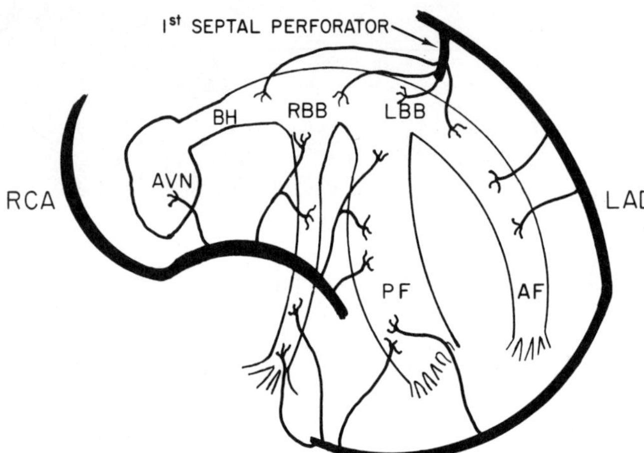

Figure 7–1. A schematic diagram of the anatomy and arterial blood supply of the ventricular specialized conduction system. *AVN* = AV node, *BH* = bundle of His, *RBB* = right bundle branch, *LBB* = left bundle branch, *AF* = anterior fascicle, *PF* = posterior fascicle, *RCA* = right coronary artery, *LAD* = left anterior descending coronary artery.

duction system, and corresponding variation in the clinical presentation of patients with disease in this area.

It has long been recognized that the rate of spontaneous depolarization of conduction system cells (a property known as automaticity) decreases with "descent" of the pacemaker along the conduction system. Thus, under ordinary circumstances, the sinoatrial node has the fastest rate of spontaneous depolarization, whereas the distal Purkinje fibers have a very slow rate that may be incompatible with life. On the basis of this premise, it is not surprising that AV nodal block is usually a more benign entity than a block within the His-Purkinje system. The work of Scherlag et al. is of particular relevance to an understanding of the pathophysiology of AV block.[63] Utilizing microelectrode studies, these authors were able to divide the AV node into three separate regions based on distinct membrane action potentials, which they labeled AN (upper), N (middle), and NH (lower). They found that the AN region had a higher intrinsic heart rate than the NH region, and the N region had no automaticity. In corresponding clinical studies, they were able to divide patients with "junctional" rhythm into two groups, one with a rate of 45 to 60 beats per minute that increased following atropine administration, and the other with a rate of 35 to 45 beats per minute that was unresponsive to atropine. Complete AV block within the bundle of His was verified by intracardiac electrophysiologic studies in several patients in the latter group, confirming the His bundle location of the pacemaker.

Bradyarrhythmias may be caused by one or both of two general mechanisms: (1) an abnormality in the generation or conduction of impulses out of the sinus node; (2) failure of an impulse that has depolarized the atria to propagate to the ventricles. Regardless of the mechanism, bradyarrhythmias result in symptoms by reducing cardiac output, either acutely or on a chronic basis. The clinical spectrum of symptoms ranges from infrequent episodes of mild lightheadedness to life-threatening episodes of cardiac arrest.

In this chapter, we review the management of patients who have bradyarrhythmias due to sinus node dysfunction, hypervagotonia, and AV block. In addition, bradyarrhythmias that occur in the setting of acute myocardial infarction are reviewed. The discussion will cover both the acute and chronic management of patients with bradyarrhythmia and bundle branch block.

THE SICK SINUS SYNDROME

The sick sinus syndrome refers to bradyarrhythmias that result from abnormal function of the sinus node. The sinus node may fail to generate impulses normally, or there may be an abnormality in conduction of impulses out of the sinus node (sinoatrial exit block). These abnormalities may become manifest as a marked sinus bradycardia, sinus pauses, or sinoatrial exit block (Fig. 7–2). Because of associated atrial abnormalities, the patient with abnormal sinus node function may have supraventricular tachyarrhythmias that alternate with bradyarrhythmias ("brady-tachy" syndrome).

Symptoms in the sick sinus syndrome are related to either an abrupt decrease in cerebral perfusion or a chronic decrease in car-

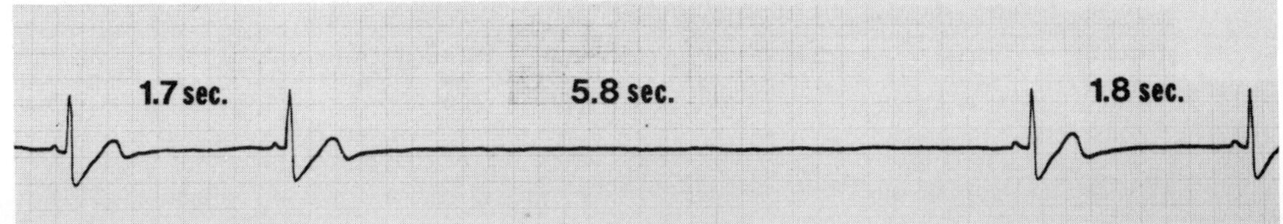

Figure 7–2. Marked sinus pause, 5.8 sec in duration. Sinus pauses are a common manifestation of the sick sinus syndrome.

diac output. Prolonged sinus pauses or episodes of sinoatrial exit block can cause syncope or presyncope. An inappropriate sinus bradycardia may aggravate congestive heart failure or angina pectoris, or may result in chronic fatigue and lassitude. On the other hand, if the sinus bradycardia is not excessively slow and the episodes of asystole are brief, patients with a "sick sinus" may have no symptoms at all.

The definitive diagnosis of the sick sinus syndrome depends on electrocardiographic documentation of a marked sinus bradycardia or a period of asystole due to either sinus arrest or sinoatrial exit block. Ambulatory ECG (Holter) monitoring for 24 hours has proved an extremely helpful diagnostic tool in patients suspected of having the sick sinus syndrome (Fig. 7–3). However, bradyarrhythmias secondary to sinus node dysfunction may be intermittent and therefore difficult to document despite several 24-hour ambulatory ECG recordings. Symptoms such as syncope or presyncope may occur infrequently, making it hard to ascertain whether the patient's symptoms are attributable to a bradyarrhythmia.

When bradyarrhythmias cannot be documented in a patient suspected of having the sick sinus syndrome, it may be helpful to evaluate sinus node function by assessing the heart rate response to atropine, isoproterenol, exercise, and carotid sinus massage[73] (Table 7–1). Electrophysiologic testing may also aid the evaluation of such patients. Sinus node function is assessed by determination of the sinus node recovery time. Atrial pacing is performed at several different rates, generally between 100 and 200 beats per minute, for one minute, after which the pacing is abruptly terminated. The sinus node recovery time (the interval between the last paced

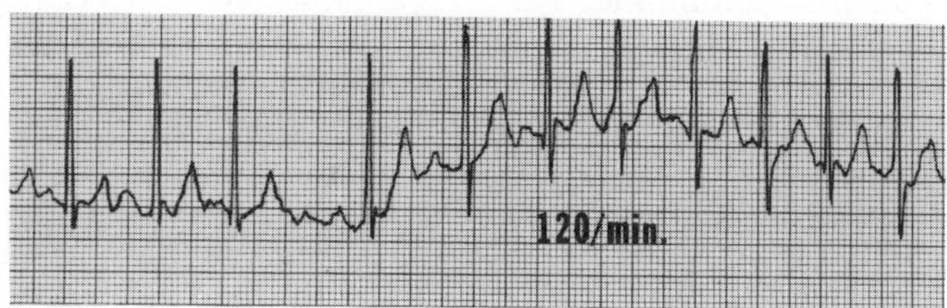

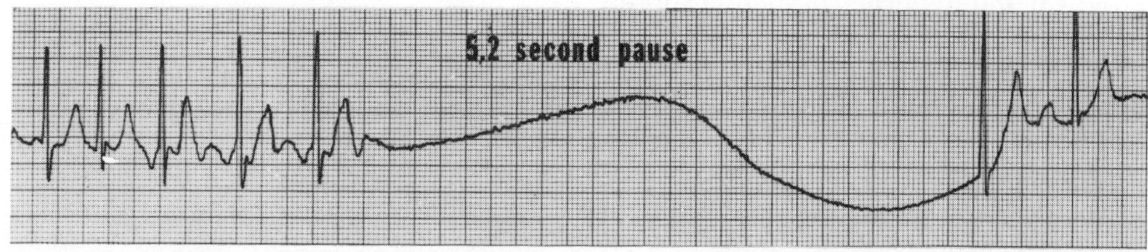

Figure 7–3. "Brady-tachy" syndrome. The patient complained of episodes of palpitations and syncope. A 24-hr ambulatory ECG recording demonstrated an episode of atrial fibrillation, during which time the patient experienced palpitations. Upon termination of the atrial fibrillation, there was a 5.2-sec pause, during which time the patient complained of presyncope.

Table 7–1. CLINICAL EVALUATION OF SINUS NODE FUNCTION

Test	Normal Response
Atropine 0.04 mg/kg IV	>50% increase in heart rate
Isoproterenol 3 μg/min IV	>25% increase in heart rate
Treadmill testing	≥90% of predicted maximal heart rate
Carotid sinus massage	Pause <3 sec

atrial beat and the first spontaneous sinus beat) has been reported to have a sensitivity of 68 to 94 per cent in the detection of abnormal sinus node function in patients with the sick sinus syndrome.[41, 59, 70]

The first consideration in the treatment of bradyarrhythmias in the sick sinus syndrome is whether the patient is symptomatic. Sinus node dysfunction tends to progress in a very slow fashion, and patients with a mild sick sinus syndrome may remain symptom-free for many years.[17, 57] In addition, sinus node dysfunction rarely is a direct cause of death, especially in those without symptoms such as syncope or presyncope.[39] Thus, bradyarrhythmias in the sick sinus syndrome generally do not require treatment unless the patient is symptomatic.

When a patient presents with a symptomatic bradyarrhythmia due to sinus node dysfunction, his list of medications should be examined. Symptomatic sinus bradycardia, sinus arrest, or sinoatrial exit block have been reported as being precipitated by the following drugs, especially in patients with underlying sinus node dysfunction: digitalis,[75] beta-adrenergic blocking agents,[71] quinidine,[46] disopyramide,[36] procainamide,[34] alpha-methyldopa,[61] guanethidine,[61] verapamil,[10] amiodarone,[7] and lithium carbonate.[23] Thus, if a patient with symptomatic bradyarrhythmias is being treated with one of these, the drug should be discontinued, if possible. If subsequent ECG monitoring demonstrates resolution of the bradyarrhythmias, no further therapy may be needed. In the patient who presents with an inappropriate sinus bradycardia, metabolic abnormalities such as hypothyroidism and hyperbilirubinemia should be ruled out.

If there is documentation that a patient's symptoms correlate with periods of asystole or bradycardia, and if no reversible cause for the bradyarrhythmia can be found, no further evaluation is necessary and a permanent cardiac pacemaker should be implanted. If the patient has been having frequent episodes of a severe bradyarrhythmia, it may be appropriate to immediately insert a temporary transvenous pacemaker to prevent further episodes before the permanent pacemaker is inserted.

In patients who have symptoms such as syncope, dizziness, or chronic fatigue but in whom there is no documentation that the symptoms correlate with episodes of sinus arrest, sinoatrial exit block, or marked sinus bradycardia, electrophysiologic testing may help decide whether a permanent pacemaker should be inserted. If the sinus node recovery time is normal or only mildly prolonged, we generally do not recommend permanent pacemaker therapy but instead continue to follow the patient with periodic ambulatory ECG recordings. On the other hand, if the sinus node recovery time is markedly prolonged, and especially if the patient's symptoms are reproduced in the electrophysiology laboratory in association with a long pause, we seriously consider implantation of a permanent pacemaker (Fig. 7–4). Ultimately, such a decision should never be based on the results of electrophysiologic testing alone, but rather on the entire clinical picture.

Implantation of a permanent pacemaker is generally very effective in relieving symptoms due to severe bradycardia or asystole.[13] However, pacemaker therapy appears to have little impact on long-term survival. Chronic follow-up of patients with the sick sinus syndrome who have been treated with a permanent pacemaker indicates that the mortality rate remains a function of the underlying heart disease.[67]

HYPERVAGOTONIA

Vagal discharge at times may cause a marked slowing of the sinus rate, which may result in vasovagal syncope, i.e. the simple faint. In the patient who has had a syncopal episode, there may be historical clues that suggest a vasovagal etiology. There may be an identifiable trigger such as emotional upset, pain, or the sight of blood. There is usually a prodrome of epigastric discomfort, weakness, lightheadedness, nausea, pallor, and diaphoresis. Consciousness is regained within a few seconds to a few minutes after the patient has assumed a horizontal position. After consciousness is regained, there may be residual symptoms of nausea, dizziness, headache, or diaphoresis. Carotid sinus massage may also be helpful; if this procedure induces a pause of greater than 3 seconds, it indicates an abnormal sensitivity to vagal stimulation and suggests a vasovagal etiology of the syncope.

In the patient who has an isolated episode of vasovagal syncope, no therapy may be needed other than instructing him to avoid future exposure to the triggering event. However, if there have been recurrent episodes of syncope, insertion of a permanent cardiac pacemaker should be considered. The pacemaker will prevent the marked bradycardia that occurs as part of the cardioinhibitory response to vagal discharge. At times, however, the patient may continue to have syncope despite artificial pacing, owing to a vasodepressor response to vagal discharge.[74] Hypotension results from peripheral vasodilation and may cause syncope despite maintenance of a normal heart rate. Unlike the cardioinhibitory response, the vasodepressor component of vagal hypersensitivity is not blocked by atropine. Patients with vasodepressor syncope typically present a very difficult management problem.

In patients with recurrent vasovagal syncope, it may at times be possible to avert the need for a permanent pacemaker by a trial of an oral anticholinergic agent such as propantheline bromide (Pro-Banthine). However, although propantheline bromide may effectively blunt the cardioinhibitory response to vagal discharge, side effects such as dry mouth, visual blurring, and urinary hesitancy often preclude chronic treatment with this drug. Another agent that may be useful in the treatment of vasovagal syncope is aminophylline, which is usually better tolerated than propantheline bromide. In a preliminary report, eight patients who had frequent episodes of vasovagal syncope were treated chronically with oral aminophylline;[4] there was an excellent response in five patients over a follow-up period of ten months.

It is important to recognize transient hypervagotonia as a cause of bradyarrhythmias in hospitalized patients who are acutely ill or are undergoing instrumentation. Vomiting, coughing, or procedures such as pericardiocentesis, tracheal intubation, or sigmoidoscopy may trigger an episode of asystole due to sinus slowing with or without associated transient AV block (Fig. 7–5). A vagotonic etiology for a bradyarrhythmia should be suspected whenever AV block is associated with slowing of the sinus rate, reflecting simultaneous vagal effects on the AV and sinus nodes.[43] Vagotonic bradyarrhythmias usually respond promptly to the rapid administration of atropine, 0.4 to 0.6 mg intravenously. At times, intense vagal discharge may cause a prolonged period of asystole, necessitating closed-chest cardiac massage until atropine is administered. Pacemaker therapy is rarely necessary in the treatment of vagotonic bradyarrhythmias that occur in hospitalized patients who are acutely ill or undergoing instrumentation, since the bradyarrhythmia usually does not recur once they have recovered from the illness and in the absence of instrumentation.

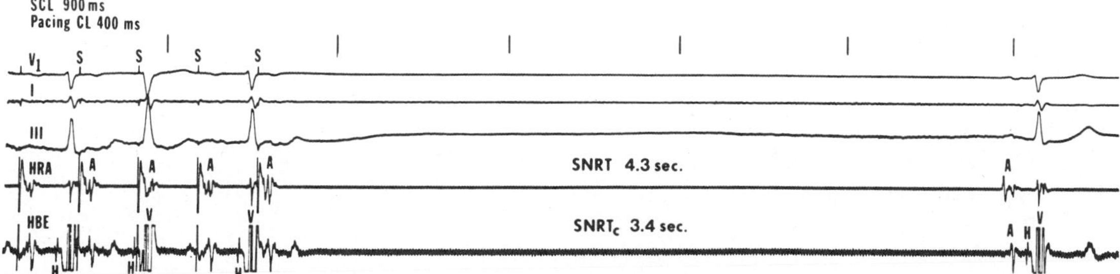

Figure 7–4. Markedly prolonged sinus node recovery time *(SNRT)*. From top to bottom are ECG leads V_1, I, and III; an intracardiac recording from the high right atrium *(HRA)*; and the His bundle electrogram *(HBE)*, consisting of atrial *(A)*, His *(H)*, and ventricular *(V)* depolarizations. Atrial pacing was performed for 1 min, at a cycle length *(CL)* of 400 ms (*S* = pacing stimuli). The SNRT is the interval between the last paced atrial beat and the first spontaneous sinus beat, in this case 4.3 sec. Corrected SNRT *(SNRTc)* is equal to SNRT minus the spontaneous CL, in this case 3.4 sec (normal up to 0.45 sec). During this pause, the patient experienced presyncope, which reproduced his clinical symptoms. On the basis of this finding, a permanent pacemaker was implanted. There has been no recurrence of presyncope. Time lines = 1 sec.

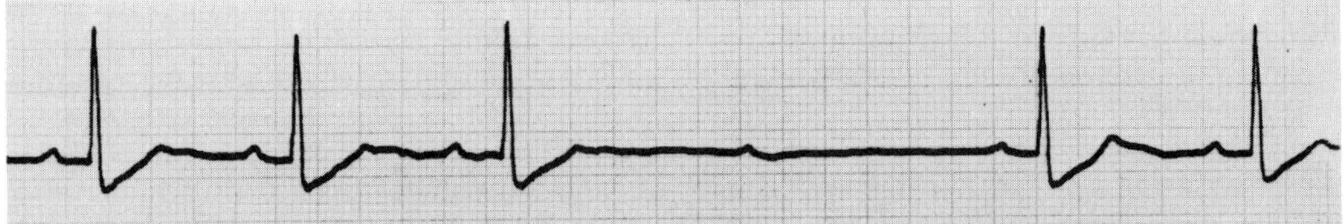

Figure 7–5. Vagotonic atrioventricular (AV) block, the hallmark of which is a slowing of the sinus rate in association with AV block. This is due to simultaneous depression of the sinus and AV nodes by increased vagal output. The condition is usually benign and does not require implantation of a permanent pacemaker unless the patient has recurrent symptomatic episodes.

BRADYARRHYTHMIAS IN ACUTE MYOCARDIAL INFARCTION

Sinus Bradycardia

Sinus bradycardia in the setting of acute myocardial infarction is thought to be secondary to stimulation of vagal nerve endings in the lower posterior portion of the interatrial septum, between the ostium of the coronary sinus and the posterior margin of the AV node.[29] In addition, sinus bradycardia during acute myocardial infarction may be related to ischemia or infarction of the sinoatrial node,[3] or may be caused by the release of substances that have a negative chronotropic effect, such as adenosine.[28] Since the blood supply to the AV node most often originates from the right coronary artery, sinus bradycardia is more often associated with inferior myocardial infarction than with anterior or lateral myocardial infarction. In studies in which patients with acute myocardial infarction have been monitored, sinus bradycardia has been reported to occur in 25 to 44 per cent of these with inferior infarction and 6 to 14 per cent of those with anterior infarction.[1, 18, 31] The incidence of sinus bradycardia is greatest in the early hours after the onset of symptoms, and is very uncommon after the first day.[1]

Overall, the occurrence of sinus bradycardia during acute myocardial infarction is not associated with an increase in mortality.[18, 26, 31] However, treatment may be necessary if the sinus bradycardia is associated with complications such as hypotension, heart failure, or frequent ventricular ectopy. The treatment of choice is atropine, which is very effective in reversing the bradycardia and improving the blood pressure, as well as in decreasing the frequency of ventricular ectopy.[11, 62] However, atropine must be administered carefully since it can cause an inappropriate sinus tachycardia that may result in angina or an increase in ventricular ectopy. Most patients respond to an initial 0.6 mg administered as an intravenous bolus;[11, 62] with this dose, there is only a 5 per cent incidence of inappropriate tachycardia.[62] In contrast, with an atropine dose of ≥0.8 mg, as many as 57 per cent of patients may develop an inappropriate sinus tachycardia.[12] On the other hand, an inappropriately small dose of atropine can actually accentuate the sinus bradycardia. In a series of ten patients given an atropine dose of 0.3 mg, nine of the ten had a decrease in heart rate of 4 to 5 beats per minute.[35] Atropine-induced bradycardia has been thought to be due either to stimulation of the medullary vagal nuclei or to a direct effect on the sinus node.

Thus, the most appropriate dose of atropine for treating sinus bradycardia in the setting of acute myocardial infarction appears to be 0.6 mg, as a single intravenous bolus. If the bradycardia does not improve within ten minutes, an additional dose of 0.4 to 0.6 mg should be administered. The duration of action of atropine when used to treat sinus bradycardia has been observed to range between ten minutes and six hours. Following an initial response, additional doses should be given as needed if the bradycardia returns. However, the cumulative dose should not exceed 2.5 mg over 2.5 hours, since this dose has been found to be frequently associated with major adverse effects.[62] Patients with symptomatic sinus bradycardia are at times unresponsive to repeated boluses of atropine; an infusion of a sympathomimetic agent, such as isoproterenol or dopamine, or insertion of a temporary pacemaker may be necessary in such cases.

Sinus Pauses

The blood supply to the sinus node originates from the proximal portion of the right coronary artery in 55 per cent of cases, and from a proximal branch of the left circumflex coronary artery in the remaining 45 per cent. Thus, sinus pauses due to sinus arrest or sinoatrial exit block can occur as a complication of either inferior or lateral myocardial infarction. Postmortem examination in a patient who had sinus pauses in association with a lateral wall infarction has documented that occlusion of the proximal left circumflex coronary artery can result in infarction of the sinus node.[27] In series in which large numbers of patients with acute myocardial infarction have been monitored, sinus pauses have been noted in approximately 1 to 4 per cent of patients.[54, 56] For example, in a series of 1665 patients with acute myocardial infarction, 32 (1.9%) were noted to have episodes of sinus arrest.[54] Such episodes usually occurred within the first four days of hospitalization and generally resolved after one to two days. Seven of the 32 patients had syncope. Patients were treated with either atropine, isoproterenol, or a temporary pacemaker. Of three individuals who received 0.5 mg of atropine intravenously, only one had resolution of the sinus pauses. On the other hand, the episodes of sinus arrest did appear to be effectively suppressed in 14 of 17 patients who were treated with a continuous infusion of isoproterenol (1–2 μg/min). A temporary pacemaker was successfully employed in the three patients who did not respond to isoproterenol. A permanent pacemaker was needed in only one patient, because of recurrent symptomatic sinus arrest 2.5 months postinfarction.

In other series of cases of acute myocardial infarction and sinus pauses, 35 to 54 per cent of patients required insertion of a temporary pacemaker, usually for two to four days, but sometimes for as long as 16 days.[56, 68] The proportion of patients who have undergone insertion of a permanent pacemaker because of persistent episodes of symptomatic sinus arrest has ranged from none to 10 per cent.[56, 68]

Thus, although pauses due to sinus arrest or sinoatrial exit block are relatively uncommon in patients with acute myocardial infarction, such pauses can at times be associated with significant symptoms such as syncope. The small amount of available evidence indicates that although atropine may at times be effective in suppressing the sinus pauses, better results are generally attained with either isoproterenol or a temporary pacemaker. If isoproterenol is used, a continuous infusion of 1 to 2 μg per min is usually needed; patients should be carefully monitored and the dose of isoproterenol adjusted as needed to avoid an inappropriate tachycardia, which can precipitate angina or ventricular ectopy. Treatment with isoproterenol or a temporary pacemaker should be maintained for approximately two to four days. If episodes of symptomatic sinus pauses persist for more than two weeks following the acute myocardial infarction, consideration should be given to insertion of a permanent pacemaker.

Atrioventricular Block

Atrioventricular block traditionally has been divided into three general types: first-degree, characterized by a prolonged P-R interval; second-degree, characterized by intermittently nonconducted P waves; and complete, in which none of the P waves are conducted to the ventricles (Table 7–2). Second-degree AV block is further subdivided into Type I, or Wenckebach block, in which gradual P-R interval prolongation precedes the nonconducted P wave, and Type II, in which the nonconducted P wave occurs abruptly and is not preceded by P-R interval prolongation (Fig. 7–6). This classification is not entirely satisfactory because the anatomic

Table 7–2. ATRIOVENTRICULAR BLOCK

Type	ECG Manifestation	Location
First-degree	↑ P-R	AV node or His-Purkinje system
Second-degree		
Type I	Gradual P-R ↑ precedes nonconducted P wave	Usually AV node
Type II	Nonconducted P wave without previous P-R	His-Purkinje system
Third-degree		
Narrow QRS	All P waves not conducted	AV node
Wide QRS	All P waves not conducted	Usually His-Purkinje system

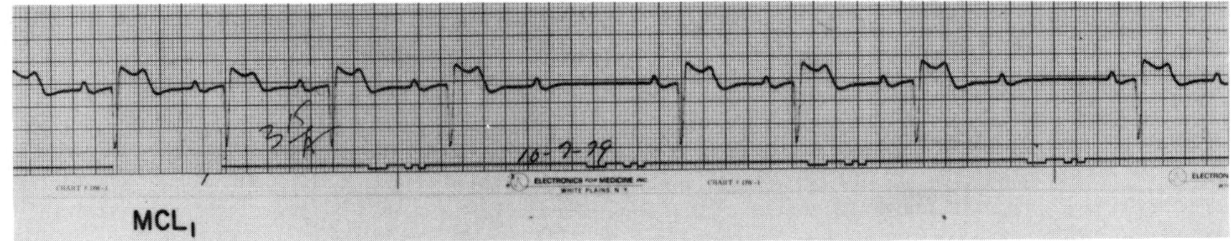

Figure 7–6. An example of Type I second-degree AV block (Wenckebach phenomenon).

level of block is not specified and, in fact, may not always be identifiable on clinical grounds alone. Thus, when AV block is associated with a narrow QRS complex, this implies that the level of block is above the branching of the common bundle of His. However, when the QRS complex is wide, the block may be anywhere in the conduction system if there is a coexisting bundle branch block. Similarly, although the Wenckebach phenomenon typically occurs in the AV node, it can also occur at times in other areas of the conduction system.

The recent introduction of intracardiac electrophysiologic techniques has provided a powerful tool for the evaluation of patients with conduction system disease. The His bundle electrogram is of particular value in the evaluation of patients with AV block in that it allows the area of block or conduction delay to be definitively localized (Fig. 7–7). It has also permitted identification of delay or block within the His bundle itself, characterized by a split His potential, a type of conduction system disorder that cannot be identified by the surface ECG alone.[5, 66]

As is the case in patients who develop AV block outside the setting of an acute myocardial infarction, the most appropriate management of AV block in association with an acute myocardial infarction depends on the level in the conduction system at which the block occurs.

Since the blood supply to both the AV node and the inferior wall of the left ventricle usually originates from the right coronary artery, AV block that accompanies an inferior wall infarction is usually due to block within the AV node. The AV block may be first degree, Mobitz I (Wenckebach), or third degree. AV block that results from ischemia of the AV node is usually transient. Even in the presence of third-degree AV nodal block, there is often no hemodynamic compromise, since the escape rhythm that originates in the AV junction usually has a rate of 40 to 60 per minute, which is adequate to maintain cardiac output. Treatment for AV nodal

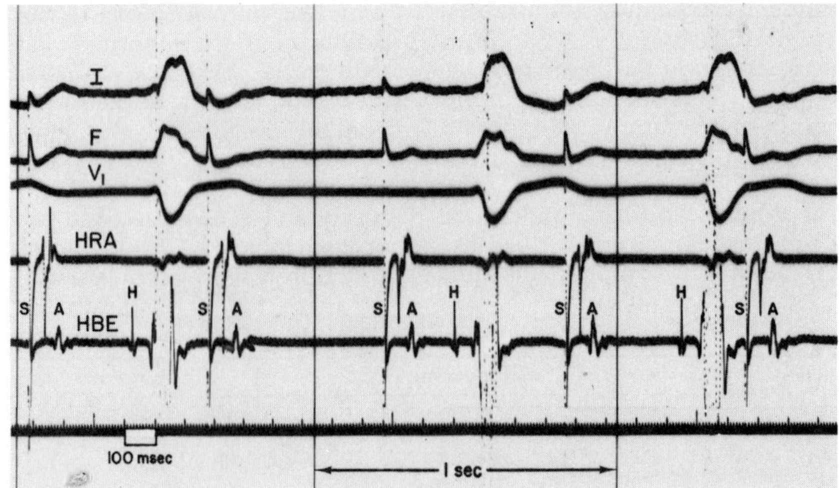

Figure 7–7. Type I second-degree AV block induced by atrial pacing in a patient with bundle branch block. At the top of the tracing are surface leads I, aVF, and V$_1$ and underneath are the high right atrial electrogram *(HRA)* and His bundle electrogram *(HBE)*. Note the gradual A to H prolongation followed by an atrial depolarization that is blocked in the AV node (above the common bundle of His). *S* = pacing artifact, *A* = atrial depolarization, *H* = His bundle depolarization. Paper speed = 100 mm/sec.

block in the setting of an acute myocardial infarction is necessary only if there is evidence of hemodynamic compromise due to a slow heart rate.

Since the blood supply to both the anterior wall of the left ventricle and a large portion of the His-Purkinje system originates from the left coronary artery, AV block that is associated with an anterior wall myocardial infarction is usually localized below the AV node. Infranodal block is generally characterized by the occurrence of Mobitz II AV block, or third-degree AV block. The idioventricular escape rhythm that occurs in high-degree infranodal block is slow (25–45 per min) and often inadequate to maintain a normal cardiac output. In contrast to escape rhythms that arise in the AV junction, idioventricular escape rhythms are often erratic and are prone to causing life-threatening periods of asystole.[8, 50] Thus, therapeutic measures are usually indicated in any patient who develops infranodal AV block in the setting of an acute myocardial infarction.

In light of the above consideration, the rational management of AV block in the setting of myocardial infarction depends on the ability to localize the level of the AV block accurately. This can usually be done at the bedside without having to resort to invasive testing. When AV block occurs in the AV node, the QRS complexes on ECG are usually narrow with a duration of less than 0.12 seconds, unless there is a pre-existing bundle branch block. If there is second-degree AV block, this will be manifest as either 2:1 AV block or a Wenckebach pattern. Since the AV node is subject to cholinergic input, the administration of atropine often improves AV conduction. If there is third-degree AV nodal block, the escape rhythm usually has a rate of 40 to 60 per minute. Atropine increases the rate of AV junctional pacemakers, and may also improve AV conduction and lessen the degree of AV block.

On the other hand, in the presence of infranodal AV block, the QRS complexes are usually wide (>0.12 sec). The escape rate is generally 25 to 45 per minute. Atropine neither improves AV conduction nor increases the rate of the escape pacemaker.

If AV nodal block results in hemodynamic compromise of a mild nature, treatment should be attempted with an intravenous bolus of atropine, 0.6 mg, which can be repeated two or three times as needed. If the AV block is persistent and the patient is hemodynamically compromised because of a slow heart rate, a temporary transvenous pacemaker should be inserted. Pacing should be continued until AV conduction returns to normal; this usually occurs within one hour to six days, the mean duration of second- or third-degree AV block being approximately 36 hours.[49] An alternative mode of therapy is the use of a beta-adrenergic stimulating agent such as isoproterenol. This has the potential disadvantage of an increase in myocardial oxygen demand related to an increase in myocardial contractility or an excessive increase in heart rate; in addition, isoproterenol may increase myocardial irritability. If isoproterenol is used rather than a temporary pacemaker, the infusion rate should be low (0.5–1.5 μg/min) and the patient should be carefully monitored. If angina or an increase in ventricular ectopy is precipitated by isoproterenol, the infusion should be discontinued and a temporary pacemaker placed.

In the patient who develops second- or third-degree infranodal block, a temporary pacemaker should be inserted immediately even if he remains asymptomatic. If the patient becomes hypotensive owing to a marked bradycardia, a bolus of epinephrine (5–10 ml of a 1:1000 dilution) or an intravenous infusion of isoproterenol (2–4 μg/min) should be administered to increase the rate of the escape rhythm until a temporary pacemaker can be inserted. The transvenous pacemakers should be left in place until the AV block resolves; in one series, the mean duration of AV block in patients with anteroseptal infarction was one day (range two hours to 2.5 days).[50] Unfortunately, despite treatment with a temporary pacemaker, patients who develop infranodal AV block in association with an anterior wall infarction may continue to have a high mortality rate owing to severe heart failure secondary to extensive myocardial infarction.[20, 51, 52] The decision to insert a permanent pacemaker in a patient with transient infranodal block who survives the acute phase of infarction depends on whether there is a persisting bundle branch block.

Bundle Branch Block

The occurrence of various types of bundle branch block during myocardial infarction is associated with an increased risk of the development of high-grade infranodal AV block. The prophylactic use of a temporary transvenous pacemaker may therefore be helpful in avoiding the life-threatening episodes of asystole or severe bradycardia, which may herald the onset of high-degree AV block. The decision to prophylactically insert a temporary pacemaker in patients with an acute myocardial infarction who have a bundle branch block should be based on the magnitude of risk of their developing high-grade AV block.

The largest series to examine the risk of progression to high-degree AV block in patients with myocardial infarction and bundle branch block is by Hindman et al.[24, 25] This risk was reported to be dependent on three variables: (1) the presence or absence of first-degree AV block; (2) whether the bundle branch block was a pre-existing condition or developed during the myocardial infarction; and (3) whether the bundle branch block was bilateral (right bundle branch block plus left anterior or left posterior hemiblock, alternating right and left bundle branch block).

A considerable risk of developing high-degree AV block was found in patients who had the new onset of bilateral bundle branch block: 38 per cent if there was also a first-degree AV block and 31 per cent if not. Thus, a temporary transvenous pacemaker should be inserted in patients with a new bilateral bundle branch block regardless of the P-R interval. The risk of progression in patients who had a first-degree AV block in combination with a new bundle branch block was 20 per cent. A prophylactic temporary pacemaker therefore should also be inserted in patients with these types of bundle branch block. In contrast, a low risk of progression to high-degree AV block (10–11%) was found in patients who had an isolated new bundle branch block or a pre-existing bilateral bundle branch block. In view of the relatively low risk of development of complete AV block, a prophylactic pacemaker is not mandatory in such patients. However, if the patient is not under close surveillance with continuous ECG monitoring, it may be decided to insert a prophylactic pacemaker to eliminate the risk (albeit small) of a sudden, life-threatening bradyarrhythmia.

Permanent Cardiac Pacing Following a Myocardial Infarction

A permanent cardiac pacemaker is clearly indicated in patients who develop high-degree AV block that is persistent. On the other hand, patients with bundle branch block who are at high risk of developing complete AV block in the course of a myocardial infarction, but who do not do so, do not have an increased risk of sudden death or high-degree AV block and therefore do not require a permanent pacemaker.[24, 25]

Some patients with bundle branch block in the course of a myocardial infarction have transient high-degree AV block with return of normal AV conduction and resolution of the bundle branch block. There are no data indicating that such patients benefit from implantation of a permanent pacemaker.

There is an alarmingly high incidence of sudden death during the follow-up period in patients who have a myocardial infarction complicated by a transient episode of high-degree AV block and by a persistent bundle branch block (Table 7–3). Several series have reported a 14 to 83 per cent incidence of sudden death over a follow-up period of six to 49 months, with a pooled incidence of 46 per cent.[2, 9, 25, 48, 58] In similar patients who do undergo pacemaker implantation before discharge from the hospital, a 10 to 17 per cent

Table 7–3. SUDDEN DEATH FOLLOWING ACUTE MYOCARDIAL INFARCTION IN PATIENTS WITH BUNDLE BRANCH BLOCK AND TRANSIENT HIGH-DEGREE ATRIOVENTRICULAR BLOCK

Series	No. Patients	No. Sudden Death (%)	Months of Follow-up
		Patients Without a Permanent Pacemaker	
Scanlon et al.[58]	6	5 (83)	8
Atkins et al.[2]	6	5 (83)	6
Nimetz et al.[48]	13	4 (31)	21
Ginks et al.[19]	14	2 (14)	49
Hindman et al.[25]	20	11 (85)	12
Pooled	59	27 (46)	
		Patients With a Permanent Pacemaker	
Ritter et al.[53]	12	2 (17)	20
Hindman et al.[25]	30	3 (10)	12
Pooled	42	5 (12)	

incidence of sudden death over 12 to 20 months has been reported.[25, 53] The lower incidence of sudden death in patients who receive a permanent pacemaker suggests that at least some of the deaths of those who are not paced may be due to the abrupt onset of high-degree AV block. Permanent cardiac pacing should therefore be considered in patients with acute myocardial infarction, persisting bundle branch block, and transient complete AV block.

One must be aware of the limitations of the available data relating to permanent pacing in patients with acute myocardial infarction. The studies summarized in Table 7–3 do not control for variables that are known to affect survival, e.g., ventricular ectopy, left ventricular function, and the degree of ischemic response during exercise. In addition, in a series of 47 patients with acute anteroseptal myocardial infarction and bundle branch block, 17 (36%) were found to have late in-hospital ventricular fibrillation.[38] This suggests that, in addition to complete AV block, malignant ventricular arrhythmias are an important cause of sudden death in this patient cohort.

CHRONIC ATRIOVENTRICULAR NODAL DISEASE

Chronic second- or third-degree AV nodal block may have a number of causes. It may be congenital or secondary to hypervagotonia or a variety of disease processes including viral myocarditis, rheumatic heart disease, sarcoidosis, neoplasms, infiltrative disease, vascular disease, or trauma.[30, 42] The underlying disease process strongly influences the clinical presentation of patients with chronic AV nodal block, although in some cases a specific etiology cannot be determined. Chronic second-degree AV nodal block is frequently asymptomatic and is considered by some to be a normal variant in children, young adults, and trained athletes.[40, 45] Thus, Brodsky et al. found transient second-degree AV block in three of 50 (6%) apparently healthy medical students undergoing 24-hour ambulatory electrocardiography.[6] On the other hand, Young et al. described a group of 16 children and adolescents with chronic second-degree AV nodal block of unknown etiology and found that two required permanent pacemakers because of recurrent syncope, even in the absence of clinically apparent organic heart disease.[76] However, it is not clear from the latter report whether syncope was directly attributed to periods of high-grade or complete AV block. Since the relationship of chronic second-degree AV nodal block to complete heart block is not well understood, it is of particular importance that seven of these 16 patients (44%) progressed to third-degree AV block during the course of their follow-up. Strasberg et al., reporting on a large group of adults with chronic second-degree AV nodal block, found that the presence and severity of underlying heart disease was the most important determinant of prognosis.[69] Thus, in the 19 patients without organic heart disease there were only two deaths (both nonsudden) and one patient who received a permanent pacemaker, whereas of the 37 patients with organic heart disease, pacemakers were implanted in ten, and there were 16 deaths. The prognosis of patients who present initially with complete block at the AV node is also uncertain. Campbell and Emanuel[9] and Hatle et al.[22] followed small numbers of patients with presumed congenital complete (narrow QRS complex) AV block over relatively long periods, and found no mortality and only rare syncope. In contrast, James and Galakhov described two cases of sudden death associated with third-degree AV nodal block resulting from a benign polycystic tumor of the conduction system.[30] Recently, Karpawich et al. presented their results of follow-up of 24 children with congenital complete AV block and narrow QRS complexes.[32] They found that ten patients (37%) required pacemakers over a one- to ten-year follow-up because of recurrent syncope and/or congestive heart failure, and that resting heart rate was the most powerful predictor of symptoms.

Therapy of chronic second- or third-degree block at the AV node consists primarily of permanent pacemaker implantation, and appears to be indicated for treatment of transient neurologic symptoms or when the slow rate contributes to congestive heart failure. The chronic use of anticholinergic or sympathomimetic agents such as propantheline bromide, ephedrine, and sublingual isoproterenol has been relatively ineffective and associated with a high incidence of side effects. Since the risk of sudden death appears to be low and since many people with AV nodal block are asymptomatic, it seems important to document that transient neurologic symptoms are, in fact, caused by the bradyarrhythmia. In situations in which there is doubt, repeated 24-hour ambulatory electrocardiography should be performed.

In summary, chronic AV nodal block is an uncommon entity of diverse etiologies. It is often benign but may be associated with recurrent syncope and, rarely, with sudden death. The resting heart rate and the severity of underlying heart disease are major determinants of the prognosis. Effective therapy of the condition usually involves permanent pacemaker insertion.

CHRONIC BUNDLE BRANCH BLOCK OR INFRANODAL BLOCK

Chronic bundle branch block occurs in between 0.2 and 1.0 per cent of the adult population.[37, 55, 64, 65] In general, there is a strong correlation between the presence of bundle branch block and underlying cardiovascular disease, even in asymptomatic individuals.[64, 65] People with bundle branch block have also been shown to have an increased incidence of spontaneous progression to high-grade AV block and sudden death. Thus, the development of syncope or recurrent dizzy spells has potentially ominous implications. It has become apparent that the standard 12-lead ECG has serious limitations in the evaluation of patients with bundle branch block. Even P-R interval prolongation, when present, is nonspecific since it fails to differentiate between AV nodal and infranodal disease.

There is currently a wealth of clinical evidence to show that patients with second- or third-degree AV block associated with a slow, wide-complex escape rhythm warrant permanent pacing; medical therapy (sympathomimetic agents) has been almost uniformly unsuccessful. However, the issue is less clear in asymptomatic patients with high-grade block in whom the site of block is in doubt (for example, 2:1 block in a patient with pre-existing bundle branch block). The His bundle electrogram provides a reliable means of demonstrating the level of AV block in this group (Fig. 7–8).[47] Patients with infranodal block should receive permanent pacemakers.

There is considerable controversy regarding the proper therapeutic approach to the patient with bundle branch block and recurrent neurologic symptoms in whom high-grade block has not been documented.[21, 33, 72] Treadmill stress testing and 24-hour ambulatory electrocardiography have unfortunately proved to be a relatively insensitive means of evaluating these patients. The His bundle electrogram can provide considerable additional information about the conduction system of patients with bundle branch block in that it permits direct assessment of the functional status of the unblocked bundle or His bundle. Prolongation of the infranodal conduction time (HQ) indicates the presence of infranodal disease, and individuals with lengthened HQ might be expected to have a more malignant clinical course.

We and several other groups initiated large prospective studies in the early 1970s to examine this hypothesis.[15, 44, 60] Up to the present, a total of 367 patients with chronic bundle branch block have undergone His bundle electrography and have been followed by our group subsequently.[60] We specifically excluded patients with documented pre-existing second- or third-degree AV block and those who had permanent pacemakers inserted for sinus node disease or second- or third-degree AV nodal block during the course of follow-up. Table 7–4*A* shows the clinical features of our population groups according to HQ. Our patients are fairly representative of those ordinarily seen by the clinician in that they are elderly and have a very high incidence of organic heart disease and transient neurologic symptoms. Table 7–4*B* shows the follow-up data. We have found that HQ <70 msec identified a group at relatively low risk, whereas at an HQ of 70 msec or greater the chances of progression to spontaneous high-grade AV block increased progressively. Similar trends were seen in overall mortality and sudden death although these trends did not attain statistical significance. Of particular note is that four of 17 patients (24%) with HQ ≥100 msec progressed to high-grade AV block and that this 24 per cent represents a minimal figure since almost half of this group had prophylactic pacemakers inserted and may have had undetected progression.

It is pertinent to compare our data with those of the two other similarly conducted large prospective studies. Dhingra et al. in 1981 reported their results in 517 patients with chronic bifascicular block followed for a mean of 3.5 years.[15] They found that a prolonged infranodal conduction time was an independent risk factor for progression to high-degree AV block, although the predic-

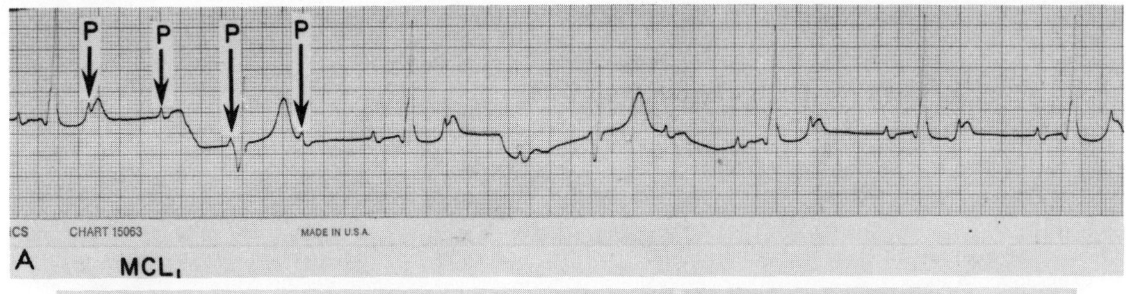

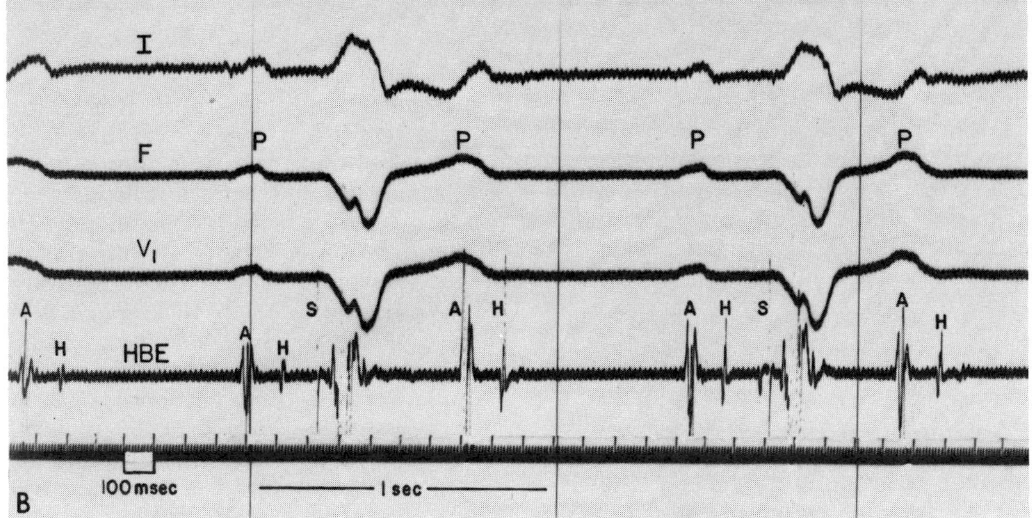

Figure 7–8. *A,* A rhythm strip showing high-grade AV block in a patient with right bundle branch block. *B,* A His bundle electrogram in the same patient, obtained during temporary pacemaker insertion, shows a left bundle branch block pattern and frequent atrial complexes blocked below the His bundle (compare with Fig. 7–7). This finding is diagnostic of high-degree block within the His-Purkinje system. Abbreviations are as in Figure 7–7. P = P wave.

Table 7–4A. PATIENTS WITH CHRONIC BUNDLE BRANCH BLOCK: CLINICAL AND ELECTROPHYSIOLOGIC DATA

Parameter	Group I H–Q 30–54 msec No. (%)	Group II H–Q 55–69 msec No. (%)	Group III H–Q 70 msec No. (%)	P Value
No. of patients	97	99	117	
Age (mean ± SD) (years)	66 ± 13	66.6 ± 14	66.5 ± 11	NS
Coronary artery disease	63 (65)	68 (67)	78 (69)	NS
Organic cardiac disease	49 (56)	65 (66)	98 (84)	0.001*
Transient neurologic symptoms	58 (60)	58 (59)	68 (56)	NS
Syncope	38 (39)	40 (40)	46 (40)	NS
Congestive heart failure (Class III or IV)	19 (18.5)	22 (22)	38 (32)	0.05*

*Group III greater than groups I or II.
NS = not significant.

Table 7–4B. PATIENTS WITH CHRONIC BUNDLE BRANCH BLOCK: FOLLOW-UP DATA

Parameter	Group I H–Q 30–54 msec No. (%)	Group II H–Q 55–69 msec No. (%)	Group III H–Q 70 msec No. (%)	P Value
Follow-up (months)	34 ± 24	34.5 ± 27	28 ± 23	NS
Progression to second-degree or third-degree block	4 (4)	2 (2)	14 (12)	0.01*
Sudden deaths	12/41 (29)	12/50 (24)	19/57 (33)	NS
Cardiac deaths	14/41 (34)	15/50 (30)	28/57 (49)	NS
Total deaths	41 (42)	50 (51)	57 (49)	NS

*Group III greater than groups I or II.
NS = not significant.

Table 7–5*A*. PATIENTS WITH AND WITHOUT PROPHYLACTIC PACEMAKERS: CLINICAL AND ELECTROPHYSIOLOGIC DATA

	Paced No. (%)	Unpaced No. (%)	P Value
No. of patients	62	231	
Age (mean ± SD) (years)	67 ± 10	22 ± 14	NS
Congestive heart failure (Class III or IV)	16 (26)	80 (35)	<0.001
Transient neurologic symptoms	47 (76)	134 (55)	<0.001
H–Q (mean ± SD) (msec)	72 ± 24	59 ± 16	<0.001

NS = not significant.

tive value of HQ was not as great as in our series. The differences may be due to the fact that their population was younger than ours and had a lower incidence of organic heart disease and transient neurologic symptoms. Similar considerations may explain the differences between our findings and those of McAnulty et al.[44] In 1979 Dhingra et al. reported that infranodal block induced by atrial pacing during electrophysiologic study in their patients was strongly predictive of subsequent high-grade block or sudden death.[16]

Inherent in the identification of a high-risk group of patients with bundle branch block is the hope that the judicious use of permanent pacemakers may decrease mortality and the incidence of sudden death. Accordingly, we compared the clinical course of patients who had permanent pacemakers inserted prophylactically (no documented second- or third-degree block) at the discretion of the referring physician with that of patients who were unpaced (Table 7–5*A*). Table 7–5*B* summarizes the follow-up data. Neurologic symptoms were relieved more frequently in the paced patients, but there was no significant difference between groups in overall mortality or the incidence of sudden death. It is noteworthy that approximately 50 per cent of unpaced patients had spontaneous resolution of symptoms, a finding similar to that of Dhingra et al.,[14] emphasizing the unreliability of using symptoms alone as an indication for permanent pacemaker insertion. It is possible to explain these seemingly contradictory findings by postulating that episodic AV block is one cause of neurologic symptoms in these patients, but that idioventricular escape rhythms emerge to sustain life. Sudden death, on the other hand, is probably due to ventricular tachycardia or fibrillation, a not unlikely event in an elderly population with a high incidence of coronary artery disease. In support of this hypothesis, two of our paced patients who died suddenly were undergoing 24-hour ambulatory electrocardiography at the time of death and both were found to have ventricular fibrillation without antecedent AV block.

In summary, patients with chronic bundle branch block are predisposed to high-grade AV block and sudden death, but the overall incidence of these complications is low and does not justify routine prophylactic permanent pacemaker insertion. Patients with documented second- or third-degree infranodal block should receive pacemakers, even in the absence of symptoms. Patients with chronic bundle branch block without either high-grade block or symptoms need not be evaluated further. Those with recurrent neurologic symptoms of unknown cause in whom chronic high-grade block has not been documented electrocardiographically should undergo Holter monitoring and detailed

Table 7–5*B*. PATIENTS WITH AND WITHOUT PROPHYLACTIC PACEMAKERS: FOLLOW-UP DATA

	Paced No. (%)	Unpaced No. (%)	P Value
Relief of syncope	36/41* (88)	43/80* (53)	0.001
Relief of any neurologic symptoms	32/47* (70)	64/134* (48)	0.05
Sudden deaths	12/62 (19)	30/231 (13)	NS
Cardiac deaths	12/62 (19)	44/231 (19)	NS
Total deaths	31 (50)	108 (40)	NS

NS = not significant.
*Denominator refers to number of patients with symptoms prior to pacing.

electrophysiologic studies, which should include evaluation of sinus node function as well as AV conduction. In addition, both atrial and ventricular stimulation studies are indicated in the attempt to exclude tachycardia as a cause of symptoms. Our preliminary evidence suggests that episodic ventricular arrhythmias may be an important cause of symptoms in these patients. Permanent pacemaker implantation is definitely indicated if high-degree block is seen on the Holter, if the HQ is ≥100 msec, or if infranodal block is induced by atrial pacing. Permanent pacing should be considered if the HQ is ≥70 msec. Although pacemaker insertion can be expected to relieve symptoms, it will not necessarily prolong life.

References

1. Adgey, A. A. J., Geddes, J. S., Mulholland, H. C., et al.: Incidence, significance, and management of early bradyarrhythmia complicating acute myocardial infarction. Lancet 2:1097, 1968.
2. Atkins, J. M., Leshin, S. J., Blomqvist, G., and Mullins, C. B.: Ventricular conduction blocks and sudden death in acute myocardial infarction. Potential indications for pacing. N. Engl. J. Med. 288:281, 1973.
3. Baba, N., Leighton, R. F., and Weissler, A. M.: Experimental cardiac ischemia. Observation of the sinoatrial and atrioventricular nodes. Lab. Invest. 23:168, 1970.
4. Benditt, D. G., Kriett, J. M., Haugland, J. M., et al.: Effects of aminophylline on sinus and atrioventricular node function in young adults with vasovagal syncope. Circulation 64:IV-134, 1981.
5. Bharati, S., Lev, M., Wu, D., et al.: Pathophysiologic correlations in two cases of split His bundle potentials. Circulation 49:615, 1974.
6. Brodsky, M., Wu, D., Denes, P., et al.: Arrhythmias documented by 24-hour continuous electrocardiographic monitoring in 50 male medical students without apparent heart disease. Am. J. Cardiol. 39:390, 1977.
7. Brown, A. K.: Use of amiodarone in bradycardia-tachycardia syndrome. Am. Heart J. 42:369, 1979.
8. Brown, R. W., Hunt, D., and Sloman, J. G.: The natural history of atrioventricular conduction defects in acute myocardial infarction. Am. Heart J. 78:460, 1969.
9. Campbell, M., and Emanuel, R.: Six cases of congenital complete heart block followed for 34–40 years. Br. Heart J. 29:577, 1967.
10. Carrasco, H. A., Fuenmayor, A., Barboza, J. S., and Gonzalez, G.: Effect of verapamil on normal sinoatrial node function and sick sinus syndrome. Am. Heart J. 96:760, 1978.
11. Chadda, K. D., Lichstein, E., Gupta, P. K., and Choy, R.: Bradycardia-hypotension syndrome in acute myocardial infarction. Reappraisal of the overdrive effects of atropine. Am. J. Med. 59:158, 1975.
12. Chadda, K. D., Lichstein, E., Gupta, P. K., and Kourtesis, P.: Effects of atropine in patients with bradyarrhythmia complicating myocardial infarction. Usefulness of an optimum dose for overdrive. Am. J. Med. 63:503, 1977.
13. Chokshi, D. S., Mascarenhas, E., Samet, P., and Center, S.: Treatment of sinoatrial rhythm disturbances with permanent cardiac pacing. Am. J. Cardiol. 32:215, 1973.
14. Dhingra, R. C., Denes, P., Wu, D., et al.: Syncope in patients with chronic bifascicular block; significance, causative mechanisms and clinical implications. Ann. Intern. Med. 81:302, 1974.
15. Dhingra, R. C., Palileo, E., Strasberg, B., et al.: Significance of the HV interval in 517 patients with chronic bifascicular block. Circulation 64:1265, 1981.
16. Dhingra, R. C., Wyndham, C., Bauernfeind, R., et al.: Significance of block distal to the His bundle induced by atrial pacing in patients with chronic bifascicular block. Circulation 60:1455, 1979.
17. Ferrer, M. I.: The sick sinus syndrome. Circulation 47:635, 1973.
18. George, M., and Greenwood, T. W.: Relation between bradycardia and the site of myocardial infarction. Lancet 2:739, 1967.
19. Ginks, W. R., Sutton, R., Oh, W., and Leatham, A.: Long-term prognosis after acute myocardial infarction with atrioventricular block. Br. Heart J. 39:186, 1977.
20. Godman, M. J., Alpert, B. A., and Julian, D. G.: Bilateral bundle branch block complicating acute myocardial infarction. Lancet 2:345, 1971.
21. Haft, J. I.: Editorial: The HV interval and patients with bifascicular block. J. Electrocardiol. 10:1, 1977.
22. Hatle, L., Saeterhau, S., and Rokseth, R.: Long-term conservative therapy of chronic AV block. Acta Med. Scand. 196:411, 1974.
23. Hayman, A., Arnman, K., and Ryden, L.: Syncope caused by lithium treatment. Report on two cases and a prospective investigation of the prevalence of lithium-induced sinus node dysfunction. Acta Med. Scand. 205:467, 1979.
24. Hindman, M. C., Wagner, G. S., JaRo, M., et al.: The clinical significance of bundle branch block complicating acute myocardial infarction. 1. Clinical characteristics, hospital mortality, and one-year follow-up. Circulation 58:679, 1978.
25. Hindman, M. C., Wagner, G. S., JaRo, M., et al.: The clinical significance of bundle branch block complicating acute myocardial infarction. 2. Indications for temporary and permanent pacemaker insertion. Circulation 58:689, 1978.
26. Imperial, E. S., Carballo, R., and Zimmerman, H. A.: Disturbances of rate, rhythm, and conduction in acute myocardial infarction. A statistical study of 153 cases. Am. J. Cardiol. 5:24, 1960.
27. James, T. N.: Myocardial infarction and atrial arrhythmias. Circulation 24:761, 1961.
28. James, T. N.: The chronotropic actions of ATP and related compounds studied by direct perfusion of the sinus node. J. Pharmacol. Exp. Ther. 149:233, 1965.
29. James, T. N.: The coronary circulation and conduction system in acute myocardial infarction. Prog. Cardiovasc. Dis. 10:410, 1968.

30. James, T. N., and Galakhov, I.: De subitaneis mortibus. XXVI. Fatal electrical instability of the heart associated with benign congenital polycystic tumor of the atrioventricular node. Circulation 56:667, 1977.
31. Julian, D. G., Valentine, P. A., and Miller, G. G.: Disturbances of rate, rhythm, and conduction in acute myocardial infarction. Prospective study of 100 consecutive unselected patients with the aid of electrocardiographic monitoring. Am. J. Med. 37:915, 1964.
32. Karpawich, P. P., Gilette, P. C., Garson, A., et al.: Congenital complete atrioventricular block: clinical and electrophysiologic predictors of need for pacemaker insertion. Am. J. Cardiol. 48:1098, 1981.
33. Kastor, J. A.: Editorial: Cardiac electrophysiology and stopped hearts. N. Engl. J. Med. 299:249, 1978.
34. Kim, H. G., and Friedman, H. S.: Procainamide-induced sinus node dysfunction in patients with chronic renal failure. Chest 76:699, 1979.
35. Kounis, N. G., and Chopra, R. K.: Atropine and bradycardia after myocardial infarction. Ann. Intern. Med. 81:117, 1974.
36. LaBarre, A., Strauss, H. C., Scheinman, M. M., et al.: Electrophysiologic effects of disopyramide phosphate on sinus node function in patients with sinus node dysfunction. Circulation 59:226, 1979.
37. Lasser, R. P., Haft, J. I., and Friedberg, C. K.: Relationship of right bundle branch block and marked left axis deviation (with left parietal or peri-infarction block) to complete heart block and syncope. Circulation 47:429, 1968.
38. Lie, K. I., Liem, K. L., Schuilenburg, R. M., et al.: Early identification of patients developing late in-hospital ventricular fibrillation after discharge from the coronary care unit. Am. J. Cardiol. 41:674, 1978.
39. Lien, W. P., Lee, Y. S., Chang, F. Z., et al.: The sick sinus syndrome. Natural history of dysfunction of the sinoatrial node. Chest 72:628, 1977.
40. Lightfoot, P. R., Sasse, L., Mandel, W. J., et al.: His bundle electrograms in healthy adolescents with persistent second degree AV block. Chest 63:358, 1973.
41. Mandel, W. J., Hayakawa, H., Allen, H. W., et al.: Assessment of sinus node function in patients with the sick sinus syndrome. Circulation 66:761, 1972.
42. Marriott, H. J. L., and Myerburg, R. J.: Recognition and treatment of cardiac arrhythmias and conduction disturbances. *In* Hurst, J. W. (ed.): The Heart, 4th ed. New York, McGraw-Hill Book Co., 1978, pp. 679–680.
43. Massie, B., Scheinman, M. M., Peters, R., et al.: Clinical and electrophysiologic findings in patients with paroxysmal slowing of the sinus rate and apparent Mobitz type II atrioventricular block. Circulation 58:305, 1978.
44. McAnulty, J. H., Rahimtoola, S. H., Murphy, E. S., et al.: A prospective study of sudden death in "high-risk" bundle branch block. N. Engl. J. Med. 299:209, 1978.
45. Meytes, I., Kaplinsky, E., Yakini, J. H., et al.: Wenckebach AV block: a frequent feature following heavy physical training. Am. Heart J. 90:426, 1975.
46. Moss, A. J., and Davis, R. J.: Brady-tachy syndrome. Prog. Cardiovasc. Dis. 16:439, 1974.
47. Narula, D. S., Scherlag, B. J., Samet, P., and Jacier, R. P.: Atrioventricular block: localization and classification by His bundle recordings. Am. J. Med. 50:146, 1971.
48. Nimetz, A. A., Shubrooks, S. J., Hutter, A. M., and DeSanctis, R. W.: The significance of bundle branch block during acute myocardial infarction. Am. Heart J. 90:439, 1975.
49. Norris, R. M.: Heart block in posterior and anterior myocardial infarction. Br. Heart J. 31:352, 1969.
50. Norris, R. M., and Mercer, C. J.: Significance of idioventricular rhythms in acute myocardial infarction. Prog. Cardiovasc. Dis. 16:455, 1974.
51. Norris, R. M., Mercer, C. J., and Croxson, M. S.: Conduction disturbances due to anteroseptal myocardial infarction and their treatment by endocardial pacing. Am. Heart J. 84:560, 1972.
52. Paulk, E. A., and Hurst, J. W.: Complete heart block in acute myocardial infarction. Am. J. Cardiol. 17:695, 1966.
53. Ritter, W. S., Atkins, J. M., Blomqvist, C. G., and Mullins, C. B.: Permanent pacing in patients with transient trifascicular block during acute myocardial infarction. Am. J. Cardiol. 38:205, 1976.
54. Rokseth, R., and Hatle, L.: Sinus arrest in acute myocardial infarction. Br. Heart J. 33:639, 1971.
55. Rotman, M., and Triebwasser, J. H.: A clinical and follow-up study of right and left bundle branch block. Circulation 51:477, 1975.
56. Rotman, M., Wagner, G. S., and Wallace, A. G.: Bradyarrhythmias in acute myocardial infarction. Circulation 45:703, 1972.
57. Rubenstein, J. J., Schulman, C. L., Yurchak, P. M., and DeSanctis, R. W.: Clinical spectrum of the sick sinus syndrome. Circulation 46:5, 1972.
58. Scanlon, P. J., Pryor, R., and Blount, S. G.: Right bundle branch block associated with left superior or inferior intraventricular block associated with acute myocardial infarction. Circulation 42:1135, 1970.
59. Scheinman, M. M., Kunkel, F. W., Peters, R. W., et al.: Atrial pacing in patients with sinus node dysfunction. Am. J. Med. 61:641, 1976.
60. Scheinman, M. M., Peters, R. W., Modin, G., et al.: Prognostic value of infranodal conduction time in patients with chronic bundle branch block. Circulation 56:240, 1977.
61. Scheinman, M. M., Strauss, H. C., Evans, G. T., et al.: Adverse effects of sympatholytic agents in patients with hypertension and sinus node dysfunction. Am. J. Med. 64:1013, 1978.
62. Scheinman, M. M., Thorburn, D., and Abbott, J. A.: Use of atropine in patients with acute myocardial infarction and sinus bradycardia. Circulation 52:627, 1975.
63. Scherlag, B. J., Lazzara, R., and Helfant, R. H.: Differentiation of "AV junctional rhythms." Circulation 48:304, 1973.
64. Schneider, J. F., Thomas, H. E., Jr., Kreger, B. E., et al.: Newly acquired left bundle branch block: the Framingham Study. Ann. Intern. Med. 90:303, 1979.
65. Schneider, J. F., Thomas, H. E., Jr., Kreger, B. E., et al.: Newly acquired right bundle branch block: the Framingham study. Ann. Intern. Med. 92:37, 1980.
66. Schuilenburg, A. M., and Durrer, D.: Conduction disturbances located within the His bundle. Circulation 45:612, 1972.
67. Simon, A. B., and Zloto, A. E.: Symptomatic sinus

node diseases. Natural history after permanent ventricular pacing. PACE 2:305, 1979.

68. Simonsen, E., Nielsen, B. L., and Nielsen, J. S.: Sinus node dysfunction in acute myocardial infarction. Acta Med. Scand. 208:463, 1980.
69. Strasberg, B., Amat-Y-Leon, F., Dhingra, R. C., et al.: Natural history of chronic second degree atrioventricular nodal block. Circulation: 63:1043, 1981.
70. Strauss, H. C., Bigger, J. T., Saroff, A. L., and Giardina, E. G. V.: Electrophysiologic evaluation of sinus node function in patients with sinus node dysfunction. Am. J. Med. 53:763, 1976.
71. Strauss, H. C., Gilbert, M., Svenson, R. H., et al.: Electrophysiologic effect of propranolol on sinus node function in patients with sinus node dysfunction. Circulation 54:452, 1976.
72. Surawicz, B.: Editorial: Prognosis of patients with chronic bifascicular block. Circulation 60:40, 1979.
73. Talano, J. V., Euler, D., Randall, W. C., et al.: Sinus node dysfunction. An overview with emphasis on autonomic and pharmacologic considerations. Am. J. Med. 64:773, 1978.
74. Walter, P. E., Crawley, I. S., and Dorney, E. R.: Carotid sinus hypersensitivity and syncope. Am. J. Cardiol. 42:396, 1978.
75. Wan, S. H., Lee, S. G., and Toh, C. C. S.: The sick sinus syndrome. A study of 15 cases. Br. Heart J. 34:942, 1972.
76. Young, D., Eisenberg, R., Fish, B., and Fisher, J. D.: Wenckebach atrioventricular block (Mobitz type I) in children and adolescents. Am. J. Cardiol. 40:393, 1977.

8

Pacemaker Emergencies

NORA GOLDSCHLAGER

and BONNIE SUDDUTH

In the United States 100,000 patients will have permanent pacing systems implanted this year, and additional thousands will undergo temporary cardiac pacing for various reasons such as drug toxicity, electrolyte abnormalities, sinus node dysfunction, and bradycardia occurring during acute myocardial infarction. In view of the frequency with which the physician is expected to encounter patients with pacemakers, and in recognition of the increasing complexity of pacemaker generator design, it is well to become familiar with certain features of normal and abnormal pacemaker function. This chapter, although not intended as an exhaustive review of cardiac pacing, addresses several common and specific circumstances in which permanent and temporary pacemaker-related emergencies may arise.

The seriousness of pacing system malfunction depends on its consequences for the patient's rhythm. Cessation of output or failure to capture are potentially the most dangerous abnormalities encountered in pacemaker-dependent patients, and in all patients in whom bradycardias cause symptoms. Failure to sense is a problem of lesser consequence, although the cause makes investigation mandatory. Rarely, the pacemaker generator can accelerate its rate ("runaway"), causing a life-threatening tachycardia or ventricular asystole due to inability of the ventricles to be stimulated at such rapid rates.

Although some instances of pacemaker malfunction are obvious, correct diagnosis may require precise knowledge of the type and specific design features of the implanted pulse generator. This is especially true today as so many permanent pacemaker generators have programmable functions, i.e., functions that can be transiently and reversibly altered (Table 8–1). Most patients have been instructed to carry their pacemaker identification cards with them at all times; however, the information contained therein is often insufficient to answer all the problems at hand. The pacemaker manufacturer's representative can be called to obtain the pulse generator characteristics if these are unfamiliar to the physician. If neither history nor identification card is available, a highly penetrated x-ray film of the generator may reveal a particular radiographic appearance and code by which the generator may be identi-

Table 8–1. PACEMAKER PROGRAMMABLE FUNCTIONS

- Rate
- Energy output
  - Volts
  - Amperes
  - Pulse duration
- Refractory period
- Sensitivity
- Mode of function
  - Asynchronous (fixed rate)
  - Hysteresis
  - Triggered
  - Synchronous (demand)
- AV delay (in dual chamber units)
- Rate limit (in dual chamber units)
  - Upper
  - Lower

fied. The standard electrocardiographic machine remains the main tool in the assessment of pacemaker function. It should be recognized that owing to paper drag, however, estimations of pacing rates may be incorrect; an inexpensive digital counter applied to the body surface provides more accurate rate measurements.

PACEMAKER RATES

A permanent pacemaker generator may have up to three rates or intervals, depending on the particular generator design. The escape interval is that interval between a spontaneous complex and the first paced complex that follows it. The automatic interval is the

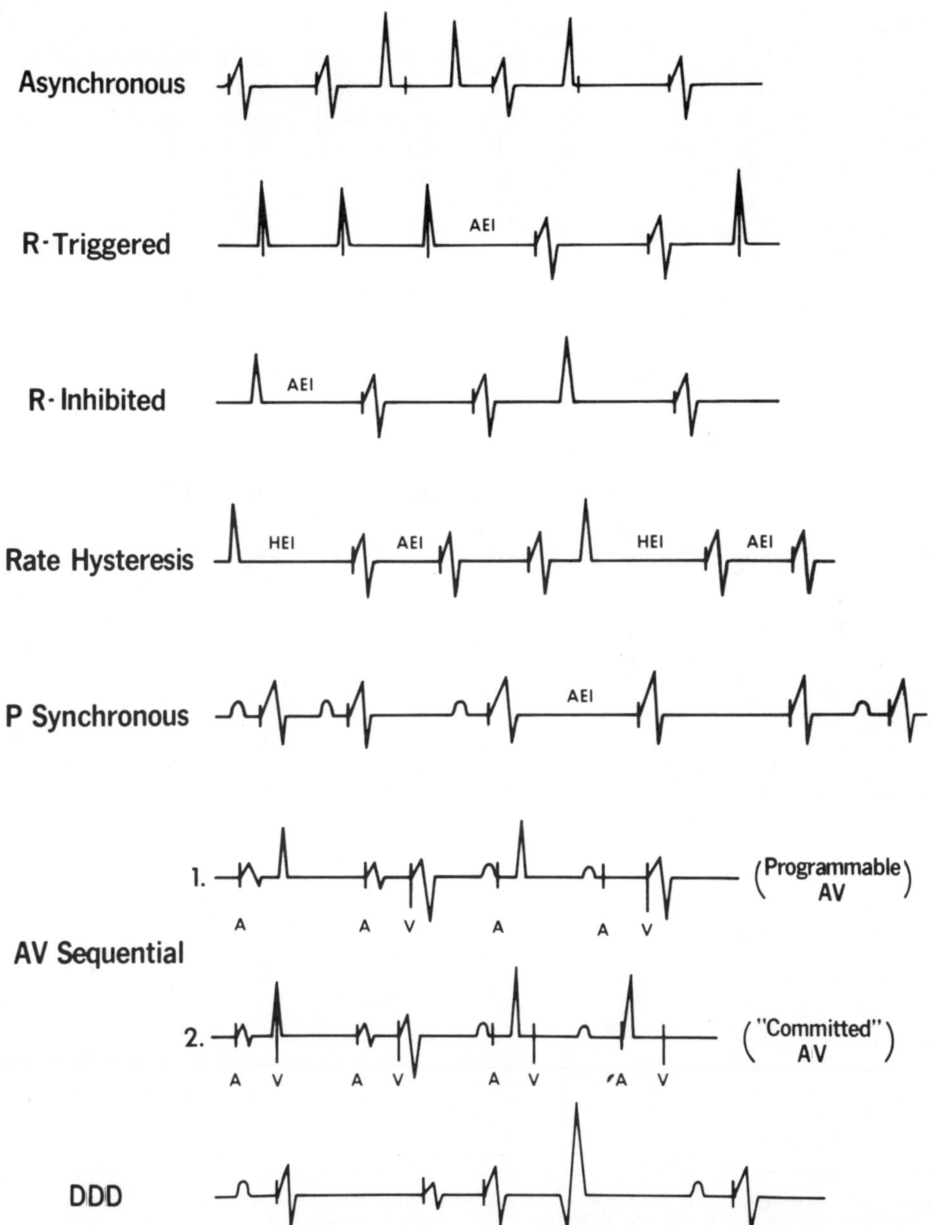

Figure 8–1. Schema of modes of function of different pacemaker generators. *AEI* = automatic escape interval; *HEI* = hysteresis escape interval; *A* = atrial stimulus; *V* = ventricular stimulus. See text for explanation.

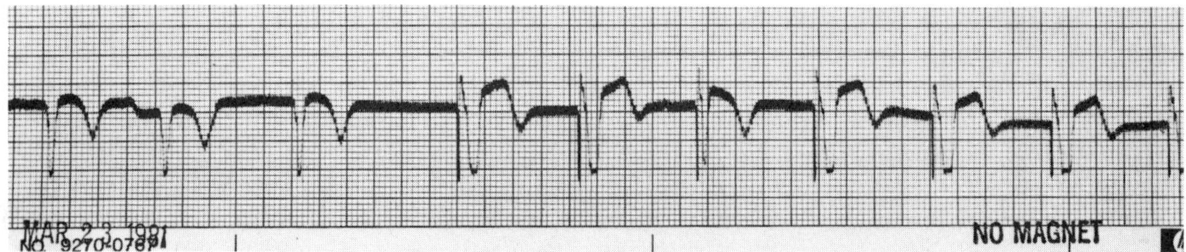

Figure 8–2. Rate hysteresis. The escape interval of the pacemaker generator is 1.2 sec and the automatic interval is 0.84 sec. The hysteresis mode of function was originally developed in order to allow maximal opportunity for a spontaneous P wave and QRS complex to occur, before ventricular pacing ensued. In some pacemaker generators currently in use, both the hysteresis mode of function and the hysteresis escape interval are programmable features.

interval between consecutive pacing artifacts. Often, but not always, the escape and automatic intervals are the same. However, several generators are designed to have the escape interval exceed the automatic interval, thus theoretically optimizing the opportunity for a spontaneous QRS complex to occur. These generators are said to show rate hysteresis (Figs. 8–1, 8–2). Awareness of rate hysteresis may obviate a mistaken diagnosis of inappropriately long pauses in paced rhythm.

The magnet rate of a pacemaker generator is the rate resulting from placement of the appropriate magnet over the generator. The properly aligned magnet closes the reed switch and inactivates the sensing mechanism of the pacemaker, converting it to an asynchronous (fixed-rate) pacemaker. Often, but again not always, the magnet rate is the same as the automatic rate (Fig. 8–3). The rationale for a difference between magnet and automatic rates lies in the assurance that the pacemaker generator has in fact been engaged by the magnet and is functioning asynchronously; magnet pacemaker rates are more accurate than automatic rates in assessing generator end-of-life.

It is important to remember that the automatic rate of a pacemaker may have been programmed to a low value. Verification that this has taken place will preclude a mistaken diagnosis of generator end-of-life, oversensing, or circuitry malfunction manifested by slow rate.

FAILURE OF OUTPUT

One of the most serious manifestations of pacing system malfunction is failure of output. Regular or irregular pauses in paced

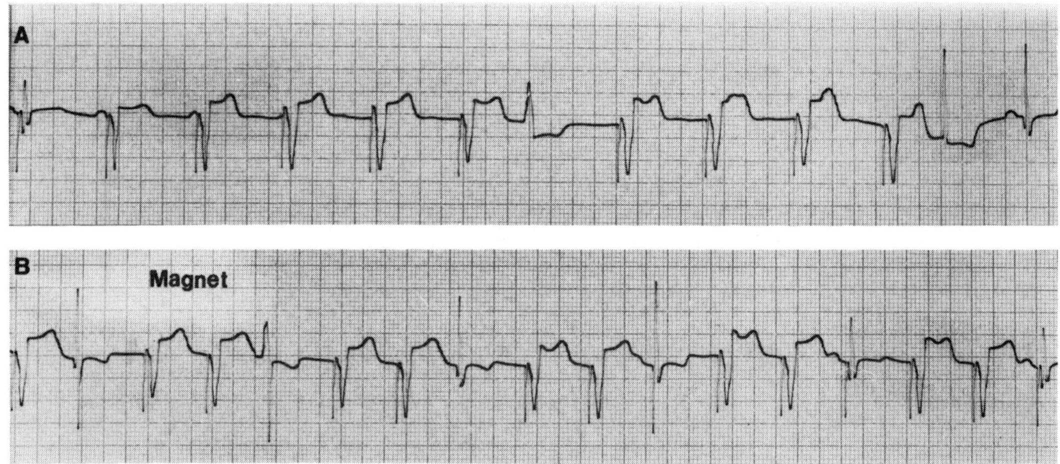

Figure 8–3. Automatic *(A)* and magnet *(B)* rates of a pacemaker generator. In *A*, the pacing rate is about 72 per min and represents the rate of the pacemaker when it is emitting stimuli "on demand." In *B*, a magnet is placed over the generator, whose rate is now about 100 per min. As not all pacemaker generators have different automatic and magnet rates, the identification card carried by the patient should be checked in order to verify these differences in pacing rates.

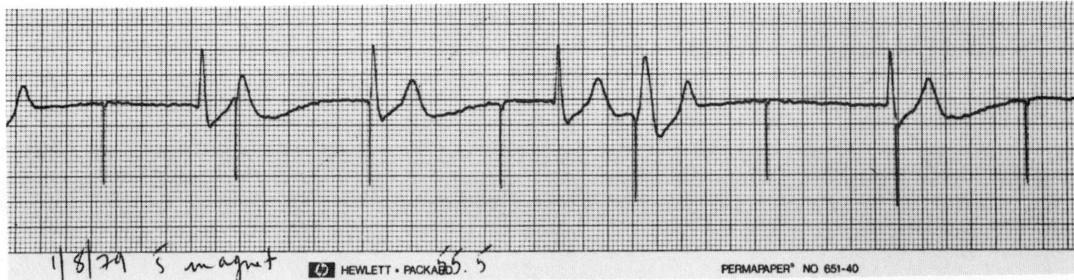

Figure 8–4. This tracing was obtained from a patient whose pulse generator was at end-of-life. Failure to capture is virtually complete, with the exception of a single instance (5th QRS complex) where capture occurs when the pacing stimulus is emitted 650 msec after a spontaneous QRS complex. When capture occurs only in a particular temporal relationship to a spontaneous QRS complex, it is considered to be related to the supernormal period of excitability of ventricular tissue, and indicates that the energy output of the pulse generator is very close to the myocardial stimulation threshold (see text).

rhythm or total cessation of pacing impulses may occur (Fig. 8–4). Symptoms of dizziness or syncope depend on the emergence, origin, rate, and stability of a spontaneous escape rhythm.

Absence of pacing artifacts can indicate normal demand pacemaker inhibition by a faster spontaneous rate, interruption of the pacing system that may be due to loose connections, lead fracture (Fig. 8–5), or battery depletion (Fig. 8–6). Only this last represents true output failure. Application of the appropriate magnet over the generator converts it to an asynchronous (fixed-rate) mode of function (Figs. 8–1, 8–3), thus allowing pacing impulses to be seen; capture occurs outside the refractory period of ventricular tissue. It should be emphasized again that a programmed rate of 50 to 60 pulses per minute is not at all unusual; recognition of this fact will obviate the mistaken diagnosis of slow rate due to battery depletion.

When the rate of a pacemaker generator slows by 7 to 10 per cent or increases by more than a few beats per minute (Fig. 8–6), elective generator replacement should be undertaken. Many programmable pulse generators indicate battery end-of-life by a fall in the magnet rate only, making routine application of a magnet mandatory during the

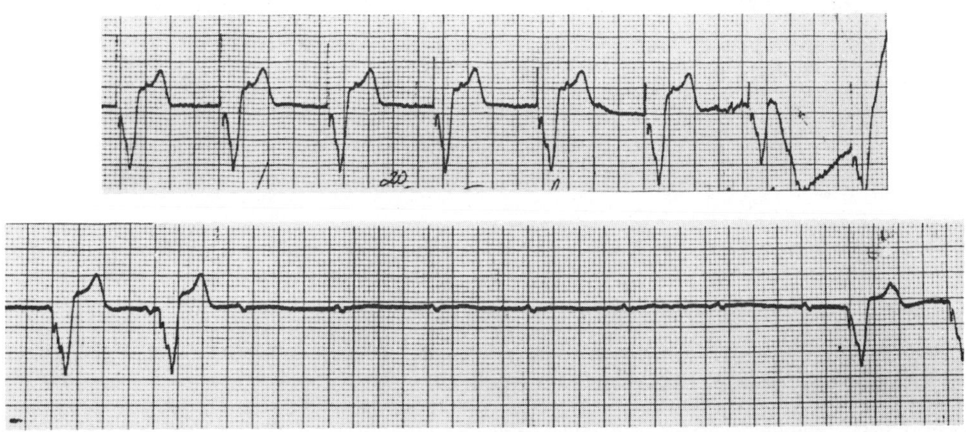

Figure 8–5. These continuous rhythm strips were taken from an ambulatory ECG recording in a patient complaining of syncopal and presyncopal spells. His pacing system had been in place for three years and had always functioned normally. All QRS complexes are paced, and there is no instance in which a pacing artifact occurs but is not followed by a QRS complex; thus, failure to capture is not present. Since spontaneous QRS complexes do not occur, sensing function is not demonstrated. Note the changing amplitude and polarity of the pacing artifacts, a finding that has been observed to occur in lead fracture. In the bottom strip, pacing artifacts abruptly disappear, resulting in ventricular asystole. The pause is not equal to a multiple of the basic pacing rate, but the potential variation in recording tape speed and/or writeout equipment preclude definitive measurements. At the time of operative revision, measurements of lead resistance and pulse generator function were normal. The course of the problem was found to be unexpected loosening and erosion of the setscrew that secured the lead to the generator. (Tracing courtesy of S. Mendelsohn, M.D.)

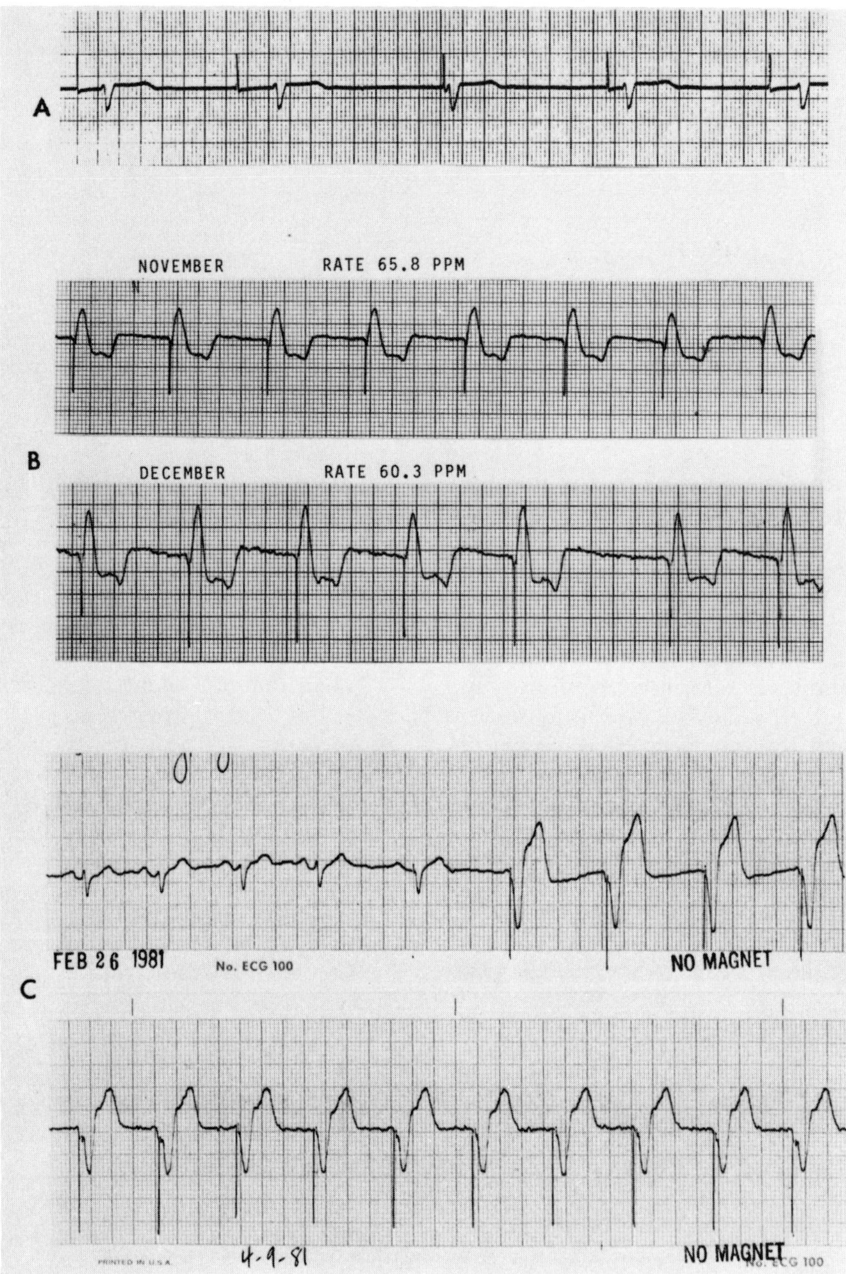

Figure 8–6. These tracings illustrate some of the manifestations of energy source depletion. The pulse generator in strip *A* had an automatic rate of 72 per min at implant. Four years later, its rate is 39 per min and no ventricular capture occurs; note that sensing function is preserved. The two strips in *B* were recorded one month apart. Not only has there been a substantial decline in automatic rate, but unexplained pauses are now occurring. The strips in *C,* taken about 5 wk apart, illustrate that generator end-of-life may present as an increase in automatic rate, in this case from a rate of about 67 per min to one of 82 per min. This was an unexpected mode of depletion, which may have represented runaway. These tracings serve to emphasize that the physician must be familiar with the end-of-life characteristics of particular pulse generators and aware that unusual modes of failure do occur.

battery check. The slowing of the magnet rate can be precipitous or gradual, depending on the power source; often the physician's manual or the manufacturer's representative must be consulted in order to provide information on the specific end-of-life characteristic of particular generators.

Random component failure can also cause a lack of pacer output. This is unpredictable in occurrence and should be diagnosed only

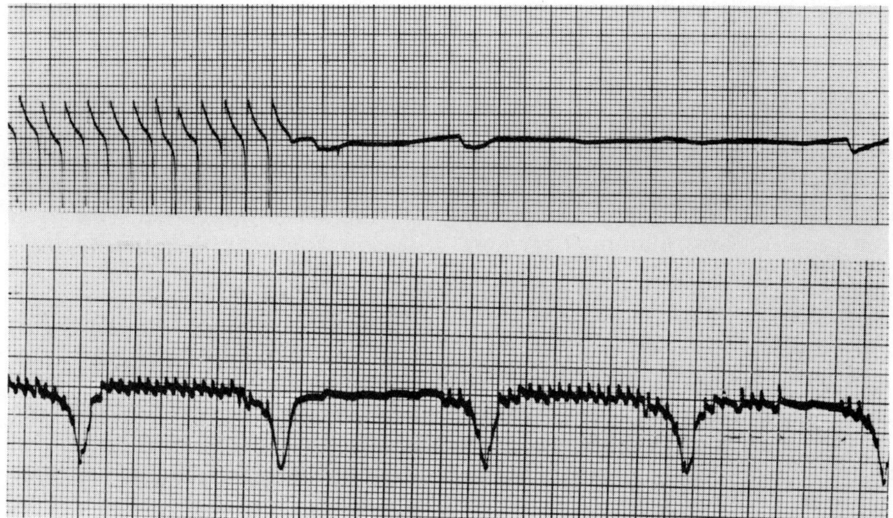

Figure 8–7. These tracings illustrate the relatively uncommon but potentially lethal "runaway pacemaker" due to electronic circuitry malfunction. In the top strip, the pacing stimuli are being emitted at a rate of about 300 per min; no ventricular capture is apparent. When pacing abruptly ceases, ventricular asystole results. In the bottom strip, pacing stimuli occur at a rate of about 800 per min, but the QRS rhythm is spontaneous and probably ventricular in origin, in view of its rate and morphology. (Tracings courtesy of S. Furman, M.D.)

after other causes have been investigated and excluded. A particular model generator may be especially suspected if like models have displayed similar features.

RUNAWAY PACEMAKER

Fortunately, runaway pacemaker due to battery depletion or electronic circuitry malfunction is relatively rare, but it still occurs.[11, 20, 32, 73, 76, 100] As it is potentially life-threatening, having an associated mortality of 40 to 60 per cent,[73] immediate recognition and rectification are required. Runaway pacemaker is present when pacing stimuli occur at rates exceeding 120 per minute; rates up to 1500 per minute have been reported[20] (Fig. 8–7). Runaway may occur in temporary or permanent pulse generators.

In instances in which the pacing stimuli occur at reasonable, albeit abnormally high, rates it is important to distinguish runaway pacemaker from spontaneous wide–QRS complex tachycardia in a patient with an R-triggered pacing system. In the latter (Figs. 8–1, 8–8), a pacing stimulus falls *within* each *sensed* QRS complex, rather than at its onset. Attention to the timing of the pacing artifacts relative to the onset of the QRS complexes and to the morphology of the wide-complex tachycardia (which may be different from the expected left bundle branch block pattern that occurs during right ventricular apical

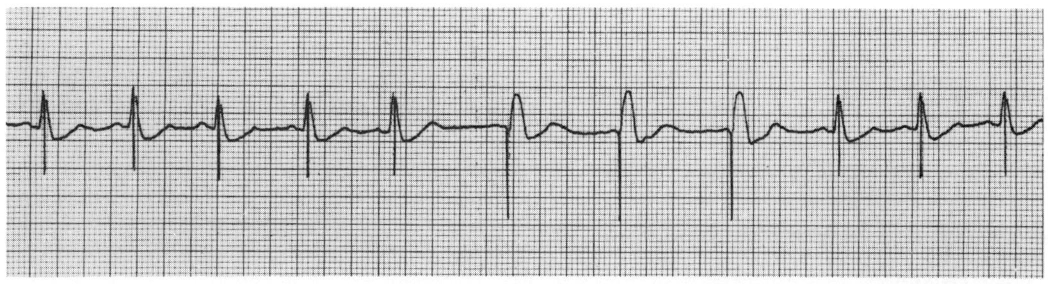

Figure 8–8. This rhythm strip illustrates the function of an R-triggered demand ventricular pacemaker generator with an automatic (pacing) rate of 72 per min (840-msec interval). An R-triggered pulse generator emits an impulse upon sensing electrical signals of a given magnitude, whether they originate within or outside of the heart. In this tracing, the first five and last three QRS complexes are spontaneous and contain pacing artifacts within them, indicating that they have been sensed by the pulse generator. As the pacing stimuli fall *within* the QRS complex, they do not contribute to ventricular activation. A pause after the fifth spontaneous QRS complex is terminated by a paced QRS complex at an escape interval of about 0.84 sec. The R-triggered mode of function may be particularly helpful in the analysis of sensing problems.

stimulation) will help to distinguish runaway from R-triggered pacemakers. Application of a magnet will convert an R-triggered generator to an asynchronous mode of function at a specific rate, thus allowing a wide-complex tachycardia to be recognized as occurring spontaneously. Finally, the pacemaker identification card carried by the patient should provide the required information regarding pacemaker generator type and, in programmable units, the programmed mode of function.

The ventricular response to stimuli delivered extremely rapidly is variable. Capture may not occur at all, resulting in ventricular asystole or the emergence of a spontaneous QRS rhythm (Fig. 8–7). Ventricular responses may occur at variable rates or at divisible intervals of the pacing cycle length; in the latter instance, exit block of the rapidly delivered impulses, or their occurrence within the refractory period of ventricular tissue, is the probable cause.

Management of runaway pacemaker consists of interrupting cardiac stimulation. The rapidity with which this must be done depends on the pacemaker rate and the hemodynamic state of the patient; however, it should be stressed that runaway pacemakers can unpredictably increase their rates within seconds to minutes,[76] necessitating prompt and aggressive treatment. If the implanted pulse generator is a programmable one, programming it to its lowest energy output may be effective in interruption of capture, provided that myocardial stimulation does not occur at the low output. Use of a magnet to convert runaway pacemakers to their slower asynchronous mode of function is usually unsuccessful. An attempt may be made to inhibit the implanted pacemaker generator temporarily by means of chest wall stimulation; this maneuver is not always successful, and failure of a spontaneous cardiac rhythm to emerge is common. On occasion, emergency bedside transection of the pacing catheter from the generator must be performed, and a new pacing system implanted at a different site at a later time. Interim temporary pacing, if required, may be accomplished either by placing a temporary pacing catheter or by connecting the wire(s) of the permanently implanted lead to an external pacemaker generator by means of alligator clamps.

FAILURE TO CAPTURE

Failure to capture may be intermittent or complete, and may be accompanied by failure to sense. In cases of failure to capture, pacing artifacts are recorded but QRS complexes are not produced. Failure to capture requires rapid diagnosis of cause, and early correction (Table 8–2). A common cause of early failure to capture is lead dislodgement, including myocardial penetration or perforation; the consequent loss of contact between the electrode(s) and the endocardium results in stimulation of insufficient heart muscle to produce ventricular activation.

Failure to capture may also be due to elevation in myocardial stimulation threshold so that energy output of the pulse generator is insufficient to depolarize ventricular tissue. Myocardial stimulation threshold depends on the interface between the stimulating electrodes and the myocardium; the duration of the emitted pacing stimulus; the size, shape, and surface area of the electrode; the presence of drugs; electrolyte balance; intercurrent cardiac events such as myocardial infarction (*see below*); and the age of the implant.[35, 84] It is now well recognized that myocardial stimulation threshold may vary considerably within the first two months after implant, before stable (chronic) stimulation thresholds are reached. Chronic stimulation thresholds are usually two to three times

Table 8–2. CAUSES AND MANAGEMENT OF LOSS OF CAPTURE

Diagnosis	Management
Electrode catheter displacement	Reposition
Generator end-of-life	Replace generator
Increased myocardial stimulation threshold	Reposition; replace generator with high-output unit; reprogram output; treat underlying clinical condition
Lead fracture	Convert to unipolar; replace
Insulation break	Repair; convert to unipolar; replace
Cardiac perforation	Reposition; replace
Loose connections	Repair; replace

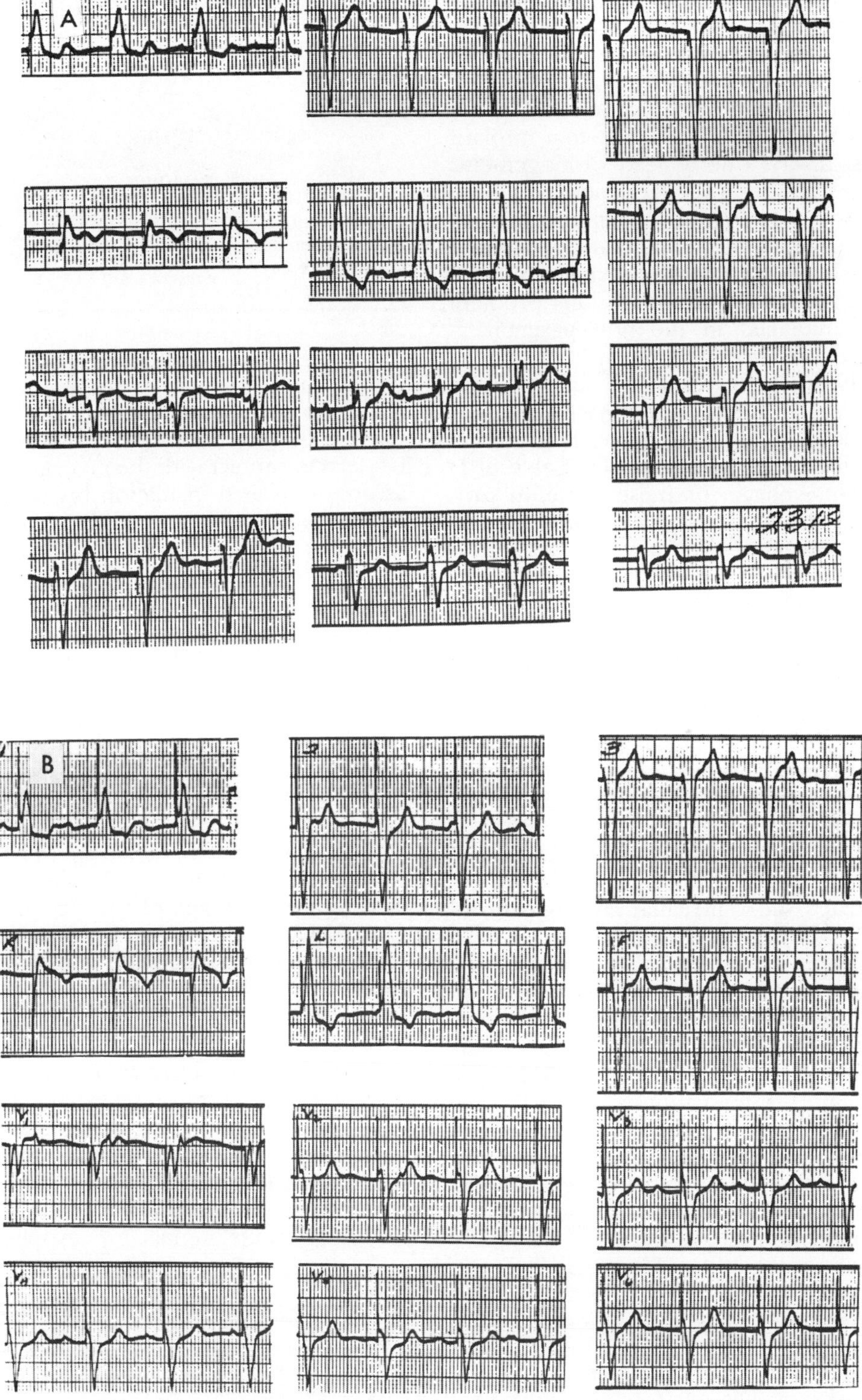

Figure 8–9. These 12-lead ECGs were recorded several weeks apart in an 87-year-old woman who had had a normally functioning bipolar pacemaker generator for five years. The QRS rhythm is paced and the QRS morphology is identical in the two tracings. In *A*, the pacing artifacts are positively directed in leads I, aVL, and aVR, and negatively directed in leads II, III, and aVF. In *B*, there has been a marked increase in pacing artifact amplitude, and reversal of polarity in the inferior leads. The preoperative diagnosis of insulation break was confirmed at the time of operative revision, when a break encompassing the entire circumference of the cathodal insulation was found.

higher than acute stimulation thresholds, although there is a small group of patients in whom stimulation threshold continues to rise with time.[64]

Failure to capture that occurs during the first two weeks after pacing system implant is almost always due to lead dislodgement; lead repositioning is the treatment of choice (Table 8–2). The most common cause of capture problems occurring between two and eight weeks after implant is elevation of myocardial stimulation threshold. This problem may be managed in the non–pacemaker-dependent patient by administration of steroids, although the results of such therapy are variable.[101] Patients who have programmable pulse generators can have their energy outputs increased noninvasively (Table 8–1) by current, voltage, or pulse duration programming; when chronic thresholds have stabilized, the energy output can be reprogrammed to a lower value. Finally, failure to capture that occurs years after pacing system implant is almost always due to energy source depletion, and generator replacement is required. Output programming can serve as a temporizing measure while arrangements are made for definitive management. If at surgery the chronic stimulation thresholds are found to be high, replacement with a high-output unit may be required.

When the energy output of a pulse generator is barely sufficient to stimulate myocardial tissue, ventricular capture may occur only during the supernormal period of excitability[14, 25, 26, 35, 42, 58, 78, 89, 94] (Fig. 8–4). The supernormal period of excitability of cardiac tissue is a specific time interval toward the end of the repolarization process when membrane potential is closest to threshold, allowing subthreshold stimuli to evoke a response, and has been defined in patients with failing pacemakers.[14, 25, 26] The supernormal period has been measured to begin 370 to 450 msec after the onset of a spontaneous QRS complex, and its duration has been determined to be 40 to 175 msec.[78, 94] Thus, the supernormal period has both variable onset after a spontaneous complex and variable duration. These characteristics have been shown to depend, at least in part, on the strength of the stimuli being applied or delivered.[94] If consistent capture occurs *only* in the supernormal period of excitability, it reflects stimulation threshold elevation and/or decreased pacemaker output voltage,

Table 8–3. CAUSES OF PAUSES IN PACED RHYTHM

A. *Oversensing*
P waves
T waves
Electromagnetic interference
Voltage transients
Electrode catheter fracture
Insulation leak
Myopotentials
Afterpotentials
B. *Rate hysteresis*
C. *Battery depletion*

but not circuit malfunction such as loose connections or lead fracture.

Failure to capture may be due to loss of energy output before it reaches the electrode(s) in contact with the myocardium, such as occurs in lead insulation break (Fig. 8–9) or wire fracture. In insulation break, current leaks out into body tissues, taking the path of least resistance to the anode. Because of this current leakage, insufficient energy may reach cardiac tissue to activate it. Comparative ECGs often offer useful clues to the diagnosis of insulation break, as pacing artifact amplitude will be noticeably larger (in bipolar pacing systems), reflecting the larger amount of current reaching body fluids. Changes in pacing artifact polarity may also occur.

Lead fracture may be partial (make-break) with normal pacing and sensing occurring during the "making" of the circuit, or total. Occasionally, two ends of a fractured wire separate totally during certain body movements and reappose during others, making diagnosis difficult. The ends of the broken wires can cause spurious ("false") signals due to abrupt changes in resistance as they move against each other; these voltage transients may be sensed, resulting in inhibition of the pulse generator (Table 8–3). In these cases, the pacemaker spike-to-spike intervals are irregular, owing to the intermittent sensing of the spurious signals.[22, 105] Application of

Table 8–4. ECG MANIFESTATIONS OF ELECTRODE FRACTURE

Absence of pacing artifacts with magnet applied
Attenuation of pacing artifacts
Occurrence of pacing artifacts at multiples of basic interstimulus interval
Alteration of vectorial characteristics of pacing artifacts
Visible voltage transients
Loss of capture

Table 8–5. UNDERSENSING OF INTRACARDIAC SIGNALS

Causes
Inadequate signal voltage
Slow rate of change of voltage (slew)
Prolonged signal duration
Clinical Situations in Which It May Occur
Acute myocardial ischemia and/or infarction
Poor electrode position
Impulse originating in ventricular tissue
Pacemaker component failure

Table 8–6. LOSS AND APPARENT LOSS OF SENSING FUNCTION

Diagnosis	Management
Generator malfunction	Replace generator
Inadequate signal	Reposition; convert to unipolar; reprogram sensitivity
Malposition	Reposition
Electrode fracture	Convert to unipolar; replace lead
Electromagnetic interference	Reprogram sensitivity; convert to asynchronous or triggered pacing if required; change pacing catheter
Spontaneous complexes falling within pacemaker refractory period	Reprogram sensitivity; reprogram refractory period; no treatment

the appropriate magnet will eliminate all sensing; should interstimulus intervals occur that are multiples of the basic pacing rate, lead fracture is documented.[4] The ECG features of wire fracture are listed in Table 8–4.

SENSING PROBLEMS

Sensing problems can be of two kinds: undersensing, or lack of sensing; and oversensing, or sensing of unwanted signals, whether arising in the heart, in the pacing system itself, or in the environment (Tables 8–3, 8–5, and 8–6).

Undersensing

Undersensing occurs when the pacemaker generator does not see an intrinsic signal and thus does not recycle, when it might be expected to do so. To meet the sensing criteria of a pulse generator (which are determined by its bandpass filter), intrinsic signals must have sufficient amplitude and rate of change of voltage (slew). Under normal circumstances, P waves and T waves do not meet these criteria and are filtered out, and therefore not sensed. Some intrinsic ventricular signals, particularly those originating in ventricular tissue, do not meet the requirements for sensing and thus are not sensed (Figs. 8–10, 8–11). Occasionally, spontaneous complexes are sensed some time after their onset as determined from the surface ECG; this "late sensing" results in the subsequent pacer impulse being emitted a few milliseconds after its expected escape interval (Fig. 8–12).[101] This phenomenon is not infrequently observed in patients with right bundle branch

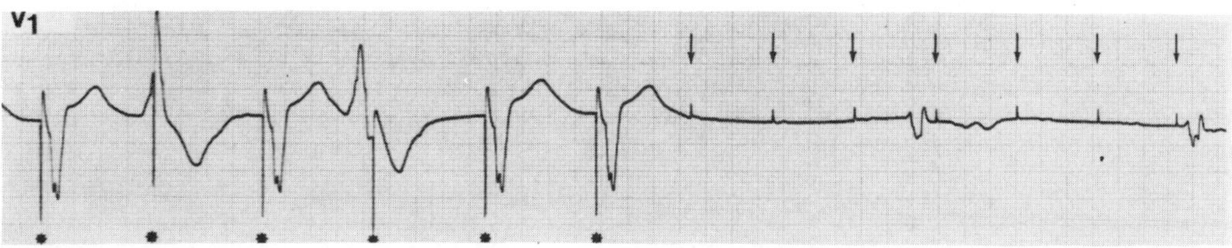

Figure 8–10. This rhythm strip was recorded in a patient with a demand pacemaker generator in place. In the left-hand portion of the tracing, pacing stimuli are being emitted asynchronously despite the occurrence of premature ventricular complexes, which therefore have not been sensed. As failure to sense the ventricular beats may be due to the suboptimal nature of the intracardiac signal or to pulse generator malfunction, integrity of the sensing function of the generator requires evaluation. In this patient, this was accomplished by means of chest wall stimulation. Chest wall stimuli *(arrows)* at a current strength of 1 mA inhibit the implanted generator, and a slow ventricular escape rhythm emerges. Because chest wall stimuli of only 1 mA effectively inhibit the generator, sensing malfunction is not present; the premature ventricular beats are not sensed because of their signal characteristics (see Table 8–5).

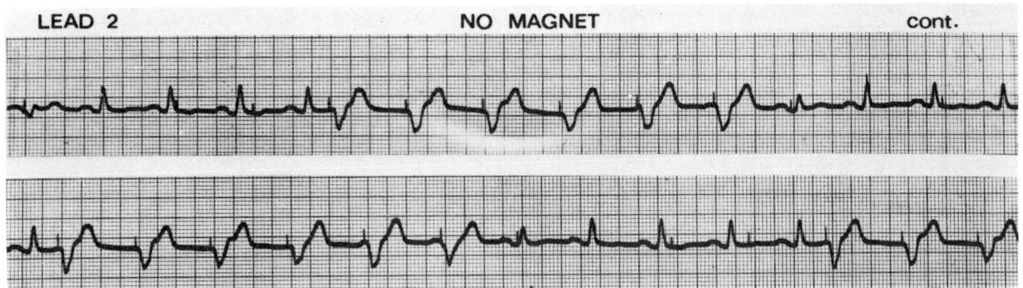

Figure 8–11. The patient is a 52-year-old man with chronic renal failure, paroxysmal complete AV block, and a permanent programmable demand pacemaker. The tracings show sinus rhythm and normal AV conduction. Pacing stimuli are occurring at regular intervals of about 0.82 sec, despite the presence of a spontaneous rhythm; thus, failure to sense is present. QRS complexes 1, 12, 22, 23 and 24 are *fusion* complexes, in which the ventricles are activated via both sinus and pacing impulses. QRS complexes 2 and 13 are *pseudofusion* complexes, in which pacing artifacts fall on a QRS complex but do not contribute to ventricular activation. In this patient, the failure to sense was corrected by noninvasive programming that enabled the generator to sense cardiac signals of boderline amplitude (sensitivity programming).

block,[103] in whom the impulse reaches the catheter electrodes (positioned in the apex of the right ventricle) after some delay, relative to the onset of inscription of the complex on the surface ECG, and in patients with inferior and/or right ventricular infarction, in whom delay in impulse conduction can be caused by ischemic or scar tissue.

A relatively common misdiagnosis of failure to sense may be made if the physician is unfamiliar with the refractory period that all pulse generators are designed to have (Fig. 8–13). After each output pulse or sensed spontaneous complex, the pacemaker generator is refractory for 200 to 400 msec (a programmable time period in some generators), during which it does not sense any signal. If an intrinsic beat occurs during this time, the pulse generator does not sense it and thus does not recycle; therefore, the interval between pacing artifacts is shorter than expected. The purpose of the refractory period is to prevent pacemaker recycling on T waves or late parts of QRS complexes, resulting in a rate that is slower than desired.

If failure to sense is detected, the possibility of lead malposition or wire fracture should be explored. If no apparent reason for the sensing failure is found, and there is no accompanying failure to capture, a patient who is asymptomatic may be closely followed without pacing system revision. If the pulse generator in place is programmable, programming it to "see" signals of lesser magnitude by increasing its sensitivity should be performed. Transient loss of sensing may be caused by intercurrent events such as myocardial infarction and congestive heart failure. Watchful waiting is indicated in such circumstances. If, however, the failure to sense causes symptoms of palpitations or repetitive ventricular beating, the pacing system requires revision. It should be noted that pacemaker-induced sustained ventricular tachycardia or fibrillation is rare with current pulse generators under the usual clinical circumstances in which they are implanted. The risk for pacemaker-induced arrhythmias does increase, however, during acute myocardial infarction[10, 15, 39, 41] and as a result of drug toxicity or electrolyte imbalance.[48, 55, 63, 79]

Rarely, failure to sense may be due to malfunction of the sensing circuit or to a sticky reed switch (the opening of which is mandatory for proper sensing function). A check of the sensing circuit can be made using the technique of chest wall stimulation[6] (Fig. 8–10). To perform this technique, surface or subcutaneous electrodes (suction cup or monitoring electrodes, or metal needles) are placed over the implanted electrodes. In bipolar pacing systems, the surface electrodes should be positioned close together (but not touching) at the lower end of the sternum, approximating the presumed position of the intracardiac electrodes in the apex of the right ventricle. In unipolar systems, one surface electrode is placed over the presumed intracardiac location of the cathode, and the other surface electrode over the pulse generator, which serves as the anode. The surface electrodes are then connected by means of cables to the pins of an external pacemaker generator. The rate of the external generator is then set to exceed that of the implanted generator, and asynchronous (fixed-rate) pacing mode is selected. The external generator is then turned on and its output gradually increased. When the chest wall stimuli are of sufficient magnitude to be sensed by the implanted generator, it will inhibit. Inhibition of the implanted generator ensures the integrity of the sensing function of the unit. At the current outputs used during chest wall stimulation, the patient suffers no discomfort.

Oversensing

Oversensing occurs when unwanted signals cause inhibition of the pulse generator (Table 8–3). Intrinsic P waves and T waves are usually filtered out by the bandpass filter of the sensing amplifier and are not sensed. P-wave sensing can occur, however, if the electrode catheter is positioned close to atrial tissue (near the tricuspid valve or in the coronary sinus), and the resulting pulse generator inhibition can have serious consequences if the patient has an inadequate intrinsic ventricular rhythm.

T-wave sensing is more common, and occurs more frequently with paced than with spontaneous QRS complexes. It is not infrequently observed just after pacing system implant and probably reflects sensing of a profound current of injury. Sensing of T waves may be difficult to distinguish from sensing of "afterpotentials," the charged energy that is present at the electrode(s) after a pacing stimulus, particularly one of high-energy output, is delivered.[8] If afterpotential sensing is occurring and if the generator is a programmable one, the pacemaker energy output can be decreased, which should result in restoration of desired sensing function. If T-wave sensing is occurring, the problem may be solved by programming the generator to lower sensitivity so that it will "see" signals of larger amplitude. Another way of abolishing T-wave sensing noninvasively is to program the generator to a longer refractory period; the T wave then falls within the refractory period and is therefore incapable of being sensed. In temporary pacing, T-wave sensing is managed by decreasing the sensitivity of the external pulse generator by turning its sensitivity setting away from "demand" toward "asynchronous."

Myopotentials generated by contraction of the pectoralis major muscles can achieve an amplitude of 0.5 to 3.0 mv. These signals may be sensed by pacemaker generators, es-

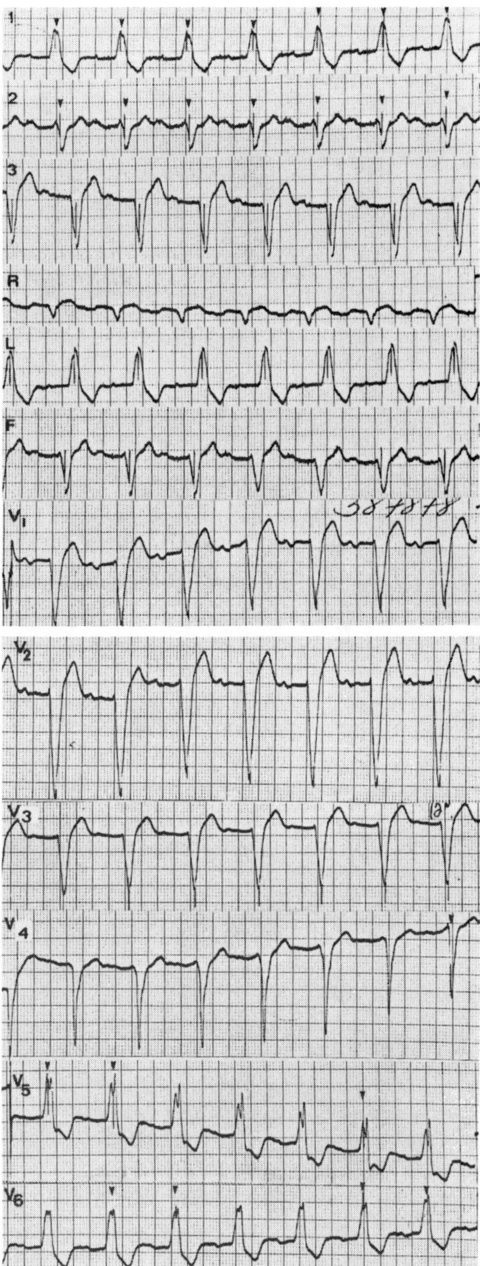

Figure 8–12. This 56-year-old woman had an epicardial pacing lead implanted on the left ventricle at the time of aortic valve replacement. The 12-lead ECG shows sinus rhythm, first-degree AV block, and left bundle branch block pattern. Within some of the QRS complexes are pacing artifacts (*arrows* point to some of these), which do not contribute to ventricular activation. The reason for the occurrence of pacing artifacts within the QRS complexes is that the left ventricular epicardial lead "sees" the spontaneous ventricular signal late relative to its onset of inscription, owing to the delay in impulse conduction over left ventricular myocardium (and thence to the electrode catheter). This is not pacemaker generator malfunction but reflects the time, relative to the beginning of ventricular depolarization, that the impulse takes to reach the sensing electrode.

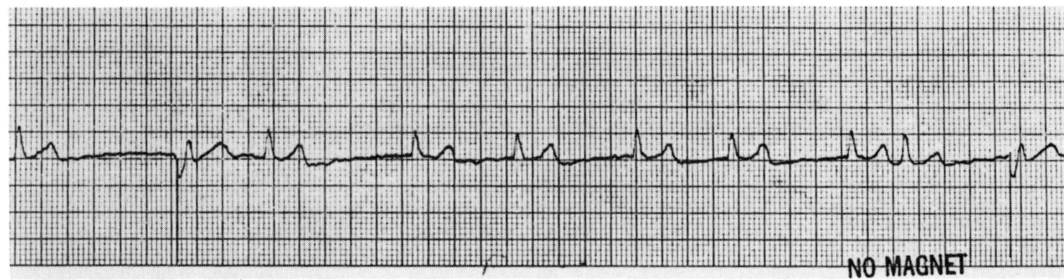

Figure 8–13. This rhythm strip was obtained in a patient whose pacemaker generator had been programmed to a rate of 50 beats per min and whose refractory period was about 400 msec. The first paced complex follows the previous spontaneous QRS complex at a normal escape interval of about 1280 msec (rate about 47 per min). The second paced complex (last complex on strip) follows the previous spontaneous complex by only about 880 msec, corresponding to a rate of about 68 per min. As the escape interval of this pulse generator is 1280 sec, the generator has not sensed the last spontaneous QRS complex. It has, however, sensed the one before it, since the interval between the second-to-last spontaneous QRS complex and the subsequent paced complex is 1280 msec. The unsensed spontaneous QRS complex follows the previous one by about 400 msec; thus, it has fallen in the refractory period of the pulse generator and is not expected to be sensed.

pecially unipolar ones, since the potential difference of the signal is augmented in unipolar units by the distance between the cathodal (intracardiac) electrode and the anode (the pulse generator). Bipolar pacemaker generators are only rarely inhibited by myopotentials, since the potential difference of the signal sensed between the distal and proximal electrodes, both intracardiac, is much smaller. Myopotentials are related to activity, and pulse generator inhibition can be avoided if required by application of the appropriate magnet, which eliminates all sensing. Patients with unipolar pacing systems who exhibit inhibition during activity should have their pacing system evaluated during several sorts of torso and upper arm activity, including pushing against a resistance, pulling, and deep breathing.[80, 82] Not rarely, only one of several types of muscle movement will cause inhibition. Management of myopotential inhibition includes changing the pacing system to a bipolar one, or, if the generator is programmable, decreasing the sensitivity to preclude sensing of low-amplitude signals. Another, less desirable option is to program the generator to an asynchronous (fixed-rate) or triggered mode of function. In the latter mode of function the generator will deliver an output pulse upon sensing any electrical activity; thus, long pauses in paced rhythm will be avoided.

Spurious ("false") signals that arise from abrupt changes in resistance in the pacing lead itself can be sensed by the pacemaker generator. False signals occur when the apposed ends of a fractured wire are intermittently in contact, when a previously implanted electrode is left in place and a new lead placed,[105] and when a temporary pacing catheter makes contact with a permanent pacing lead. Application of a magnet eliminates unwanted pauses due to sensing of spurious signals. Proper management consists of recognizing the problem and removing the source of its generation.

Electromagnetic interference from the environment, in the form of pulsed electrical energy, can inhibit demand pacemaker generators.[49] Arc welders, car or lawn mower engines, electrocautery devices, and radiofrequency transmitting systems have been reported to interfere with cardiac pacemakers. Another response of a pacemaker generator to strong electromagnetic interference is conversion to a fixed-rate mode of function, which usually is not perceived by the patient. In the hospital setting, radiofrequency signals and use of electrocautery devices are potential causes of ventricular asystole due to pulse generator inhibition. The appropriate magnet should always be available to convert the generator to a fixed-rate mode of function, thus ensuring stable pacing.

CARDIAC PACING IN DRUG TOXICITY AND ELECTROLYTE ABNORMALITIES

The most frequently encountered drug and electrolyte disturbances associated with pacemaker-related problems are hyperkalemia and Type I antiarrhythmic (quinidine, procainamide, disopyramide) drug toxicity, although hypokalemia can cause problems on occasion.

Hyperkalemia has been well documented as causing an increase in myocardial stimulation threshold, resulting in failure to capture.[96] In the experimental setting, the increase in stimulation threshold is related directly but nonlinearly to increases in serum

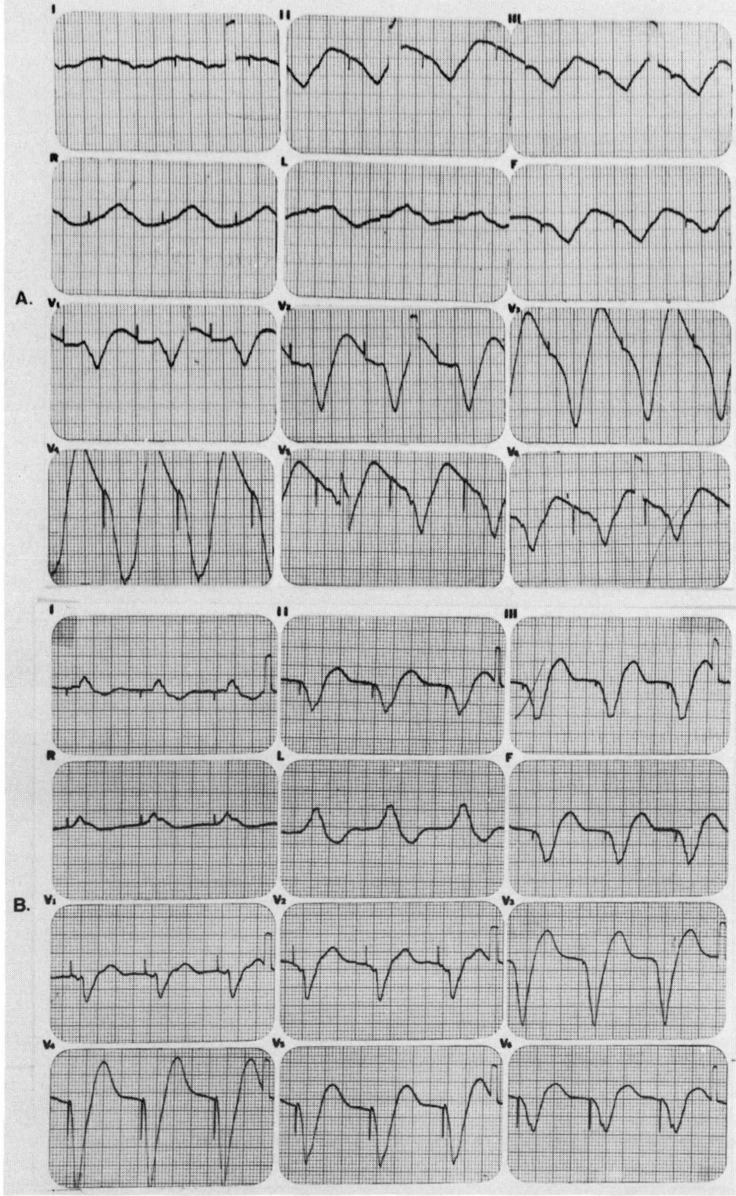

Figure 8–14. These 12-lead ECGs were recorded from a patient with severe congestive heart failure, renal failure, metabolic acidosis (pH 7.2), and profound hyperkalemia (serum K^+ = 7.8Eq/l). Tracing *A* was obtained on admission, and tracing *B* about 30 min later after intravenous administration of sodium bicarbonate, glucose, and insulin. Atrial activity is not discerned in either tracing. In *A*, the paced QRS complexes have markedly long duration of about 0.40 sec, and the T waves merge with the QRS complexes in a sine-wave pattern, compatible with the diagnosis of hyperkalemia. In several of the precordial leads, the pacemaker spike-to-QRS complex exceeds 0.20 sec, raising the possibility of first-degree pacemaker exit block, in which there is delay in conduction of the pacing impulses from the electrodes to surrounding ventricular muscle. In *B*, (serum K^+ = 5.8 mEq/l), the paced QRS complexes are narrower and better defined and the sine-wave pattern is resolving. The precordial leads now show a shorter spike-to-QRS interval, suggesting some improvement in the previously marked local conduction delay between the pacing electrodes and myocardial tissue.

concentration of potassium, and occurs independently of pH, Po_2, Pco_2, and sodium and calcium concentrations.[96] This last point deserves particular emphasis since, in the clinical setting of hyperkalemia, treatment directed specifically at lowering the serum potassium must be carried out urgently, regardless of any additional therapeutic maneuvers to correct accompanying abnormalities in pH or Po_2.

In clinical situations in which intermittent failure to capture occurs, hyperkalemia as the underlying cause can be suspected from a prolonged P-wave duration or total absence of atrial activity, and from the morphology of spontaneous or paced QRS complexes[45] (Figs. 8–14 to 8–16). These complexes are markedly prolonged in duration, often exceeding 200 msec; loss of QRS-complex definition occurs, with merging of the QRS "wave" into the ST–T "wave," producing a sine-wave appearance (Fig. 8–14). Treatment of the hyperkalemia is associated with narrowing of the QRST complex and improved morphologic features (Fig. 8–14). Restoration of stable pacing occurs and stimulation threshold progressively decreases.

The mechanism for failure to capture in hyperkalemia relates to the effect of high potassium concentrations on the action potentials of cardiac tissue. High potassium concentration reduces the resting membrane potential toward zero, slows the rate of depolarization (phase 0), and shortens the action potential duration, all of which contribute to the requirement for greater stimulus intensity to initiate a response. Interestingly, sensing function of a pacemaker generator in patients with hyperkalemia is often preserved despite pacing problems, suggesting that the effects of high potassium concentration on intracardiac electrical signal quality is not detrimental, at least in the usual ranges of clinical hyperkalemia.

Management of failure to capture in the setting of hyperkalemia is directed toward restoring normal serum levels of potassium and improving the intra- and extracellular potassium relationship. If a programmable pulse generator is in place, energy output can be increased by noninvasive programming; in our experience, however, the myocardial stimulation threshold almost always exceeds the maximal output of the pacemaker generator.

On occasion, temporary cardiac pacing has been employed successfully in patients with hyperkalemia and life-threatening bradycardia.[88, 98] Despite associated marked prolongation of QRS duration, ventricular capture may occur at acceptable pacing stimulus strengths.

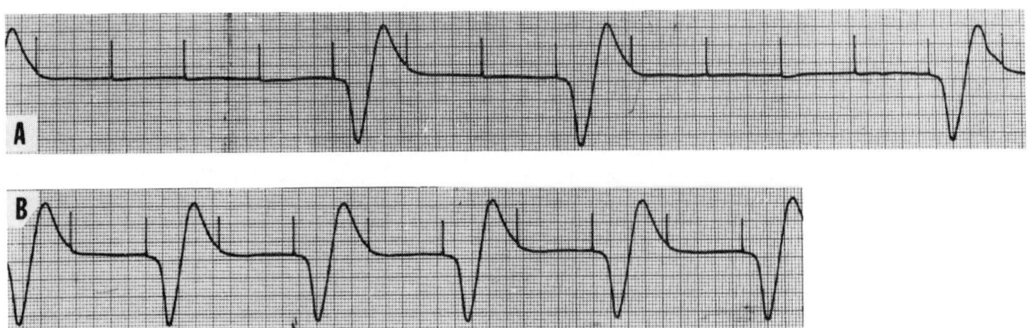

Figure 8–15. Exit block from a pacemaker generator in a patient with hyperkalemia and end-stage congestive heart failure. In *A*, the QRS complexes are paced at a long spike-to-QRS interval of 0.14 sec. Most pacing stimuli are not followed by a QRS complex, indicating that myocardial stimulation threshold has exceeded the output of the pacemaker generator. In *B*, recorded during an intravenous infusion of isoproterenol, 2:1 pacemaker exit block is present. The improved conduction ratio between pacemaker and ventricular myocardium could not be sustained and the patient expired.

In cases of pacemaker exit block, temporizing measures to lower myocardial stimulation threshold include intravenous use of steroids and isoproterenol; optimization of arterial blood gases, pH, electrolyte concentraiton, and ventricular function; and avoidance of pharmacologic agents that produce local conduction blocks such as Type I antiarrhythmic agents. Temporizing measures that increase pacemaker generator output consist of programming the generator to deliver stimuli of greater intensity, if this is possible. Despite these measures, the outcome remains dismal owing to the underlying clinical state.

It is important to recognize that the failure to capture illustrated in this tracing is due not to pacemaker generator malfunction, but to an abnormally elevated myocardial stimulation threshold resulting from myocardial disease and electrolyte disturbance.

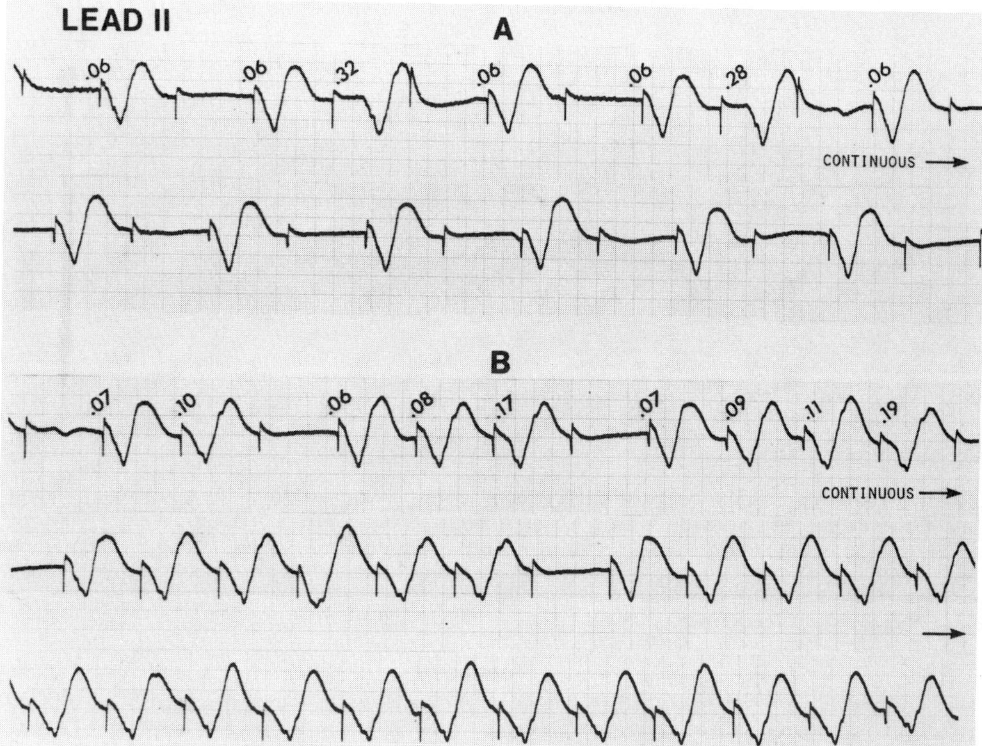

Figure 8–16. These tracings were recorded before *(A)* and after *(B)* the correction of severe metabolic acidosis and hyperkalemia related to end-stage congestive heart failure. The QRS rhythm is paced and no spontaneous cardiac activity is seen. The tracings demonstrate varying degrees of pacemaker exit block, in which the threshold for myocardial stimulation exceeds the energy output of the generator. At these times a pacing stimulus will be delivered but does not activate the ventricles, and therefore no QRS complex is inscribed. In *A,* the exit block between pacing stimuli and QRS complexes has ratios of 2:1 and 3:2; the increasing stimulus-to-QRS durations indicate a Wenckebach type of conduction delay between delivery of pacing stimuli and activation of ventricular tissue. In *B,* 2:1 exit block is no longer present and the Wenckebach block is resolving; 1:1 conduction of pacing stimuli to ventricular tissue is present in the last strip. This response, unfortunately, was short-lived (see Fig. 8–17).

Increases in myocardial stimulation threshold have also been reported in the presence of hypokalemia[104] and have been effectively treated with intravenously administered potassium. The mechanism(s) for the threshold rise in this clinical circumstance is/are not known. On occasion, intravenous potassium has been used to restore myocardial capture by the pulse generator when other pharmacologic agents such as isoproterenol and calcium have been ineffective.[104] It therefore appears that myocardial stimulation threshold is optimal within certain ranges of serum potassium concentration, both hypo- and hyperkalemia being associated with failure to capture.

Pacing and sensing functions of a pacemaker generator may become abnormal in patients with high plasma concentrations of antiarrhythmic agents, notably Type I agents such as quinidine and procainamide, and (more rarely) lidocaine.[36, 67] Pacemaker malfunction in these clinical circumstances may result in life-threatening rhythm disturbances, including total electromechanical dissociation. Failure to capture appears to occur more commonly than failure to sense. As in hyperkalemia (which, with metabolic acidosis, often accompanies drug toxicity in the clinical setting of myocardial failure), failure to capture may be intermittent or complete and may take the form of fixed exit block or Wenckebach periodicity; often, both forms alternate with each other in the same individual (Figs. 8–16, 8–17).

The mechanism by which Type I antiarrhythmic agents exert their effects in patients with pacemakers is probably an extension of their therapeutic effects of increasing myocardial fiber refractoriness, decreasing conduction velocity, and increasing excitability threshold by depressing membrane respon-

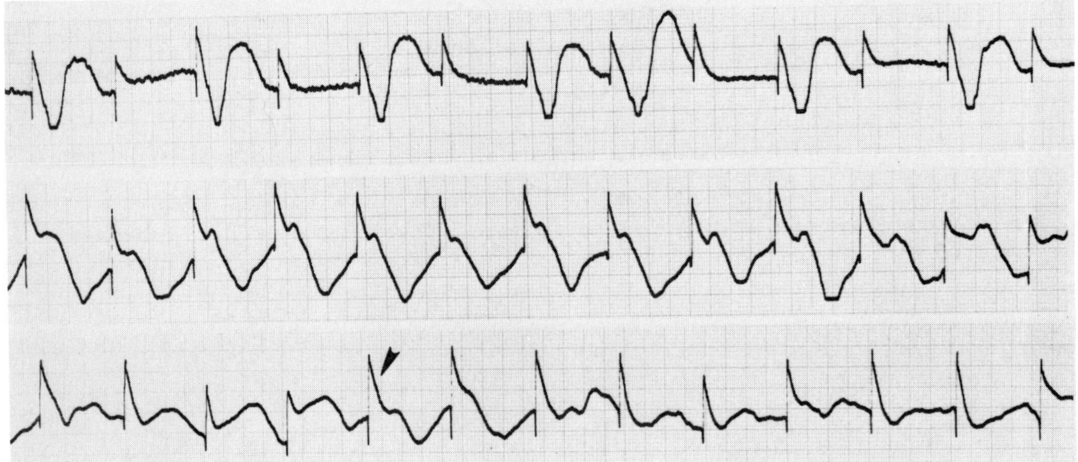

Figure 8–17. These continuously recorded MCL_1 rhythm strips in a patient with end-stage congestive heart failure show progressive degrees of exit block between pacing stimuli and ventricular activation (see also Fig. 8–16). In the *top* strip, 2:1 and 3:2 stimuli-to-QRS ratios are present. In the *middle* strip, 1:1 stimulus-to-QRS ratios are seen but there is marked delay between the inscription of the pacing artifacts and the very broad and bizarre QRS complexes they produce. In the *bottom* strip, the pacing stimuli and their decay curve artifacts are clearly seen *(arrow)* but no ventricular complexes follow (electromechanical dissociation). The patient expired.

siveness and reducing resting membrane potential. The surface ECG reflects these changes in prolongation of the QRS duration and Q-T interval, increase in delay between the pacing stimulus and the QRS complex ("latency"),[53] and periods of noncapture.[36, 72, 84]

Management of pacemaker-related problems due to antiarrhythmic agent toxicity can be difficult and includes rapid correction of pH and electrolyte and blood gas abnormalities when these are present. In this regard, it is well to remember that the effects of some Type I antiarrhythmic agents (specifically quinidine) are exaggerated by high serum potassium concentration.[12] Sodium lactate or sodium bicarbonate have been reported to reverse the toxic effects of quinidine or procainamide,[7, 36] possibly by increasing the serum sodium, which acts to restore membrane potential toward normal and to increase the rate of rise of phase 0 of myocardial fibers. Acceleration of quinidine or procainamide removal by any method, including hemodialysis and hemoperfusion, has not been particularly successful owing to their extensive tissue distribution; disopyramide toxicity, on the other hand, may be effectively treated by these methods. Increasing the pacing stimulus strength and, if required, the sensitivity threshold by noninvasive programming of appropriate permanent pulse generators could conceivably improve the clinical situation, although documentation is lacking. In the setting of temporary cardiac pacing, increasing the stimulus strength does not necessarily result in restoration of normal pacing function, in view of other variables such as impulse propagation and the amount of tissue that must be depolarized in order to generate a ventricular contraction.

Considering the widespread use of high doses of Type I antiarrhythmic agents in patients with significant heart disease, the occurrence of pacemaker-related capture and sensing problems must be relatively infrequent. This suggests that accompanying conditions such as myocardial ischemia, congestive heart failure, or multiple drug interactions constitute the prerequisites for these problems.

CARDIAC PACING IN ACUTE MYOCARDIAL INFARCTION

Sensing Problems

Acute myocardial infarction provides a setting for potential problems related to both sensing and pacing. Sensing problems may be due to malposition of a temporary electrode catheter, pulse generator malfunction, or undersensing resulting from poor intracardiac signals characterized by inadequate

Table 8–7. GUIDE TO POSITION OF TRANSVENOUS PACING CATHETERS

Electrode Catheter Position	X-Ray Appearance	Morphology of Paced Complexes
Right ventricular apex	Anterior, inferiorly directed, well to left of spine near left cardiac border	Superior frontal plane axis, LBBB pattern
Right ventricular inflow tract	Overying spine	Normal frontal plane axis, LBBB pattern
Right ventricular outflow tract	Anterior, directed superiorly	Vertical frontal plane axis, LBBB pattern
Coronary sinus	Posterior, superior, and leftward	Atrial pacing with inverted P waves in ECG leads 2, 3, and aV_F; ventricular pacing with RBBB pattern, vertical frontal plane axis
Middle coronary vein	Resembles right ventricular apical position but less anterior	Superior frontal plane axis; both axis and pattern of intraventricular conduction may be variable, depending on site of initiation of ventricular activation

voltage, slow rate of change of voltage (slew), or prolonged signal duration (Table 8–5).[2, 3, 34]

Temporary transvenous electrode catheter position may be evaluated by noting its location on posteroanterior and lateral chest radiographs and comparing it with previous films when available (Table 8–7). Right ventricular apical position of a transvenous pacing lead is suggested by an anteriorly and inferiorly directed lead tip, which lies well to the left of the spine near the left cardiac border (Table 8–7). A more sensitive evaluative technique is afforded by analysis of a paced 12-lead ECG and comparison of the QRS morphology with that seen in previous tracings; right ventricular apical location as well as significant migration of the pacing catheter tip can be determined by changes in paced QRS morphology and axis.

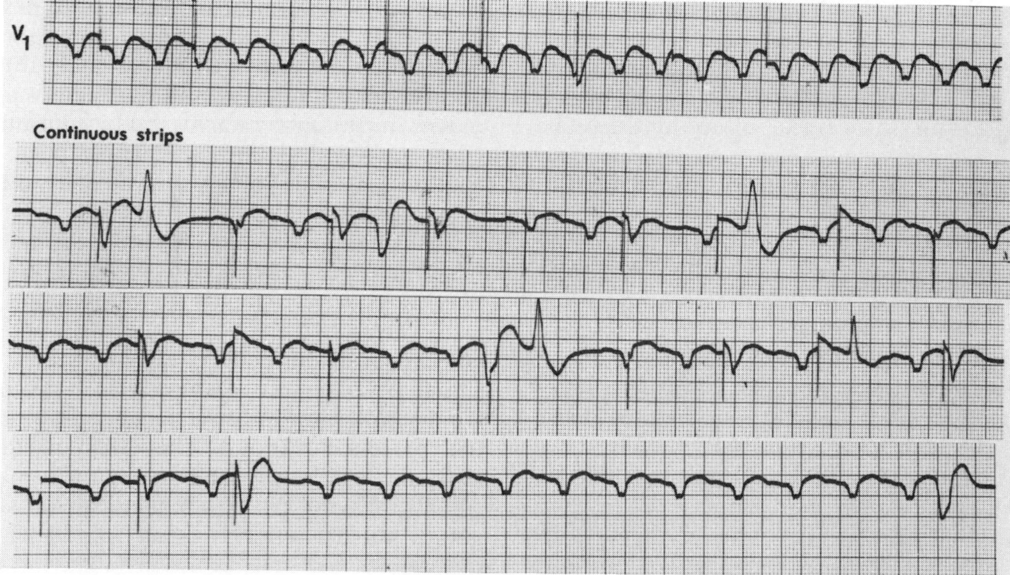

Figure 8–18. Behavior of a permanent pacemaker shortly after cardiac arrest due to ventricular fibrillation. The spontaneous rhythm is sinus tachycardia. In the *top* strip, the pacemaker is emitting stimuli asynchronously at its programmed rate of 60/min; thus, failure to sense is present. Failure to capture is also present as pacer stimuli falling outside the refractory period of ventricular tissue do not produce or contribute to a QRS complex. Failure to pace and/or capture during and just after cardiac arrest is not rare; it is contributed to by local pH and electrolyte imbalances, and ischemia or infarction. The three continuously recorded V_1 rhythm strips were obtained several minutes after the *top* strip. They illustrate the restoration of normal pacing function (present throughout the strips) and, finally (*bottom* strip), normal sensing function. Return of normal pacemaker function accompanies restoration of electrical and hemodynamic stability after resuscitation from cardiac arrest.

Table 8–8. PACEMAKER-RELATED ARRHYTHMIAS: CONDITIONS DECREASING V_T–V_F THRESHOLD*

Ischemia
Vagal stimulation
Digitalis
Epinephrine
Anesthesia
Hypoxia

*V_T = ventricular tachycardia; V_F = ventricular fibrillation.

Pulse generator malfunction resulting in sensing problems may be evaluated in permanent units by the technique of chest wall stimulation[6] and in temporary pacing situations by means of a pacing system "analyzer". Oversensing of P waves, T waves, or voltage transients caused by electrode catheter fracture or environmental electromagnetic interference should be recognized and corrected.

The most common cause of sensing problems in patients with acute myocardial infarction is the suboptimal nature of the intracardiac signal, which, falling below the sensing threshold of a pacemaker generator, is sensed intermittently or not at all[2, 3, 34] (Fig. 8–18). Sensing problems resulting from poor signals should not be called sensing "failure," since pulse generator malfunction is not the cause. Borderline intracardiac signals occurring during myocardial infarction may be due to ischemia and necrosis of tissue, and to local or more widespread disturbances in impulse conduction.[103] In the latter situation, the electrodes, located at the tip of the pacing lead, "see" the impulse well after ventricular activation has begun. Impulses arising in ventricular tissue often are not sensed because of their poor quality, a circumstance that can lead to repetitive ventricular beating[39] (Table 8–8). Because of the dynamic nature of the infarction process, sensing problems are often transient, and unless life-threatening pacemaker-related arrhythmias occur as a result of unsensed spontaneous beats they can be managed by careful observation only.

During temporary cardiac pacing, turning the generator's sensitivity setting to full demand position optimizes its ability to sense signals of low amplitude. Unipolarization of a bipolar temporary pulse generator in order to augment the intracardiac signal may also be tried; this is accomplished by connecting one of the lead's electrodes to the negative terminal of the pulse generator and a surface (skin) electrode to the positive terminal of the generator by means of double alligator clamps. The remaining lead electrode should be encased in nonconducting material such as a rubber glove, so that stray currents cannot be conducted down the lead to the heart. It has been well documented that intracardiac signals sensed by unipolar and bipolar electrode catheters are not always identical.[24] The signal sensed by a bipolar pacing lead reflects the potential difference between the distal (tip) and proximal (ring) electrodes, the interelectrode distance and thus the time taken by the impulse to travel from one electrode to the other, and the orientation of the electrodes relative to the depolarization wavefront.[24] In contrast, the electrical signal sensed by a unipolar lead reflects electrical activity present only at the cathodal (intracardiac) electrode, the anode being extracardiac in location and therefore serving as an indifferent electrode. In individual patients, the unipolar signal may be larger than the bipolar signal.

In permanent pacemakers with programmable features, increased sensitivity may be achieved by programming the generator to "see" intracardiac signals of low voltage. If, owing to unsensed spontaneous beats, lethal pacemaker-induced arrhythmias occur,[39] total suppression of permanent pacemaker output may be achieved by continuous chest wall stimulation; if cardiac pacing is required, it may be accomplished by means of a temporary pacing catheter.

The changing quality of intracardiac signals that occurs during myocardial infarction may be due to ischemia, acidosis and alkalosis, ventricular dilation, myocardial cellular edema, local conduction delay with failure of signal propagation to the area of the electrodes, and alterations in local drug or electrolyte concentrations. The effect of metabolic acidosis and alkalosis on intracardiac signals has not been systematically investigated, but it is entirely conceivable that pH derangements, such as are seen during and after cardiac arrest or in association with cardiogenic shock, may distort electrical signals, making them suboptimal for sensing. Myocardial cellular edema and ventricular dilation have been shown to produce such signal distortion.[17, 18]

It is important to note that the surface

ECG gives no clue as to the nature of the intracardiac signal as "seen" by the pacing catheter electrodes. Thus, sensed and unsensed events may not appear electrocardiographically to be different from each other. The only means of assessing the quality of intracardiac signals is to record them from the intracardiac electrodes, which is, of course, feasible only in the setting of temporary cardiac pacing.

Pacing Problems

Failure to capture during acute myocardial infarction may be due to malposition of the lead during temporary cardiac pacing or to an increase in myocardial stimulation threshold, which can occur during either temporary or permanent pacing. Changing stimulation thresholds resulting in failure to capture are common during infarction and often, but not always, arise concomitantly with sensing problems. Underlying causes for failure to capture due to increased stimulation threshold include local hyperkalemia associated with tissue necrosis, severe acidosis, shock, and high concentrations of Type I antiarrhythmic agents (quinidine, procainamide, and disopyramide). As previously described, failure to capture may be intermittent or complete and may take the form of Type I (Wenckebach) or Type II exit block[53, 79] (Figs. 8–16, 8–17). Although this is frequently a harbinger of electromechanical dissociation, normal pacing function can be restored with appropriate pharmacologic therapy and correction of hemodynamic abnormalities.

Failure to capture in temporary pacing situations may be managed by repositioning the lead, increasing the current output of the external pulse generator, or unipolarizing the system if the tip or ring unipolar stimulation thresholds have been shown to be lower than bipolar stimulation thresholds. If a permanent pacemaker generator without programmable features is in place and pacing is required, temporary pacing must be instituted. Occasionally, stimulation thresholds remain elevated after myocardial infarction and the pulse generator must be changed to a unit with ability to deliver higher energy output. If the permanent pacemaker generator is programmable, energy output can be increased by programming higher current, voltage, or pulse duration.

DIRECT CURRENT CARDIOVERSION AND DEFIBRILLATION IN PATIENTS WITH CARDIAC PACEMAKERS

The necessity for DC cardioversion or defibrillation arises quite frequently in patients with tachyarrhythmias causing hemodynamic compromise. Pacemaker generators are designed so that the circuitry is protected from excessive electrical energy, but on occasion the protective mechanism(s) may fail, resulting in generator malfunction.

General guidelines for electroversion or defibrillation in patients with pacemakers include adequate separation between defibrillator paddles, avoidance of paddle placement within 3 to 5 inches of the pulse generator, and ensuring that the dipole created by the defibrillator paddles is perpendicular to that between the electrode catheter tip and generator in unipolar pacing systems, or to that between the electrodes of the lead in bipolar pacing systems.

Despite these precautions, abnormalities of pulse generator function following defibrillation have been reported and include failure to capture due to current drain, myocardial burns caused by high current flow along the pacing lead, and unwanted programming of automatic rate function in some programmable units.[1, 3] The reasons for defibrillator-produced reprogramming of permanent pacemaker generators are not entirely explained, but have been considered to involve the interaction between the generator circuitry and electrical noise artifacts and static discharges occurring during placement of the paddles on the body surface. The pacemaker generator malfunction may be transient, normal function being restored in a short time,[37] or more permanent, warranting pulse generator replacement.

Sensing problems that develop after defibrillation may be due to pulse generator malfunction, but are more likely to be related to the electromechanical effects of the dysrhythmia itself or defibrillation-related myocardial injury resulting in distortion of intracardiac signals.

It is well to test all parameters of pacemaker generator function, including automatic and magnetic rates, and the integrity of programmable parameters, as soon as the patient is stabilized. Failure of function to return to normal necessitates generator replacement.

ACUTE COMPLICATIONS OF PACING SYSTEM IMPLANTATION*

Lead Dislodgement

The most common surgical approach for the placement of permanent pacing leads is the transvenous one. Access to the venous system can be achieved either by cephalic or jugular venous cutdown approach, or by the newer subclavian vein puncture method.[60, 61] Regardless of the vein used, the most common immediate postprocedure complication is lead dislodgement, which usually occurs within the first 48 hours and tapers off by the second week. Occasional cases of dislodgement have been observed as long as one year after pacing system implant.[46] The advent of newer lead designs such as the tined lead has reduced considerably the incidence of electrode catheter displacement.[44]

After pacing system implant and upon the patient's arrival in a monitored unit, good-quality anteroposterior and lateral chest radiographs should be obtained in order to check the placement of the pacing system. A paced 12-lead ECG should be taken to verify pacing artifact axis and the morphology of paced QRS complexes. If lead displacement is suspected (usually because of loss of pacing or sensing), the chest films and paced ECG should be repeated and compared with the immediate postoperative ones. It should be mentioned that slight changes in position of the pacing catheter on the x-ray film often reflect differences in radiographic technique rather than actual catheter dislodgement. A change in the axis of the pacing artifacts or morphology of the paced QRS complexes helps to verify the diagnosis of lead dislodgement.

With the increasing use of dual-chambered pacemaker generators, the electrocardiographic diagnosis of lead dislodgement will become more difficult. For example, an atrial synchronous pacemaker generator (Fig. 8–1) may cease its P-wave tracking function, and function in a ventricular-inhibited (VVI) mode. The uncommitted AV sequential pulse generator (Fig. 8–1) may evince "crosstalk" if the ventricular lead becomes displaced toward the atrium, so that ventricular signals are sensed by the atrial lead and vice versa, causing undesired pacemaker inhibition.

*See Table 8–9.

Table 8–9. INTRA- AND PERIOPERATIVE COMPLICATIONS OF PACING SYSTEM IMPLANTATION

Transvenous	Epicardial
Lead dislodgement	Myocardial laceration
Cardiac perforation with tamponade	Pericarditis
Air embolism	Pericardial effusion
Arterial bleeding	Late pericardial constriction
Pneumothorax	

Subclavian Venipuncture

In recent years the use of a modified Seldinger technique for introduction of a pacing catheter into the subclavian vein by direct puncture has achieved great popularity.[21, 30, 43, 59–61, 66, 102] The method provides a simple and usually quite safe approach that considerably reduces operative time. The method may be used for placement of atrial, ventricular, or dual-chambered pacing systems, as two leads may be placed through the same sheath.

The complications of pneumothorax, hemopneumothorax, arterial bleeding, and air embolism are real, but not especially frequent. Rarely, cases of arteriovenous fistula, thoracic duct injury, cardiac tamponade, and brachial plexus injury have been reported.[66, 68]

Pneumothorax, Hemothorax

If the pleural space is entered by a needle that is then disconnected from the syringe, air can be introduced, causing pneumothorax. Although this is not common, major morbidity may be encountered when it occurs. Confirmation of pneumothorax may be made by fluoroscopic visualization and by inspection of the postoperative chest radiographs. Small pneumothoraces may be expected to resolve spontaneously, whereas larger ones require aspiration with chest tubes. Hemothorax can occur if blood from a lacerated vessel oozes into the pleural cavity; thoracentesis may be required.

Use of small-gauge needles in performing pacing system implant lessens the danger of both these complications.

Air Emboli

During the pacing system implant procedure, especially when direct subclavian venipuncture is being used, air may be introduced into the venous system when the aspirating syringe is removed from the needle, when the guidewire is placed into the vein, and if negative pressure is created. Before venipuncture, the patient should be placed in the supine position with the head flat; the Trendelenburg position may be utilized in order to distend the venous system. To guard against entry of air into the venous system, a small amount of back-bleeding is advisable, and the patient should be instructed to exhale and hold his breath during the venipuncture; he should be cautioned against deep breathing or coughing.

If air emboli do occur, vital signs must be carefully monitored while location of the air embolism is followed fluoroscopically. If necessary, the patient should be placed on his side until the air bubble is absorbed; rarely, it may require the breaking up of a large air embolus with a catheter.

Arterial Bleeding

Occasionally, the subclavian artery rather than the subclavian vein is lacerated or punctured. This complication should be suspected if the blood aspirated is bright red in color and has a high pressure head. The problem is minimized by the use of small-caliber needles. The possibility of arterial puncture is lessened if a rolled sheet or towel is placed between the shoulder-blades in order to hyperextend the back and prop the shoulders. This maneuver pushes the subclavian vein superiorly to a more accessible position under the clavicle.[66] If the artery is inadvertently entered, the needle should be withdrawn and pressure applied to the site for ten minutes while vital signs are monitored. Venipuncture can then be attempted again or tried from the other side.

Hematomas

Hematomas of the pacemaker pocket occur most frequently in the anticoagulated or hypertensive patient.[93] Any contribution to hematoma formation made by oozing around the venipuncture site is thought to be minimal because of the pressure exerted by the pectoral fascia.[60,61] In our experience, hematoma formation can be minimized by applying a pressure dressing over the incision site for 24 hours; keeping the patient in a semi-Fowler's position for the first several hours after implant may also be helpful.

MYOCARDIAL PENETRATION AND PERFORATION

Myocardial penetration after pacemaker insertion reportedly occurs in 5 to 10 per cent of patients.[9] It is important to note that this complication is not usually an acute event occurring at the time of implant and associated with cardiac tamponade, but is more commonly detected within the first postoperative month.[9] The cited incidence of cardiac perforation accompanied the use of older pacing leads, which often were stiffer and required stiffer stylets to achieve proper placement; newer designs in both passive and active fixation leads could conceivably be associated with a lower incidence of this complication.

Cardiac perforation with the tip of the pacing lead lying free in the pericardial space or totally extracardiac is quite rare; most instances represent penetration of the pacing catheter tip into the myocardium. In our experience, when epicardial leads are placed after cardiac "perforation" has occurred, the lead is not visible in the pericardial space and only mild, if any, pericardial reaction is observed, despite the presence of a pericardial friction rub, loss of normal pacing function, and the pain of pericarditis. In bipolar pacing catheters the distal (tip) electrode may lie within the myocardium or in the epimyocardial area and the proximal (ring) electrode at the endocardial surface. The portion of myocardium that has been penetrated and thus activated early determines the ECG features of paced QRS complexes, and may reflect initial activation of interventricular septum or left ventricular myocardium.

Myocardial penetration usually manifests itself as intermittent or complete failure to sense or capture; the patient's symptomatic complaints therefore depend, at least in part, on his degree of pacemaker dependence. The failure to sense is likely due to attenuation of the intracardiac signal as the myocardium is penetrated; failure to capture is related to stimulation threshold differences between endocardium and myocardium. Occasionally, diaphragmatic pacing occurs. If a programmable pacemaker generator is in place, increasing the energy output may offer

Table 8–10. CAUSES OF RIGHT BUNDLE BRANCH BLOCK PATTERN DURING CARDIAC PACING

Distal coronary sinus (left ventricular epicardial) pacing
Apposition of pacing lead to interventricular septum with early activation of left bundle branch
Cardiac perforation
Normal finding

temporary protection against bradycardia, but the situation remains unstable and definitive management may be urgently required.

A pericardial friction rub is often, but not always, present. Although its presence is helpful in leading to the correct diagnosis, it is neither sensitive nor specific for cardiac perforation, since friction rubs may occur in the absence of diagnosable perforation,[38] and perforation may be unaccompanied by pericardial rubs. It is important to distinguish the pericardial rub due to myocardial penetration from murmurs that may follow pacing system implantation and might suggest tricuspid regurgitation or have no identifiable cause; most have no significant hemodynamic consequences.[92] It is also important to distinguish a pericardial rub from a pacemaker "sound" or "click," which does not necessarily portend pacing system problems but probably reflects movement of the pacing catheter against cardiac structures.[54, 69]

The ECG manifestations of cardiac perforation depend on the direction the pacing lead takes. Shift in axis of the pacing artifacts may be observed, as well as changes in paced QRS complex morphology. Thus, the proper magnet should be applied in order to record paced QRS complexes. Although a change in paced QRS complex morphology from the expected left bundle branch block pattern to that of right bundle branch block pattern is highly suggestive of perforation of the interventricular septum or pacing catheter location against left ventricular epicardium, a right bundle branch block pattern does not per se indicate perforation (Table 8–10). Other techniques that verify the diagnosis of cardiac perforation include comparison of highly penetrated chest radiographs with those obtained immediately after pacemaker implant (often not helpful), and two-dimensional echocardiography to locate the tip of the catheter. The latter may be especially useful in patients who have pacemaker malfunction but neither chest pain nor pericardial rub. In temporary cardiac pacing, recording of unipolar electrograms from the tip and ring electrodes will help document the diagnosis.[70, 99]

The management of myocardial penetration consists of repositioning or removal of the lead and implantation of epicardial leads. Withdrawal of the lead is not itself usually associated with complications, although ventricular extrasystoles are common as the catheter enters the cavity of the right ventricle. Simple withdrawal of the pacing lead to the endocardium without repositioning is a frequently performed maneuver, but reperforation may occur at the original site. We recommend withdrawal to the right atrium and complete repositioning as the procedure of choice. Recording of the intracardiac electrogram during pacing lead withdrawal confirms the diagnosis of perforation and may also be used as a guide in repositioning.[70, 99]

THROMBOEMBOLISM

Clinical recognition of clot formation around a transvenous pacing catheter is infrequent. The patient may present with signs and symptoms of venous obstruction, right ventricular inflow obstruction, and pulmonary embolism.[106] Unexplained heart failure, tachycardia, chest pain, dyspnea, and nonspecific systemic symptoms such as weakness and malaise without cause warrant consideration of these complications.

The true incidence of venous thrombosis is underestimated clinically.[47, 75, 95] Consecutively performed venographic studies have demonstrated venous obstruction (usually proximal to the superior vena cava, but occasionally involving the innominate or subclavian veins) in from 25 to 80 per cent of patients with pacing systems in place for two years or longer;[16, 95] most such individuals have no clinical evidence of venous obstruction. The relative rarity of major venous thrombosis is noteworthy[23, 91] and suggests that thrombus propagation does not occur. Temporary transvenous cardiac pacing has been reported to cause asymptomatic local thrombosis in up to 25 per cent of patients studied by radioisotopic techniques[77] and 34 per cent of patients studied by venography.[75] In addition to contrast or isotope venography, other methods of verifying suspected venous thrombosis include computerized tomography, Doppler ultrasonography, and two-dimensional echocardiography.

Patients with symptomatic venous thrombosis present with arm or neck and facial edema, pain, redness, absence or diminution of ipsilateral venous pulsations, and a prominent subcutaneous venous pattern due to collateral channel formation if the obstruction is chronic. Treatment consists of elevation of the involved extremity, and parenteral and oral anticoagulation.

Venous thrombosis due to local vascular factors must be distinguished from that due to clot formation around the intracardiac portion of the electrode catheter, as the latter is a more dangerous situation and often more difficult to manage. Intracardiac clot, if of sufficient size, may be demonstrated by contrast or radionuclide angiography, and non-invasively by two-dimensional echocardiography. Clinical features that predispose to clot formation include congestive heart failure, previous myocardial infarction, low cardiac output, and atrial fibrillation, but these are neither sensitive nor specific for the condition. The onset of clinical signs and symptoms of intracardiac clot formation is extremely variable, ranging from the day of implant[62, 86] to seven years after implant,[52] with an average of several months. Autopsy series suggest that many cases are clinically unrecognized.[47, 87]

Right atrial thrombi range in size from less than 1 cm to several centimeters in diameter;[74] in one reported case, the clot occupied 80 per cent of the right cavity, extending superiorly into the superior vena cava and inferiorly across the tricuspid valve.[62]

While serving as a nidus for embolization to the pulmonary bed, large right atrial thrombi can also lead to disorders of atrial rhythm if they involve the sinoatrial area, malfunction of the tricuspid valve (functional stenosis or insufficiency, much like an atrial myxoma), and right ventricle inflow obstruction. The latter situation results in impairment of hemodynamic function, which may be difficult to distinguish from progression of the intrinsic disease. The diagnosis of intra-atrial clot should be considered in patients with pacemakers who have "refractory" heart failure.

Clinically recognizable pulmonary embolism from a transvenous pacing catheter is rare,[85] occurring in from 0.6 to 3.5 per cent of patients.[9, 29] However, clinical recognition again underestimates the actual incidence.[75, 87] In a review of autopsied cases, Bernstein and colleagues found a 33 per cent incidence of pulmonary emboli in patients with permanent pacemakers;[9] and in a series of temporarily paced patients undergoing lung scans, Nolewajka and co-workers demonstrated pulmonary embolism in 60 per cent.[75] As most of these patients do not have evidence of pulmonary infarction or pulmonary hypertension due to the pulmonary emboli, it is likely that most emboli are not of sufficient magnitude to be clinically significant.

The treatment for pacemaker-related thromboembolism is anticoagulation with heparin followed by warfarin. In patients with pulmonary embolism, the use of streptokinase is warranted only when active clot formation is considered to be occurring. If pulmonary emboli are recurrent, thoracotomy with clot and pacing catheter removal under cardiopulmonary bypass may be required.[52]

A very rare occurrence is embolization of the electrode catheter itself, which usually follows its transection as a result of inability to remove it from the right ventricle.[97] Embolization into the inferior venous system, as well as into the pulmonary circulation, have been described. Often the patient suffers no consequences of this event; however, if clinical sequelae such as vessel perforation or infection result, attempts to remove the embolized catheter by snare devices or laparotomy or thoracotomy need to be considered.

INFECTION

The reported incidence of generalized sepsis in patients with permanent pacing systems averages about 1 to 3 per cent in large series.[65, 71] However, the incidence of localized infections that involve the pacemaker pocket or the site of entry of the pacing catheter into the vein has been reported to be as high as 19 per cent. Infection of an epicardial pacing system is particularly dangerous, since purulent pericarditis can result. The prophylactic use of antibiotics at the time of pacing system implant has not affected the incidence of infection. Infection has been noted as early as the day of implant and as late as eight years after implant,[71] with an average of four to eight weeks. Previous procedures such as pulse generator changes have been indicted as predisposing to pocket infections,[19, 51] as have systemic illnesses such as diabetes mellitus.

The usual infecting organism is coagulase-positive staphylococcus, although *Staphylococcus epidermidis* has also been identified, especially in more indolent infections. Tricuspid valve endocarditis with valve destruction, as well as abscess formation in the atrial or right ventricular mural endocardium adjacent to the pacing lead, have been described.[71, 90]

Treatment of pacemaker-related infections consists of parenteral antibiotics and removal of the entire pacing system. Early experience with removal of only that part of the pacing system considered to be involved in the infection was uniformly poor, with continuing infection resulting.[13, 31] The new pacing system should be implanted on the contralateral side or epicardially, and may be accomplished either at the same time as removal of the infected pacing system or after a period of antibiotic treatment and temporary cardiac pacing, with little discernible difference in results. In several reported cases, reimplantation of a new pacing system transvenously despite previous septicemia has not resulted in infection of the new lead, suggesting that intracardiac abscess formation had not occurred.

TRICUSPID VALVE INJURY

Acute tricuspid valve injuries produced by temporary or permanent pacing leads include laceration, fenestration, and partial avulsion.[27, 40, 56, 81] Fenestration of valve tissue, if significant, may produce a murmur of tricuspid regurgitation and clinical signs compatible with right heart failure. The need to reposition or remove the pacing lead may result in avulsion of tissue. Often, however, the diagnosis of iatrogenic tricuspid valve perforation is not made ante mortem; clues

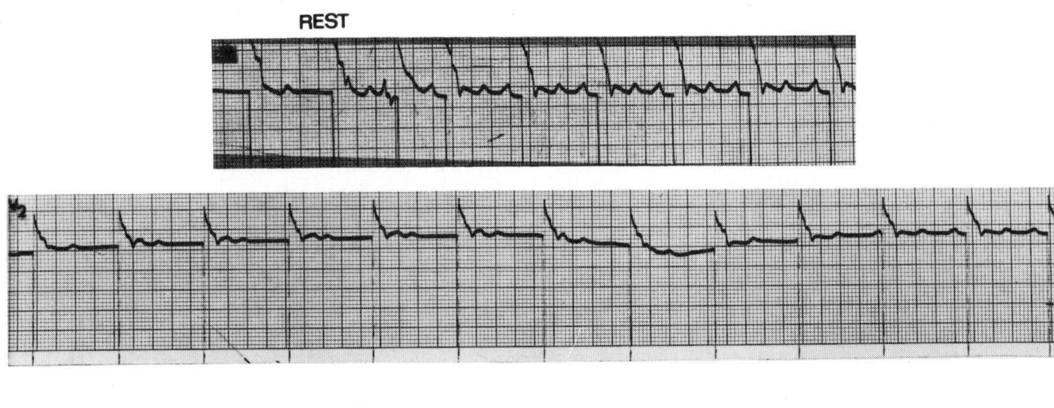

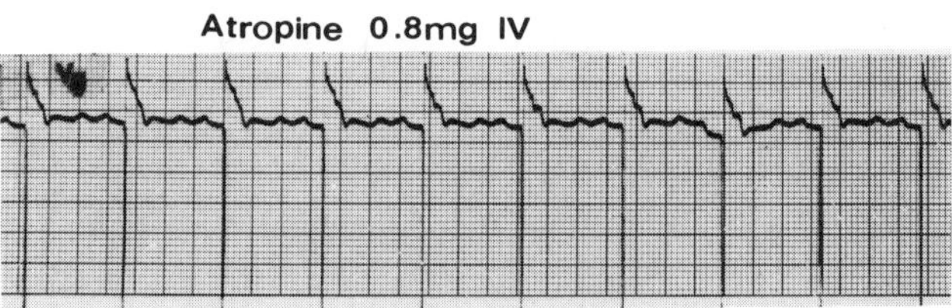

Figure 8–19. These noncontinuous lead V_2 rhythm strips illustrate the function of one type of atrial synchronous pacing system (Cordis Atricor). Sensing function is limited to signals "seen" by an atrial or coronary sinus electrode catheter; atrial pacing does not occur. Pacing does occur in the ventricles, following a programmable time delay after a sensed atrial event (the "AV interval"). When no atrial signals are sensed, the ventricles are paced asynchronously.

In the *top* strip, fixed rate ventricular pacing occurs for the first two complexes, following which an atrial premature beat and then sinus rhythm appear and result in ventricular pacing at the prevailing sinus rate. In the *middle* strip, the sinus rate has slowed below the automatic rate of the generator, and fixed-rate ventricular pacing occurs. Sinus rhythm resumes toward the end of the strip but has not accelerated above the asynchronous ventricular pacing rate. The *bottom* strip was recorded after the sinus rate had been increased by intravenous atropine. Ventriculcar pacing is occurring at the sinus rate, following the AV delay.

The changes in paced ventricular rates often lead to confusion regarding pacemaker generator function unless this type of pacing system is recognized. In general, in P-synchronous units, faster-paced ventricular rates are preceded by P waves and have varying spike-to-spike intervals. If the sinus rate slows, the ventricular paced rate will be constant unless recycled by a sensed spontaneous QRS complex.

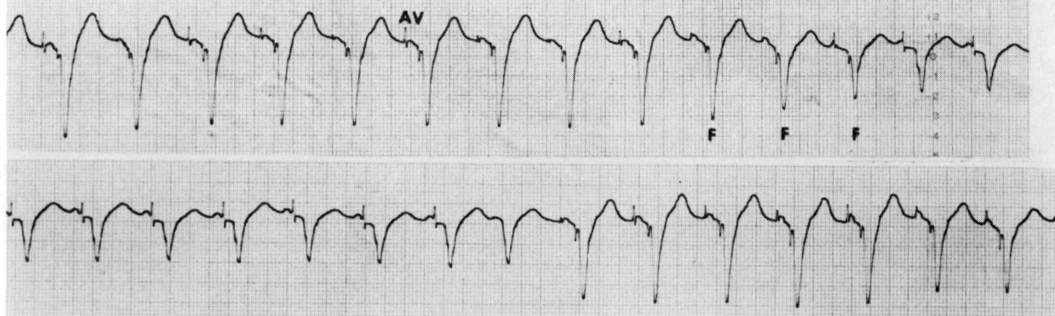

Figure 8–20. These continuous MCL_1 rhythm strips were recorded from a patient with an AV sequential pacing system (see also Fig. 8–1). This particular system senses only in the ventricle and, after a programmable time period after a sensed or paced QRS complex (called the "VA interval"), an atrial stimulus is delivered. It is important to note that the atrial stimulus is delivered regardless of presence or type of spontaneous atrial activity. Since sensing does occur in the ventricle, the delivery of a ventricular pacing stimulus will depend on whether a spontaneous QRS complex has occurred.

In the *top* strip, ventricular stimuli are delivered 0.12 sec after atrial stimuli (the "AV interval"). It is difficult to tell whether the atria are in fact being paced. Toward the end of the *top* strip and throughout the *bottom* strip, sinus rhythm is clearly present and atrial stimuli are being delivered within the spontaneous P waves, 0.60 sec after QRS complexes (the "VA interval"). The superimposition of a pacing stimulus upon a spontaneous complex without contributing to activation of the chamber is called a *pseudofusion* complex. The ventricles are paced at the beginning and at the end of the rhythm strips, with several examples of fusion *(F)* complexes. When the programmed AV interval exceeds the spontaneous PR interval, spontaneous QRS complexes occur; when the PR interval exceeds the programmed AV interval, paced QRS complexes occur.

to its presence may be found in the description of the implant procedure itself, during which excessive force may have been necessary to "cross" the valve.

Avulsion of tricuspid valve leaflet tissue has accompanied attempts to remove infected electrodes with traction,[56] as well as efforts to achieve optimal right ventricular apical placement that require extensive catheter manipulation. Electrode catheter entrapment of chronic leads may result from adhesion formation to right atrial or ventricular endocardium and tricuspid valve apparatus including chordae tendineae,[87] making catheter removal difficult and potentially dangerous.[23, 81] Newer insulating materials may help to reduce the potential problem of fibrous adhesion formation.

Despite these acute mechanical complications, symptomatic or hemodynamically significant tricuspid regurgitation is extremely unusual.

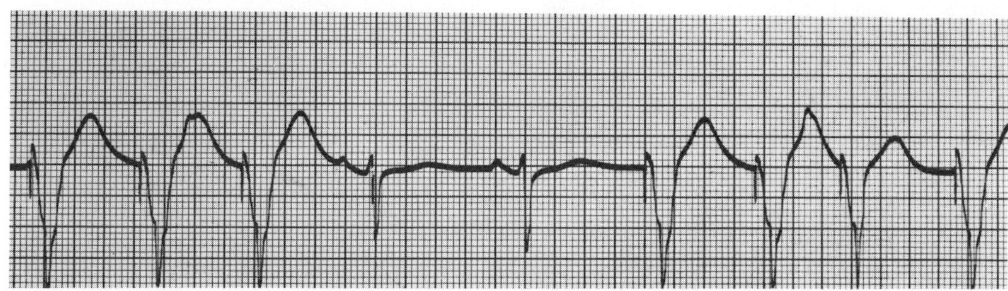

Figure 8–21. This rhythm strip was recorded from a patient with an atrial synchronous, ventricular inhibited pacemaker (VDD), which senses atrial activity and then paces the ventricles after a variable, rate-dependent AV delay, provided that no ventricular depolarization occurs within that interval. It will track P waves at rates of 60 to 118 per min; if no P waves (or intrinsic QRS complexes) occur, it will pace the ventricles asynchronously. The automatic interval of this generator is about 750 msec (corresponding a rate of 80 per min). If P waves occur, an AV interval of approximately 200 msec ensues, allowing for an intrinsic QRS to occur. If none does occur, it will pace the ventricles; thus, the *maximal* ventricular pacing interval becomes 950 (750 + 200). In this tracing, the first two QRS complexes are paced and occur at the automatic interval of 750 msec. The third paced QRS complex occurs early, as it follows a sensed spontaneous P wave by the AV interval. The fourth P-QRS complex is spontaneous (the QRS complex containing within it a pacing artifact—a *pseudofusion* complex). A spontaneous P wave then occurs and an intrinsic QRS falls within the AV delay, inhibiting ventricular pacing. Because no intervening P wave occurs after this complex, the next paced QRS complex occurs at the usual interval of about 750 msec. The remainder of the QRS complexes are paced, the second from the last occurring early in response to a sensed spontaneous P wave. Clearly, familiarity with this type of pacemaker generator is required in order not to diagnose malfunction.

PACEMAKER ELECTROCARDIOGRAPHIC MISINTERPRETATION: A POTENTIAL CAUSE OF MISTAKEN DIAGNOSIS OF MALFUNCTION

Owing to the complexity of newer pacemaker design and the availability of dual chamber systems, pacemaker electrocardiography has become difficult and confusing. Figures 8–1 and 8–19 to 8–21 illustrate just a few examples of normal pacemaker generator function that could easily be misinterpreted as malfunction.

Clearly, before such a diagnosis is made and acted upon, physicians are obliged to familiarize themselves with the design features of the pulse generator.

References

1. Aylward, P., Blood, R., and Tonkin, A.: Complications of defibrillation with permanent pacemaker in situ. PACE 2:462, 1979.
2. Barold, S. S., and Gaidula, J. J.: Failure of demand pacemaker from low-voltage bipolar ventricular electrograms. J.A.M.A. 215:923, 1971.
3. Barold, S. S., Gaidula, J. J., Lyon, J. L., et al.: Irregular recycling of demand pacemakers from borderline electrographic signals. Am. Heart J. 82:477, 1971.
4. Barold, S. S., Ong, L. S., Falkoff, M., et al.: Complex demand pacemaker arrhythmias: the differential diagnosis of pacemaker pauses. *In* Thalen, J. T., and Harthorne, J. W. (eds.): To Pace Or Not To Pace: Controversial Subjects on Cardiac Pacing. The Hague, Martin Mijhoff Medical Division, 1978, p. 302.
5. Barold, S. S., Ong, L. S., Scovil, J., et al.: Reprogramming of implanted pacemaker following external defibrillation. PACE 1:514, 1978.
6. Barold, S. S., Pupillo, G. A., Gaidula, J. J., et al.: Chest wall stimulation in evaluation of patients with implanted ventricular-inhibited demand pacemakers. Br. Heart J. 32:783, 1970.
7. Bellet, S., Hamden, G., Somlyo, A., et al.: A reversal of the cardiotoxic effects of procaine amide by molar sodium lactate. Am. J. Med. Sci. 237:177, 1959.
8. Berman, M.: T-wave sensing with a programmable pacemaker. PACE 3:656, 1980.
9. Bernstein, V., Rotem, C. E., and Peretz, D. I.: Permanent pacemakers: 8-year follow-up study. Incidence and management of congestive cardiac failure and perforations. Ann. Intern. Med. 74:361, 1971.
10. Bilitch, M., Crosby, R. S., and Cafferky, E. A.: Ventricular fibrillation and competitive pacing. N. Engl. J. Med. 276:598, 1967.
11. Bramowitz, A. D., Smith, J. W., and Eber, L. M.: Runaway pacemaker. A persisting problem. J.A.M.A. 228:340, 1974.
12. Brandfonbrener, M., Kronholm, J., and Jones, H. R.: The effect of serum potassium concentration on quinidine toxicity. J. Pharmacol. Exp. Ther. 131:212, 1966.
13. Bryan, C. S., Sutton, J. P., Saunders, D. E., et al.: Endocarditis related to transvenous pacemakers. Syndromes and surgical implications. J. Thorac. Cardiovasc. Surg. 75:758, 1978.
14. Burchell, H. B.: Analogy of electronic pacemaker and ventricular parasystole with observations on refractory period, supernormal phase, and synchronization. Circulation 27:878, 1963.
15. Burgess, M. J., Grossman, M., and Abildskov, J. A.: Fibrillation threshold of a patient with myocardial infarction treated with a fixed-rate pacemaker: case report. Am. Heart J. 80:112, 1970.
16. Chamorro, H., Rao, G., and Wholey, M. H.: Superior vena cava obstruction syndrome. A complication of transvenous pacemaker implantation. Radiology 126:377, 1978.
17. Chatterjee, K., Davies, G., and Harris, A.: Fall of endocardial potentials after acute myocardial infarction. Lancet 1:1308, 1970.
18. Chatterjee, K., Sutton, R., and Davies, J. G.: Low intracardiac potentials in myocardial infarction as a cause of failure of inhibition of demand pacemakers. Lancet 1:511, 1968.
19. Choo, M. H., Holmes, D. R., Jr., Gersh, B. J., et al.: Permanent pacemaker infections: characterization and management. Am. J. Cardiol. 48:559, 1981.
20. Chudasama, L., Ernest, A. C., Greif, E., et al.: Runaway temporary pacemaker: case report of a runaway temporary pacemaker with a rate over 1500/min. PACE 1:529, 1978.
21. Corwin, J. H., and Moseley, T.: Subclavian venipuncture and central venous pressure, technic and application. Am. Surg. 32:413, 1966.
22. Coumel, P., Mugica, J., and Barold, S. S.: Demand pacemaker arrhythmias caused by intermittent incomplete electrode fracture. Am. J. Cardiol. 36:105, 1975.
23. Crook, B. R. M., Gishen, P., Robinson, C. R., et al.: Occlusion of the subclavian vein associated with cephalic vein pacemaker electrodes. Br. J. Surg. 64:329, 1977.
24. DeCaprio, V., Hurzeler, P., and Furman, S.: A comparison of unipolar and bipolar electrograms for cardiac pacemaker sensing. Circulation 56:750, 1977.
25. Dolara, A., and Cammilli, L.: Supernormal excitation and conduction. Electrocardiographic observations during subthreshold stimulation in two patients with implanted pacemaker. Am. J. Cardiol. 21:746, 1968.
26. Dressler, W., Jonas, S., and Schwartz, E.: Supernormal phase of myocardial excitability in man. Circulation 31-32(Suppl. II):79, 1965.
27. Fishenfeld, J., and Lamy, Y.: Laceration of the tricuspid valve by a pacemaker wire. Chest 61:697, 1972.
28. Friedberg, H. D., and D'Cunha, G. F.: Adhesions of pacing catheter to tricuspid valve. Adhesive endocarditis. Thorax 24:498, 1969.
29. Friedman, S. A., Berger, N., Cerutti, M. M., et al.: Venous thrombosis and permanent cardiac pacing. Am. Heart J. 85:531, 1973.
30. Friesen, A., Klein, G. J., Kostuk, W. J., et al.: Percutaneous insertion of a permanent transvenous pacemaker electrode through the subclavian vein. Can. J. Surg. 20:131, 1977.

31. Furman, S.: Letter to the Editor: Cardiac pacemaker wound infection. Ann. Thorac. Surg. 14:328, 1972.
32. Furman, S.: Pacemaker emergencies. Med. Clin. North Am. 63:113, 1979.
33. Furman, S., and Escher, D. J. W.: Retained endocardial pacemaker electrodes. J. Thorac. Cardiovasc. Surg. 55:737, 1968.
34. Furman, S., Hurzeler, P., and DeCaprio, V.: Cardiac pacing and pacemakers III. Sensing the cardiac electrogram. Am. Heart J. 93:794, 1977.
35. Furman, S., Hurzeler, P., and Mehra, R.: Cardiac pacing and pacemakers IV. Threshold of cardiac stimulation. Am. Heart J. 94:115, 1972.
36. Gay, R. J., and Brown, D. F.: Pacemaker failure due to procainamide toxicity. Am. J. Cardiol. 34:728, 1974.
37. Giedweyn, J. O.: Pacemaker failure following external defibrillation. Circulation 44:293, 1971.
38. Glassman, R. D., Noble, R. J., Tavel, M. E., et al.: Pacemaker-induced endocardial friction rub. Am. J. Cardiol. 40:811, 1977.
39. Goldschlager, N., and Andrews, B.: Protracted chest wall stimulation in the management of permanent pacemaker-induced ventricular tachycardia and fibrillation occurring during acute myocardial infarction. West. J. Med., 138:569, 1983.
40. Gould, L., Reddy, R., Yacub, U., et al.: Perforation of the tricuspid valve by a transvenous pacemaker. J.A.M.A. 230:86, 1974.
41. Han, J., DeJalon, P. D. G., and Moe, G. K.: Fibrillation threshold of premature ventricular responses. Circ. Res. 14:516, 1964.
42. Hernandez-Pieretty, O., Morales-Rocha, J., and Barcelo, J. E.: Supernormal phase of conduction in human heart demonstrated by subthreshold pacemakers. Br. Heart J. 31:553, 1968.
43. Hess, D. S., Gertz, E. W., Morady, F., et al.: Permanent pacemaker implantation in the cardiac catheterization laboratory: the subclavian approach. J. Cath. Cardiovasc. Diag. 8:453, 1982.
44. Holmes, D. R., Jr., Nissen, R. G., Maloney, J. D., et al.: Transvenous tined electrode systems. An approach to acute dislodgement. Mayo Clin. Proc. 54:219, 1979.
45. Howard, J. A., and Kosowsky, B. D.: Electrocardiographic diagnosis of hyperkalemia in the presence of ventricular pacing and atrial fibrillation. Chest 78:491, 1980.
46. Hsu, Y. H., Guzman, L. G., Lau, S. H., et al.: Surgical aspects of transvenous endocardial pacemakers. Milit. Med. 146:254, 1981.
47. Huang, T. Y., and Baba, N.: Cardiac pathology of transvenous pacemakers. Am. Heart J. 83:469, 1972.
48. Hughes, H. C., Tyers, F. O., and Torman, H. A.: Effects of acid-base imbalance on myocardial pacing thresholds. J. Thorac. Cardiovasc. Surg. 69:743, 1975.
49. Irnich, W., deBakker, J. M. T., and Bispring, H. J.: Electromagnetic interference in implantable pacemakers. PACE 1:52, 1978.
50. Kaulbach, M. G., and Krukonis, E. E.: Pacemaker electrode-induced thrombosis in the superior vena cava with pulmonary embolization: a complication of pervenous pacing. Am. J. Cardiol. 26:205, 1970.
51. Kennelly, B. M., and Piller, L. W.: Management of infected transvenous permanent pacemakers. Br. Heart J. 36:1133, 1974.
52. Kinney, E. L., Allen, R. P., Weidner, W. A., et al.: Recurrent pulmonary emboli secondary to right atrial thrombus around a permanent pacing catheter: a case report and review of the literature. PACE 2:196, 1979.
53. Klein, H. O., DiSegni, E., Kaplinsky, E., et al.: The Wenckebach phenomenon between electric pacemaker and ventricle. Br. Heart J. 38:961, 1976.
54. Korn, M., Schoenfeld, C. D., Ghahramani, A., et al.: The pacemaker sound. Am. J. Med. 49:451, 1970.
55. Ku, D. D., and Lucchesi, B. R.: Ischemic-induced alterations in cardiac sensitivity to digitalis. Eur. J. Pharmacol. 57:135, 1979.
56. Lee, M. E., Chaux, A., and Matloff, J. M.: Avulsion of a tricuspid valve leaflet during traction on an infected, entrapped endocardial pacemaker electrode. J. Thorac. Cardiovasc. Surg. 74:433, 1977.
57. Lekven, J., Chatterjee, K., Tyberg, J. V., et al.: Pronounced dependence of ventricular endocardial QRS potentials on ventricular volume. Br. Heart J. 40:891, 1978.
58. Lewis, T., and Master, A. M.: Supernormal recovery phase, illustrated by two clinical cases of heart block. Heart 11:371, 1924.
59. Linos, D. A., Mucha, P., Jr., van Heerden, J. A., et al.: Subclavian vein. A golden route. Mayo Clin. Proc. 55:315, 1980.
60. Littleford, P. O., Parsonnet, V., and Spector, S. D.: Method for the rapid and atraumatic insertion of permanent endocardial pacemaker electrodes through the subclavian vein. Am. J. Cardiol. 43:980, 1979.
61. Littleford, P. O., and Spector, S. D.: Device for the rapid insertion of a permanent endocardial pacing electrode through the subclavian vein: preliminary report. Ann. Thorac. Surg. 27:3;265, 1979.
62. London, A. R., Runge, P. J., Balsam, R. F., et al.: Large right atrial thrombi surrounding permanent transvenous pacemakers. Circulation 40:661, 1969.
63. Lown, B., Klein, M. D., Barr, I., et al.: Sensitivity to digitalis drugs in acute myocardial infarction. Am. J. Cardiol. 30:388, 1972.
64. Luceri, R. M., Furman, S., and Hurzeler, P.: Threshold behavior in long-term ventricular pacing. Circulation 54:11, 1976.
65. Ma, P.: Incidence of septicemia in patients with cardiac pacemakers. Crit. Care Med. 2:3, 1974.
66. McNeill, G. P., and Taylor, N. C.: Use of subclavian vein for permanent cardiac pacing. Br. Heart J. 40:114, 1978.
67. Mehta, J., and Khan, A. H.: Pacemaker Wenckebach phenomenon due to antiarrhythmic drug toxicity. Cardiology 61:189, 1976.
68. Miller, F. A., Holmes, D. R., Gersh, B. J., et al.: Permanent transvenous pacemaker implantation via the subclavian vein. Mayo Clin. Proc. 55:309, 1980.
69. Misra, K. P., Korn, M., Ghahramani, A. R., et al.: Auscultatory findings in patients with cardiac pacemakers. Ann Intern. Med. 74:245, 1971.
70. Mond, H. G., Stuckey, J. G., and Sloman, G.: The diagnosis of right ventricular perforation by an endocardial pacemaker electrode. PACE 1:62, 1978.
71. Morgan, G., Ginks, W., Siddons, H., et al.: Septicemia in patients with an endocardial pacemaker. Am. J. Cardiol. 44:221, 1979.
72. Moss, A. J., and Goldstein, S.: Clinical and phar-

macological factors associated with pacemaker latency and incomplete pacemaker capture. Br. Heart J. 31:112, 1969.
73. Nasrallah, A., Hall, R. J., Garcia, E., et al.: Runaway pacemaker in seven patients. J. Thorac. Cardiovasc. Surg. 69:365, 1975.
74. Nicolosi, G. L., Charmet, P. A., and Zanuttini, D.: Large right atrial thrombus. Rare complication during permanent transvenous endocardial pacing. Br. Heart J. 43:199, 1980.
75. Nolewajka, A. J., Goddard, M. D., and Brown, T. C.: Temporary transvenous pacing and femoral vein thrombosis. Circulation 62:646, 1980.
76. Obadashian, H. C., and Brown, D. F.: "Runaway" in a modern generation pacemaker. PACE 2:152, 1979.
77. Pandian, N. G., Kosowsky, B. D., and Gurewich, V.: Transfemoral temporary pacing and deep vein thrombosis. Am. Heart J. 100:847, 1980.
78. Parker, D. P., and Kaplan, M. A.: Demonstration of the supernormal period in the intact human heart as a result of pacemaker failure. Chest 59:461, 1971.
79. Peter, T., Harper, R., Hunt, D., et al.: Wenckebach phenomenon in the exit area from a transvenous pacing electrode. Br. Heart J. 38:201, 1976.
80. Peter, T., Harper, R., and Sloman, G.: Inhibition of demand pacemakers caused by potentials associated with inspiration. Br. Heart J. 38:211, 1976.
81. Petterson, S. R., Singh, J. B., Reeves, G., et al.: Tricuspid valve perforation by endocardial pacing electrode. Chest 63:125, 1973.
82. Piller, L. W., and Kennedy, B. M.: Myopotential inhibition of demand pacemakers. Chest 66:418, 1974.
83. Preston, T. A.: Electrocardiographic diagnosis of pacemaker catheter displacement. Am. Heart J. 85:445, 1973.
84. Preston, T. A., Fletcher, R. D., Lucchesi, B. R., et al.: Changes in myocardial threshold. Physiologic and pharmacologic factors in patients with implanted pacemakers. Am. Heart J. 74:235, 1967.
85. Prozan, G. B., Shipley, R. E., Madding, G. F., et al.: Pulmonary thromboembolism in the presence of an endocardial pacing catheter. J.A.M.A. 206:1564, 1968.
86. Reynolds, J., Anslinger, D., Yore, R., et al.: Transvenous cardiac pacemaker, mural thrombosis, and pulmonary embolism. Am. Heart J. 76:688, 1969.
87. Robboy, S. J., Harthorne, J. W., Leinbach, R. C., et al.: Autopsy findings with permanent pervenous pacemakers. Circulation 39:495, 1969.
88. Rosenberg, A. S., Furman, S., and Escher, D. T. W.: Emergency cardiac pacing in hyperkalemia. Arch. Intern. Med. 126:658, 1970.
89. Scherf, D., and Schott, A.: The supernormal phase of recovery in man. Am. Heart J. 17:357, 1939.
90. Schwartz, I. S., and Pervez, N.: Bacterial endocarditis associated with a permanent transvenous cardiac pacemaker. J.A.M.A. 218:736, 1971.
91. Sethi, G. K., Bhayana, J. N., and Scott, S. M.: Innominate venous thrombosis. A rare complication of transvenous pacemaker electrodes. Am. Heart J. 87:770, 1974.
92. Shirato, C., and Ishikawa, K.: Newly developed systolic murmur in patients with a transvenous pacemaker. Am. Heart J. 99:722, 1980.
93. Smyth, N. P.: Techniques of implantation: atrial and ventricular, thoracotomy and transvenous. Prog. Cardiovasc. Dis. 23:435, 1981.
94. Soloff, L. A., and Fewell, J. W.: The supernormal phase of ventricular excitation in man; its bearing on the genesis of ventricular premature systoles, and a note on atrioventricular conduction. Am. Heart J. 59:869, 1960.
95. Stoney, W. S., Addlestone, R. B., Alford, W. C., et al.: The incidence of venous thrombosis following long-term transvenous pacing. Ann. Thorac. Surg. 22:166, 1976.
96. Surawicz, B., Chlebus, H., Reeves, J. T., et al.: Increase in ventricular excitability threshold by hyperpotassemia. J.A.M.A. 191:1049, 1965.
97. Theiss, W., and Wirtzfeld, A.: Pulmonary embolization of retained transvenous pacemaker electrode. Br. Heart J. 39:326, 1977.
98. Udall, J. A.: Cardiac pacing for cardiac arrest due to hyperkalemia plus digitalis and quinidine toxicity. West. J. Med. 124:497, 1976.
99. Van Durme, J. P., Heyndrickx, G., Snoeck, J., et al.: Diagnosis of myocardial perforation by intracardiac electrograms recorded from the indwelling catheter. J. Electrocardiol. 6:97, 1973.
100. Van Gelder, L. M., and El Gamal, M. I. H.: Externally induced irreversible runaway pacemaker. PACE 4:578, 1981.
101. Varriale, P., and Swa, R. P.: Pacemaker electrocardiography. *In* Varriale, P., and Naclerio, E. A. (eds.): Cardiac Pacing. A Concise Guide to Clinical Practice. Philadelphia, Lea & Febiger, 1979, pp. 283–305.
102. Vazquez, R. M.: Subclavian catheterization using the peel-away sheath. Surg. Gynecol. Obstet. 153:852, 1981.
103. Vera, Z., Mason, D. T., Awan, N. A., et al.: Lack of sensing by demand pacemakers due to intraventricular conduction defects. Circulation 51:815, 1975.
104. Walker, W. J., Elkins, J. T., Jr., and Wood, L. W.: Effect of potassium in restoring myocardial response to a subthreshold cardiac pacemaker. N. Engl. J. Med. 271:597, 1964.
105. Widmann, W. O., Mangiola, S., Lubow, W. A., and Dolan, F. M.: Suppression of demand pacemakers by inactive pacemaker electrodes. Circulation 45:319, 1972.
106. Williams, E. H., Tyers, G. F. O., and Shaffer, C. W.: Symptomatic deep venous thrombosis of the arm associated with permanent transvenous pacing electrodes. Chest 73:613, 1978.
107. Wohl, B., Peters, R. W., Carliner, N., et al.: Late unheralded pacemaker pocket infection due to *Staphylococcus epidermidis:* a new clinical entity. PACE 5:190, 1982.
108. Yarnoz, M., Attai, L. A., and Furman, S.: Infection of pacemaker electrode and removal with cardiopulmonary bypass. J. Thorac. Cardiovasc. Surg. 68:43, 1974.

9

Hypertensive Emergencies

DOROTHEE PERLOFF

A hypertensive crisis is a condition characterized by very high or rapidly rising arterial pressure in which prompt lowering of the pressure is beneficial. Failure to lower the pressure can lead to irreversible damage to the brain, heart, kidneys, and vasculature, whereas successful therapy can relieve the clinical symptoms and signs and arrest the underlying pathologic condition. A hypertensive crisis is defined not so much by the specific level of the blood pressure as by the rate of rise of the pressure and development of associated symptoms. Most hypertensive crises could have been prevented, being the result of inadequate management of patients with known hypertension. Occasionally, however, such an emergency develops in a previously normotensive patient and may signal the presence of secondary hypertension.

Table 9–1 lists conditions in which hypertension is a primary feature, and in which the rise in blood pressure results directly in rapid deterioration of vital functions. Table 9–2 lists conditions that are not primarily due to hypertension but which are aggravated by associated high arterial pressure. The urgency with which the blood pressure must be lowered in these conditions varies from minutes to hours, or at most to days, depending on the level of the blood pressure, the severity and rate of development of symptoms, the age of the patient, and the underlying pathology. In each situation the physician must promptly recognize the problem, formulate a reasonable differential diagnosis, and, with the use of available procedures, make a diagnosis and initiate appropriate therapy.

Most hypertensive crises can be prevented by the treatment of chronic hypertension and by the avoidance of drug interactions or abrupt withdrawal of antihypertensive drugs. These measures have successfully reduced the frequency with which hypertensive crises occur now as compared with the incidence before effective drugs were available. As a result, the average practitioner rarely sees patients with hypertensive emergencies and does not gain experience in their management. The problem of the hypertensive crisis is interdisciplinary, involving internists and surgeons, pediatricians and gerontologists. This chapter deals with the mechanisms and manifestations of hypertensive emergencies and the clinical management of the hypertension contributing to them.

CONDITIONS IN WHICH HIGH ARTERIAL PRESSURE IS A PRIMARY FACTOR

Hypertensive Encephalopathy

Hypertensive encephalopathy is an acute, reversible clinical syndrome characterized by progressive cerebral dysfunction resulting from marked blood pressure elevation or from abrupt increase in blood pressure from any cause. It usually develops in a patient with previous uncontrolled hypertension, either primary or secondary, such as chronic

Table 9–1. HYPERTENSIVE CRISES: CONDITIONS IN WHICH HIGH ARTERIAL PRESSURE IS A PRIMARY FACTOR

1. Hypertensive encephalopathy complicating:
   a. Primary hypertension
   b. Secondary hypertension
2. Malignant hypertension complicating:
   a. Primary hypertension
   b. Secondary hypertension
3. Acute stimulation of sympathetic nervous system due to
   a. Pheochromocytoma or other chromaffin cell tumor
   b. Administration of sympathomimetics directly or contained in other drugs
   c. Interaction of monoamine oxidase inhibitors with catecholamine or tyramine-containing drugs or foods
   d. Induction of anesthesia, laryngoscopy, intraoperative manipulations
   e. Rebound hypertension after abrupt withdrawal of antihypertensive drugs acting on sympathetic nervous system
   f. Release of stored catecholamines by injection of drugs such as guanethidine or reserpine
   g. Autonomic hyperreflexia in patients with transverse lesions of spinal cord
4. Acute expansion of extracellular fluid volume
5. Eclampsia or preeclampsia of pregnancy
   a. Superimposed on pre-existing hypertension or renal disease
   b. Arising de novo in pregnancy
6. Miscellaneous conditions

renal parenchymal disease or renovascular hypertension; however, it may develop when previously normotensive patients become acutely hypertensive, such as in children with acute glomerulonephritis, oliguric renal failure, lead poisoning, or acute fluid overload. The level of blood pressure at which symptoms develop is much lower in the latter than in the former group. The reason for the progressive increase in pressure is not always apparent, but discontinuation of antihypertensive medication, major emotional stress, induction of anesthesia, acute expansion of extracellular fluid volume, certain drug interactions or toxins, preeclampsia, or acute renal failure can initiate the clinical syndrome.

Hypertensive encephalopathy is postulated to be due to either excessive autoregulation of cerebral blood flow leading to exaggerated vasospasm and cerebral ischemia, or failure of autoregulation of cerebral blood flow leading to "breakthrough" overperfusion of the brain.[21] Cerebral blood flow is normally maintained constant over a wide range of blood pressures, except as modified by changes in acid-base balance, owing to the mechanism of *autoregulation.*[27] A fall in systemic pressure or low pH results in vasodilatation of the cerebral resistance vessels in order to maintain cerebral perfusion, whereas an increase in blood pressure or high pH results in vasoconstriction, preventing overperfusion and rupture of blood vessels. In the normal adult, cerebral blood flow is constant from a mean pressure of 60 to 120 mm Hg. If the pressure falls below that level, cerebral blood flow decreases, the brain is underperfused, and cerebral anoxia results. If the blood pressure rises above the level at which the arterioles can constrict no further, failure of autoregulation occurs.[21, 27] Some arterioles or portions of arterioles dilate, so that cerebral blood flow increases suddenly, while other arterioles and capillaries are injured or ruptured, so that transudation of fluid, cerebral edema, and petechial hemorrhages result.[10] In patients with previously uncontrolled hypertension, blood pressure is maintained relatively constant between a mean pressure of 120 and 220 mm Hg. This adaptive mechanism protects the brain against chronically high levels of blood pressure. Hypertensive encephalopathy occurs when blood pressure exceeds the upper limit of the body's ability to autoregulate, whatever that level may be. This explains why normotensive patients who suddenly become hypertensive develop symptoms at much lower pressures than do patients with chronic hypertension.[13]

Table 9–2. HYPERTENSIVE CRISES: CONDITIONS AGGRAVATED BY COEXISTENCE OF HIGH ARTERIAL PRESSURE

1. Acute left ventricular failure or pulmonary edema
2. Acute myocardial ischemia with prolonged pain
3. Intracranial, subarachnoid, or epidural hemorrhage; cerebral infarction
4. Dissecting or leaking aneurysm of aorta
5. Hypertension or bleeding associated with renal, vascular, cardiac, or neurosurgical procedures or severe epistaxis

The clinical manifestations of hypertensive encephalopathy usually develop over the course of 24 to 48 hours and include severe headache and vomiting (especially in children); confusion and drowsiness progressing to coma; irritability, agitation, muscle twitching, myoclonus, and focal or generalized seizures; blurred vision, diplopia, nystagmus, and cortical or retinal blindness; and pareses, aphasia, and abnormal reflexes.[13] On physical examination the optic fundi often show papilledema, hemorrhages, cotton wool patches (formerly known as soft or fluffy exudates, and representing ischemic infarcts and edema of the retina), or generalized arteriolar spasm. The neurologic defects fluctuate in intensity and usually suggest a diffuse rather than a focal lesion. Bradycardia is common.

Conditions that must be differentiated from hypertensive encephalopathy include brain tumor or other intracranial mass lesion; encephalitis; vasculitis; subarachnoid, intracerebral, or subdural hemorrhage; thrombotic stroke; metabolic causes of coma; and postictal state. The distinctive characteristic of hypertensive encephalopathy is the complete reversibility of the signs and symptoms following reduction of blood pressure, unless severe cerebral edema, herniation of the cerebellum through the foramen magnum, and multiple petechial hemorrhages have already occurred. The rapid response to therapy is thus a useful tool in the differential diagnosis. In a patient with thrombotic stroke, reduction of blood pressure may actually worsen the condition and increase the neurologic deficit.[10] The differential diagnosis can usually be suspected from the clinical history, if available, the mode of onset and evolution of symptoms, and the physical examination. Nuchal rigidity is not present in hypertensive encephalopathy as it is in subarachnoid hemorrhage. The neurologic findings do not conform to the pattern of distribution of a single arterial hemorrhage or occlusion, but vary in distribution and intensity. The cerebrospinal fluid may be under increased pressure but is otherwise clear with normal, or only slightly elevated, protein, and does not contain abnormal red or white cells. The electroencephalogram is diffusely abnormal but the abnormalities are nonspecific and nonlocalizing. The computed tomography (CT) or isotope brain scan is usually normal.[13]

Patients with hypertensive encephalopathy should be promptly hospitalized in an intensive care unit for close monitoring and titration of medication. Initiating factors, when recognized, should be corrected. Blood pressure reduction should be initiated promptly after the diagnosis is suspected, and the patient should be watched closely for changes in neurologic status. The pressure can be rapidly reduced to normal levels in young patients who have not been previously hypertensive. However, in patients with chronic hypertension, especially in older individuals with cerebrovascular disease or angina, rapid reduction of blood pressure to normal levels is not only unnecessary but hazardous.[23]

In the selection of antihypertensive drugs, it is important to avoid centrally acting agents that cloud the sensorium or produce drowsiness, so as not to interfere with the ongoing assessment of neurologic status. Clonidine, methyldopa, and reserpine should therefore be avoided, especially since their onset of action is unpredictable and may be delayed. Hydralazine, which can produce nausea and vomiting, should not be used in semicomatose patients, to avoid the risk of vomiting and aspiration, nor in patients with underlying coronary insufficiency.[20] Diazoxide, which produces hyperglycemia, may complicate the differentiation from and management of diabetic acidosis. However, diazoxide, followed by a loop diuretic and beta-adrenergic blocking agent if needed, is very effective in producing a sustained reduction of blood pressure in conscious, nondiabetic patients, especially if close monitoring is not feasible.[11] This combination is particularly useful in patients with underlying renal or renovascular disease. Nitroprusside and trimethaphan camsylate are rapidly effective drugs but require very careful titration and close monitoring of vital signs. Trimethaphan inactivates pupillary reflexes and so can interfere with evaluation of neurologic signs. Nifedipine,[4] the new calcium channel antagonist, has been used successfully, both orally and sublingually, for the treatment of hypertensive emergencies and promises to be a useful drug in the conscious patient.*

In patients with underlying primary hypertension, a transition to longer acting oral drugs for long-term therapy should be made as soon as feasible. Persons with such severe

*Nifedipine has not yet been approved for the treatment of hypertension in the United States.

hypertension usually require triple drug therapy with a diuretic, a vasodilator, and a sympathetic blocking agent. Every effort should be made to prevent a recurrence of encephalopathy by adequate control of the blood pressure, education of the patient, and correction of underlying causes of hypertension when possible.

Malignant Hypertension

Malignant hypertension is characterized clinically by the presence of very high blood pressure levels, diastolic pressures often greater than 130 mm Hg, and papilledema with hemorrhages, cotton wool patches, and arteriolar spasm in the optic fundi (Keith-Wagener Grade IV changes).[18] The characteristic pathologic condition is a necrotizing arteriolitis that rapidly leads to deterioration of renal function with death from uremia, congestive heart failure, cerebral hemorrhage, or aortic dissection within weeks to months after onset of symptoms.[19,45] The malignant phase of hypertension usually develops in a patient with long-standing primary hypertension, but may develop in a previously normotensive individual as a complication of end-stage renal parenchymal disease, collagen vascular disease, or renovascular or other forms of secondary hypertension.[38] In children, malignant hypertension usually occurs as a result of renal or endocrine hypertension.[30] The term "malignant" hypertension is used in contrast to "benign" hypertension because in the days before effective hypotensive drugs were available the condition was rapidly fatal, especially once renal function had begun to deteriorate.[38] The term "accelerated" hypertension is applied to an earlier stage of the syndrome when hemorrhages and exudates but not papilledema are present in the optic fundi (Keith-Wagener Grade III).[18] However, the differentiation of accelerated from malignant hypertension is only one of degree; the eventual outcome is the same unless the process is arrested or reversed by reduction of blood pressure.[38] Since the widespread use of antihypertensive drugs, malignant hypertension occurs in less than 1 per cent of hypertensive patients. However, in certain population groups such as black men, the incidence is still relatively high.[35]

The development of malignant hypertension appears to be triggered by a rapid rise in blood pressure in the presence of increased vascular reactivity.[19] This leads to arteriolar constriction, especially in the afferent arterioles of the kidney, with activation of the renin-angiotensin-aldosterone system and increase in other vasoactive pressor substances. The profound vasoconstriction and increased level of angiotensin II result in the typical vascular lesions of necrotizing arteriolitis, characterized by intimal proliferation and fibrinoid necrosis of the media, especially in the glomerular arterioles.

The symptoms of malignant hypertension, which may develop over the course of several weeks or manifest themselves abruptly, include headache, often diffuse and severe, especially in the morning, associated occasionally with projectile vomiting; visual impairment, blurring, diplopia, even blindness due to papilledema, macular edema, and focal retinal hemorrhages; weight loss, nausea, vomiting, weakness, and fatigue due to uremia and sodium wasting with dehydration; painless gross hematuria; and central nervous system symptoms including confusion, transient or permanent focal neurologic deficits, and uremic encephalopathy. Patients with malignant hypertension occasionally present a picture of hypertensive encephalopathy with myoclonus, convulsions, and coma.[38]

The characteristic findings on physical examination include very high blood pressure, often 250 to 300 mm Hg systolic and 150 to 180 mm Hg diastolic in patients with previous hypertension, but as low as 160 to 180/110 mm Hg in those who were previously normotensive. The optic fundi show characteristic changes: papilledema, which may be unilateral in the early stages; elongated, flame-shaped hemorrhages located in the nerve cell layer of the retina and radiating from the optic nerve; and cotton wool patches.[18] Patients with malignant hypertension of some duration often have localized retinal edema residues distributed radially around the macula, giving the appearance of a "macular star."

The characteristic laboratory abnormalities include a hypokalemic, hypochloremic alkalosis due to stimulation of the renin-angiotensin-aldosterone system, and microangiopathic hemolytic anemia manifested by fragmentation of red cells and the appearance of schistocytes in the blood smear, increase in fibrin split products, thrombocytopenia, hemolysis, prolongation of the prothrombin time, and contracted plasma volume.[12] Hematuria and proteinuria (usually less than 2 gm/24 hr) are common findings. The degree of impairment of renal function depends on the stage of the disease.

Patients with accelerated or malignant hypertension should be hospitalized if they are symptomatic, but can be followed closely as outpatients if asymptomatic, especially before papilledema has developed. Blood pressure should be lowered over the course of one to two days (although not immediately to normal levels), using oral medication. Symptomatic patients with encephalopathy, congestive failure, increased cerebrospinal fluid pressure, nausea, and vomiting or patients with vascular catastrophes or pre-existing impairment of renal function should be hospitalized, and the blood pressure should be lowered more rapidly with parenteral medication.[2, 30, 32] Patients should be weaned to oral antihypertensive drugs for maintenance therapy as soon as possible. In persons with long-standing hypertension or chronic renal disease, the combination of a vasodilator (hydralazine, prazosin, minoxidil, captopril, nifedipine) and a diuretic (furosemide, ethacrynic acid, metolazone, or thiazide) with a sympathetic blocking agent is particularly effective and may prevent further deterioration of renal function.[11, 46] In older patients, or those with angina or cerebrovascular insufficiency, blood pressure must be lowered slowly and moderately with close observation to avoid hypoperfusion of vital organs.[23] As blood pressure is lowered, renal perfusion pressure is also reduced and renal function may deteriorate temporarily. Occasionally, patients require hemodialysis or peritoneal dialysis during this initial period of blood pressure control.[32] Dialysis is also required in volume-overloaded patients with pulmonary edema who do not respond to intravenous diuretics, and in those with severe hyperkalemia and acidosis unresponsive to therapy. Once sustained blood pressure reduction is achieved, renal function usually improves, but some patients require chronic dialysis.[26]

All the available antihypertensive drugs can be used in patients with malignant hypertension: sodium nitroprusside, diazoxide, and most recently nifedipine for immediate blood pressure reduction; and minoxidil, prazosin, clonidine, methyldopa, and beta-adrenergic blocking agents with hydralazine for more gradual reduction.[3] Captopril is often very effective, for both immediate and chronic oral therapy, especially in conjunction with a diuretic and beta-adrenergic blocking agent.[7, 41] However, since hyperreninemia, vasoconstriction, and a contraction of plasma volume are common features, a diuretic is not indicated as primary therapy; diuretics are used as an adjunct treatment with such drugs as diazoxide or other vasodilators that result in secondary retention of sodium and water. If renal function is impaired, thiazide diuretics are relatively ineffective and loop diuretics such as furosemide or ethacrynic acid must be employed. Further, in patients with impaired renal function who are treated with nitroprusside, the thiocyanate levels must be checked frequently and a lower dose employed.[8] When a direct arteriolar vasodilator such as hydralazine, diazoxide, or minoxidil is used, the reflex tachycardia and increase in cardiac output must be avoided or minimized by coadministration of an intravenous or oral beta-adrenergic blocking agent such as propranolol.

In spite of the microangiopathic hemolytic anemia with evidence of intravascular coagulation, anticoagulants are not advisable. Bilateral nephrectomy followed by chronic hemodialysis was formerly used by some groups for the treatment of malignant hypertension in patients with uncontrollable renin-dependent hypertension due to uncorrectable end-stage renal disease.[22] With the availability of beta-adrenergic blocking drugs that block the release of renin, converting enzyme inhibitors, and minoxidil, nephrectomy is now rarely necessary. Once blood pressure has been controlled, further diagnostic studies to rule out curable forms of secondary hypertension should be initiated, especially in children and in patients not previously known to be hypertensive.[30]

Acute Stimulation of the Sympathetic Nervous System

Acute stimulation of the sympathetic nervous system can result in an alarming increase in blood pressure and distressing, potentially lethal, cardiovascular and cerebral complications. The hypertension can be difficult to control unless the underlying mechanism is suspected and specific catecholamine antagonists are administered.

Although the best recognized example of hypertension due to excessive levels of the catecholamines epinephrine and norepinephrine is the paroxysmal hypertension seen in patients with a pheochromocytoma, several other conditions produce hypertension by a similar mechanism (see Table 9–1). Patients with thyrotoxicosis, manic psychosis, severe pain, or acute anxiety attacks are often quite hypertensive when first seen, but blood pressure is rarely elevated sufficiently or over a long enough time to produce symptoms requiring rapid blood pressure reduction. Pheochromocytomas are benign and operable in 90 per cent of patients, and the major conditions mimicking these tumors can also be completely prevented or corrected. The prompt and appropriate management of the acute crisis and prevention of recurrent crises is thus particularly rewarding.

Pheochromocytomas. These are tumors, composed of chromaffin tissue derived from primitive neuroectoderm, which occur in the adrenal medulla and in association with sympathetic ganglia (paraganglioma).[28] Other tumors of similar origin include ganglioneuromas and neuroblastomas; the latter are especially common in children. These tumors occur in perhaps 0.1 per cent of patients with hypertension. Pheochromocytomas are found predominantly in the adrenal medulla (60%), and 90 per cent occur within the abdomen, in the para-aortic ganglia and organ of Zuckerkandl or bladder wall. Less than 2 per cent occur in the chest, and even fewer arise at the carotid bifurcation or along the arch of the aorta (glomus tumors). Less than 10 per cent are truly malignant. However, pheochromocytomas may be multicentric in origin (10%) and, when familial, occur in both adrenals in 70 per cent of patients. They occur in association with neurofibromatosis and with other endocrine tumors such as medullary carcinoma of the thyroid and parathyroid adenoma (MEN-2, multiple endocrine neoplasia) or with von Hippel-Lindau disease (cerebellar hemangioblastoma and retinal angioma).[6] Pheochromocytomas secrete both norepinephrine and epinephrine, but more often predominantly the former.[28]

Patients with a pheochromocytoma characteristically have paroxysms of hypertension and symptoms associated with excess secretion of catecholamines.[39] These may be so severe as to constitute a hypertensive crisis. Some patients have sustained hypertension between attacks; others are normotensive. The frequency and duration of the attacks vary widely, as does the severity of symptoms. An occasional patient is first seen with severe circulatory collapse during anesthesia, surgery, or delivery, as a result of hemorrhagic necrosis of the tumor. Some individuals have symptoms for many years, often misdiagnosed as anxiety attacks, before the correct diagnosis is made; in others, the first attack results in an acute hypertensive crisis. Attacks can arise spontaneously or be precipitated by massage or compression of the tumor; by a shift in position or exercise; by ingestion of various foods; by pain or change in temperature; or by increase in intra-abdominal pressure such as from a Valsalva maneuver, straining, voiding, or parturition; or by hypotension. Many drugs can precipitate release of catecholamines, as can laryngoscopy, induction of anesthesia, diagnostic tests, and manipulation of the tumor at surgery.

Table 9–3. SYMPTOMS AND SIGNS OF INCREASED PLAMSA LEVELS OF CATECHOLAMINES

Hypertension
Palpitations—tachycardia
Tachyarrhythmias—atrial and ventricular ectopy
Headache—often severe and pulsating
Chest pain—abdominal pain
Blurred vision—dilated pupils
Heat intolerance—sweating
Pallor or flushing
Fatigue, weakness
Anxiety, apprehension
Tremor
Constipation or diarrhea
Dizziness, syncope, postural hypotension
Glucose intolerance, glycosuria
Weight loss

The symptoms common during the acute attack and the findings on examination are listed in Table 9–3. Patients with this tumor can develop a cerebrovascular accident, myocardial infarction, congestive heart failure, catecholamine-induced myocarditis, malignant hypertension, life-threatening arrhythmias, and ischemic enterocolitis as a direct result of the excessive levels of circulating catecholamines.[28] The diagnosis should be suspected especially when patients present with sudden onset of hypertension, tachycardia, and sweating. However, the list of conditions that must be differentiated is long and includes anxiety, thyrotoxicosis, migraine headaches, coronary insufficiency, hypertensive disease of pregnancy, hypoglycemia, acute porphyria, and many others.

When a patient is seen during an attack with very high blood pressure, a cautious trial of intravenous phentolamine (Regitine) is both diagnostic and therapeutic. However, false-positive phentolamine tests do occur if the patient has received antihypertensive drugs before arriving in the emergency room. Phentolamine should be given intravenously beginning with 1 mg followed sequentially by 3-mg, 5-mg, or larger doses, if necessary, until a fall in blood pressure is observed. At the start of the procedure, a timed urine specimen should be initiated to be completed at the termination of the hypertensive crisis for assay of urinary catecholamines and their metabolites, metanephrines and vanillylmandelic acid.[14, 39] Blood samples for plasma catecholamines should be obtained if the procedure can be readily performed. Sodium nitroprusside can also be used for rapid control of blood pressure if phentolamine is not readily available or not rapidly effective. Once a diagnosis is strongly suspected, blood pressure control should be maintained with oral phentolamine, 5 to 20 mg every two to four hours, or intravenous phentolamine, 0.2 to 0.5 mg per minute, alternately with oral phenoxybenzamine (Dibenzyline), 10 to 30 mg, or even more, twice daily. Once alpha-blockade is achieved with these drugs, beta-adrenergic blocking agents can be added to control the tachycardia. However, beta-blockers should not be used alone as initial therapy since they may result in increased arterial pressure.

Hypertensive and hypotensive crises can recur during diagnostic tests such as angiography or CT scanning performed for localization of the tumor, as well as during induction of anesthesia and removal of the tumor. Patients must therefore be handled with great care; no unnecessary procedures should be performed and phentolamine should be readily available for intravenous use at all times. Plasma volume depletion should be corrected before surgery by treating the patient for several days with phenoxybenzamine. During the operation, pressor agents as well as phentolamine and parenteral beta-adrenergic blocking agents should be available to maintain a stable blood pressure. Following removal of the tumor, repeat urinary catecholamines should be measured to ensure complete removal of the tumor or of multiple tumors, especially in familial pheochromocytoma or in children.

Sympathomimetic Drugs. Such agents, which stimulate peripheral postsynaptic alpha-receptors directly or by releasing stored catecholamines, invariably raise blood pressure. These drugs include norepinephrine, metaraminol bitartrate, phenylephrine hydrochloride, methoxamine hydrochloride, mephentermine sulfate, amphetamines and derivatives, ephedrine, and phencyclidine hydrochloride (Sernylan, or "angel dust"). The effects of sympathomimetic drugs are exaggerated in patients with depletion of catecholamine stores from nerve endings due to chronic treatment of hypertension with reserpine or guanethidine.[29]

Sympathomimetic amines are used widely in the treatment of asthma, allergy, and hypotension; for weight reduction; and as vasoconstrictors and decongestants in nasal sprays and cold remedies, in local anesthetics, and in ophthalmic solutions. Although these drugs do not produce a hypertensive crisis in most patients, some individuals are particularly sensitive to alpha-receptor stimulation and a crisis may be precipitated in severely hypertensive patients.

Tricyclic Antidepressants. These agents usually produce orthostatic hypotension but occasionally cause marked blood pressure elevation in addition to interfering with the uptake and hypotensive action of such drugs as guanethidine, and maybe also of alphamethyldopa and clonidine. Tricyclic antidepressants in common use are listed in Table 9–4.[29]

A careful history regarding the use of prescribed and over-the-counter drugs should be obtained when a patient develops a hypertensive crisis without other obvious precipitating factors. Discontinuation of the offending drug may be sufficient. However, if symptoms persist or serious complications

Table 9–4. COMMONLY USED TRICYCLIC ANTIDEPRESSANTS*

Imipramine (Tofranil)
Desipramine (Pertofrane)
Amitriptyline (Elavil)
Nortriptyline (Aventyl)
Protriptyline (Vivactil)
Doxepin (Sinequan)

*Trade names in parentheses.

Table 9–5. MONOAMINE OXIDASE (MAO) INHIBITORS*

Phenelzine (Nardil)
Isocarboxazid (Marplan)
Nialamide (Niamid)†
Pargyline (Eutonyl)
Tranylcypromine (Parnate)
Iproniazid (Marsilid)†

*Trade names in parentheses.
†Not marketed in the United States.

appear imminent, alpha-adrenergic blockers such as phentolamine followed by a beta-blocker such as propranolol are the therapy of choice. Sodium nitroprusside, however, is also effective.

Monoamine Oxidase (MAO) Inhibitors. Table 9–5 lists the MAO inhibitors, which were used extensively for patients with psychiatric and neurotic problems before the tricyclic antidepressants became available. One of these, pargyline, was also used to treat hypertension. MAO inhibitors interfere with the normal oxidative metabolism of catecholamines and therefore increase the storage of these substances at nerve endings. The use of catecholamine-releasing drugs, amphetamine, ephedrine, and phenylpropanolamine together with MAO inhibitors can produce a syndrome resembling a pheochromocytoma crisis. A similar crisis can result when a person on chronic treatment with MAO inhibitors eats foods containing large amounts of tyramine, a precursor of catecholamines (Table 9–6). Other drugs that produce a hypertensive crisis when used together with MAO inhibitors include methionine, methoxamine, dopamine, and levodopa. Now that MAO inhibitors are no longer widely used and their potential interaction with drugs and foods is recognized, this problem rarely arises.

The treatment for hypertensive crisis is primarily one of prevention by avoidance of the offending foods and drugs. Alpha-adrenergic blocking drugs such as phentolamine are immediately effective and can be followed by oral alpha-adrenergic blockers until the symptoms subside. In the acute situation, intravenous nitroprusside can also be used. Beta-adrenergic blocking agents should not be used until after alpha-blockade is achieved, since unopposed stimulation of the alpha-receptors can actually aggravate the symptoms.

Table 9–6. FOODS CONTAINING RELATIVELY LARGE AMOUNTS OF TYRAMINE

Avocado	Chocolate
Beer	Game
Broad beans	Meat extracts
Canned figs	Pickled herring
Cheddar cheese	Ripe bananas
Chianti or other red wines	Yeast
Chicken or beef liver	Yogurt

Anesthesia and Surgery in Hypertensive Patients. Patients with chronic hypertension present special problems during induction of anesthesia, and both during and after surgery. The difficulties are those of exaggerated increases in blood pressure and heart rate, which result in increased cardiac work, and of hypotension due to the use of antihypertensive drugs that interfere with normal homeostatic mechanisms and sympathetic reflexes.[36] The anesthetist should be fully informed about all drugs used by a hypertensive patient and the time of discontinuation.[42] Antihypertensive agents should not routinely be discontinued before surgery, although a drug such as clonidine can be tapered and discontinued and replaced with another medication.[44] There is no advantage in having a patient's blood pressure uncontrolled at the time of surgery. Certain anesthetics such as ketamine hydrochloride, cyclopropane, and pancuronium bromide can produce hypertension in susceptible patients. Anxiety, fear, pain, laryngoscopy, and endotracheal intubation can also raise blood pressure excessively in hypertensive individuals.

Drugs that deplete catecholamines, such as reserpine and guanethidine, increase the responsiveness to exogenous pressor amines, norepinephrine, metaraminol, phenylephrine, and methoxamine, but decrease the response to catecholamine-releasing drugs such as ephedrine. Patients on large doses of beta-adrenergic blocking agents are less sensitive to the chronotropic and inotropic effects of sympathetic agonists such as isoproterenol, and have a reduced chronotropic response to atropine.[44] Hypertensives on medication also respond sluggishly to hemorrhage and other causes of hypotension owing to the suppression of their autonomic reflexes. The hypokalemia resulting from chronic diuretics, especially when exaggerated by the hypocapnia seen with artificial ventilation, can increase the risk of cardiac arrhythmias. In patients with hypertension and ischemic heart disease, the problems are again compounded by the need to avoid increased work for the heart, which can further aggravate the ischemia.[42] Patients who undergo spinal, subarachnoid, or extradural anesthesia occasionally have an excessive fall in blood pressure and an unpredictable response to pressor amines.[36] With manipulation of the gallbladder, crossclamping of the aorta, or sternum-splitting procedures, reflex sympathetic activity may produce a drastic rise in heart rate and blood pressure, increasing the work of the heart.

Hypertensive patients should be carefully monitored during and after surgery. This should include, when indicated, direct monitoring of arterial pressure, central venous pressure, pulmonary capillary wedge pressure (using a Swan-Ganz balloon-tipped catheter), and urine output. With careful preoperative evaluation, plus a full understanding of the drugs used before surgery and of the anticipated effects of those used during the procedure, hypotensive and hypertensive crises can be largely prevented.[42] Intravenous nitroprusside is the drug of choice when rapid reduction of an excessive rise in blood pressure is necessary in the operating room.

Rebound Hypertension After Withdrawal of Antihypertensive Drugs. A marked rise in pressure is occasionally seen when patients who have been receiving large doses of clonidine especially, but also methyldopa or propranolol, abruptly discontinue their medication.[15] The blood pressure may rebound to pretreatment levels or to alarmingly high levels, and a pattern of excess catecholamine release is observed. The picture is often encountered in hypertensive patients immediately following cardiac or other surgery if the usual antihypertensive medication is withheld on the morning of the operation.[31] The treatment of choice is reinstitution of the previously discontinued drug. Methyldopa and propranolol are available for intravenous use. Clonidine must be given orally in the United States although an intravenous form is available in Europe. If the reinstitution of previous therapy is not feasible, an alpha-adrenergic blocking agent such as intravenous phentolamine reduces blood pressure rapidly and can be followed by a beta-adrenergic blocking agent.[17] Again, intravenous nitroprusside has been used successfully. Preoperative reduction of medication with tapering and discontinuation of the sympatholytic drug, or continuation of the drug during and after surgery, is recommended for prevention of this type of crisis.

Reserpine and guanethidine (and similar drugs such as bethanidine) interfere with reuptake and storage of catecholamines at nerve endings. When given intravenously they cause an initial release of stored catecholamines, which can produce a sudden pressor effect before the hypotensive action begins. This transient, although occasionally rapid, rise in blood pressure rarely needs therapy. Neither reserpine nor guanethidine is used intravenously in the United States at this time.

Attacks of Autonomic Hyperreflexia. Such attacks can occur in quadriplegic patients with transverse lesions of the spinal cord at or above the 5th thoracic vertebral level.[16] The attacks are characterized by sudden onset of severe pulsating headache, sweating and flushing of the face, piloerection, blood pressure elevation, and bradycardia. The crises are caused by stimulation of nerves below the spinal cord lesion from distention or manipulation of the bladder, rectum, or viscera. The result is excess stimulation of preganglionic sympathetic neurons in the distal spinal cord stump and activation of supraspinal baroreceptor reflexes. Sympathetic and parasympathetic activity both increase, and both dopamine beta-hydroxylase and prostaglandin (PGE_2) levels increase in the plasma.[33] Paraplegic patients undergoing surgery on the abdomen and bladder are especially at risk. A similar acute hypertensive crisis is occasionally seen in Guillain-Barré syndrome and acute poliomyelitis.[9]

Management hinges primarily on speedy recognition and correction or discontinuation of the precipitating factors. Cautious use of intravenous phentolamine is recommended if bladder emptying, for instance, fails to relieve the symptoms promptly. Nitroprusside and trimethaphan are also very effective, especially during an operation when close monitoring is available.

Acute Expansion of Extracellular Fluid Volume

Acute expansion of vascular volume can produce a marked rise in blood pressure with symptoms of encephalopathy and left ventricular failure plus pulmonary edema. In addition, expansion of plasma volume reduces the effectiveness of most antihypertensive drugs and makes control of the hypertensive crisis more difficult. Patients with hypertension can rapidly excrete a large load of sodium and water unless their renal function is impaired. However, patients with end-stage renal disease, those on chronic dialysis, and children with acute nephritis can be easily precipitated into a hypertensive crisis when the critical extracellular fluid volume is exceeded.[30]

Expansion of plasma volume can result from rapid intravenous infusion of saline, especially during and after a surgical procedure and especially in infants and children. Large amounts of sodium can be ingested with salty foods such as pickles, potato chips, salted peanuts, and salted fish and with the hidden sources of sodium such as sodium bicarbonate and other sodium-containing antacids. Mineralocorticoids (11-desoxycorticosterone and fluorocortisone) and glucocorticoids, when used in the treatment of Addison's disease or congenital adrenal insufficiency, lupus erythematosus, arthritis, allergies, and asthma, result in the retention of sodium and water and can produce marked rises in blood pressure.[29] These patients develop a picture similar to primary aldosteronism with suppressed plasma renin activity. The possibility of unexpected uses of steroids, such as in nasal sprays and topical preparations, must not be overlooked in hypertensive patients. Ginseng has a corticosteroid-like action and can produce hypertension.[29] Oral contraceptives, estrogens, and anabolic steroids, especially when used in large doses for the treatment of malignancy, can cause marked fluid retention. Other compounds that result in fluid retention include licorice, owing to its content of glycyrrhizic acid; its derivatives, which are used to promote healing for gastric ulcers in Europe and Canada; and nonsteroidal anti-inflammatory agents such as aspirin, phenylbutazone (Butazolidine), and indomethacin (Indocin), owing to their antagonism of prostaglandin synthetase.

A first step in treatment is to discontinue the causative agent. Patients with chronic renal failure should be dialyzed promptly. In individuals with good renal function and urine output, a diuretic such as furosemide is rapidly effective.[30] Furosemide has the added advantage that it can be given parenterally in postoperative patients and in patients with nausea and vomiting. Diazoxide is contraindicated owing to the fluid retention it causes. However, all other antihypertensive agents, except perhaps the beta-adrenergic blocking agents, also result in fluid retention and therefore should be used only with a diuretic. A careful review of the clinical history to determine the precipitating factors, and education of the patient to prevent these in the future, are key elements in the management of this type of hypertensive crisis.

Preeclampsia/Eclampsia of Pregnancy

Preeclampsia/eclampsia is a condition unique to pregnancy characterized by the development of hypertension, retinal edema, proteinuria (greater than 300–500 mg/day) and edema (preeclampsia), progressing in some patients to convulsions (eclampsia), the development of which is a medical and obstetric emergency.[24] This condition develops after 22 weeks of gestation (usually after 30 wk) and can occur in a previously normotensive woman, usually during the first pregnancy, especially in a teenager or in a woman with multiple gestation or hydatidiform mole. The incidence is 4 to 6 per cent in the United States but is higher in some countries where malnutrition may be a factor. Women with pre-existent hypertension, diabetes mellitus, or renal disease are at increased risk for developing superimposed preeclampsia/eclampsia and do so earlier in pregnancy and during subsequent pregnancies, not only the first.

The rapid rise in blood pressure can lead to the development of hypertensive encephalopathy and convulsions, left ventricular failure and pulmonary edema, cerebral hemorrhage, coma, and even death, as well as acute hepatic necrosis and subcapsular hemorrhage. The associated nephrosclerosis results in massive proteinuria, edema, rapidly deteriorating renal function, and anuria. Uteroplacental blood flow is impaired, in association with premature arteriosclerosis and aging of the uteroplacental arteries, resulting in infarction of the placenta. Abruptio placentae can also occur and can result in massive hemorrhage, thrombocytopenia, and diffuse intravascular coagulation. Meanwhile the fetus is at increased risk of intrauterine growth retardation and intrauterine demise.

Preeclampsia thus constitutes an imminent, and eclampsia an actual, emergency for both the mother and fetus.

Early in a normal pregnancy the blood pressure falls below the levels present in the nonpregnant state, rising slightly during the last trimester. The hemodynamic changes during pregnancy include retention of 900 mEq of sodium and 6 to 8 liters of total body water, resulting in a 30 to 40 per cent increase in blood volume, cardiac output, and creatinine clearance. There is generalized vasodilatation and decreased total peripheral resistance. The hormonal changes include increased secretion of the vasodilator prostaglandin (PGE_2) as well as renin, aldosterone, and progesterone, with decreased vascular sensitivity to exogenous angiotensin. In women with preeclampsia, on the other hand, plasma renin activity decreases, angiotensin sensitivity increases, and plasma volume contracts. There is generalized vasospasm and it is postulated that synthesis of vasodilator prostaglandins decreases.[24]

The management of hypertension in a woman with preeclampsia is controversial since there is no evidence that lowering the blood pressure arrests the underlying process or improves fetal salvage. There is, however, general agreement that prevention of preeclampsia by regular prenatal care and good nutrition, and of eclampsia by timely delivery, are most important.

Patients at risk should be followed at regular intervals to assess blood pressure, degree of proteinuria, renal function, as well as fetal growth and fetal heart rate responsiveness. Baseline renal function should be assessed by creatinine clearance, and fetal age by sonography. Patients with previous hypertension may continue their usual antihypertensive medication when they become pregnant; however, some obstetricians prefer that patients discontinue antihypertensive drugs at onset of pregnancy. Beta-adrenergic blocking agents, although used widely in the United Kingdom, Australia, and New Zealand, are avoided in the United States because of reports of adverse effects on the fetus.[24] Methyldopa and hydralazine, in the usual doses, are the preferred drugs, although prazosin has been used successfully outside the United States. Women not on treatment who are found to have significant hypertension early in pregnancy should be treated similarly.

If blood pressure rises above 135/85 mm Hg for the first time after the 20th week of gestation (or increases more than 30 mm Hg systolic and 15–20 mm Hg diastolic above the level in early pregnancy), this may represent unmasking of underlying mild hypertension or the onset of toxemia. At this stage, sodium intake should not be restricted and diuretics should not be used because sudden decrease in plasma volume could further reduce the already compromised uterine blood flow. However, the degree to which uterine blood flow can autoregulate is not known. Antihypertensive drugs (methyldopa and hydralazine) and bed rest, in the left lateral decubitus position at home or in the hospital, often control blood pressure at this stage. If conservative medical management does not control blood pressure and if the mother becomes symptomatic from the hypertension and her renal function deteriorates, delivery (by cesarean section if necessary) is the definitive therapy, even if the fetus is immature. Fetal indications for early delivery include evidence of placental failure determined by decreasing urinary estriol levels, intrauterine growth retardation, and fetal distress determined by regular nonstress or oxytocin contraction tests. Close cooperation between obstetrician and neonatologist is important for maximal fetal salvage.

When delivery or cesarean section appears imminent, the mother's central venous or pulmonary capillary wedge pressure and urine output should be monitored to determine the degree to which the plasma volume is contracted, and the deficit should be corrected with plasma expanders. Intravenous hydralazine in doses of 5 to 20 mg can be given intermittently for diastolic blood pressures greater than 110 mm Hg. Magnesium sulfate should be administered to prevent cerebral irritability and convulsions. An intravenous loading dose of 4 gm given over 20 minutes or an intramuscular loading dose of 10 gm is followed by an intravenous infusion of 1 to 2 gm per hour, using an infusion pump. Plasma levels of 4 to 6 mg per dl should be maintained; higher levels can suppress respiration. If the blood pressure remains elevated following delivery, intravenous diazoxide or hydralazine can be given. Occasionally, furosemide (20 mg intravenously) is useful for initiating a postpartum diuresis. Although a rare patient becomes hypertensive for the first time during or immediately following delivery, emptying the uterus reverses the pathologic process completely in most patients.

Miscellaneous Conditions

Conditions in which blood pressure can rise to alarming levels, although the mechanism is not always understood, include the following: extensive body burns;[5] poisoning with heavy metals such as mercury, barium, or lead; chronic alcohol abuse; a combination of disulfiram (Antabuse) and alcohol; ingestion or injection of ergot alkaloids after parturition (ergonovine [Ergotrate]) or for migraine headaches (ergotamine tartrate [Gynergen, Cafergot, Ergomar]); the use of large doses of lithium carbonate in a manic hypertensive, especially when thiazide diuretics are also given; hypertensive reaction during hypoglycemia in a patient on nonselective beta-adrenergic blocking agents; acute anxiety with hyperventilation; postictal state; tetanus; thyroid storm; and acute porphyria.[29] A sudden rise in blood pressure is often seen when the competitive antagonist of angiotensin II, saralasin, is injected intravenously as a diagnostic test for renovascular hypertension. The weakly agonist properties of saralasin are apparent before the interference with the action of angiotensin II reduces the blood pressure, especially in patients who do not have high plasma renin levels.

Discontinuation of the offending drug or precipitating factor is a rational first step in management. The hypertension is usually transient and does not require rapid reduction. When rapid reduction of pressure is necessary, however, a cautious trial of intravenous phentolamine followed by a beta-adrenergic blocking agent or intravenous sodium nitroprusside is justified.

CONDITIONS AGGRAVATED BY COEXISTENT HYPERTENSION

Conditions that are not primarily due to hypertension but are aggravated by coincident high blood pressure are largely discussed elsewhere in this book. Below we review only the specific "do's" and "dont's" of antihypertensive drug therapy that apply to these conditions.

Acute Left Ventricular Failure

In this condition a decrease in myocardial performance results in decreased renal perfusion, activation of the renin-angiotensin system with retention of sodium and water, and expansion of plasma volume. As cardiac output falls and perfusion is reduced, peripheral vessels constrict. The rise in total peripheral resistance results in a rise in blood pressure. Even a small increase in "afterload," not necessarily to the level seen in hypertensive crises, adds a further burden on the failing heart. Therapy should therefore be directed at reduction of "afterload," reduction of plasma volume, and, in the patient who has pulmonary edema, reduction of "preload" also.

When patients are acutely ill and cared for in an intensive care unit where close monitoring is possible, intravenous nitroprusside is rapidly effective. The rate and degree of blood pressure reduction can be closely titrated to avoid cerebral and cardiac hypoperfusion while cardiac function is improved. Diazoxide is contraindicated because it produces fluid retention. Hydralazine and minoxidil (both direct arterial vasodilators) have been used orally for reduction of afterload in chronic congestive failure, but must be used with caution in the presence of myocardial ischemia because of the reflex tachycardia that increases the work of the heart. Beta-adrenergic blocking agents, however, can be used to counteract the tachycardia, although alone they are contraindicated because of their myocardial depressant effect. Parenteral diuretics such as furosemide act as vasodilators and reduce plasma volume, and can therefore be used effectively in pulmonary edema but not in low cardiac output states. The centrally acting sympathetic blocking agents clonidine, reserpine, and methyldopa are rarely used in the management of acute left ventricular failure unless a previously hypertensive patient has responded well to these drugs in the past.

Myocardial Ischemia with Prolonged Pain

The patient with acute coronary artery insufficiency and ischemic pain, whether previously hypertensive or not, may develop a rise in blood pressure in part due to the emotional and physical strain of the condition. The rise in blood pressure further increases the work of the heart, thereby aggravating the imbalance between coronary blood flow and myocardial oxygen demands. The aim of therapy therefore is to reduce the work of the heart by reducing wall tension and afterload. This may be beneficial both in preventing the evolution of a myocardial infarction and in reducing infarct size. In choosing an antihypertensive drug it is important to avoid those that produce a reflex tachycardia and increase cardiac output, such as the direct arterial vasodilators hydralazine, diazoxide, and minoxidil, unless coadministered with a beta-adrenergic blocking agent. As in acute left ventricular failure with hypertension, blood pressure should be reduced cautiously to avoid abrupt hypotension that could aggravate the ischemia. Nitroprusside intravenously is very effective because of its rapid onset of action and controlled effect; it decreases myocardial oxygen demands, decreases venous return, decreases left ventricular volume, and decreases left ventricular wall tension, thereby decreasing myocardial ischemia. Nifedipine is effective in patients with coronary artery spasm, but may produce sufficient reflex tachycardia to require the coadministration of a beta-adrenergic blocking agent. Reduction of plasma volume with diuretics is indicated if central venous and pulmonary capillary wedge pressures are elevated. Reserpine should be avoided because of its delayed and unpredictable onset of action. Methyldopa and clonidine likewise should be avoided unless used as maintenance treatment in a previously treated hypertensive patient.

Cerebral Hemorrhage

The desirability of lowering blood pressure in a patient with subarachnoid hemorrhage due to a ruptured congenital aneurysm of the circle of Willis, or with intracranial hemorrhage due to a ruptured Charcot-Bouchard aneurysm, is controversial.[10, 23, 37] Although marked blood pressure elevation may be associated with prolonged bleeding and a rapidly expanding hematoma, the arterial spasm in the area of the hemorrhage may lead to cerebral ischemia that would be aggravated by reducing the perfusion pressure.[1, 10] The injury to the brain caused by the expanding hematoma results in vasomotor paralysis and loss of the ability to autoregulate. Cerebral blood flow is then directly related to blood pressure. Persistent high pressure could lead to breakthrough, as in hypertensive encephalopathy, and aggravate the edema. Abrupt or excessive blood pressure reduction, on the other hand, could result in hypoperfusion and further cerebral ischemia.

Many neurologists recommend that the hypertension not be treated. If the pressure is alarmingly high, however, a cautious reduction of pressure may be attempted using rapidly acting and easily titrated parenteral medications that do not act on the central nervous system directly. If the neurologic status worsens, the blood pressure should be allowed to rise again. If reduction of blood pressure appears to be beneficial, with lessening of the neurologic deficit, longer acting drugs should be initiated and the patient weaned off intravenous therapy to maintain long-term blood pressure control.

Sodium nitroprusside and trimethaphan can be titrated accurately to allow for controllable blood pressure reduction while the patient's neurologic status is closely observed. Trimethaphan, however, produces inactivation of pupillary reflexes, interfering with ongoing neurologic evaluation of the patient. Centrally acting drugs such as methyldopa, clonidine, and reserpine are contraindicated because the sedation they produce can interfere with the evaluation of neurologic status. However, once the latter has stabilized, the centrally acting drugs can be used safely if severe hypertension persists. Parenteral diuretics such as furosemide are particularly useful in patients with cerebral edema and increased intracranial pressure, especially when steroids are used and overhydration with parenteral medication has occurred.

Patients with cerebellar hemorrhage usually have a sudden onset and rapid progression of neurologic abnormalities with loss of consciousness, sometimes heralded by a severe headache. With the aid of CT scanning the diagnosis can usually be made rapidly.[25] In patients with cerebellar hemorrhage, rapid diagnosis is crucial since early surgical decompression and evacuation of the hematoma can be life-saving and is the treatment of choice.

Cerebral Infarction

Patients with cerebral infarction must be differentiated from those with hypertensive encephalopathy by the rate of onset of symptoms and the persistence or progression of the localizing neurologic defects. Blood pressure usually does not rise excessively. Owing to the vasomotor paralysis that often accompanies infarction, patients may be very sensitive to minor fluctuations in blood pressure, and many neurologists recommend that blood pressure not be reduced.[23] If diastolic blood pressure is greater than 120 mm Hg, however, a cautious trial of gradual blood pressure reduction may be justified. Rapidly acting, controllable, and predictable parenteral drugs such as nitroprusside or trimethaphan can be used to reduce blood pressure, keeping in mind that trimethaphan inactivates pupillary reflexes. If the initial blood pressure reduction is tolerated, further reduction can be attempted. If the patient does not tolerate the reduced perfusion pressure, and if the neurologic deficit increases, blood pressure should be allowed to return to higher levels. Again, centrally acting drugs and longer acting drugs that cannot be titrated such as diazoxide, clonidine, reserpine, and methyldopa should be avoided until the initial situation stabilizes.

Epidural Hemorrhage

In a patient with epidural hemorrhage the definitive management is rapid surgical intervention. Although coexistent hypertension can accelerate the rate of bleeding, antihypertensive medication is rarely used in this situation.

Dissecting or Leaking Aneurysm of the Aorta

The pathophysiology and management of aortic dissection are discussed elsewhere in this book. In Type I proximal dissection, the development of acute aortic valve insufficiency and dissection into the pericardium with development of tamponade requires prompt surgical intervention. Likewise, when circulation to major vessels is compromised by the dissection or when aortic rupture into the thorax or abdomen is suspected or imminent, surgery is the definitive therapy.[40] However, even in these patients, lowering of blood pressure reduces the shearing forces on the aortic wall and reduces the upstroke of the arterial pulse, thereby slowing the progression of the dissection and allowing for stabilization of the patient before surgery. In patients with Type III distal dissection in whom aortic rupture is not imminent and renal function is maintained, blood pressure reduction is often the definitive therapy.[43]

The drugs of specific value in aortic dissection are those that reduce myocardial contraction and reduce the first derivative of the maximal aortic pressure rise (aortic dP/dt max). These include intravenous trimethaphan, intramuscular reserpine, and intravenous beta-adrenergic blocking agents. The pure arterial vasodilators (hydralazine, diazoxide, and minoxidil) increase heart rate and cardiac output as well as the shearing forces on the aorta. Even nitroprusside, although effective in reducing blood pressure rapidly, may produce some increase in cardiac output and is not recommended alone unless combined with beta-blockers.[34] Trimethaphan is thus the best single drug for immediate blood pressure reduction. This may be supplemented by a diuretic and beta-adrenergic blocking agent as needed. Blood pressure should be reduced as low as tolerated while urine output and central nervous system status are monitored. Since tachyphylaxis may develop with trimethaphan after a few days, a diuretic and longer acting drug such as methyldopa or a beta-adrenergic blocking agent should be added early to maintain blood pressure control.

Hypertension or Bleeding Associated With Surgical Procedures

When hypertensive patients bleed during or following operations on the brain, heart, kidneys, or major vessels, the amount of blood loss and damage to surrounding tissues can be reduced by lowering the pressure. In addition, patients with renovascular surgery or renal transplantation, coronary artery bypass grafting, and repair of a coarctation may develop acute postoperative blood pressure rises that require urgent management to avoid development of cerebral edema, acute tubular necrosis, or rupture at the arterial suture lines. In anesthetized or unconscious patients, immediate and controlled blood pressure reduction is best accomplished with intravenous nitroprusside or trimethaphan. Drugs such as diazoxide, which cannot be titrated, and intramuscular agents, the absorption of which is unpredictable, should be avoided. Intravenous methyldopa can be used when a more sustained reduction of blood pressure is desirable in patients who cannot take oral medication. Intravenous hydralazine is often used intraoperatively, but may produce nausea, vomiting, and sinus tachycardia, which can complicate the management of a semicomatose patient or an elderly patient with coronary artery insufficiency.

Epistaxis results from erosion of, or irritation of, superficial arteries in the nasal septum. Patients with hypertension do not necessarily have more frequent epistaxes than normotensive patients, but when they bleed, they do so more vigorously. The anxiety produced by the very visible exsanguination further increases the blood pressure. This is especially aggravated in a patient who has precipitated the epistaxis by inhalation of cocaine, which produces profound vasoconstriction with ischemic necrosis of the nasal septum while raising total peripheral resistance. A similar aggravation of hypertension can be seen in patients who use sympathomimetic amines in nasal sprays. When such persons are seen in the emergency room, their blood pressure is often found to be alarmingly high. Packing the nose, sedation with diazepam (Valium), and reassurance are usually sufficient, together with resumption of previous antihypertensive medications. Parenteral treatment with nitroprusside or diazoxide is rarely required.

INITIAL MANAGEMENT OF PATIENTS WITH HYPERTENSIVE CRISIS

Patients with a hypertensive crisis should be hospitalized in an acute or intensive care unit where close observation and expert nursing care are available. In comatose patients it is essential to establish an airway, an intravenous line, and, depending on the severity of the crisis, an arterial line, a central venous pressure gauge or Swan-Ganz catheter for determining pulmonary capillary wedge pressure, and a Foley catheter for measuring urine output.

The initial history-taking should include the following: history of previous hypertension, diabetes mellitus, renal disease, epilepsy, trauma, other major medical illnesses, or recent surgery; previous hospitalizations, chronic illnesses, and medications; recent ingestion of drugs or toxins; events leading up to the current crisis; and medication or treatment received at other hospitals, emergency rooms, or clinics immediately prior to admission.

On physical examination attention should be paid to the following: measurement of blood pressure in both arms, inspection for evidence of trauma or ecchymoses; estimation of jugular venous pressure; palpation of peripheral pulses and auscultation for bruits; palpation of the thyroid; auscultation of the lungs; careful cardiovascular examination; examination of the abdomen for evidence of acute distention, rebound tenderness, organomegaly, or masses; careful neurologic examination; and inspection of the optic fundi.

Initial laboratory studies should include: hemoglobin, hematocrit, leukocyte count with differential, examination of the peripheral smear, urinalysis with microscopic examination, serum electrolytes, serum glucose, urea, and creatinine. A coma profile should be performed if indicated, including testing for alcohol, acetone, and ammonia. The cerebrospinal fluid should be obtained cautiously, when indicated, and examined for the presence of cells, protein, and bacteria. In patients in whom a pheochromocytoma is suspected, a timed urine specimen should be initiated and plasma catecholamine levels determined. Electrocardiography, portable chest radiography, brain scan, or other more specialized procedures should be carried out as indicated.

Following the rapid initial evaluation, the physician must formulate a working differential diagnosis and plan of action, determining the rate at which blood pressure must be reduced and which associated problems are to be anticipated. In patients with symptoms suggesting a cerebellar hemorrhage or a proximal aortic dissection, the surgical members of the team should be alerted and blood submitted for typing and crossmatching.

ANTIHYPERTENSIVE DRUGS

Table 9–7 lists the drugs available for rapid lowering of blood pressure.

Table 9–7. DRUGS USED IN HYPERTENSIVE EMERGENCIES

Drug	Mechanism of Action	Route	How Supplied	Initial Dosage	Onset of Action	Duration of Action	Maintenance Dosage	Major Side Effects
sodium nitroprusside (Nipride)	vasodilator, arterial and venous	continuous IV infusion	50 mg in 5-ml vial; dilute in 500 ml D5W = 100 μg/ml	0.5–1.5 μg/kg/min; increase rate every 2–3 min to desired response	immediate	3–5 min	0.5–10.0 μg/kg/min infusion	thiocyanate[1] toxicity, nausea, vomiting, twitching, psychosis, restlessness
diazoxide (Hyperstat)	vasodilator, arterial	rapid IV bolus (20–30 sec) or slow infusion	20-ml ampule containing 300 mg = 15 mg/dl	2.5–5 mg/kg or 100-, 200-, 300-mg sequential injections at 10-min intervals or 15–30 mg/min	1–2 min	3–12 hr	repeat effective dosage every 6–12 hr	hypotension, hyperglycemia, flushing, nausea, vomiting, tachycardia, sodium retention
hydralazine hydrochloride (Apresoline)	vasodilator, arterial	IM or IV injection or continuous infusion	1-ml ampule containing 20 mg; dilute to 50 or 100 mg/l in saline	10–25 mg IV bolus or in 20 ml over 10 min or 50–150 μg/min infusion	10–20 min	2–6 hr	repeat effective dose every 3–6 hr or 50–150 μg/min infusion	nausea, vomiting, tachycardia, headache, flushing, angina
captopril (Capoten)	vasodilator, arterial, inhibitor of conversion of angiotensin I to II	oral	25-, 50-, 100-mg tablets	25 mg every 6–8 hr	15–30 min	4–6 hr	25–150 mg every 6–8 hr	maculopapular rash, proteinuria, agranulocytosis, ageusia, neutropenia
minoxidil (Loniten)	vasodilator, arterial	oral	2.5- and 10-mg tablets	5 mg PO or 0.2 mg/kg under age 12 yr	30–60 min	12–24 hr	5–20 mg every 12 hr	reflex tachycardia, headache, flushing, angina, fluid retention, hirsutism
nifedipine (Procardia, Adalat)[2]	vasodilator, arterial, calcium channel antagonist	oral or sublingual[3]	10-mg capsules	10 mg PO every 6 hr; 10 mg sublingual	30 min (PO); 5–10 min (sublingual)	4–6 hr	10–20 mg every 6–8 hr	tachycardia, flushing, headache
furosemide (Lasix)	diuretic vasodilator	oral, or IV	2-ml and 10-ml ampules; 10 mg/ml	20–80 mg IV over 1–2 min; 0.5–1.0 mg/kg	1–5 min	2–4 hr	40–160 mg every 12 hr IV or PO	hyponatremia, hypokalemia, dehydration
ethacrynic acid (Edecrin)	diuretic	oral or IV	50-mg vial; dilute in 50 ml D5W	50–100 mg IV or 0.5–1.0 mg/kg	1–5 min	2–4 hr	50–100 mg every 12 hr	local irritation, hypokalemia, hyponatremia

camsylate (Arfonad)	parasympathetic ganglion blocking agent	infusion	ampule of 50 mg; dilute in 500 ml D5W	mg/min; increase infusion rate every 5–8 min			infusion	ileus, constipation, orthostatic hypotension, tachyphylaxis, cycloplegia, xerostomia
methyldopa (Aldomet)	central and peripheral sympathetic blocking agent	IV	5-ml vial of 250 mg; dilute in 100 ml D5W	250–500 mg in 100 ml IV over 30 min	½–2 hr	2–8 hr	250–500 mg every 6–8 hr	sedation, somnolence, fever, liver function abnormalities
reserpine (Serpasil)	central and peripheral sympathetic blocking agent	IM	2-ml ampule containing 5 mg; multiple-dose vial; 10 ml = 25 mg	0.25–5 mg IM; 0.07 mg/kg IM in children	1–4 hr (may be delayed)	6–24 hr	0.25–5 mg every 8–12 hr	prolonged hypotension, nasal stuffiness, increased gastric acidity and gastrointestinal, motility, sedation, somnolence
clonidine (Catapres)	central alpha-adrenergic stimulant, decreasing sympathetic outflow	oral[4]	0.1-, 0.2-, 0.3-mg tablets	0.2 mg or previously effective (discon-tinued) dose	60–90 min	6–10 hr	0.1–0.4 mg every 8 hr	sedation, somnolence, xerostomia
propranolol[5] (Inderal)	beta-adrenergic receptor blocking agent	IV	1-ml ampule = 1 mg	1–3 mg IV; repeat after 2 min if needed	2–5 min	2–6 hr	1–3 mg every 4–6 hr	bradycardia, asthma, heart block, CNS effects
prazosin (Minipress)	postsynaptic alpha-adrenergic blocking agent, vasodilator	oral	1-, 2-, 5-mg capsules	1–2 mg PO	60–90 min	3–6 hr	1–10 mg every 8–12 hr	postural hypotension, rarely tachycardia, flushing, headache
phentolamine (Regitine)	competitive inhibitor of norepinephrine	IV	5-mg ampule	1 mg; repeat with 3- or 5-mg IV injection until desired effect is achieved	½–2 min	5–30 min	25–100 mg every 2–4 hr or repeat effective IV dose as needed or 0.2–2.0 mg/min infusion	tachycardia, dizziness, angina, flushing

[1]Toxic plasma levels of thiocyanate occur at a level of 10 mg/dl or greater.
[2]Nifedipine marketed in Mexico and Europe as Adalat; not yet approved by FDA for treatment of hypertension.
[3]Nifedipine not yet available in sublingual form in USA, but capsule can be chewed rather than swallowed for rapid effectiveness.
[4]Clonidine available for IV use in Europe.
[5]Propranolol, listed as the prototype beta-blocker, is the only parenteral beta-blocker available in the USA at this time; alprenolol, atenolol, and oxprenolol available in parenteral form in other countries.

Sodium Nitroprusside

Sodium nitroprusside (Nipride) is the most effective drug available for rapid and controlled reduction of blood pressure.[2] A vascular smooth muscle relaxant, it dilates both arteries and veins and reduces both preload and afterload. It is effective almost immediately after initiation of intravenous infusion and permits blood pressure to be lowered to any desired level, but the effect lasts only three to five minutes after the infusion is stopped. This drug must therefore be administered with a constant infusion pump to allow for careful regulation of the rate of infusion, since minor changes in dosage lead to wide swings in pressure. Blood pressure must be monitored at one- to two-minute intervals until an effective reduction of blood pressure has occurred and the maintenance rate of infusion is determined. In a critically ill patient, blood pressure should be monitored with an intra-arterial catheter.

Nitroprusside is metabolized in the red blood cells to cyanide and conjugated to form thiocyanate in the plasma. In patients with impaired renal function especially, prolonged infusion can result in toxic levels of thiocyanate (greater than 10 mg/dl). The symptoms of toxicity, which result from tissue anoxia and acidosis, include sweating, weakness, nausea, vomiting, abdominal cramps, tinnitus, muscle twitching, apprehension, disorientation, and psychosis. The potential use of the antidotes hydroxycobalamine and sodium thiosulfate is being investigated.[8] Extravasation at the infusion site causes severe local skin and tissue reactions. Since the solution of nitroprusside is photosensitive, the infusion bottle must be wrapped in foil to retard deterioration and a new solution must be prepared every four hours. The effect of nitroprusside is augmented by coadministration of a diuretic such as furosemide.

Nitroprusside can be effectively used in all forms of hypertensive crisis when careful monitoring of the blood pressure is feasible. It is especially valuable in hypertensive encephalopathy, acute cerebral hemorrhage or edema, postoperative hypertension or hemorrhage, and acute left ventricular failure, and can be used to initiate blood pressure control in malignant hypertension, acute glomerulonephritis, chronic renal failure with accelerated hypertension, severe body burns, and crises due to excess circulating catecholamines.

Diazoxide

Diazoxide (Hyperstat) is a benzothiadiazine derivative that acts as a direct arteriolar smooth muscle relaxant, perhaps by inhibition of transcellular calcium fluxes. Since diazoxide dilates only arterioles without affecting the venous capacitance vessels, it produces reflex activation of the sympathetic nervous system with tachycardia, increased left ventricular ejection velocity, and increased cardiac output. Although it is a thiazide-like compound, diazoxide produces retention of sodium and water by a direct tubular antidiuretic action. When injected intravenously, 90 per cent of the drug is rapidly bound to serum albumin and effectively neutralized. Diazoxide has therefore been traditionally given as a single bolus injection of 5 mg per kg or 300 mg in the average-sized adult over 10 to 20 seconds. Since the response is unpredictable and blood pressure may fall excessively, it is preferable to begin with a dose of 100 mg followed at five- to 15-minute intervals by increasing doses of 200 and 300 mg until an effect is achieved. Recent reports indicate that a slower infusion, 15 to 30 mg per minute over 20 to 30 minutes, is both effective and safe.[11] Because of the fluid retention, the initial injection should be followed in 30 to 60 minutes by an intravenous injection of furosemide. The reflex tachycardia can be counteracted with intravenous propranolol. In addition to the reflex tachycardia and increased cardiac output resulting from diazoxide, flushing, nausea, vomiting, fluid retention, and hyperglycemia are also observed. The solution is alkaline (pH of 11), and therefore extravasation of the intravenous solution into the subcutaneous tissues must be scrupulously avoided.

Diazoxide is of particular use in patients with hypertensive encephalopathy who are not comatose, since it does not produce central nervous system side effects; in patients with malignant hypertension in whom a sustained rather than transient fall in blood pressure is desirable; and in patients with end-stage renal disease who have developed resistant hypertension. Although used in toxemia of pregnancy, it is not recommended since it crosses the placenta, resulting in bilirubinemia and hyperglycemia in the fetus, and reduces uterine contractions. Diazoxide should be avoided in patients with acute myocardial ischemia, left ventricular failure, and aortic dissection because of the reflex stimulation of the sympathetic nervous system and the fluid retention. The hyperglycemia rarely becomes a problem unless the drug is used over the course of many days, but plasma glucose and acetone should be checked daily and urinary glucose and acetone at six-hour intervals in patients treated with diazoxide. Because of the nausea and vomiting and relatively unpredictable response, the drug is not recommended for postoperative patients and those with cerebrovascular accidents who are not fully alert.

Hydralazine

Hydralazine (Apresoline) is a direct arteriolar vasodilator that has no effect on venous capacitance vessels; the fall in blood pressure therefore activates the baroreceptors, resulting in reflex tachycardia and an increase in cardiac output.[20] It also produces headache, nausea, vomiting, and flushing. The drug can be given intramuscularly or by intermittent or continuous intravenous infusion. Since the rate of absorption from intramuscular injection is unpredictable, the intravenous route is preferred in patients with true hypertensive emergencies. The reflex increase in heart rate can be counteracted with concomitant use of an intravenous beta-adrenergic blocking agent such as propranolol.

Hydralazine is especially useful in patients with acute glomerulonephritis, hypertension of pregnancy, and intraoperative and postoperative hypertension. It can produce nausea and vomiting, however, and should be avoided in unconscious patients who might aspirate their vomitus. It is contraindicated in acute myocardial ischemia and aortic dissection because of the reflex increase in cardiac output and heart rate. Since sodium nitroprusside became generally available, hydralazine has been less commonly used, although it is still the drug of choice in acute hypertension of pregnancy.

Captopril

Captopril (Capoten) is an oral inhibitor of the enzyme kininase II that promotes the conversion of inactive angiotensin I to the active pressor substance angiotensin II, and the inactivation of the vasodilator bradykinin, which also releases vasodilator prostaglandins.[41] Captopril is rapidly but incompletely absorbed after oral ingestion, reaching a peak blood level in 30 to 90 minutes; 30 to 75 per cent is absorbed from the gastrointestinal tract, it is rapidly metabolized, and more than one third is excreted unchanged by the kidneys in 24 hours. This agent is widely distributed in the body but does not cross the blood-brain barrier. In patients with impaired renal function, the dose and frequency of administration must be decreased. Since captopril has some venodilator effects (decreasing venous return), the reflex increase in cardiac output and heart rate seen with pure arteriolar vasodilators is usually not seen. Following the initial blood pressure fall, which is particularly dramatic in patients with high plasma renin levels such as those with malignant hypertension, renovascular hypertension, or end-stage renal disease, blood pressure tends to rise again unless a diuretic is added.[7] With the decrease in angiotensin II, there is also a decrease in aldosterone production and a rise in serum potassium levels. The serious side effects include rare neutropenia or agranulocytosis with myeloid hypoplasia, which have been reported in 0.3 per cent of patients and which occur within a few months of initiation of therapy. Proteinuria and occasionally even nephrotic syndrome, probably due to an immune-complex glomerulopathy, occur in 1 to 2 per cent of patients. A pruritic rash with eosinophilia occurs in 10 per cent and loss of taste (ageusia) in about 6 per cent of patients.

Captopril should be given one half-hour before meals in a dose of 25 to 150 mg three times daily, except in patients with renal failure in whom the dose should be halved. Captopril is of particular use in patients with severe hypertension due to renovascular disease unresponsive to other medications, in whom sustained reduction of blood pressure is desirable.

Minoxidil

Minoxidil (Loniten) is a direct arterial vasodilator that causes reflex stimulation of the sympathetic nervous system, with resulting tachycardia and an increase in cardiac output. It is available only for oral use, but is rapidly effective in reducing blood pressure, especially in patients with resistant hypertension from renovascular disease, end-stage renal parenchymal disease, and malignant hypertension.[46] The marked retention of sodium and water produced can be counteracted with a loop diuretic such as furosemide, and the reflex tachycardia with a beta-adrenergic blocking agent. Minoxidil should not be used in acute myocardial infarction, acute congestive heart failure, or cerebral vascular disease, nor in aortic dissection.

Nifedipine*

Nifedipine (Procardia, Adalat) is a newly released calcium channel antagonist that acts as a direct arterial vasodilator by interfering with excitation-contraction coupling in the vascular smooth muscle.[4] Unlike other calcium channel blockers, it has very little effect on the heart, so the decrease in blood pressure results in reflex tachycardia, flushing, and increased cardiac output. The drug can be given in 10 to 20 mg doses three times a day orally; the maximal blood pressure effect is noted within one hour, and blood pressure returns to baseline in eight to ten hours. Nifedipine can be combined effectively with sympathetic blocking agents such as methyldopa and beta-adrenergic blocking agents, as well as diuretics, for the long-term treatment of severe hypertension. It can also be given sublingually in a 10- or 20-mg dosage.[4] Blood pressure under these circumstances falls within one to five minutes, reaching a maximal fall in 20 to 30 minutes and returning to baseline after four to five hours. Although nifedipine is not available in the intravenous form in the United States, the oral capsule can be chewed to yield an effective "sublingual" dose.

References

1. Adams, H. P., Jr., Jergenson, D. D., Kassell, N. F., et al.: Pitfalls in the recognition of subarachnoid hemorrhage. J.A.M.A. 244:794, 1980.
2. Ahearn, D. J., and Grim, C. E.: Treatment of malignant hypertension with sodium nitroprusside. Arch. Intern. Med. 133:187, 1974.
3. Anderson, R. J., Hart, G. R., Crumpler, C. P., et al.: Oral clonidine loading in hypertensive urgencies. J.A.M.A. 246:848, 1981.
4. Beer, N., Gallegos, I., Cohen, A., et al.: Efficacy of sublingual nifedipine in the acute treatment of systemic hypertension. Chest 79:571, 1981.

---

*Not yet approved for the treatment of hypertension in the United States.

5. Brizio-Molteni, L., Molteni, A., Cloutier, L. C., et al.: Incidence of post burn hypertensive crisis in patients admitted to two burn centers and a community hospital in the United States. Scand. J. Plast. Reconstr. Surg. 13:21, 1979.
6. Carney, J. A., Sizemore, G. W., and Sheps, S. G.: Adrenal medullary disease in multiple endocrine neoplasia, type 2: pheochromocytoma and its precursors. Am. J. Clin. Pathol. 66:279, 1976.
7. Case, D. B., Atlas, S. A., Sullivan, P. A., et al.: Acute and chronic treatment of severe and malignant hypertension with the oral angiotensin-converting enzyme inhibitor captopril. Circulation 64:765, 1981.
8. Cottrell, J. E., Casthely, P., Brodie, J. D., et al.: Prevention of nitroprusside-induced cyanide toxicity with hydroxocobalamin. N. Engl. J. Med 298:809, 1978.
9. Davidson, D. L. W., Jellinek, E. H.: Hypertension and papilledema in the Guillain-Barré syndrome. J. Neurol. Neurosurg. Psychiatry 40:144, 1977.
10. Dinsdale, H. B., Robertson, D. M., Haas, R. A., et al.: Cerebral blood flow in acute hypertension. Arch. Neurol. 31:80, 1974.
11. Garrett, B. N., and Kaplan, N. M.: Efficacy of slow infusion of diazoxide in the treatment of severe hypertension without organ hypoperfusion. Am. Heart J. 103:390, 1982.
12. Gavras, H., Brown, W. C., Brown, J. J., et al.: Microangiopathic hemolytic anemia and the development of the malignant phase of hypertension. Circ. Res. 28 (Suppl. 2):127, 1971.
13. Gifford, R. W., Jr., and Westbrook, E.: Hypertensive encephalopathy: mechanisms, clinical features, and treatment. Prog. Cardiovasc. Dis. 17:115, 1974.
14. Gitlow, S. E., Mendlowitz, M., and Bertani, L. M.: The biochemical techniques for detecting and establishing the presence of a pheochromocytoma. Am. J. Cardiol. 26:270, 1970.
15. Goldberg, A. D., Raftery, E. B., and Wilkinson, P.: Blood pressure and heart rate and withdrawal of antihypertensive drugs. Br. Med. J. 1:1243, 1977.
16. Guttman, L., and Whitteridge, D.: Effects of bladder distension on autonomic mechanisms after spinal cord injuries. Brain 70:361, 1947.
17. Hansson, L., Hunyor, S. N., Julius, S., et al.: Blood pressure crisis following withdrawal of clonidine (Catapres, Catapresan), with special reference to arterial and urinary catecholamine levels, and suggestions for acute management. Am. Heart J. 85:605, 1973.
18. Keith, N. M., Wagener, H. P., and Barker, N. W.: Some different types of essential hypertension: their course and prognosis. Am. J. Med. Sci. 197:332, 1939.
19. Kincaid-Smith, P., McMichael, J., and Murphy, E. A.: The clinical course and pathology of hypertension with papilloedema (malignant hypertension). Q. J. Med. 27:117, 1958.
20. Koch-Weser, J.: Hydralazine. N. Engl. J. Med. 295:320, 1976.
21. Lassen, N. A., and Agnoli, A.: The upper limit of autoregulation of cerebral blood flow—on the pathogenesis of hypertensive encephalopathy. Scand. J. Clin. Lab. Invest. 30:113, 1972.
22. Lazarus, J. M., Hampers, C. L., Bennett, A. H., et al.: Urgent bilateral nephrectomy for severe hypertension. Ann. Intern. Med. 76:733, 1972.
23. Ledingham, J. G. G., and Rajagopalan, B.: Cerebral

complications in the treatment of accelerated hypertension. Q. J. Med. 48:25, 1979.

24. Lindheimer, M. D., Katz, A. I., and Zuspan, F. P. (ed.): Hypertension in Pregnancy. New York, John Wiley & Sons, 1976.
25. Little, J. R., Tubman, D. E., and Ethier, R.: Cerebellar hemorrhage in adults: diagnosis by computerized tomography. J. Neurosurg. 48:575, 1978.
26. Luft, F. C., Bloch, R., Szwed, J. J., et al.: Minoxidil treatment of malignant hypertension: recovery of renal function. J.A.M.A. 240:1985, 1978.
27. MacKenzie, E. R., Strandgaard, S., Graham, D. I., et al.: Effects of acutely induced hypertension in cats on pial arteriolar caliber, local cerebral blood flow, and the blood-brain barrier. Circ. Res. 39:33, 1976.
28. Manger, W. M., and Gifford, R. W., Jr.: Pheochromocytoma. New York, Springer-Verlag, 1977.
29. Messerli, F. H., and Frohlich, E. D.: High blood pressure: a side effect of drugs, poisons, and food. Arch. Intern. Med. 139:682, 1979.
30. McLain, L. G.: Therapy of acute severe hypertension in children. J.A.M.A. 239:755, 1978.
31. Miller, R. R., Olson, H. G., Amsterdam, E. A., et al.: Propranolol-withdrawal rebound phenomenon: exacerbation of coronary events after abrupt cessation of antianginal therapy. N. Engl. J. Med. 293:416, 1975.
32. Mroczek, W. J., Davidov, M., Gavrilovich, L., et al.: The value of aggressive therapy in the hypertensive patient with azotemia. Circulation 40:893, 1969.
33. Naftchi, N. E., Demeny, M., Lowman, E. W., et al.: Hypertensive crises in quadriplegic patients: changes in cardiac output, blood volume, serum dopamine-β-hydroxylase activity, and arterial prostaglandin PGE_2. Circulation 57:336, 1978.
34. Palmer, R. F., and Lasseter, K. C.: Nitroprusside and aortic dissecting aneurysm. N. Engl. J. Med. 294:1403, 1976.
35. Pitcock, J. A., Johnson, J. G., Hatch, F. E., et al.: Malignant hypertension in blacks: malignant intrarenal arterial disease as observed by light and electron microscopy. Hum. Pathol. 7:333, 1976.
36. Prys-Roberts, C., and Meloche, R.: Management of anesthesia in patients with hypertension or ischemic heart disease. Int. Anesthesiol. Clin. 18:181, 1980.
37. Russell, R. W. R.: How does blood-pressure cause stroke? Lancet 2:1283, 1975.
38. Schottstaedt, M. F., and Sokolow, M.: The natural history and course of hypertension with papilledema (malignant hypertension). Am. Heart J. 45:331, 1953.
39. Sjoerdsma, A., Engleman, K., Waldman, T. A., et al.: Pheochromocytoma: current concepts of diagnosis and treatment. Ann. Intern. Med. 65:1302, 1966.
40. Slater, E. E., and DeSanctis, W. W.: The clinical recognition of dissecting aortic aneurysm. Am. J. Med. 60:625, 1976.
41. Tifft, C. P., Gavras, H., Kershaw, G. R., et al.: Converting enzyme inhibition in hypertensive emergencies. Ann. Intern. Med. 90:43, 1979.
42. Wells, P. H., and Kaplan, J. A.: Optimal management of patients with ischemic heart disease for noncardiac surgery by complementary anesthesiologist and cardiologist interaction. Am. Heart J. 102:1029, 1981.
43. Wheat, M. W., Jr., Palmer, R. F., Bartley, T. D., et al.: Treatment of dissecting aneurysms of the aorta without surgery. J. Thorac. Cardiovasc. Surg. 50:364, 1965.
44. Whelton, P. K., Flaherty, J. T., MacAllister, N. P., et al.: Hypertension following coronary artery bypass surgery: role of preoperative propranolol therapy. Hypertension 2:291, 1980.
45. Wilson, C., and Byrom, F. B.: Renal changes in malignant hypertension. Lancet 1:136, 1939.
46. Wood, B. C., Sharma, J. N., and Crouch, T. T.: Oral minoxidil in the treatment of hypertensive crisis. J.A.M.A. 241:163, 1979.

10

Aortic Dissection

ROBERT M. DOROGHAZI,

EVE E. SLATER, and

ROMAN W. DESANCTIS

Few diseases are more dramatic in onset or pursue a more ominous course than aortic dissection. If untreated, 20 per cent of patients die within 24 hours and over 90 per cent within the first week.[13] Fortunately, recent advances in medical and surgical therapy have markedly improved this grim prognosis. Early diagnosis and prompt institution of therapy are especially important in aortic dissection, since events that influence survival generally occur early in the course of the disease.

PATHOGENESIS

Definition. The term dissecting aneurysm, or "aneurysme disséquant," was originally proposed by the French physician René Laennec. Because the dissection represents neither a true nor a false aneurysm, the simple term "aortic dissection" is now widely used to describe this disease.

Some form of degeneration of the aortic media is generally considered a basic prerequisite for the development of spontaneous aortic dissection.[35] Aortic dissection is characterized by a hematoma in the aortic media that results in a longitudinal cleavage of the aortic wall. In most cases, the hematoma originates at the site of a tear in the aortic intima and media. In a small percentage, the intimal tear cannot be identified pathologically.[13]

Predisposing Factors. Factors predisposing to spontaneous aortic dissection include hypertension, Marfan's syndrome, a congenitally bicuspid aortic valve, and coarctation of the aorta. Hypertension is the most common of these and coexists with aortic dissection in 75 to 90 per cent of patients in most series.[18, 20 37] It is especially prevalent in dissections originating in the descending thoracic aorta. Marfan's syndrome, bicuspid aortic valve, and coarctation are predisposing factors especially in younger patients. Aortic dissection has also been reported during pregnancy, occurring most frequently in the third trimester. This association is believed to be the consequence of circulatory changes that take place during pregnancy and humoral factors that alter the integrity of connective tissue.

Iatrogenic aortic dissection can be divided into two categories: cannulation induced and incision induced.[33] Cannulation-induced dissection can occur during insertion of an intra-aortic balloon pump, or during angiography or cannulation for cardiopulmonary bypass. Incision-induced aortic dissection can complicate aortic valve replacement and aortic crossclamping or placement of aortocoronary bypass grafts. Rarely, aortic dissection may result from blunt chest or abdominal trauma;[30] in such cases, pathologic degeneration of the aortic media is usually found to coexist.

Classification. The most widely used classification of aortic dissection is that of DeBakey et al.,[8] who identify three types of dissection based on the site of the intimal tear and the extent of the dissecting hematoma.[8] In Types I and II, the intimal tear is located in the ascending aorta, within a few centimeters of the aortic valve. In Type I dissection, the hematoma extends for variable distances beyond the ascending aorta, whereas Type II dissections are confined to the ascending aorta. Type III dissections originate in the descending aorta, usually just beyond the origin of the left subclavian artery; these usually propagate antegrade into the descending thoracic aorta or, rarely, retrograde into the aortic arch and ascending aorta. Because Types I and II behave similarly, they are usually referred to as "proximal" or "ascending" dissections. Type III lesions are termed "distal" or "descending" dissections. Subsequently, Daily et al.[6] and Miller et al.[25] have proposed a simpler classification based only on the presence or absence of involvement of the ascending aorta.[6, 25] In their classification, Type A refers to all dissections that involve the ascending aorta, regardless of the point of origin of the dissection. All other dissections are classified as Type B. This classification appropriately emphasizes the importance of the involvement of the ascending aorta in the clinical behavior of, and approach to therapy for, these patients.

Dissections are considered to be "acute" if less than two weeks have elapsed from the onset of clinical symptoms, and "chronic" if more than two weeks have passed.

Aortic dissection is two to three times more common in men than in women, with a peak incidence in the sixth and seventh decades. Patients with proximal dissection tend to be younger than those with distal dissection.

SYMPTOMS

The most common presenting symptom of aortic dissection is severe pain, which is present in over 90 per cent of patients.[37] Other presentations, with or without associated chest pain, include syncope and congestive heart failure. Aortic dissection may also simulate any type of vascular accident and present as an acute neurologic deficit or pulse loss.

The pain of aortic dissection is usually sudden in onset and of unbearable intensity. It may cause the patient to writhe in bed or pace to obtain relief. The pain often is aptly described by the patient as having a "ripping" or "tearing" quality. Migration of the pain from its initial location along the course of the dissecting hematoma as it extends to other sites occurs in almost three quarters of patients.[37] Unlike the pain of ischemic heart disease, that of aortic dissection is often maximal at onset.

The location of pain may be of some help in suggesting the site of origin of the dissection. Pain felt simultaneously anteriorly and posteriorly can be present with a dissection originating in either the ascending or descending aorta. Pain felt exclusively in the anterior chest, however, is significantly more frequent with proximal origin. Similarly, pain that is exclusively posterior is more common with distal origin. Posterior pain is characteristically in the interscapular area. The absence of any back pain strongly militates against a dissection originating in the descending aorta, since 90 per cent of patients with distal dissection report some back pain.[37] Other sites of pain include the throat and jaw, abdomen, low back, or suprapubic area. The sudden onset, intensity, peculiar quality, location, and patterns of migration of the pain serve as important clues in distinguishing aortic dissection from other causes of chest pain such as myocardial infarction, pulmonary embolism, pneumothorax, or pleurisy. Rarely, aortic dissection can be painless.[4, 5]

In our series, six of 124 patients with aortic dissection presented with syncope.[37] In each case, they were later found to have rupture of the dissection into the pericardial cavity, resulting in cardiac tamponade.

Congestive heart failure almost invariably results from involvement of the ascending aorta and is due to acute severe aortic insufficiency. A soft or absent first heart sound and an abbreviated diastolic decrescendo murmur are important clues to the diagnosis of acute aortic insufficiency when it is complicated by congestive heart failure. Rarely, dissection involving a coronary artery may result in myocardial infarction.

Aortic dissection may precipitate several types of neurologic syndromes, the most significant of which are cerebrovascular accidents and spinal cord ischemia.[40] Clues that a cerebrovascular accident may be due to

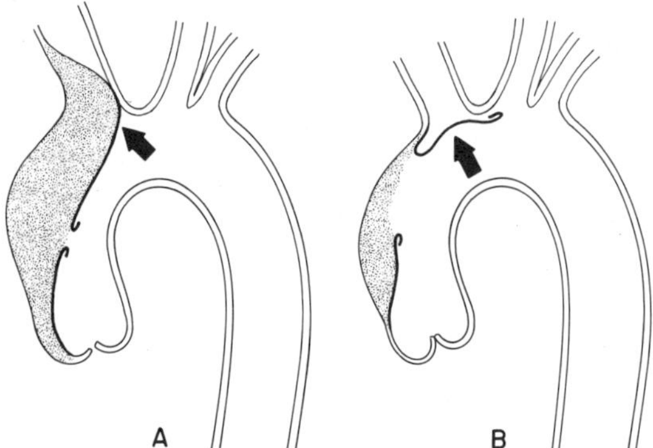

Figure 10–1. In aortic dissection, pulse loss can occur by one of two mechanisms: *A*, obliteration of the vessel lumen by the hematoma, or *B*, obliteration of the vessel lumen by the intimal flap.

aortic dissection include chest pain, pulse deficit, a new murmur of aortic insufficiency, or a widened mediastinum on chest radiograph. Other neurologic syndromes include paraplegia from spinal cord injury or ischemic peripheral neuropathy.

Aortic dissection can simulate arterial embolism and should be sought in any patient presenting with acute pulse loss. The pulse deficits associated with aortic dissection can result from compromise of the true lumen by the dissecting hematoma or intimal flap (Fig. 10–1). They are occasionally transient owing to fluctuations of the flap.

PHYSICAL FINDINGS

Findings on physical examination are frequently sufficient to enable the diagnosis of aortic dissection to be made with reasonable assurance. Patients with aortic dissection may appear to be in shock with diaphoresis and restlessness, but the blood pressure is often elevated.[20, 37] This is especially true in distal or Type B dissection, in which one half to two thirds of the patients in two large series were hypertensive when originally seen.[20, 37] Hypotension, usually due to aortic rupture into the pericardial, pleural, or peritoneal cavities, is more common in patients with proximal or Type A dissection.

Those physical findings most typically associated with aortic dissection, namely, pulse deficits, aortic regurgitation, and neurologic deficit, are more characteristic of proximal (Type A) than of distal dissection. Pulse deficits were found in over one half of our patients with dissections of the ascending aorta or arch, with the brachiocephalic vessels most frequently compromised. Pulse deficits are much less common in patients with distal dissection, and more commonly involve the left subclavian and femoral vessels, although these latter vessels are equally affected by the distal propagation of a proximal dissection.

The murmur of aortic insufficiency likewise predominates in dissections originating in the ascending arch and occurs in more than 50 per cent of these patients in most series. When aortic insufficiency is present in patients with a distal dissection, it is imperative to consider retrograde involvement of the ascending aorta. However, pre-existing aortic insufficiency from another cause, for example, long-standing hypertension or Marfan's syndrome, may be present in these patients. The mechanisms of aortic insufficiency in aortic dissection derive from one of three mechanisms (Fig. 10–2). First, the dissection may dilate the root of the aorta, widening the annulus and making it impossible for the leaflets to coapt in diastole. Second, with an asymmetric dissection, the pressure of the dissecting hematoma may depress one aortic cusp substantially below the level of the others, thus rendering the valve incompetent. Third, the annular support of the leaflets or the leaflets themselves may be torn by the hematoma to the extent that they are unable to support the column of blood in the aorta during diastole.

The principal neurologic deficits associated with aortic dissection include cerebrovascular accident, ischemic peripheral neuropathy, paraplegia, and disturbances of consciousness.[40] These deficits are found more commonly in patients with proximal or Type A dissection. In distal or Type B dissection, the deficits principally involve the lower extremities. Additional neurologic lesions include Horner's syndrome, caused by compression of the superior cervical sympathetic ganglion, and vocal cord paralysis with hoarseness, due to stretching of the left recurrent laryngeal nerve by the hematoma.

Additional complications may result from aortic rupture or compromise of circulation to a vital organ. A hemorrhagic pleural effusion, usually on the left, may occur from aortic rupture or exudation of blood from the involved aorta. Compromise of circulation to a vital organ may result in mesenteric, myocardial, or renal ischemia or actual infarction.

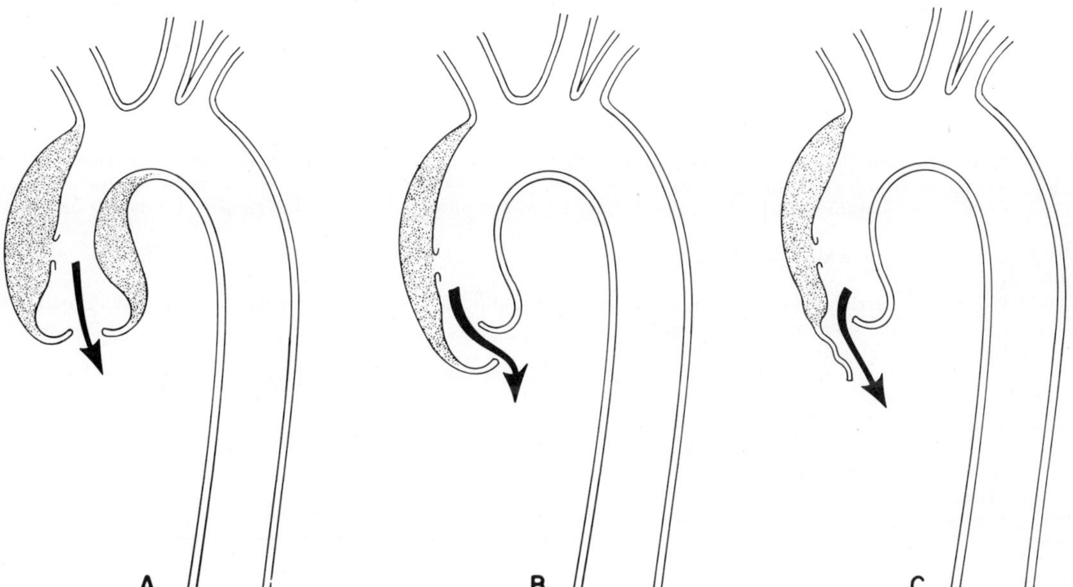

Figure 10–2. Mechanism of aortic regurgitation in dissecting aortic aneurysm. *A,* Circumferential tear with widening of aortic root and separation of the aortic cusps. *B,* Displacement of one aortic cusp substantially below the level of the others by pressure of the dissecting hematoma. *C,* Actual disruption of the annular leaflet support leading to a flail cusp.

Other complications reported in patients with aortic dissection include reduplicated pulses, pulsatile sternoclavicular joint,[22] superior mediastinal syndrome from superior vena cava obstruction, pulsatile neck masses, superficial bruises in the neck and abdomen, tracheal compression, hemorrhage into the tracheobronchial tree or gastrointestinal tract,[34] fever of unknown origin,[27] and disturbances of cardiac rhythm conduction from extension of a proximal dissection into the interatrial septum and the AV node.[42]

LABORATORY FINDINGS

Except for chest roentgenography and aortic angiography, the laboratory is not of great help in establishing the diagnosis of aortic dissection. Both the electrocardiogram and cardiac enzymes are helpful in a negative sense, by failing to show evidence of myocardial infarction in a patient whose history may suggest that possibility. However, left ventricular hypertrophy is common because of preexisting hypertension in many patients. Elevated lactic dehydrogenase levels occur and presumably result from hemolysis within the false lumen, which may also elevate the serum bilirubin. Leukocytosis is present in almost two thirds of patients, and anemia may result from leakage or sequestration of blood in the hematoma. Electrolytes show no consistent abnormalities, although elevated blood urea nitrogen and creatinine levels should suggest the possibility of renal involvement by the dissecting process.

The routine chest roentgenogram is usually abnormal in patients with aortic dissection. The most frequent aberrancy is an abnormally widened aorta. Other fndings include a double density due to superimposed posterior aortic enlargement, deviation of the trachea to the right, and a left pleural effusion.[12] A localized bulge in the aorta may suggest the site of origin of the dissection.[21] The "calcium sign," which represents the displacement of the calcified intima greater than 1 cm from the outer aortic wall, is virtually pathognomonic of aortic dissection but is found in only 10 to 15 per cent of patients.

Echocardiography[3, 15, 26] and computerized tomography (CT) may be of help in establishing the diagnosis of aortic dissection. The criteria for M-mode echocardiographic diagnosis of dissection involving the aortic root include: (1) enlargement of the external diameter of the aortic root (42 mm or more); (2) widening of the anterior and posterior

Table 10–1. APPROACH TO THE PATIENT WITH ACUTE AORTIC DISSECTION

Initial

1. Immediate monitoring and stabilization of vital signs including pulse, blood pressure, cardiac rhythm, central venous pressure, urinary output, and pulmonary capillary wedge pressure.
2. Reduce systolic blood pressure to 100 to 120 mmHg or lowest possible level commensurate with adequate organ perfusion. Use nitroprusside, 50–100 mg in 500 ml D5W, infused at 25–50 μg/min; or trimethaphan, 500 mg to 2 gm in 500 ml D5W, infused at 1 mg/min; and titrate against blood pressure response.
3. Effect beta-blockade with propranolol, 1.0 mg IV over 5 min, and repeat until pulse ≤ 60 or to a total of 0.15 mg/kg.
4. Once stable, proceed to definite diagnosis by angiography. Decide on medical or surgical therapy.

Definitive

1. Proximal dissection—Surgical unless definite contraindication (if associated with myocardial infarction or cerebrovascular accident, surgical results are poor).
2. Distal dissection—Medical unless:
   a. Rupture or impending rupture (large dilated and opacified false lumen and/or late development of saccular aneurysm).
   b. Progression with vital organ compromise.
   c. Inability to control pain or blood pressure medically.
   d. Marfan's syndrome.
3. Regardless of type of dissection or ultimate therapy, medical therapy, both initial and long-term, should control blood pressure and dp/dt, and thus diminish risk of hematoma progression or redissection.

aortic wall above 16 and 10 mm, respectively; and (3) maintenance of parallelism between the separated margins of the aortic walls. These findings, however, are not specific and occur in a variety of other clinical settings. Diastolic fluttering of the septum or anterior leaflet of the mitral valve or mitral valve preclosure suggests aortic insufficiency. The accuracy of echocardiographic diagnosis is improved by the use of two-dimensional echocardiography.[23] The findings of aortic dissection suggested on CT scan include a localized increase in aortic caliber, the presence of a displaced intimal calcification or flap, and demonstration of the false lumen.[17] Despite the utility of these noninvasive techniques, contrast angiography (as discussed below) is still currently required to confirm the diagnosis and to determine the origin and extent of the dissecting process.

TREATMENT

Initial Management

The management of all patients whose clinical presentation strongly suggests acute aortic dissection includes initial medical stabilization followed by definitive diagnosis using retrograde aortic angiography (Table 10–1). Patients should be immediately admitted to an intensive care unit where vital signs including blood pressure, cardiac rhythm, and urine output can be monitored continuously. Accurate and continuous blood pressure measurement, preferably with an intraarterial cannula, is required because of the need for precise blood pressure control during the administration of potent hypotensive agents. A pulmonary artery catheter is also recommended to measure cardiac filling pressures.

The goals of medical therapy of acute aortic dissection were originally outlined by Wheat and Palmer and associates.[31, 41] These are to decrease the velocity of ventricular contraction (dp/dt), reduce blood pressure, and control pain. Therapy to control dp/dt is begun in all patients, including those who are normotensive or pain-free upon presentation. The objective of hypotensive therapy is to reduce systolic blood pressure to 100 to 120 mm Hg or to the lowest level that will sustain adequate cerebral, cardiac, and renal perfusion. Urinary output should be maintained at or above 20 ml per hour. The pain of acute aortic dissection is often difficult or impossible to control with narcotics, but occasionally subsides once the progression of the hematoma is halted by the reduction of dp/dt and control of blood pressure.

Drugs for the first several days should be administered parenterally. In this way it is possible to gain immediate antihypertensive effect and also to minimize the possibility of "overshoot" hypotension. In addition, absorption of oral medications in acutely ill patients may be unreliable and surgery may be imminent for many.

The most effective agent for the immediate reduction of blood pressure is sodium nitroprusside, given with concomitant beta-adrenergic blockade. A solution of 50 to 100 mg in 500 ml D5W is infused at an initial rate of 25 to 50 μg per min, and the dosage is titrated against blood pressure up to a maximum of approximately 3 μg per kg per min. Not more than 1 mg per kg should be given during the first three hours, and a maximum of 0.2 to 0.3 mg per kg per hr thereafter. The solution, which must be prepared immediately before use, is light sensitive so that the bottle containing it should be covered with aluminum foil. Blood pressure reduction occurs within seconds and "overshoot" hypotension can occur.

Cyanide and thiocyanate toxicity may develop after more than 48 hours and are the most important complications of high-dose nitroprusside therapy. Metabolic acidosis is the earliest sign of cyanide toxicity. Neurologic symptoms are the first signs of thiocyanate toxicity and include confusion, hyperreflexia, and convulsions. Blood thiocyanate levels can be monitored, and levels below 10 mg per dl are generally well tolerated.

Sodium nitroprusside decreases platelet adhesiveness in vitro, but clinically apparent difficulties with hemostasis have not been reported. By inhibiting hypoxically mediated pulmonary vasoconstriction, sodium nitroprusside may worsen ventilation-perfusion defects. However, the resulting hypoxia is usually of little consequence unless the patient is severely hypoxemic prior to therapy. Methemoglobinemia occurs rarely. Other side effects of nitroprusside therapy include nausea, restlessness, and somnolence.

Sodium nitroprusside alone or in combination with inadequate doses of propranolol can cause reflex tachycardia and an increase in dp/dt, which might conceivably promote the extension of the dissection.[28] Therefore, adequate beta-adrenergic blockade is mandatory when sodium nitroprusside is used.

The ganglionic blocker trimethaphan, which can both lower blood pressure and reduce dp/dt, is used when sodium nitroprusside is poorly tolerated or ineffective, or when intravenous beta-blockade is contraindicated. Trimethaphan is mixed as a solution of 500 mg to 2 gm in 500 ml D5W and infused initially at 1 mg per min, titrating the dose against the blood pressure response. The head of the bed must be elevated to gain orthostatic effect.

The toxicities of trimethaphan include overshoot hypotension, respiratory arrest, and ganglionic blockade manifested by urinary retention, paralytic ileus, and pupillary dilatation with blurred vision. In spite of its initial success in the therapy of aortic dissection, trimethaphan has now become our drug of second choice because of its short duration of action, its unpleasant and serious side effects, and the development of tachyphylaxis that usually occurs within 48 hours.

The hypotensive effect of both sodium nitroprusside and trimethaphan can be blunted by fluid retention, which may necessitate the concomitant administration of an intravenous diuretic such as furosemide.

Therapy to reduce dp/dt is mandatory in all patients, including those who are normotensive or pain free on presentation. Beta-adrenergic blockade with intravenous propranolol is the treatment of choice to achieve this effect: propranolol usually has only a minimal hypotensive effect when administered intravenously. In the acute setting, an initial dose of 0.5 mg is given intravenously, followed by incremental doses of 1 mg every five minutes up to a total intravenous dose of 0.15 mg per kg or until there is evidence of adequate beta-blockade.

Although a heart rate of 50 to 60 beats per minute usually indicates sufficient beta-blocking effect, higher rates may be acceptable in patients who are in pain or critically ill, or when maximal doses of propranolol have been given. Contraindications to the use of propranolol include pre-existing sinus bradycardia of 45 beats per minute or less, congestive heart failure (cardiac index 2 l/min/m^2), second- or third-degree AV block, and severe bronchospastic pulmonary disease.

Reserpine can both lower blood pressure and reduce dp/dt, and can be substituted for propranolol if necessary. Reserpine is given in doses of 0.5 to 2 mg intramuscularly every four to eight hours, with effects beginning after one to three hours. Side effects include drowsiness, depression, and gastric ulceration, which can be minimized by the use of nasogastric suction and the concomitant administration of cimetidine and antacids.

Methyldopa is another agent that may be used for the semiacute reduction of blood pressure in patients with acute aortic dissection. Like reserpine, methyldopa reduces both blood pressure and dp/dt. It is administered intravenously in doses of 100 to 500

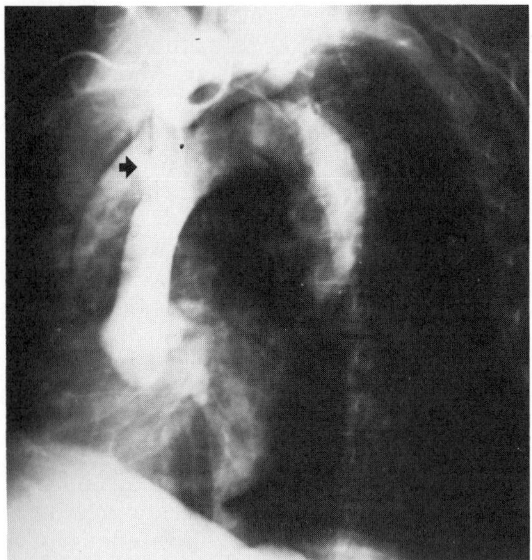

Figure 10–3. Angiogram of a Type I or "proximal" dissection with site of origin just proximal to the right innominate artery (*arrow*). The dissecting hematoma extends up into the innominate artery, antegrade through the aortic arch and descending thoracic aorta, and retrograde into the ascending aorta, producing mild aortic regurgitation. This patient also had subdiaphragmatic extension of the dissection occluding the left artery (*not pictured*).

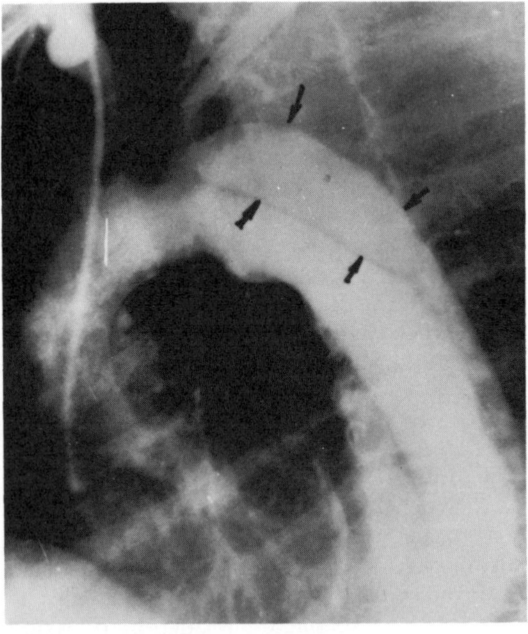

Figure 10–4. Angiogram of a Type III or "distal" dissection with its site of origin just beyond the left subclavian artery and antegrade extension. There is prompt angiographic filling of a large false lumen (*arrows*).

mg every six to 12 hours. However, this drug may not begin to work for several hours and it causes considerable somnolence when initially given. In addition, methyldopa occasionally results in problems with blood pressure regulation in patients who subsequently undergo surgery. We therefore tend to avoid it in the early treatment of acute dissection.

Hydralazine is another powerful hypotensive agent, but it is a direct vasodilator that causes a reflex tachycardia and increase in dp/dt. As with nitroprusside, these reflex changes can be largely counteracted by adequate beta-blockade. However, we continue to recommend agents other than direct vasodilators for the management of hypertension in acute aortic dissection.

When hypertension is refractory to large amounts of hypotensive agents, the possibility of dissection involving the renal arteries with resultant renovascular hypertension must be considered. Either angiography or a renal scan can be used to document renal artery occlusion. Surgical intervention to decompress the hematoma is almost always required in such patients to achieve blood pressure control.

Adequate sedation is important in the management of acute aortic dissection. Blood pressure may be adequately controlled when patients are quiet and asleep, only to rise dramatically when they are awake and agitated. Sedatives with minimal cardiovascular effects are preferred, such as haloperidol, 1 to 10 mg intravenously every eight hours.

When the patient is hemodynamically stable, retrograde aortic angiography should be performed as soon as possible to confirm the diagnosis. This procedure also provides essential information regarding subsequent medical or surgical management,[9] including the site of origin and extent of the dissecting hematoma, and the anatomy and patency of the branches of the aorta. The most common angiographic findings of aortic dissection include opacification of the false lumen, visualization of an intimal tear, and deformity of the true lumen.[12] The presence of aortic insufficiency can also be confirmed. Several pitfalls, however, may occur, including faint opacification of the false lumen, unusual tearing of the intima, and equal simultaneous opacification of both channels.[36] Nevertheless, the procedure is well tolerated by even the critically ill patient and provides definitive diagnosis in almost every case. If a life-threatening complication develops such as aortic rupture, severe aortic insufficiency, cardiac tamponade, or compromise of the circulation to a vital organ, surgery may have to be undertaken without angiography. Examples of angiograms of a proximal and distal dissection are presented in Figures 10–3 and 10–4.

Definitive Therapy

Following initial stabilization and diagnosis by angiography, a decision is made either to continue medical therapy or to proceed to surgery.

Despite the lack of any truly controlled series, a relatively uniform approach to the subsequent treatment of aortic dissection has developed as experience with medical and surgical therapy has accumulated.[1, 2, 7, 14, 19, 24, 29, 32, 39]

Surgical Therapy

The modern surgical treatment of aortic dissection was pioneered by DeBakey et al. in 1955.[7A] Their approach involves excision of the intimal tear, oversewing of the aortic layers, and reconstruction of the aorta with or without the use of a synthetic graft to replace the excised aortic segment. Aortic valve replacement is required in proximal dissection only when decompression of the hematoma is insufficient to restore valve competence, or when there has been direct damage to the valve ring or valve itself.

Surgery is the therapy of choice in acute proximal or Type A dissections because of the high incidence of immediately life-threatening complications, many of which are surgically remediable. These include acute aortic insufficiency, loss of a major arterial pulse, and cardiac tamponade. Surgical intervention is advised in distal dissection complicated by rupture, reversible compromise of the blood supply to a vital organ, inability to control pain or blood pressure medically, extension of the dissecting hematoma as manifest by recurrent pain or the appearance of a new complication, localized expansion of the aorta, or evidence of retrograde dissection into the aortic arch or ascending aorta (Type A). Patients with Marfan's syndrome, with either proximal or distal dissection, should also be treated surgically. Survival rates from surgery for acute aortic dissection are 60 to 70 per cent at most centers.

The principal complications of surgical intervention in aortic dissection include bleeding, renal failure, hypotension or myocardial dysfunction, respiratory failure, and central nervous system deficit.[10]

Medical Therapy

Long-term continuation of medical therapy is indicated mainly in patients with uncomplicated stable distal or Type B dissection. A recent series from the Massachusetts General Hospital demonstrated significantly better hospital survival of medically treated patients with uncomplicated distal dissection than of those treated surgically.[11] Definitive medical treatment is also advised in uncomplicated distal or proximal dissection when patients are poor surgical candidates (e.g., those with severe emphysema or a major neurologic deficit). Medical therapy is also recommended for dissections originating in the aortic arch, because surgical correction is associated with an extremely high mortality and is most difficult to perform.[16]

In the past it has been the policy to treat medically patients with stable proximal dissection in whom the site of origin cannot be identified. In contrast, Miller et al. do not insist on identification and excision of the intimal tear as a requisite for definitive surgical repair.[25] In their series of 125 consecutive patients with Types A and B dissections, immediate and long-term survival did not appear to be adversely influenced in the 14 patients with acute dissection and 14 with chronic dissection in whom the origin could not be identified. Thus, these authors advise surgery in all patients with Type A dissection regardless of the site of origin. This result has not yet been confirmed by other groups.

Semielective surgery is still considered for some patients with uncomplicated distal dissection following a period of initial medical stabilization, and in particular for those in whom there is evidence of the possibility of subsequent localized aneurysm formation (e.g., if there is wide filling of the false lumen on angiography). In general, such surgery should be undertaken only for such patients with otherwise normal cardiac, renal, and pulmonary function, because long-term survival in distal dissection is influenced as much by complications associated with advanced age and atherosclerosis as by late complications of the dissection itself.

In addition to the side effects from individual drugs,[38] the major complications of medical therapy are related to the rapid reduction of blood pressure in patients who often are elderly or were previously hypertensive. Mental status changes such as somnolence and agitation are most commonly observed. These are more properly considered side effects of therapy rather than complications, and should not result in discontinuation of medical therapy if other signs of vital organ perfusion are maintained.[10] Overzealous reduction of blood pressure, however, can result in acute tubular necrosis or may precipitate myocardial or cerebral infarction.

Whatever the mode of definitive treatment, all patients require long-term chronic medical therapy, including those who have undergone successful surgical intervention. Medically treated patients can be transferred to oral medications after two to five days.

Regardless of whether hypertension is present, all patients require ongoing therapy to reduce dp/dt. The agent of choice is the beta-adrenergic blocking drug propranolol (Inderal), 40 to 320 mg per day in four divided doses. Metoprolol (Lopressor), a cardioselective beta-blocking agent, may be preferable in patients with bronchospastic pulmonary disease, the usual dose being 50 to 100 mg three times daily. This property of more cardioselective beta-1-adrenergic receptor blockade is shared by atenolol (Tenormin), recently approved for use in the United States; the usual dose is 50 to 100 mg once daily. Three other beta-blocking drugs are available: nadolol (Corgard), a longer acting drug given in doses of 40 to 320 mg once daily, and timolol (Blocadren) administered in initial doses of 10 mg twice daily to a maximum of 30 mg twice daily, are both similar pharmacologically to propranolol. Pindolol (Visken), a nonselective beta-blocker with intrinsic sympathomimetic activity, is administered in initial doses of 10 mg twice daily to a maximum of 60 mg per day. Although experience with these new beta-blocking drugs in aortic dissection is so far limited, there is reason to believe that they will be as effective as propranolol.

If therapy with propranolol and a diuretic is insufficient to maintain systolic blood pressure at 130 mm Hg or less, another drug that can reduce both blood pressure and dp/dt should be added; preferred agents include methyldopa or clonidine. Direct vasodilators, such as hydralazine, prazosin, or minoxidil, should probably be avoided because of the reflex tachycardia and effect of increased dp/dt; however, if they are needed because of otherwise refractory hypertension, adequate concomitant beta-blockade is essential. There is no specific experience with SQ 14225 (Captopril) in lowering blood pressure in patients with chronic aortic dissection; its potential inotropic properties would necessitate concomitant beta-blockade.

Some degree of postural hypotension is commonly observed when patients begin to ambulate, methyldopa being an especially frequent cause. Adjustments in medications and dosage should overcome this problem.

Long-Term Follow-Up

All patients who survive hospitalization must be followed closely for late complications. These include redissection, progressive aortic insufficiency, or localized saccular aneurysm formation, the last-named being most prevalent in medically treated patients.[10] A routine chest radiograph should be obtained every three months after hospital discharge for the first year, every four months during the second year, and every six months thereafter. More frequent x-ray examinations may be warranted if there is evidence of progressive aortic enlargement. In dissections that involve the descending aorta, serial CT scans may provide more accurate follow-up information. In ascending aortic dissections, echocardiography may be of value. Experience with digital subtraction angiography in aortic dissection is only now accruing but we are optimistic that it will prove of great value in follow-up and possibly in diagnosis of this disease.

Patients in whom the dissection extends into the abdominal aorta must be watched for the development of abdominal aortic aneurysms. Baseline measurement of the abdominal aorta with ultrasound is advisable in such cases.

Chronic Dissection

Chronic dissection, as previously defined, is associated with a better prognosis than acute dissection. This presumably reflects the survival of these patients through the highly lethal initial two weeks during which 75 per cent of all deaths from untreated aortic dissection occur.

Initial therapy can be administered orally. All patients should be treated with a beta-blocking agent, an antihypertensive being added if required. Patients with chronic proximal dissection may require surgical intervention either because of localized aneurysm formation or, more commonly, for a significant aortic insufficiency. Medical therapy may be continued for patients with chronic distal dissection if there is no evidence of saccular aneurysm formation, although surgery may be necessary for the removal of localized aneurysms.

References

1. Anagnostopoulos, C. E., Prabhakar, M. J. S., and Kittle, C. F.: Aortic dissection and dissecting aneurysms. Am. J. Cardiol. 30:263, 1972.
2. Applebaum, A., Karp, R. B., and Kirklin, J. W.: Ascending vs descending aortic dissections. Ann. Surg. 183:296, 1976.
3. Brown, O. R., Popp, R. H., and Kloster, F. E.: Echocardiographic criteria for aortic root dissection. Am. J. Cardiol. 36:17, 1975.
4. Case Records of the Massachusetts General Hospital (Case 32-1974). N. Engl. J. Med. 291:350, 1974.
5. Cohen, S., and Litman, D.: Painless dissecting aneurysm of the aorta. N. Engl. J. Med. 291:143, 1964.
6. Daily, P. O., Trueblood, H. W., Stinson, E. B., et al.: Management of acute aortic dissections. Ann. Thorac. Surg. 10:237, 1970.
7. Dalen, J. E., Alpert, J. J., Cohn, L. H., et al.: Dissection of the thoracic aorta. Medical or surgical therapy? Am. J. Cardiol. 34:803, 1974.

7A. DeBakey, M. E., Cooley, D. A., and Creech, O., Jr.: Surgical considerations of dissecting aneurysm of the aorta. Ann. Surg. 142:586, 1955.

8. DeBakey, M. E., Henly, W. S., Cooley, D. A., et al.: Surgical management of dissecting aneurysms of the aorta. J. Thorac. Cardiovasc. Surg. 49:130, 1965.
9. Dinsmore, R. E., Willerson, J. T., and Buckley, M. J.: Dissecting aneurysm of the aorta. Aortographic features affecting prognosis. Radiology 150:567, 1972.
10. Doroghazi, R. M., Slater, E. E., Austen, W. G., et al.: Early and late complications of medical and surgical therapy for aortic dissection. Circulation 62:111, 1980 (abstr.)
11. Doroghazi, R. M., Slater, E. E., DeSanctis, R. W., et al.: Long-term survival for 184 patients with treated aortic dissection. Am. J. Cardiol. 45:489, 1980 (abstr.)
12. Earnest, F., IV, Muhm, J. R., and Sheedy, P. F., II: Roentgenographic findings in thoracic aortic dissection. Mayo Clin. proc. 54:43, 1979.
13. Hirst, A. E., Jr., Johns, V. J., Jr., and Kime, S. W., Jr.: Dissecting aneurysm of the aorta: a review of 505 cases. Medicine 37:217, 1958.
14. Kidd, J. N., Reul, G. J., Jr., Cooley, D. A., et al.: Surgical treatment of aneurysms of the ascending aorta. Circulation (Suppl. III) 54:118, 1976.
15. Kloster, F. E.: Echocardiographic criteria for aortic root dissection. Am. J. Cardiol. 36:17, 1975.
16. Kolff, J., Bates, R. J., Balderman, S.C., et al.: Acute aortic arch dissection: re-evaluation of the indications for medical and surgical therapy. Am. J. Cardiol. 39:727, 1977.
17. Large, D., Beloir, C., Vasile, N., et al.: Computed tomography of aortic dissection. Radiology 136:147, 1980.
18. Leonard, J. C., and Hasleton, P. S.: Dissecting aortic aneurysms: a clinicopathological study. Q. J. Med. 189:55, 1979.
19. Liddicoat, J. E., Bekassy, S. M., Rubio, P. A., et al.: Ascending aortic aneurysms. Review of 100 consecutive cases. Circulation (Suppl. I) 51 and 52:202, 1975.
20. Lindsay, J., Jr., and Hurst, J. W.: Clinical features and prognosis in dissecting aneurysm of the aorta. A re-appraisal. Circulation 35:880, 1967.
21. Lodwich, G. S.: Dissecting aneurysms of the thoracic and abdominal aorta; report of 6 cases, with a discussion of roentgenologic findings and pathologic changes. Am. J. Roentgenol. 69:907, 1953.
22. Logue, R. B., and Sikes, C.: New sign in dissecting aneurysm of the aorta; pulsation of sternoclavicular joint. J.A.M.A. 148:1209, 1952.
23. Matsumoto, M., Matsuo, H., Ohara, T., et al.: A two-dimensional echoaortocardiographic approach to dissecting aneurysms to prevent false-positive diagnosis. Radiology 127:491, 1978.
24. McFarland, J., Willerson, J. T., Dinsmore, R. E., et al.: The medical treatment of dissecting aortic aneurysms. N. Engl. J. Med. 286:115, 1972.
25. Miller, D. C., Stinson, E. B., Oyer, P. E., et al.: Operative treatment of aortic dissections. J. Thorac. Cardiovasc. Surg. 78:365, 1979.
26. Moothart, R. W., Spangler, R. D., and Blount, S. G., Jr.: Echocardiography in aortic root dissection and dilatation. Am. J. Cardiol. 36:11, 1975.
27. Murray, H. W., Mann, J. J., Genecin, A., and McKusick, V. A.: Fever with dissecting aneurysm of the aorta. Am. J. Med. 61:140, 1976.
28. Palmer, R. F., and Lasseter, K. C.: Nitroprusside and aortic dissecting aneurysm. N. Engl. J. Med. 294:1403, 1976.
29. Parker, F. B., Jr., Neville, F. F., Jr., Hanson, E. L., et al.: Management of acute aortic dissection. Ann. Thorac. Surg. 19:436, 1975.
30. Parmley, M. C., Mattingly, T. W., Manion, W. C., et al.: Nonpenetrating traumatic injury of the aorta. Circulation 17:1086, 1958.
31. Prokop, E. K., Palmer, R. F., and Wheat, M. W., Jr.: Hydrodynamic forces in dissecting aneurysms. In-vitro studies in a Tygon model and in dog aortas. Circ. Res. 27:121, 1970.

32. Reul, G. J., Jr., Cooley, D. A., Hallman, G. L., et al.: Dissecting aneurysm of the descending aorta. Improved surgical results in 91 patients. Arch. Surg. 110:632, 1975.
33. Roberts, W. C.: Aortic dissection: anatomy, consequence and causes. Am. Heart J. 101:195, 1981.
34. Roth, J. A., and Parekh, M. A.: Dissecting aneurysms perforating the esophagus. N. Engl. J. Med. 299:776, 1978.
35. Schlatmann, T. J. M., and Becker, A. E.: Pathogenesis of dissecting aneurysm of the aorta. Comparative histopathologic study of significance of medical changes. Am. J. Cardiol. 39:21, 1977.
36. Shuford, W. H., Sybers, R. G., and Weens, H. S.: Problems in the aortographic diagnosis of dissecting aneurysms of the aorta. N. Engl. J. Med. 280:225, 1969.
37. Slater, E. E., and DeSanctis, R. W.: Clinical recognition of dissecting aortic aneurysm. Am. J. Med. 60:625, 1976.
38 Slater, E. E., and Haber, E.: High blood pressure. *In* Rubenstein, E., and Federman, D. D. (eds.): Scientific American Medicine: "Principles and Progress for Practicing Physicians." New York, Scientific American, Inc., 1978.
39. Strong, W. W., Moggio, R. A., and Stansel, H. C., Jr.: Acute aortic dissection. Twelve-year medical and surgical experience. J. Thorac. Cardiovasc. Surg. 68:85, 1974.
40. Weisman, A. D., and Adams, R. D.: Neurological complications of dissecting aortic aneurysm. Brain 67:69, 1944.
41. Wheat, M. W., Jr., Palmer, R. F., Bartley, T. D., et al.: Treatment of dissecting aneurysms of the aorta without surgery. J. Thorac. Cardiovasc. Surg. 50:364, 1965.
42. Yacoub, M. H., Schottenfeld, M., and Kittle, C. F.: Hematoma of the interatrial septum with heart block secondary to dissecting aneurysm of the aorta. A clinicopathologic entity. Circulation 46:537, 1972.

11

Acute Diseases of Native and Prosthetic Cardiac Valves

PAUL SIMPSON
and J. DAVID BRISTOW

Valvular heart disease is most often a chronic illness. When the patient is first seen, the specific lesion must be identified and its severity assessed. Subsequently, prophylactic antibiotics, anticoagulants, digitalis, diuretics, and vasodilators are used as indicated until the time when symptoms and evidence of hemodynamic significance indicate the need for surgical intervention.

Table 11–1. PRESENTING SYMPTOMS OF VALVE EMERGENCIES

Respiratory Distress Due to Pulmonary Congestion
1. Aortic stenosis with superimposed ischemia, arrhythmia, or altered loading conditions
2. Mitral stenosis with atrial fibrillation and rapid ventricular rate
3. Acute mitral regurgitation (all causes)
4. Acute aortic regurgitation (all causes)
5. Prosthetic valve disease (all causes)

Chest Pain
1. Aortic stenosis with myocardial ischemia, with or without coronary artery disease
2. Myocardial infarction with acute mitral regurgitation due to ruptured papillary muscle head
3. Aortic dissection with acute aortic regurgitation
4. Prosthetic valve obstruction

Syncope or Shock Due to Low Cardiac Output
1. Aortic stenosis
2. Prosthetic valve obstruction
3. Mitral stenosis with atrial fibrillation or due to "ball-valve" thrombus or atrial myxoma
4. Aortic dissection with acute aortic regurgitation

Fever
1. Acute mitral regurgitation due to infective endocarditis
2. Acute aortic regurgitation due to infective endocarditis
3. Prosthetic valve endocarditis

On some occasions, however, valvular heart disease is an acute illness, and the physician's diagnostic and therapeutic decisions must be accomplished rapidly. In this chapter, the most important of these urgent problems in valvular heart disease are discussed: critical valvular aortic stenosis, mitral stenosis with atrial fibrillation and rapid ventricular rate, acute aortic regurgitation, and acute mitral regurgitation. In addition, the difficulties encountered in the patient with a prosthetic valve are reviewed, since prosthetic valve complications always require prompt assessment.

Proper recognition and management of the emergencies in valvular heart disease can be particularly gratifying. In many cases ventricular function is normal or nearly so and the patient may improve remarkably.

GENERAL CONCEPTS

The major presenting symptoms of urgent valve disorders are listed in Table 11–1. Respiratory distress, chest pain, and syncope or shock are the common symptoms of cardiovascular disease, and fever is nonspecific. Initial recognition that one of these symptoms is due to valve disease usually requires detection of a pathologic murmur. With prosthetic valve disorders, there is the evidence of previous thoracotomy. Although the presence of a murmur is the major feature that directs attention to the possibility of a valve disorder, this finding is nonspecific and insensitive. For example, patients with acute respiratory distress from any cause may have a nonpathologic murmur or a murmur reflecting a hemodynamically insignificant valve lesion. On the other hand, a diagnostic murmur may not be heard if it is obscured by the rales of acute pulmonary edema or if it is absent owing to critical depression of cardiac output. In the settings to be described, the murmurs indicating significant underlying valve disease are frequently neither long nor loud; i.e., they are often less than holosystolic or holodiastolic and are grade 3/6 or less.

To further complicate matters, these emergency valve lesions are typically accompanied by a normal-sized heart on chest radiograph. Either the left ventricle does not dilate (mitral stenosis) or it dilates infrequently (aortic stenosis); alternatively, as will be discussed, the left ventricle has not had time to dilate (acute aortic or mitral regurgitation). Therefore, these valve disorders often present as acute pulmonary edema without cardiomegaly on chest radiograph. They must be distinguished from other cardiac causes (acute myocardial infarction, for example)[16] and from the numerous noncardiac causes of pulmonary edema without elevated pulmonary capillary wedge pressure (smoke inhalation, aspiration of gastric contents, neurogenic and high-altitude pulmonary edema, narcotic overdose, and others). Fortunately, emergency treatment of acute pulmonary edema with oxygen, morphine, and intravenous furosemide and/or aminophylline will be appropriate whatever the etiology. While treatment is under way, the underlying cause can be sought. A major caveat, as discussed later, is to look early for critical aortic stenosis, a lesion with unstable hemodynamics that can be greatly worsened by over-vigorous diuresis or vasodilation.

The chest radiograph usually shows cardiomegaly in two situations of emergency valve disorders. First, patients with a prosthetic valve implanted for a volume-overload lesion (chronic aortic or mitral regurgitation) have cardiac enlargement. Second, an acute valve lesion may complicate the course of a patient with a chronic underlying disease that has produced cardiomegaly; for example, infective endocarditis in an individual with chronic aortic or mitral regurgitation. For this reason, acute valve lesions, specifically acute aortic or mitral regurgitation, must be considered along with the other causes that can precipitate acute pulmonary edema in a patient with compensated chronic congestive heart failure; these causes include increased cardiac demand (due to infection or anemia, for example), arrhythmia, and pulmonary embolism.

In summary, it may not be obvious that a valve emergency is responsible for the patient's symptoms. Recognition requires consideration of the possibility, careful attention to the clinical features to be described, and selected diagnostic tests. Recognition is particularly important because therapy can be highly successful. The final therapeutic maneuver is surgical in almost all cases. Initial medical management is selected to stabilize the patient if possible, and the major decision is the timing of surgical intervention.

CRITICAL AORTIC STENOSIS

Background

At the onset of dyspnea, angina, or syncope in patients with adult valvular aortic stenosis, the valve area typically has become critically reduced, i.e., from the normal 4 cm^2 to about 0.7 cm^2 or less, with a systolic gradient of 50 mm Hg or more if the cardiac output is normal. For most patients, the average life expectancy is only a few years after the onset of symptoms;[52] for others, the prognosis is even more dismal, with hemodynamic deterioration occurring over weeks to months.[9]

In both groups of patients with critical aortic stenosis, the maintenance of normal or near-normal cardiac output and pulmonary capillary pressure requires a very delicate balance of both left ventricular preload and afterload. For example, preload (the left ventricular filling pressure reflected as the pulmonary capillary wedge pressure) must be high enough to maintain cardiac output, yet not so high that pulmonary edema results. Similarly, that part of ventricular afterload represented by systemic pressure must be high enough to support coronary perfusion, but not so high that ventricular oxygen need is increased excessively. The ranges of appropriate values of preload and afterload are more restricted in aortic stenosis than in the normal heart. The circulatory changes to be described may disturb the balance of preload or afterload and rapidly precipitate refractory pulmonary edema or shock. The physician must therefore be alert to avoid or to treat the inciting hemodynamic disturbances, and be prepared to recognized and manage the patient who has developed severe congestive failure or peripheral hypoperfusion. It is vital to remember that the patient with aortic stenosis may progress over only a few hours from a state of relative well-being to one of malignant pump failure and cardiac arrest.

Etiology of Sudden Cardiovascular Decompensation

The inciting hemodynamic disturbances that can precipitate decompensation are several. The hypertrophied, noncompliant left ventricle in aortic stenosis may require a relatively high filling pressure to sustain its stroke volume. Excessive reduction of filling pressure (preload) may occur, for example, with overvigorous diuretic treatment; with the administration of vasodilating drugs such as nitroglycerin or morphine; with the fluid loss resulting from preparation for gastrointestinal or urologic radiography; and with the osmotic diuresis following cardiac or other angiography. In addition to these iatrogenic causes, acute febrile or volume-depleting illnesses can reduce filling pressure excessively.

Atrial systole is particularly important to left ventricular preload in aortic stenosis; it contributes substantially more to left ventricular stroke volume in aortic stenosis than in the normal heart (about 40% vs. 25%).[62] The new onset of atrial fibrillation therefore may seriously compromise cardiac output.

Since the left ventricle is thick and is operating at a high systolic pressure, its oxygen demand is large. Its coronary perfusion is only marginally adequate,[7, 24] particularly the perfusion of the subendocardial region. Ischemic left ventricular dysfunction may be induced if oxygen demand is increased or if supply is reduced. Any of the above-mentioned decreases in preload may reduce supply by reducing stroke volume. Tachycardia of any type both increases oxygen demand and abbreviates the time for coronary perfusion by shortening diastole. Systemic hypotension decreases diastolic coronary flow without alleviating the high systolic pressure and oxygen demand proximal to the stenotic valve. Systemic hypertension, on the other hand, may increase oxygen need more than it increases coronary perfusion. In short, alterations in preload or afterload may intiate a vicious cycle of ischemic pump failure that has as its basis an increase in the ratio of oxygen demand to oxygen supply.

Recognition

The patient with aortic stenosis who is at risk for sudden decompensation may have been admitted to the hospital for elective evaluation of aortic valve disease, or may be awaiting replacement of the aortic valve following cardiac catheterization. In previously undiagnosed cases, recognition of severe aortic stenosis generally is not difficult if attention is paid to the harsh, grunting systolic murmur with thrill at the upper sternal border; the absent aortic component of the second sound; the reduced carotid pulse with delayed upstroke; the hypertrophied ventricle on examination and electrocardiography; and, in particular, the presence of valve calcification on lateral chest radiograph or cardiac fluoroscopy. It must be recalled, however, that the valve gradient and the murmur are dependent on flow across the valve, and thus the murmur may be unimpressive when cardiac output is severely depressed. One may also be misled in occasional cases with maximal intensity of the murmur at the cardiac apex, rather than the upper right sternal border. Even if the murmur is not loud or is atypically located, the other signs mentioned above may suggest severe aortic stenosis; the echocardiogram may be useful by demonstrating multiple, dense echoes in the aortic root, associated with a thick-walled ventricle.

This lesion must be carefully considered in the elderly male patient with unexplained pulmonary edema, especially if there is left ventricular hypertrophy on ECG and a normal-sized heart on chest radiograph, whether or not a systolic murmur is present. The diagnosis can be effectively excluded in adult patients if a high-quality lateral chest radiograph shows no calcification or if the echocardiogram reveals mobile aortic leaflets. Aortic stenosis in young people is not accompanied by prominent valve calcification.

Management

Elective replacement of the valve should be scheduled for the stable patient with symptoms who has critical aortic stenosis documented at catheterization. Many cardiologists also recommend simultaneous bypass of significant coronary stenoses shown by arteriography, especially if the patient complains of angina.

In managing the patient with critical aortic stenosis preoperatively, care should be taken to avoid the causes of sudden decompensation discussed above, or to treat them if possible should they occur. For example, electrical cardioversion of atrial fibrillation or flutter or other paroxysmal supraventricular tachycardia should be considered promptly. Similarly, systemic hypertension or hypotension accompanied by evidence of deleterious effect, such as angina, should be carefully treated. Hypotension is the more common problem, which may be corrected with volume replacement or pressor agents. However, since overcorrection with resultant pulmonary edema is a definite threat, such therapy often requires monitoring of pulmonary capillary wedge and intra-arterial pressures, as well as cardiac output.

The patient who develops peripheral hypoperfusion or more than mild pulmonary congestion requires urgent treatment. The rapidly deteriorating individual should have valve replacement on an emergent basis. The patient in extremis should be taken to the operating room without delay. In less life-threatening situations, medical therapy may temporarily stabilize the patient and permit an elective procedure. Treatment can be initiated with digitalis, dobutamine, vasopressors (dopamine, norepinephrine), and volume expanders or diuretics, depending on the results of hemodynamic measurements. Pharmacologic afterload reduction is unlikely to increase cardiac output, since the major afterload is the stenotic valve. However, the additional diastolic augmentation of coronary perfusion provided by the intra-aortic balloon pump may relieve ventricular dysfunction caused by ischemia and facilitate cardiac catheterization or the institution of cardiopulmonary bypass. If the patient also has aortic regurgitation, use of the intra-aortic balloon is contraindicated.

Medical therapy in the critically ill patient with aortic stenosis should be clearly recognized as a preparation for surgery and should not be unduly prolonged. Correction of pulmonary edema may result in systemic hypoperfusion, and treatment for hypoperfusion may re-establish pulmonary edema. Furthermore, unexpected cardiac arrest is not uncommon.[26] Ideally, cardiac catheterization should be done preoperatively to confirm the diagnosis, to exclude additional valve lesions, and to assess the coronary arteries and left ventricle. The procedure requires time and carries a greater-than-normal risk; it may be eliminated in selected cases. Replacement of the aortic valve has been accomplished in moribund patients with an in-hospital mortality rate of 0 to 45 per cent.[26, 55]

MITRAL STENOSIS WITH ATRIAL FIBRILLATION

Pathophysiology

In contrast to aortic stenosis, the natural history of mitral stenosis is usually marked by a gradual deterioration over many years after the onset of symptoms. Dyspnea generally does not appear until the valve area is reduced from the normal 4.5 cm^2 to about 1.5 cm^2 or less; a "critical" stenosis is considered to be less than 1 cm^2, at which point the left atrial pressure must be about 25 mm Hg to sustain a cardiac output at the lower limit of normal.

The symptomatic decline of patients with mitral stenosis commonly begins with the onset of atrial fibrillation.[56] In some patients this event can precipitate life-threatening pulmonary edema with or without systemic hypoperfusion. The bases for this effect are several: first, atrial systole contributes about 25 per cent of left ventricular stroke volume in patients with mitral stenosis, as is the case in normals.[62] In addition, atrial systole may sustain flow across the valve without requiring an elevated left atrial pressure throughout diastole. Finally, for a given valve area, the left atrial pressure is inversely related to the diastolic filling period. As the diastolic filling time decreases with tachycardia, left atrial and pulmonary capillary pressures rise, and cardiac output may fall.

Management

Atrial fibrillation with a rapid ventricular rate (more than about 130 beats per minute) can thus present a medical emergency. Treatment modalities include electrical cardioversion, or verapamil, propranolol, or digitalis to slow conduction through the atrioventricular node. The choice depends on the urgency of the clinical status. If the patient has severe pulmonary edema, electrical cardioversion should be done using an energy level of at least 100 watt-seconds. In most cases, however, pulmonary congestion can be alleviated with oral or intravenous diuretics; control of ventricular rate to about 110 beats per minute or less is achieved with intravenous digoxin, 0.25 to 0.5 mg intravenously at six-hour intervals to a total dose of 1.0 to 1.5 mg, followed by maintenance at 0.25 mg per day orally (if renal function is normal). This method generally establishes rate control over the first day. If not, or if more urgent therapy is required, intravenous verapamil, 5 to 10 mg over a one- to two-minute interval, will effectively reduce ventricular rate within five to ten minutes. Patients on digoxin without evidence of toxicity can safely be given verapamil.[67] Propranolol also can be given by intermittent bolus infusion at a rate of 1 mg per minute every five minutes, with a maximal total dose of about 10 mg. In this setting, pulmonary congestion is not a contraindication to the use of propranolol. If the patient remains symptomatic with a rapid ventricular rate despite digoxin and verapamil or propranolol, direct-current cardioversion should be considered. If large doses of digoxin are given over several days, the risk of digitalis-toxic arrhythmias during subsequent cardioversion is increased.

With control of ventricular rate to about 100 beats per minute or less, maintenance oral digoxin should be continued. In some cases, chronic oral verapamil or propranolol therapy may be required in addition. If sinus rhythm is restored, quinidine may be added and may forestall the return of atrial fibrillation for up to a year in one third to one half of patients. Chronic anticoagulation is indicated, particularly if atrial fibrillation persists, to reduce the risk of systemic embolization.

ACUTE AORTIC REGURGITATION

Pathophysiology

In most cases of aortic regurgitation, the disease pursues a chronic course, with the regurgitant leak increasing gradually. The left ventricle thus has time to grow and adapt to the increased load by an increase in volume, so that left ventricular diastolic and left atrial pressure may remain normal for years. Because of an increased end-diastolic volume and a normal or increased ejection fraction, total stroke volume is large, resulting in the hyperdynamic left ventricular impulse and wide pulse pressure that characterize the chronic disease. In the late stage of the chronic disease, myocardial contractility and ejection fraction are decreased. As a consequence, ventricular end-diastolic and left atrial pressure rise, and the signs of a hyperactive circulation become less obvious, being replaced by congestive failure and low cardiac output. When a large regurgitant leak develops suddenly, on the other hand, congestive failure and low cardiac output are present early. There is no time for an increase in ventricular volume in acute aortic regurgitation. End-diastolic pressure, and consequently left atrial and pulmonary capillary pressure, rise markedly. Since end-diastolic volume is not increased greatly, a large total stroke volume is not possible, even though ejection fraction may be normal. Thus, the traditional signs of chronic aortic regurgitation are not seen, and cardiac output is low despite compensatory tachycardia.

Between the two extremes just described are many gradations, dependent on the time over which regurgitation develops and the pre-existent state of the left ventricle. The following comments characterize sudden, severe regurgitation into a normal ventricle, a topic that has been comprehensively reviewed.[41]

Etiology

Four major mechanisms (Table 11–2) can produce acute, severe aortic regurgitation: infective endocarditis, proximal dissecting

Table 11–2. ETIOLOGY OF ACUTE AORTIC REGURGITATION

1. Infective endocarditis
2. Dissection of ascending aorta
3. Blunt chest or upper abdominal trauma
4. Spontaneous rupture of abnormal leaflet (uncommon)

aneurysm of the aorta, blunt chest or upper abdominal trauma, and spontaneous rupture of an abnormal aortic leaflet. Although the hemodynamic sequelae are similar for each, recognition and management differ in certain details.

Infective endocarditis is by far the most common cause, and any organism may be responsible. The infection may be present for days, weeks, or months prior to admission,[22, 35] depending on the destructive capabilities of the infecting pathogen and the presence or absence of underlying valvular disease.

Dissecting aneurysm involving the aortic root above the valve resulted in acute, severe aortic regurgitation in eight of 53 cases in one report.[59] A murmur of aortic regurgitation was present in about two thirds of the patients. It is uncommon to have dissection of the ascending aorta without either aortic regurgitation or pulse loss. A dissecting hematoma in the aortic root can produce regurgitation by three mechanisms: widening of the root with separation of the valve cusps, displacement of one cusp below the level of the others, and disruption of the valve anulus.

Blunt chest trauma during diastole, when the ventricle is distended and the aortic valve is closed, can tear or avulse an aortic leaflet. Alternatively, an aortic dissection or tear may be produced. Characteristically there is a delay from the time of injury to the appearance of aortic regurgitation, possibly reflecting progression of a leaflet tear with hemodynamic stress.[27]

On rare occasions, acute, severe aortic regurgitation can be due to spontaneous rupture of a myxomatous or fenestrated leaflet. Preoperatively this diagnosis can be entertained only if infection, dissection, and trauma have been excluded.

Recognition

The patient with acute aortic regurgitation usually is critically ill with severe congestive failure and often peripheral hypoperfusion. The historical setting may suggest the diagnosis and the etiology. Infection is usually obvious, with fever and positive blood cultures. The presence of an aortic dissection may not be apparent. Chest and/or back pain is the characteristic presenting symptom of aortic dissection, and the major differential diagnosis is acute myocardial infarction. However, pain may be absent if the dissection has produced shock (cardiac tamponade), stroke (carotid occlusion), or pulmonary edema (aortic regurgitation). In the series of Slater and DeSanctis,[59] chest pain was absent in half of the patients with aortic regurgitation and congestive failure. However, a normal chest radiograph was rare, the great majority showing an abnormal aortic contour. Valve damage consequent to blunt trauma, most often a steering-wheel injury, must not be dismissed if chest bruises or rib fractures are absent; they may not be present.

There may be a latent period of a few weeks to a few months between the onset of infection and the appearance of aortic regurgitation. On the other hand, significant valve damage usually occurs simultaneously with an aortic dissection. After chest trauma, several days may elapse before aortic incompetence becomes manifest, particularly if the patient has been hypovolemic.

The characteristic signs of acute, severe aortic regurgitation include tachycardia with a normal or even decreased pulse pressure and a left ventricular impulse that is not markedly hyperdynamic. The first sound is decreased or absent, and a fourth sound is absent. Both of these auscultatory findings are due to early mitral valve closure by the regurgitant jet and by the rapidly rising left ventricular diastolic pressure. Importantly, the aortic regurgitant murmur is short, ending in mid-diastole as left ventricular pressure rises to equal aortic pressure; it may be very faint and rarely may be absent. A systolic aortic flow murmur may be present but will not be loud.

The ECG, in the absence of pre-existing disease, usually does not show evidence of left ventricular hypertrophy, although it has been said that such evidence can develop over a two-week period.[20]

The chest radiograph demonstrates pulmonary venous hypertension or pulmonary edema with a heart size that is modestly increased or even normal. The mediastinum may be widened in aortic dissection; a normal appearance militates against the diagnosis. Portable chest films must be interpreted with caution, however.

Echocardiography furnishes much useful information. The regurgitant jet itself produces fine fluttering of the anterior mitral valve leaflet in diastole. A diagnosis of acute, severe aortic regurgitation is supported by the finding of early closure of the mitral leaflets in diastole, before the QRS on the simultaneously recorded ECG.[35] Exaggerated wall motion and a markedly dilated ventricle are not seen, in contrast to chronic aortic regurgitation. The echocardiogram may also assist in elucidating the cause. Dense, irregular echoes on one or more valve leaflets, usually best seen in diastole, may represent vegetations of endocarditis.[53, 66] Normal systolic opening should be demonstrated, to avoid confusion with the dense echoes of a heavily calcified valve. A flail leaflet prolapsing into the left ventricular outflow tract in diastole suggests valve disruption by infective endocarditis. The presence of aortic dissection may be suggested by dilation of the aortic root, with a double lumen representing the false channel.[40] The specificity of these findings is not high, however,[6] and the current procedure of choice for acute diagnosis of aortic dissection is computerized tomography.[65]

Management

The presence of acute, severe aortic regurgitation and its likely cause are established in most cases by the noninvasive evaluation described above. Cardiac catheterization and aortography are nevertheless indicated to confirm the diagnosis and to clarify pathologic conditions that may affect the surgical approach, e.g., an unsuspected dissection or a left-to-right shunt produced by extension of infection through the interatrial or interventricular septum. In rare cases, the patient's condition may be too precarious to permit this study.

Acute, severe aortic regurgitation is a surgical emergency; treatment consists of aortic valve replacement. Immediate surgical intervention is usually recommended in proximal aortic dissection, in trauma complicated by aortic regurgitation, and in life-threatening aortic incompetence resulting from endocarditis.

Pending surgery, medical therapy with digitalis, dobutamine, and diuretics should be initiated under hemodynamic monitoring. Afterload reduction with vasodilators such as nitroprusside may be particularly appropriate,[38] unless there is excessive hypotension. In the setting of dissection, antihypertensive therapy may be indicated. The intra-aortic balloon pump for afterload reduction is contraindicated, since diastolic augmentation by the balloon would increase aortic regurgitation.

In endocarditis, antibiotics should be started as early as possible, with doses sufficient to ensure that the patient's serum at a dilution of 1:8 or greater is bactericidal for the infecting organism. In the setting of refractory congestive failure from aortic endocarditis, surgery should not be delayed to allow completion of a course of antibiotic therapy, since such procrastination results in increased mortality.[22, 41] The valve should be replaced despite the infected field, with continuation of high-dose antibiotics in the postoperative period. Only less severe cases of endocarditis with easily controlled congestive failure allow the opportunity to temporize. If the patient is asymptomatic on medical management, valve replacement may be preceded by a period of antibiotic therapy; however, required surgery should not be delayed longer than about two weeks.[41] Furthermore, during this period the attending physician must be alert for the several potential complications that can result from extension of infection: e.g., coronary embolization (leading to myocardial infarction or arrhythmia); penetration of the atrial or ventricular septum (leading to atrioventricular conduction defects or left-to-right shunt); and perforation of the aorta or left ventricular free wall (producing cardiac tamponade).

Acute aortic regurgitation from whatever cause is not severe in every case. As in all valvular heart disease, the decision to undertake valve replacement is based on the patient's symptoms and evidence that the lesion is hemodynamically significant. In some cases of endocarditis, for example, antibiotic therapy may be all that is required.

ACUTE MITRAL REGURGITATION

Pathophysiology

The pathophysiology of acute mitral regurgitation is different from that of chronic mitral regurgitation, and the reason is analogous to the difference between acute and chronic aortic regurgitation. In mitral regurgitation, the compliance of the left atrium is the pathophysiologic basis for the differing manifestations of the acute and chronic diseases, rather than the left ventricle as in aortic regurgitation. Acute mitral regurgitation involves a left atrium of normal size and compliance. This increased volume load in a normally distensible chamber results in marked left atrial hypertension and subsequent pulmonary venous and pulmonary arterial hypertension; right ventricular failure may ensue. In contrast, in patients with chronic, severe mitral regurgitation, a large distensible left atrium may absorb the volume load without elevation of left atrial pressure.[4] Acute mitral regurgitation differs from acute aortic regurgitation in being generally better tolerated than acute aortic valvular disease. In many instances of acute mitral regurgitation, the course is protracted over months, with some degree of hemodynamic compensation permitting elective surgical correction. This comparatively indolent course is in part due to the systolic unloading of the left ventricle because of the incompetent mitral valve. Thus, during systole, left ventricular volume falls rapidly and markedly, because of the mitral regurgitation. Since ventricular wall tension is proportional to the ventricular radius, wall tension also diminishes greatly. With less contractile energy needed for the generation of wall tension, more is available for shortening, with the consequence that the left ventricle is able to increase its total stroke volume strikingly. In aortic regurgitation, on the other hand, the total forward and regurgitant volumes must be ejected through the same orifice, and ventricular volume does not decrease as dramatically; wall tension is therefore higher. Since the myocardium in aortic regurgitation must develop high tension, the amount it can shorten is proportionately reduced.[4]

As in aortic regurgitation, gradations exist between pure acute disease and chronic disease; the clinical manifestations depend on the size of the regurgitant leak and the rapidity with which it develops, as well as the presence or absence of underlying myocardial disease. Such mixed clinical states are particularly common when acute mitral regurgitation caused by ruptured chordae tendineae complicates chronic rheumatic disease or mitral valve prolapse. The comments that follow will focus on pure, acute, severe mitral regurgitation.

Etiology

Acute mitral regurgitation may be classified according to the part of the mitral apparatus involved and the etiology of the involvement[50] (Table 11–3). Variations in clinical manifestations are largely a function of etiology. Almost all cases of acute, severe mitral regurgitation are a consequence of rupture of either of two parts of the subvalvular mitral apparatus: the chordae tendineae or the papillary muscles.

Rupture of the chordae tendineae may occur in the following settings: in the course of chronic rheumatic mitral regurgitation;[50] with infective endocarditis of normal or abnormal valves; as a complication of the mitral valve prolapse syndrome;[13, 21] as a consequence of blunt chest trauma;[27] or spontaneously. Spontaneous rupture of the chordae tendineae[54, 58] is the purest expression of acute, severe mitral regurgitation, since it occurs in the absence of any other definite cardiac disease. Its cause is unknown, but focal dissolution of chordal connective tissue has been demonstrated.[8] Chordae to the posterior mitral leaflet are more frequently involved than those to the anterior leaflet. This syndrome typically affects men in late middle age. Although the mitral valve prolapse syndrome is more common in young women, mitral prolapse complicated by ruptured chordae tendineae may also show a preponderance in older men.[21]

The second pathologic substrate of acute, severe mitral regurgitation is rupture of the head of a papillary muscle. By far the most frequent cause is acute myocardial infarction, but it occasionally may follow chest trauma. The posteromedial papillary muscle, sup-

Table 11–3. ETIOLOGY OF ACUTE MITRAL REGURGITATION

1. Spontaneous idiopathic rupture of chordae tendineae
2. Infective endocarditis
3. Acute myocardial infarction (usually inferior) with dysfunction or rupture of papillary muscle
4. Chest trauma
5. Rupture of chordae tendineae complicating chronic mitral valve disease

plied by the posterior descending coronary artery and variably by the circumflex, has less abundant collateral vessels than the anterolateral muscle, perfused by the left anterior descending and circumflex arteries. Therefore, it is commonly the posterior muscle that ruptures, during the course of inferior myocardial infarction. Rupture occurs after necrosis has developed (a few days after myocardial infarction) and before the muscle has become fibrotic (a few weeks). Transection of an entire papillary muscle is incompatible with life, since each muscle anchors chordae to both leaflets. Immediate survivors therefore have ruptured only one or a few of the six "heads" of a muscle (two chordae orginate from each head).[50] In fact, autopsy studies have shown that the infarctions tend to be small and limited to the area of a papillary muscle.[44, 68] Acute, severe mitral regurgitation due to papillary muscle infarction without rupture has been described;[10] the clinical picture is identical.

In summary, acute mitral regurgitation can occur in the absence (rupture of chordae tendineae) or presence (rupture or dysfunction of papillary muscle) of acute myocardial infarction (Table 11–3).

Recognition of Ruptured Chordae Tendineae

The patient with ruptured chordae presents with the sudden onset of dyspnea due to the high left atrial and pulmonary venous pressure. On occasion, the acute episode is sufficiently well tolerated that the patient does not seek attention until later, but the time of onset is historically clear in most cases.[51] Depending on the etiology, there may be a history of a pre-existent murmur, or recent trauma, or symptoms of infection.

On physical examination, there is tachycardia with briskly rising but small pulses. The ventricular impulse is hyperdynamic, in contrast to acute, severe aortic regurgitation, but it is not greatly enlarged. The second sound may be widely split, owing to early closure of the aortic valve, and a third sound is present. To distinguish acute from chronic disease, a fourth sound is an important and relatively consistent finding in acute mitral regurgitation, unless atrial fibrillation is present. A fourth heart sound is absent when the left atrium is dilated and hypocontractile, as in chronic, severe mitral regurgitation. The systolic murmur of acute mitral regurgitation is audible at the apex. Commonly and importantly, the murmur is not holosystolic but is crescendo-decrescendo in early to mid-systole; the attenuation in late systole results when the left atrial pressure equals or exceeds left ventricular pressure. When the posterior leaflet is detached, the regurgitant stream is deflected toward the base of the heart; this basal radiation of the murmur and its diamond shape may suggest aortic stenosis. A thrill often accompanies the murmur. The murmur may radiate widely across the thorax and may be heard in the back on occasion. The signs of pulmonary hypertension (accentuated pulmonic second sound, right ventricular impulse) and even right ventricular failure (tricuspid regurgitation, distended neck veins) are at times present.

Electrocardiographic changes are nonspecific. Since the left atrium is not dilated, atrial fibrillation is usually absent. Left ventricular hypertrophy is unusual in the absence of preexisting disease. Both atrial fibrillation and left ventricular hypertrophy are often present in chronic regurgitation.

The chest radiograph is similar to the ECG in showing no evidence of marked chamber enlargement. As in acute aortic regurgitation, the only abnormality may be pulmonary congestion. Cardiomegaly may be found when the patient is seen weeks to months after onset.[51]

Echocardiography is a helpful noninvasive study. The echocardiographic expressions of the mitral regurgitation include exaggerated motion of the left ventricle and left atrium, and abbreviated systolic opening of the aortic valve. The left ventricular cavity may show mild-to-moderate enlargement. The flail anterior or posterior leaflet, untethered because of ruptured chordae, may be visualized moving into the left atrium in systole.[25, 63] Valvular vegetations may be identified in patients with infective endocarditis,[53, 66] but may be difficult to distinguish from the chaotic flail echoes.

Recognition of Ruptured Papillary Muscle Head

Ruptured papillary muscle head usually occurs in the first week after acute inferior myocardial infarction. It is often the patient's first infarction, so that the ventricle is not "protected" by areas of fibrosis from previous infarcts. In this setting, acute mitral regurgitation presents as an acute deterioration in the patient's clinical status, with a systolic murmur and pulmonary congestion with or without systemic hypoperfusion. Although the clinical picture at times may be similar to that in ruptured chordae, it is more likely to be modified by the accompanying depression of ventricular function due to the underlying myocardial ischemia. Thus, the briskly rising arterial pulse and hyperdynamic left ventricular impulse found in ruptured chordae are often not present. The systolic murmur is similar to that just described. However, it is important to note that rarely there may be no murmur;[68] a large regurgitant channel and an ischemic, poorly contracting ventricle may make the regurgitation inaudible. The physician must therefore consider the diagnosis of ruptured papillary muscle head in any patient who develops pulmonary congestion in the period following infarction.

The chest radiograph in ruptured papillary muscle is usually similar to that in ruptured chordae. The ECG will demonstrate a recent infarction in most instances. The echocardiographic findings may be modified by poor ventricular function; i.e., exaggerated left ventricular wall motion may not be present.

The patient who deteriorates with pulmonary edema and a systolic murmur in the setting of an acute infarction may have a perforated interventricular septum, a ruptured papillary muscle, or depression of left ventricular systolic function with papillary muscle dysfunction. These entities cannot be reliably distinguished noninvasively, but require right heart catheterization with measurement of right-sided oxygen saturations and pulmonary capillary wedge "V" waves. A significant increase in right ventricular as compared with right atrial oxygen saturation is diagnostic of a left-to-right shunt through a ventricular septal defect, while exaggerated "V" waves indicate acute mitral regurgitation. Initial medical management of congestive failure is the same for all three. The differential diagnosis of a systolic murmur in the patient with acute infarction also includes tricuspid regurgitation due to right ventricular infarction, hemodynamically insignificant mitral regurgitation from papillary muscle dysfunction, a single-component systolic pericardial friction rub, and pre-existing aortic valve disease.

Management

In most cases, urgent surgical intervention need not be considered. Congestive failure should be treated with digitalis, dobutamine, diuretics, and afterload reduction (nitroglycerin, nitroprusside, intra-aortic balloon pump), as required. Antibiotics are given in endocarditis. Following stabilization, cardiac catheterization and left ventricular and coronary angiography should be performed to confirm the diagnosis, to assess the severity of mitral regurgitation, and to document the presence and magnitude of associated coronary disease or left ventricular dysfunction. The critical distinction is between predominant mitral regurgitation and predominant left ventricular dysfunction. If regurgitation is severe and requires aggressive medical therapy and if left ventricular function is not severely depressed, elective surgery may be recommended. Treatment usually consists of mitral valve replacement, although a reparative procedure has been advocated for spontaneous rupture of the chordae to the posterior leaflet.[57] In ruptured papillary muscle, coronary bypass may also be indicated. Valve replacement usually should be postponed until some weeks or months after the acute infarction, if possible. If the patient cannot be stabilized with medical therapy, surgery may be needed more urgently. Some physicians have stressed the risk of sudden and unpredictable clinical deterioration, and have advocated consideration of early surgery in stable patients.[44] As in acute aortic regurgitation caused by endocarditis, in acute mitral regurgitation due to endocarditis necessary surgery should not be delayed for completion of a course of antibiotic therapy.[3]

PROSTHETIC VALVE DISEASE

Background

After aortic or mitral valve replacement, elevated intracardiac and pulmonary arterial pressures return to normal at rest in most patients. Cardiac output increases with exercise, although pressure may rise abnormally.[5] Most important, symptoms improve and life may be prolonged more than in those not having surgery, particularly in selected groups of patients such as those described earlier in this chapter. The results of valve replacement are best in patients with acute aortic or mitral regurgitation and with aortic or mitral stenosis, probably because left ventricular function is usually normal. Long-term results are less favorable after surgery for chronic aortic regurgitation, and least successful with chronic mitral regurgitation, in these cases probably because of impaired ventricular function at the time of surgery.[45] These factors might argue for valve replacement at a presymptomatic stage of chronic regurgitant lesions. However, the very significant problems of prosthetic valve disease suggest caution in consideration of early surgery.

Hospital mortality for initial valve replacement averages about 5 to 10 per cent, being in the higher range for mitral procedures. Surgical mortality for prosthesis re-replacement may be similar to that of the original procedure, but may double if the operation has to be done on an emergency basis.[11] There is also some evidence that the late results of re-replacement operations are not as good as for initial procedures.[30] Adequate antibiotic prophylaxis is required for all patients with prosthetic valves during procedures or with illnesses that have a potential for bacteremia, according to the guidelines of the American Heart Association.[1] Therapeutic anticoagulation (prothrombin time about twice that of control) is mandatory for all mechanical valves and for tissue valves in the mitral position in the presence of atrial fibrillation.[28] Antiplatelet drugs alone are inadequate. Anticoagulation carries the risk of hemorrhagic complications, with a rate of 1 to 5 per cent per year. The incidence of serious, prosthesis-related complications is difficult to determine, but in general 1 to 5 per cent of patients per year have a problem causing death or morbidity or requiring prosthetic valve replacement. The prosthesis may be responsible for postoperative death in 10 to 20 per cent of patients.[43]

In summary, prosthetic valve disease is a significant concern. Due consideration should be given to the timing of original implantation and to the choice of valve. Complications should be anticipated and promptly assessed, given the higher surgical mortality rate for urgent prosthesis re-replacement.

Available Prostheses and Major Complications

Table 11–4 outlines the common types of prostheses, examples of each type, and the major problems encountered. Table 11–5 lists the major complications associated with prostheses, according to the likelihood of requiring prosthetic valve replacement; the lesions most likely to demand emergency management are indicated.

Table 11–4. MAJOR COMPLICATIONS WITH DIFFERENT PROSTHETIC CARDIAC VALVES

Valve Type	Commonly Used Examples*	Major Complications†
Caged-ball	*Starr-Edwards Magovern Smeloff-Cutter Braunwald-Cutter	Systemic embolism Prosthesis-chamber disproportion
Caged-disc	Beall Kay-Shiley Cross-Jones	Thrombosis Intrinsic stenosis
Tilting-disc	*Bjork-Shiley Lillehei-Kaster St. Jude (two half-discs)	Thrombosis (Insufficient data on St. Jude)
Tissue	*Hancock *Carpentier-Edwards Ionescu-Shiley	Calcification and degeneration

*Currently the most prevalent valves.

†All valves are subject to endocarditis. Adequate anticoagulation is required with all mechanical valves and with tissue valves if the patient has atrial fibrillation, especially if the valve is in the mitral position;[28] under these conditions there is no significant difference in the rate of systemic embolization among the valves.[34, 43]

Table 11–5. MAJOR COMPLICATIONS OF PROSTHETIC CARDIAC VALVES

A. Usually requiring valve re-replacement
   1. *Valve thrombosis
   2. *Endocarditis
   3. *Mechanical prosthesis component failure
   4. Tissue valve calcification and degeneration
B. Sometimes requiring valve re-replacement
   1. *Systemic emboli
   2. Paravalvular leak not due to endocarditis
C. Rarely requiring valve re-replacement
   1. Hemolysis and cholelithiasis
   2. Intrinsic stenosis
   3. Prosthesis-chamber disproportion

*Complications that typically present acutely and require emergency diagnosis and management.

Several problems are common to all prostheses, particularly endocarditis. In addition, all prostheses are intrinsically stenotic, with average areas one half of or less than that of the native valves.[43] Prosthesis-chamber disproportion (see below) can be found with any prosthesis and contributes to stenosis.[48] Tissue valves appear to become increasingly stenotic with time after implantation. Durability is better with mechanical prostheses, but component failure includes ball or disc swelling or fracture (with resultant sticking or escape, respectively), strut fracture, and cloth wear. Significant hemolysis may accompany the wearing of cloth-covered Starr-Edwards prostheses.

Any prosthesis may be complicated by paravalvular leak producing aortic or mitral regurgitation. This problem is due to disruption of sutures between the prosthesis sewing ring and the valve anulus. Suture dehiscence can be spontaneous or a consequence of infective endocarditis. Spontaneous suture disruption usually occurs early after surgery, but it may be unrecognized until it progresses later and the murmur becomes louder. This feature serves to emphasize the requirement to perform and record very careful cardiac examinations in the immediate postoperative period. As expected, spontaneous suture disruption is more common when running sutures are used, and when the tissue of the valve anulus is pathologic, as with infective endocarditis, a heavily calcified mitral anulus or aortic root, or myxomatous degeneration. Significant hemolysis may accompany paravalvular leaks. A paravalvular leak should be considered if there is evidence for significant hemolysis in the patient with a tissue valve, since these valves are the least likely to damage red cells.

The caged-ball valve has a long record of durability and acceptable hemodynamics. Systemic emboli are a persistent and significant problem, as with all mechanical prostheses on anticoagulants and with tissue valves not on anticoagulants. Earlier valves (Braunwald-Cutter and pre-1967 Starr-Edwards) had silicone poppets that could degenerate, with swelling and sticking or loss from the cage. To reduce embolism, the metal struts of the older Starr-Edwards valves (series 1000/1200/1260 aortic and 6000/6120 mitral) were covered with cloth (series 2300/2400 aortic, 6300/6400 mitral). To minimize the problem of cloth wear, which can aggravate hemolysis or interfere with valve function, later models had a non–cloth-covered metal track on the inside of the struts. However, the 1260 and 6120 models are presently in common use. The caged ball is a bulky valve, and the apparatus can be too large for the aorta or ventricle (prosthesis-chamber disproportion). For example, a caged ball inserted for correction of mitral stenosis may obstruct the outflow tract of the nondilated left ventricle.

Although no prosthesis is immune to prosthesis-chamber disproportion,[49] disc valves with lower profiles were developed to minimize the problem. However, the caged-disc valve has proved undesirable because of thrombosis and unacceptable intrinsic stenosis,[48] as well as component malfunction. Tilting-disc valves have acceptable hemodynamics and are in wide use. The incidence of systemic emboli is similar to that of the caged-ball valves.[34] Thrombosis of the tilting disc is a major problem.

Tissue valves were introduced in an effort to avoid the need for anticoagulation, and include glutaraldehyde-fixed porcine heterografts mounted on a flexible stent (Hancock, Carpentier-Edwards) and bovine pericardium mounted on a perforated stent (Ionescu-Shiley). In general, anticoagulation can be discontinued three months after implantation, subsequent rates of embolism being similar to those of mechanical valves with anticoagulation. Unfortunately, anticoagulation is required for patients with atrial fibrillation, particularly when the tissue valve is in the mitral position.[28] Initial hemodynamics are satisfactory. The major problem with tissue valves is calcification and degeneration, with the progressive development of stenosis or regurgitation. Valve re-replacement may be required in a high proportion of patients after five to ten years.[45,49] Unfortunately, the process of valve deterioration appears to be accelerated in young patients.

Approach to Patients with Prosthetic Valves

If the patient is asymptomatic, the major requirement is to ensure that anticoagulation is adequate and that the patient has been advised regarding endocarditis prophylaxis. The physical examination should be carefully recorded. Normal auscultatory findings with the various prostheses have been summarized in Table 11–6.[61] The variability of normal findings among prostheses and with the same prosthesis should be noted. Opening sounds are not commonly heard with tilting discs, since the disc does not strike any metal structure when it opens. Although a diastolic rumble may be recorded by phonocardiography in patients with a normally functioning tilting disc in the mitral position,[61] an audible diastolic murmur should raise suspicion of valve thrombosis.[39] The presence of an opening sound ("opening snap") and diastolic rumble in asymptomatic patients with tissue valves in the mitral position presumably reflects progression of the usual prosthesis stenosis as this valve calcifies. In general, the intrinsic stenosis of prosthetic mitral valves (a resting gradient of about 5 mm Hg) does not produce a diastolic murmur. In contrast, the intrinsic stenosis of prosthetic aortic valves (resting gradient about 15 mm Hg) does result in a systolic murmur. Turbulent flow probably contributes to this murmur. Mitral prostheses also produce a systolic ejection–type murmur, most likely due to projection of the apparatus into the left ventricular outflow tract. In addition, a trace of regurgitation can often be demonstrated angiographically, reflecting the inertia of valve closure, and this regurgitation may contribute to the systolic murmur with mitral prostheses.[23] Careful examination in the asymptomatic patient may detect a hemodynamically insignificant lesion, e.g., a spontaneous paravalvular leak, or the early signs of an ultimately catastrophic complication, e.g., thrombosis of a Bjork-Shiley valve.

If the patient presents with congestive failure, chest pain, syncope, fever, or systemic embolism, immediate and thorough evaluation is mandatory to check for the complications outlined in Table 11–5. Fever may signify endocarditis, as dicussed below. Systemic embolism may indicate endocarditis or a significant lesion of the prosthesis, or may be an isolated occurrence; its management is outlined subsequently. The differential diagnosis in the patient with congestive failure, chest pain, or syncope is prosthesis disease and/or "natural" disease: i.e., ventricular dysfunction, myocardial ischemia, or uncorrected valve lesions. The most common and most difficult differential diagnosis in the patient who fails to improve after valve replacement or who later develops congestive failure is between prosthesis malfunction and impaired left ventricular function. Myocardial failure may be a consequence of long-standing pressure or volume overload, intraoperative damage, or intercurrent myocardial ischemia. Recognition that the basic problem is muscle disease, rather than prosthesis dysfunction, may be very difficult, even with cardiac catheterization and left ventric-

Table 11–6. NORMAL AUSCULTATION OF PROSTHETIC VALVES

	Valve Type		
	Ball	***Disc***	***Tissue***
Aortic Position			
Opening sound (EC)	Loud	Unusual with tilting-disc Common with caged-disc	Rare
SEM	2/6	2/6	2/6
Closing sound (S2)	Loud	Usual	Usual
Diastolic murmur	No	No	No
Mitral Position			
Closing sound (S1)	Loud	Usual	Usual
SEM	2/6	2/6	2/6
Opening sound (OS)	Loud	Unusual with tilting-disc Common with caged-disc	Present in 50%
Diastolic murmur	No	No	Present in 50%

EC = ejection click; S1 and S2 = first and second heart sounds.
SEM = systolic ejection–type murmur; OS = opening snap; 2/6 = murmur of intensity grade 2 of 6.

ular angiography. For example, abnormal loading conditions induced by valve malfunction may simulate ventricular failure as estimated by depressed ejection fraction.

Recognition of malfunction of a prosthesis may be possible with combined physical examination, echophonocardiography, and cinefluoroscopy. Echophonocardiography is potentially very useful,[18] but false-positive and false-negative results are not uncommon. In one report of 118 reoperated cases, echophonocardiograms were considered abnormal preoperatively in only 50 per cent, and diagnostic findings were often apparent only in retrospect.[14] Another study compared noninvasive techniques with catheterization findings in the evaluation of 81 patients with Bjork-Shiley aortic or mitral or Beall mitral prostheses.[39] Auscultation was found to be more sensitive and specific than echophonocardiography or cinefluoroscopy. Almost all cases of malfunction were detected by the presence of one or more of the following criteria: (1) loss of previously audible opening or closing prosthetic valve clicks; (2) with aortic prostheses, an aortic regurgitation murmur of at least grade 2/6; or (3) with mitral prostheses, a diastolic rumble of mitral stenosis or a holosystolic murmur of mitral regurgitation of at least grade 2/6.[39]

Consideration of the most likely complications (Table 11–4) and correct interpretation of auscultation (Table 11–6) depend on knowledge of the type of valve. When this historical data is lacking, the radiographic appearance is most useful, and a comprehensive guide for valve identification on chest radiograph has been published.[37] Cinefluoroscopy may detect abnormal rocking of a prosthesis with suture dehiscence,[69] but 60 to 75 per cent of the suture line must be detached. Fluoroscopy may also demonstrate abnormal motion of a radiopaque poppet or disc.

With all these noninvasive techniques, a single study may not be diagnostic because of normal variability. It may therefore be appropriate to perform baseline noninvasive studies postoperatively. A difficulty with this approach is that prosthetic valve motion may vary with myocardial contractility, loading conditions, and conduction pattern, just as with native valves.

Cardiac catheterization with very careful measurement of pressure gradients and cardiac output, and with left ventricular or aortic angiography, may be required when the clinical picture is not clear and there is a potential need for prosthesis re-replacement. This procedure should be carried out to obtain a diagnosis in the patient who fails to improve after surgery or who later manifests clinical-hemodynamic deterioration. The yield of correctable abnormalities in cases selected on this basis appears to be high enough to warrant invasive study,[42] even though measurement of the gradient across an aortic prosthesis may require puncture of the left ventricle or interatrial septum. Correctable abnormalities are most likely to be found in the patient who has deteriorated acutely.

The difficulties just reviewed in the general diagnosis of prosthetic valve complications reinforce the view that original valve replacement should be very carefully thought out. In the following sections, we review certain specific problems and their management.

Prosthetic Valve Endocarditis

Infection complicates the course of 1 to 2 per cent of patients with prostheses, being somewhat more common with multiple and aortic valves than with mitral. It is a serious emergency complication, with case-fatality rates averaging about 60 per cent in a summary of 18 reports.[36] Prosthetic valve endocarditis typically presents as does infection of native valves, with fever (over 95% of cases), a new murmur (about 50%), leukocytosis (50%), and positive blood cultures (85%).[36] Negative cultures are more common in patients receiving antibiotics, in Q-fever endocarditis, in fungal endocarditis (in which diagnosis may be made from examination of embolic material), and in endocarditis occurring within two months after surgery (early endocarditis). The most common organisms differ, depending on the time after operation.[15, 60] Infections during the first two months are most commonly due to *Staphylococcus epidermidis* (about 30%), *S. aureus* (20%), and aerobic gram-negative bacilli (20%), with diphtheroids and *Candida* or *Aspergillus* contributing 10 per cent each. The microbiology of late infections (more than two months postoperatively) is more similar to that of native endocarditis, with the prevalence of *Streptococcus viridans* (about 25%) and group D streptococci (10%) suggesting seeding from transient bacteremia with dental, genitourinary, and gastrointestinal procedures. However, many cases of late endocarditis are caused by *S. epidermidis* (about 26%), *S. aureus* (10%), and gram-negative rods and fungi (15%), raising the possibility of delayed appearance of infection acquired in the perioperative period.[36] The site of infection is usually an abscess around the sewing ring, except in the case of tissue valves, where the leaflets may be involved.[49] The site of infection explains why paravalvular leaks producing regurgitation are common and why vegetations are difficult to detect by echocardiography. Vegetations may spread onto the valve apparatus and impede its motion, producing stenosis; this is more common with mitral than with aortic prostheses.[2] The occurrence of systemic emboli is very variable (5 to 50% of cases).[36] Other peripheral stigmata of classic subacute endocarditis are infrequent, and cardiopulmonary bypass may cause conjunctival petechiae that persist for up to ten days.[70] The noninvasive techniques previously discussed may point to malfunction of the prosthesis. However, the suspicion of infection is based on the other clinical data mentioned.

Once the diagnosis has been considered and three blood cultures have been drawn over several hours, therapy should be begun with two agents, maintaining trough bactericidal levels of 1:8 or more. The combination of cephalothin (2 gm every four hours) and tobramycin (1.5 mg/kg every eight hours) has been recommended when the organism is unknown.[36]

The stable patient with prosthetic valve endocarditis should be treated for four to six weeks with appropriate parenteral antibiotics. If congestive failure caused by the prosthesis infection is not easily controlled or if it appears during therapy, immediate reoperation is indicated, with continuation of antibiotics in the postoperative period. Early surgical intervention should be carefully considered in the presence of the following risk factors for a poor outcome with medical therapy alone:[29, 36] congestive heart failure, paravalvular leak with regurgitant murmur, multiple systemic emboli, endocarditis within two months after operation, infection of an aortic or mechanical prosthesis, endocarditis not due to streptococci, fever lasting longer than ten days, and persistent or recurrent bacteremia. Conversely, patients with late-onset, uncomplicated streptococcal endocarditis, particularly of a tissue valve in the mitral position, may be most likely to have a successful outcome with medical therapy alone.[36] A more extensive discussion of specific antimicrobial therapy for infected prostheses may be found in Chapter 12.

A decision about anticoagulant management is difficult in the patient with an infected prosthesis.[29] Central nervous system embolization may result if anticoagulants are discontinued, and anticoagulation can result in hemorrhage with an emboli vegetation. It is the practice of many cardiologists carefully to maintain the prothrombin time at the lower part of the therapeutic range, i.e., at about 1.5 times the control value. This problem has been reviewed,[71] with the finding that CNS complications were much less common in patients with prothrombin times at least 1.5 times normal than in those with prosthetic endocarditis and either no or inadequate anticoagulation. If a CNS complication occurs, anticoagulants can be discontinued for three days and then restarted if there is no evidence of intracranial hemorrhage.[71]

Systemic Embolism

Systemic embolism is a distressingly frequent complication. In a 10- to 19-year follow-up of 300 patients with non–cloth-covered prostheses, 40 per cent had an embolic event after 15 years and approximately 10 per cent had recurrent emboli.[19] Of all emboli, most were cerebral, 50 per cent left a neurologic deficit, and 10 per cent were fatal. Embolic rates with current mechanical prostheses in adequately anticoagulated patients are 1 to 3 per cent per patient-year for aortic prostheses and 3 to 5 per cent per patient-year for mitral prostheses. Rates are similar with tissue valves without anticoagulants, unless there is atrial fibrillation, which greatly increases the rate, particularly with mitral prostheses.[28] The main risk factor for embolism, besides atrial fibrillation, appears to be inadequate anticoagulation. For example, with mitral Starr-Edwards prostheses, the embolic rate was doubled with inadequate anticoagulation (prothrombin time less than 1.5 times control). With aortic prostheses, the increase in emboli in poorly anticoagulated patients was less impressive (30%). It is possible that platelets are more important in emboli from aortic prostheses, whereas red cell–fibrin clots are present with mitral prostheses.[19]

Most systemic emboli are isolated events, but they can be associated with endocarditis, valve thrombosis, or component failure. If clinical evaluation of the patient with an embolus reveals no evidence of prosthesis dysfunction, cardiac catheterization is not generally indicated. A potential complication after cerebral embolization in the patient on anticoagulation is the development of a hemorrhagic infarct. Some authors have discussed stopping anticoagulants for ten days.[43] Others point to the likelihood of early recurrence of cerebral emboli and suggest that the patient be anticoagulated immediately with heparin, if there is no blood in the cerebrospinal fluid and no hematoma on CT scan.[17] Warfarin can subsequently be adjusted to maintain a prothrombin time of at least twice normal. Following an embolic event, the anticoagulation history should be carefully reviewed and consideration should be given to adding an antiplatelet agent to warfarin therapy. Some authorities recommend the routine use of this combination.[19] If there is recurrent embolization despite these measures, replacement of a mechanical prosthesis with a tissue valve can reduce the likelihood of subsequent emboli. Antiplatelet agents alone do not prevent emboli with mechanical valves. Therefore, anticipated inability to maintain adequate anticoagulation is a relative contraindication to implantation of a mechanical prosthesis. In women who plan to become pregnant, it may be appropriate to use a tissue valve to avoid the requirement to switch from warfarin to heparin during pregnancy; the problem with this approach is the high likelihood that the tissue valve will have to be re-replaced in these young women.[31, 45]

Management of the patient with a prosthesis who must undergo general surgery also presents special problems. Attention must be given to endocarditis prophylaxis. As for anticoagulation, several groups have found that the risk of hemorrhagic or embolic complications is very low if anticoagulation is stopped for one to three days before the procedure and restarted one to seven days afterward.[64] This procedure may be too dangerous with the Bjork-Shiley prosthesis, with its risk of thrombosis after short discontinuation of anticoagulants. In this case, heparin can be given after warfarin is discontinued. Heparin is then stopped a few hours before surgery and restarted as soon as possible afterward.[72]

Valve Thrombosis

Thrombosis can occur on any prosthesis. In the past it was a problem with caged-disc valves, and at present it is a major complication associated with the Bjork-Shiley tilting-disc valve. In one report, the incidence was 3 per cent at four years for aortic Bjork-Shiley prostheses and 13 per cent for mitral or double valves.[30] The true incidence may be higher, since this complication may produce sudden death. Thrombosis of the Bjork-Shiley valve is the most acute and life-threatening emergency caused by prosthetic valves in current use.

Thrombosis involves the valve hinge mechanism and obliterates the minor aperture. The tilting disc is fixed at a partially open angle, and there is both stenosis and regurgitation. Valves in the mitral position are more commonly involved than are aortic prostheses. Atrial fibrillation probably contributes additional risk. Introduction of a convexo-concave disc has not eliminated the problem. The main risk factor for thrombosis is inadequate anticoagulation, perhaps for even a brief period. Therefore, it has been suggested that heparin be used whenever warfarin must be temporarily discontinued (see above).

Reported patients have generally presented acutely and critically ill with respiratory distress and, in some cases, ischemic or pleuritic chest pain.[12] Syncope may occur with the sudden reduction of cardiac output. Systemic emboli are unusual. The thrombotic process appears to progress extremely rapidly, and patients have expired while undergoing diagnostic evaluation.

The diagnosis should be strongly suspected on the basis of the clinical presentation. There may be a new murmur of aortic regurgitation or mitral stenosis, but a new murmur is not always present, possibly because blood flow is diffuse through the thrombosed prosthesis.[12] Previously audible prosthetic sounds usually diminish or disappear, but there is variability in the auscultation of a properly functioning prosthesis (Table 11–6). If clinical evaluation raises the question of valve thrombosis, the most useful diagnostic method is fluoroscopy to show limited motion or fixation of the disc. Since 1975, there has been a radiopaque marker in the disc to facilitate visualization. High-resolution fluoroscopy may document excursion of a radiolucent disc; 33,000 of these were issued between 1971 and 1977.[46] Catheterization is usually unnecessary and is excessively time-consuming. If fluoroscopy shows impaired disc motion in the proper clinical setting, the patient should be taken immediately to surgery for thrombus removal or, more commonly, valve re-replacement, advisedly with a different prosthesis. Patients with thrombosis of a Bjork-Shiley prosthesis in the tricuspid position may have a less life-threatening course, and thrombolytic therapy may prove to be useful.[72] It appears that this prosthesis should not be implanted if constant, adequate anticoagulation cannot be confidently anticipated.

Paravalvular Leak and Hemolysis

Paravalvular regurgitation may be caused by endocarditis or may be due to spontaneous suture dehiscence. The former may present acutely, whereas the latter generally does not. The patient with paravalvular leak without congestive failure or evidence of infection can be followed without surgery. Periprosthetic regurgitation may significantly aggravate the intravascular hemolysis seen with mechanical prostheses. Paravalvular leak should be suspected if hemolysis is present in a patient with a tissue valve. Therapy with iron and folate may be necessary to prevent anemia. Iron replacement is necessary because iron is lost in the urine with the intravascular hemolytic process, and folate requirements are increased by the chronic hemolysis. Significant hemolysis in the absence of a paravalvular leak is most common in patients with cloth-covered, caged-ball prostheses in the aortic position, particularly when there is cloth tear.

References

1. American Heart Association Report on Prevention of Bacterial Endocarditis. Circulation 56:139A, 1977.
2. Arnett, E. N., and Roberts, W. C.: Prosthetic valve endocarditis. Am. J. Cardiol. 38:281, 1976.
3. Black, S., O'Rourke, R. A., and Karliner, J. S.: Role of surgery in the treatment of primary infective endocarditis. Am. J. Med. 56:357, 1974.
4. Braunwald, E.: Mitral regurgitation. N. Engl. J. Med. 281:425, 1969.
5. Bristow, J. D., and Kremkau, E. L.: Hemodynamic changes after valve replacement with Starr-Edwards prostheses. Am. J. Cardiol. 35:716, 1975.
6. Brown, O. R., Popp, R. L., and Kloster, F. E.: Echocardiographic criteria for aortic root dissection. Am. J. Cardiol. 36:17, 1975.
7. Buckberg, G., Eber, L., Herman, M., et al.: Ischemia in aortic stenosis: hemodynamic prediction. Am. J. Cardiol. 35:778, 1975.
8. Caulfield, J. B., Page, D. L., Kastor, J. A., et al.: Connective tissue abnormalities in spontaneous rupture of chordae tendineae. Arch. Pathol. 91:537, 1971.
9. Cheitlin, M., Gertz, E., Brundage, B., et al.: Rate of progression of severity of valvular aortic stenosis in the adult. Am. Heart J. 98:689, 1979.
10. Cheng, T. O., Bashour, T., and Adkins, P. C.: Acute severe mitral regurgitation from papillary muscle dysfunction in acute myocardial infarction. Circulation 46:491, 1972.
11. Cohn, L. H., Koster, J. K., Jr., Vande Vanter, S., and Collins, J. J., Jr.: The in-hospital risk of re-replacement of dysfunctional mitral and aortic valves. Circulation 66 (Suppl. 1):I-153, 1982.
12. Copans, H., Lakier, J. B., Kinsley, R. H., et al.: Thrombosed Bjork-Shiley mitral prosthesis. Circulation 61:169, 1980.
13. Corrigall, D., Bolen, J., Hancock, E. W., et al.: Mitral valve prolapse and infective endocarditis. Am. J. Med. 63:215, 1977.
14. Cunha, C. L. P., Giuliani, E. R., Callahan, J. A., and Pluth, J. R.: Echophonocardiographic findings in patients with prosthetic heart valve malfunction. Mayo Clin. Proc. 55:231, 1980.
15. Dismukes, W. E., Karchmer, A. W., Buckley, M. J., et al.: Prosthetic valve endocarditis. Circulation 48:365, 1973.
16. Dodek, A., Kassebaum, D. G., and Bristow, J. D.: Pulmonary edema in coronary artery disease without cardiomegaly: a paradox of the stiff heart. N. Engl. J. Med. 286:1347, 1972.
17. Easton, J. D., and Sherman, D. G.: Management of cerebral embolism of cardiac origin. Prog. Cerebrovasc. Dis. 11:433, 1980.
18. Feigenbaum, H.: Echocardiography, 2nd ed. Philadelphia, Lea & Febiger, 1976, pp. 199–213.
19. Fuster, V., Pumphrey, C. W., McGoon, M. D., et al.: Systemic thromboembolism in mitral and aortic Starr-Edwards prostheses: a 10–19 year follow-up. Circulation 66 (Suppl. I): I-157, 1982.
20. Goldschlager, N., Pfeifer, J., Cohn, K., et al.: The natural history of aortic regurgitation. Am. J. Med. 54:577, 1973.
21. Goodman, D., Kimbiris, D., and Linhart, J. W.: Chordae tendineae rupture complicating the systolic click–late systolic murmur syndrome. Am. J. Cardiol. 33:681, 1974.
22. Griffin, F. M., Jr., Jones, G., and Cobbs, C. G.: Aortic insufficiency in bacterial endocarditis. Ann. Intern. Med. 76:23, 1972.
23. Harthorne, J. W.: Case Records of the Massachusetts General Hospital. N. Engl. J. Med. 297:37, 1977.
24. Hoffman, J. I. E., and Buckberg, G. D.: Pathophysiology of subendocardial ischaemia. Br. Med. J. 11:76, 1975.
25. Humphries, W. C., Jr., Hammer, W. J., Mc-

Donough, M. T., et al.: Echocardiographic equivalents of a flail mitral leaflet. Am. J. Cardiol. 40:802, 1977.
26. Hutter, A. M., DeSanctis, R. W., Nathan, M. J., et al.: Aortic valve surgery as an emergency procedure. Circulation 41:623, 1970.
27. Jackson, D. H., and Murphy, G. W.: Nonpenetrating cardiac trauma. Mod. Concepts Cardiovasc. Dis. 45:123, 1976.
28. Jamieson, W. R., Janusz, M. T., Migagishima, R. T., et al.: Embolic complications of porcine heterograft cardiac valves. J. Thorac. Cardiovasc. Surg. 81:626, 1981.
29. Karchmer, A. W., Dismukes, W. E., Buckley, M. J., et al.: Late prosthetic valve endocarditis. Am. J. Med. 64:199, 1978.
30. Karp, R. B., Cyrus, R. J., Blackstone, E. H., et al.: The Bjork-Shiley valve, intermediate-term follow-up. J. Thorac. Cardiovasc. Surg. 81:602, 1981.
31. Kirklin, J. W.: The replacement of cardiac valves. N. Engl. J. Med. 304:291, 1981.
32. Kloster, F. E.: Diagnosis and management of complications of prosthetic heart valves. Am. J. Cardiol. 35:872, 1975.
33. Leachman, R. D., and Cokkinos, D. V. P.: Absence of opening click in dehiscence of mitral-valve prosthesis. N. Engl. J. Med. 281:461, 1964.
34. Macmanus, Q., Grunkemeier, G. L., Lambert, L. E., et al.: Year of operation as a risk factor in the late results of valve replacement. J. Thorac. Cardiovasc. Surg. 80:834, 1980.
35. Mann, T., McLaurin, L., Grossman, W., et al.: Assessing the hemodynamic severity of acute aortic regurgitation due to infective endocarditis. N. Engl. J. Med. 293:108, 1975.
36. Mayer, K. H., and Schoenbaum, S. C.: Evaluation and management of prosthetic valve endocarditis. Prog. Cardiovasc. Dis. 25:43, 1982.
37. Mehlman, D. J., and Resnekov, L.: A guide to the radiographic identification of prosthetic heart valves. Circulation 57:613, 1978.
38. Miller, R. R., Vismara, L. A., DeMaria, A. N., et al.: Afterload reduction therapy with nitroprusside in severe aortic regurgitation: improved cardiac performance and reduced regurgitant volume. Am. J. Cardiol. 38:564, 1976.
39. Mintz, G. S., Carlson, E. B., and Kotler, M. N.: Comparison of noninvasive techniques in evaluation of the nontissue cardiac valve prosthesis. Am. J. Cardiol. 49:39, 1982.
40. Moothart, R. W., Spangler, R. D., and Blount, S. G., Jr.: Echocardiography in aortic root dissection and dilatation. Am. J. Cardiol. 36:11, 1975.
41. Morganroth, J., Perloff, J. K., Zeldis, S. M., et al.: Acute severe aortic regurgitation. Ann. Intern. Med. 87:223, 1977.
42. Morton, M. J., McAnulty, J. H., Rahimtoola, S. H., et al.: Risks and benefits of postoperative cardiac catheterization in patients with ball valve prostheses. Am. J. Cardiol. 40:870, 1977.
43. Murphy, E. S., and Kloster, F. W.: Late results of valve replacement surgery. Mod. Concepts Cardiovasc. Dis. 48:53, 1979.
44. Nishimura, R. A., Schaff, H. V., Shub, C., et al.: Papillary muscle rupture complicating acute myocardial infarction: analysis of 17 patients. Am. J. Cardiol. 51:373, 1983.
45. Oakley, C. M.: Long-term complications of valve replacement. Br. Med. J. 284:995, 1982.
46. Olinger, G. N., Thompson, M. A., and Keelan, M. H., Jr.: Optimal management of suspected thrombosis of standard Bjork-Shiley unmarked tilting disc mitral valve prosthesis. Am. Heart J. 103:440, 1982.
47. Rahimtoola, S. H.: The problem of valve prosthesis-patient mismatch. Circulation 58:20, 1978.
48. Roberts, W. C.: Choosing a substitute cardiac valve: type, size, surgeon. Am. J. Cardiol. 38:633, 1976.
49. Roberts, W. C.: Complications of cardiac valve replacement: characteristic abnormalities of prostheses pertaining to any or specific sites. Am. Heart J. 103:113, 1982.
50. Roberts, W. C., and Perloff, J. K.: Mitral valvular disease. Ann. Intern. Med. 77:939, 1972.
51. Ronan, J. A., Jr., Steelman, R. B., DeLeon, A. C., Jr., et al.: The clinical diagnosis of acute severe mitral insufficiency. Am. J. Cardiol. 27:284, 1971.
52. Ross, J., Jr., and Braunwald, E.: Aortic stenosis. Circulation 37 and 38 (Suppl. V): 61, 1968.
53. Roy, P., Tajik, A. J., Giuliani, E. R., et al.: Spectrum of echocardiographic findings in bacterial endocarditis. Circulation 53:474, 1976.
54. Sanders, C. A., Austen, W. G., Harthorne, J. W., et al.: Diagnosis and surgical treatment of mitral regurgitation secondary to ruptured chordae tendineae. N. Engl. J. Med. 276:943, 1967.
55. Sanders, J. H., Jr., Cohn, L. H., Dalen, J. E., et al.: Emergency aortic valve replacement. Am. J. Surg. 131:495, 1976.
56. Selzer, A., and Cohn, K. E.: Natural history of mitral stenosis: a review. Circulation 45:878, 1972.
57. Selzer, A., Kelly, J. J., Jr., Kerth, W. J., et al.: Immediate and long range results of valvuloplasty for mitral regurgitation due to ruptured chordae tendineae. Circulation 46 and 47 (Suppl. I):52, 1972.
58. Selzer, A., Kelly, J. J., Jr., Vannitamby, M., et al.: The syndrome of mitral insufficiency due to isolated rupture of the chordae tendineae. Am. J. Med. 43:822, 1967.
59. Slater, E. E., and DeSanctis, R. W.: The clinical recognition of dissecting aortic aneurysm. Am. J. Med. 60:625, 1976.
60. Slaughter, L., Morris, J. E., and Starr, A.: Prosthetic valvular endocarditis. Circulation 47:1319, 1973.
61. Smith, N. D., Raizada, V., and Abrams, J.: Auscultation of the normally functioning prosthetic valve. Ann. Intern. Med. 95:594, 1981.
62. Stott, D. K., Marpole, D. G. F., Bristow, J. D., et al.: The role of left atrial transport in aortic and mitral stenosis. Circulation 41:1031, 1970.
63. Sweatman, T., Selzer, A., Kamagahi, M., et al.: Echocardiographic diagnosis of mitral regurgitation due to ruptured chordae tendineae. Circulation 46:580, 1972.
64. Tinker, J. H., and Tarhan, S.: Discontinuing anticoagulant therapy in surgical patients with cardiac valve prostheses: observations in 180 operations. J.A.M.A. 239:738, 1978.
65. Turley, K., Ullyot, D. J., Godwin, J. D., et al.: Repair of dissection of the thoracic aorta: evaluation of false lumen utilizing computed tomography. J. Thorac. Cardiovasc. Surg. 81:61, 1981.
66. Wann, L. S., Dillon, J. C., Weyman, A. E., et al.: Echocardiography in bacterial endocarditis. N. Engl. J. Med. 295:135, 1976.

67. Waxman, H. L., Myerburg, R. J., Appel, R., and Sung, R. J.: Verapamil for control of ventricular rate in paroxysmal supraventricular tachycardia and atrial fibrillation or flutter. Ann. Intern. Med. 94:1, 1981.
68. Wei, J. Y., Hutchins, G. M., and Buckley, B. H.: Papillary muscle rupture in fatal acute myocardial infarction: a potentially treatable form of cardiogenic shock. Ann. Intern. Med. 90:149, 1979.
69. White, A. F., Dinsmore, R. E., and Buckley, M. J.: Cineradiographic evaluation of prosthetic cardiac valves. Circulation 48:882, 1973.
70. Willerson, J. T., Moellering, R. C., Jr., Buckley, M. J., et al.: Conjunctival petechiae after open-heart surgery. N. Engl. J. Med. 284:539, 1971.
71. Wilson, W. R., Geraci, J. E., Danielson, G. K., et al.: Anticoagulant therapy and central nervous system complications in patients with prosthetic valve endocarditis. Circulation 57:1004, 1978.
72. Wright, J. O., Hiratzka, L. F., Brandt, B., III, and Doty, D. B.: Thrombosis of the Bjork-Shiley prosthesis. J. Thorac. Cardiovasc. Surg. 84:138, 1982.

12

Management of Infective Endocarditis and Its Complications

H. F. CHAMBERS

and JOHN MILLS

This chapter describes current opinion regarding the management of infective endocarditis and its complications. Before the availability of antimicrobial chemotherapy, the mortality rate for infective endocarditis was virtually 100 per cent. Despite antimicrobial therapy and sophisticated supportive care, mortality remains high, varying from 10 to 40 per cent in various series.[69,103,110] Death is most often caused by congestive heart failure and central nervous system complications. Further reduction in mortality requires coordination of information and advice from several consulting physicians, and skillful management of complications in patients with complex clinical courses.

PATHOGENESIS

Normal cardiac valves are quite resistant to infection even during high-grade bacteremia, but damaged or abnormal valves (from rheumatic heart disease, trauma, previous endocarditis, and possibly stress) are much more readily infected.[29,31,70,71,84] Infection is probably preceded by formation on the damaged valve of a sterile thrombus or "vegetation" composed of platelets and fibrin.[4,26] Bacteria in the blood stream (perhaps as a result of a dental or urologic procedure or from an infected intravenous catheter) attach to this thrombus and readily grow in this favorable environment. Once infection has set in, the vegetation grows by accretion of an outer layer of multiplying organisms, platelets, and fibrin over an inner layer of dead or metabolically inactive bacteria.[27] This vegetation easily fragments and embolizes to distant sites, and in chronic cases also stimulates a vigorous host-immune response.[3,35,49,58]

Once established, infection upon the valve is not affected by host defenses, probably because leukocytes cannot penetrate the overlying fibrin meshwork to reach bacteria within the vegetation. To be effective, therefore, antimicrobials must kill bacteria without assistance of host defenses (i.e., they must be bactericidal).

Infective endocarditis causes disease through four principal mechanisms: (1) destruction of valves and other cardiac or vascular structures causes valvular insufficiency, rhythm disturbances, fistulae, aneurysms, myocardial abscesses, and myocarditis; (2) persistent bacteremia establishes distant foci of infection in bones, joints, and vital organs; (3) systemic and pulmonary arterial embolism from the infected vegetation causes infarction of the brain, kidney, spleen, lung, or myocardium; (4) immune complexes formed in response to the infection deposit in blood vessels and are partly responsible for vasculitis, cutaneous manifestations, arthritis, and glomerulonephritis.

MANAGEMENT OF BACTEREMIA AND ITS COMPLICATIONS

Diagnosis of Septicemia

Diagnosis of endocarditis and subsequent therapy depend on recovery of the responsible organism, usually from blood cultures. Rarely, blood cultures are sterile and the organism is recovered from other sites (e.g., septic emboli).[99, 116] Since the bacteremia of endocarditis is continuous and on the order of 10 to 100 organisms per milliliter, three to five blood cultures recover the organism in approximately 95 per cent of cases, and all blood cultures are positive in 90 per cent or more.[33, 106, 111] Correspondingly, culture-negative endocarditis is uncommon (5–15% in published series but less than 5% in our recent experience) in the absence of previous antibiotic therapy and should raise suspicions of either nonbacterial or unusual bacterial etiologies.[18, 28, 73]

In patients with characteristic clinical findings (fever, underlying valvular disease, pathologic murmur, embolic phenomenon), blood cultures confirm the diagnosis. In patients without characteristic signs and symptoms of endocarditis, blood cultures that grow pathogens such as enterococci, viridans streptococci, or *Staphylococcus aureus* (recognized common causes of endocarditis) should prompt a search for signs of valvular infection.[67]

Septic Shock

Septic shock is rare in endocarditis because as a rule the concentration of bacteria in the blood is low, and gram-positive organisms predominate. However, acute endocarditis, caused by virulent organisms (e.g., *S. aureus*) or by gram-negative rods, may occasionally cause septic shock. Cardiogenic shock from myocardial infarction, ventricular septal defect, or acute valvular insufficiency is more common than septic shock in patients with endocarditis and must be differentiated from it. Shock due to septicemia typically is characterized by hypotension associated with a normal or high cardiac output, low systemic vascular resistance, and low pulmonary capillary wedge pressure.

In patients with shock and endocarditis, the blood pressure, urine output, level of consciousness, state of peripheral perfusion, and arterial blood pH should be monitored as guides to therapy. In the absence of evidence for a cardiogenic cause (e.g., signs of pulmonary congestion, low cardiac output, significant valvular or myocardial damage), 200 to 300 ml of normal saline or other isotonic electrolyte solution may be administered cautiously. Colloids (albumin, plasma substitutes) probably offer no special advantage over crystalloids, and the former in fact have been implicated in worsening noncardiogenic pulmonary edema.[91] Patients who promptly respond with improved perfusion, blood pressure, or urine output probably do not need more aggressive therapy. Those who fail to improve after judicious fluid resuscitation, who show signs of decreased perfusion, or who require vasopressors to maintain blood pressure should have a pulmonary arterial catheter positioned to measure cardiac output and wedge pressure. Vigorous fluid resuscitation in these patients without invasive monitoring techniques is ill advised because it risks the development of cardiogenic pulmonary edema from cardiac complications and noncardiogenic pulmonary edema from increased capillary permeability caused by shock states.[39, 94]

If blood pressure and urine output do not increase after fluids alone, an infusion of dopamine is begun, 2 μg per kg per minute. Other vasopressors are also effective. Dopamine is likewise useful in patients who have septic shock and low cardiac output. The dose is adjusted according to changes in blood pressure, cardiac output, and systemic vascular resistance but should not exceed 20 μg per kg per minute. In addition, arterial blood pH needs to be monitored for increasing metabolic acidosis, and the patient should be frequently examined for signs of ischemia of fingers and toes, especially when cardiac output remains below normal despite large doses of dopamine.

These supportive measures notwithstanding, the single most important step in the management of septic shock remains specific treatment of the infection by appropriate antibiotics. After cultures are obtained, antibiotics are selected on the basis of the clinical presentation and historical information.

Empiric Antimicrobial Therapy

Selection of empiric antimicrobial therapy depends on the duration and severity of the illness (acute, subacute, or chronic), the presence of other factors that adversely affect the outcome (e.g., aortic valvular infection, prosthetic valvular endocarditis), a history of recent antimicrobial therapy or previously treated endocarditis, and the certainty of diagnosis. Other historical information (e.g., the presence of rheumatic heart disease, a history of intravenous drug abuse) also helps in the choice of antimicrobials.

In the setting of acute endocarditis, antibiotics must be started before results of blood cultures become available so that further valvular destruction and clinical deterioration are prevented (Table 12–1). Acute endocarditis is most often caused by virulent organisms such as *S. aureus,* Group A streptococci, pneumococci, and *Neisseria gonorrhoeae,* although organisms typically associated with subacute endocarditis (e.g., viridans streptococci and enterococci) may cause an acute syndrome.[6, 49, 103] A beta-lactamase–resistant antibiotic, such as nafcillin, cephalothin, or vancomycin, should be given in combination with an aminoglycoside, such as tobramycin or gentamicin. This combination is synergistic in vitro for most of the likely pathogens, and more rapidly sterilizes vegetations than a single agent in experimental infections.[85, 86] Since the combination of a beta-lactamase–resistant penicillin or cephalosporin and an aminoglycoside is not effective for enterococci, penicillin G should be added.[2, 37, 53]

In cases of subacute endocarditis, therapy may safely be delayed until the blood cultures have shown growth, which usually occurs within two to three days. Therapy may justifiably be withheld for even longer in patients who have a clinical syndrome of endocarditis but who have recently received antibiotics, who are being evaluated for apparent relapse, or who already have a diagnosis of

Table 12–1. THERAPEUTIC REGIMENS FOR PATIENTS WITH ENDOCARDITIS BEFORE CULTURE RESULTS ARE KNOWN

Clinical Setting	Likely Pathogen	Therapy*
Acute endocarditis	*Staphylococcus aureus* Group A streptococcus *Streptococcus pneumoniae* Enterococcus	Penicillin G 2 mU q4h IV *and* Nafcillin 1.5 gm q4h IV *or* Vancomycin 500 mg q6hIV *plus* Gentamicin 1 mg/kg q8h IV *or* IM
Subacute endocarditis	Streptococcus Enterococcus	Penicillin 2 mU q4h IV *or* Ampicillin 1.5 gm q4h IV *or* Vancomycin 500 mg q6h IV *plus* Gentamicin 1 mg/kg q8h IV *or* IM
Prosthetic valve endocarditis	*Staphylococcus epidermidis* *Staphylococcus aureus* Streptococcus Gram-negative rod	Vancomycin 500 mg q6h IV *plus* Gentamicin 1 mg/kg q8h IV *or* IM *plus* Rifampin 300 mg q12h PO
Endocarditis in a parenteral drug user†	*Staphylococcus aureus* Streptococcus Enterococcus *Pseudomonas*	Nafcillin 1.5 gm q4h IV *or* Vancomycin 500 mg q6h IV *plus* Gentamicin 1 mg/kg q8h IV *or* IM

*Doses are for 70-kg adult with normal renal function.

†Vancomycin and gentamicin are preferred if methicillin-resistant *S. aureus* or enterococcus occur regionally. If *Pseudomonas* endocarditis is a possibility, ticarcillin 3 gm q4h IV should be added to the regimen.

culture-negative endocarditis. In these situations, antimicrobials begun prematurely may preclude recovery of the responsible organism and greatly complicate subsequent management. In other cases of subacute endocarditis, particularly when the diagnosis seems well established on clinical grounds and while culture results are pending, therapy may be started with either penicillin or vancomycin in combination with gentamicin.

Endocarditis of prosthetic valves, especially within two months of operation, is a special situation because *Staphylococcus epidermidis* and *S. aureus* are common pathogens and the outcome is worse than in native valve infections.[25, 46] *S. epidermidis* is often resistant to numerous antibiotics, particularly to beta-lactams; thus, vancomycin is the drug of choice.[7] Some evidence suggests that addition of an aminoglycoside or rifampin to vancomycin is more effective than single-agent therapy.[44]

Intravenous drug abusers are commonly infected with *S. aureus,* and thus the drug chosen must be effective against this organism.[48] Since 1980, an outbreak of methicillin-resistant *S. aureus* has been reported in addicts from Detroit. In cases in which this pathogen is likely, vancomycin is preferred. In addition, some centers report a high prevalence of other unusual pathogens such as *Pseudomonas, Serratia,* or enterococci.[60, 76] Initial therapy in most cases need not be directed against these organisms unless they are known to be present in a particular location.

Definitive Antimicrobial Therapy

Once the organism and results of susceptibility tests are known, therapy is altered accordingly (Table 12–2). For reasons discussed elsewhere, only bactericidal drugs should be used and these are given at high dose for four to six weeks. Bacteriostatic or weakly bactericidal drugs such as clindamycin are less consistently effective than fully bactericidal drugs and should be used only for patients who cannot tolerate standard therapy.[16, 30]

Culture-negative endocarditis should be managed as enterococcal endocarditis after other causes have been excluded (Table 12–3).[49] Every attempt should be made to identify the infective agent. Nutritionally deficient streptococci may grow if thiols or other nutrients are added to the culture media.[56] *Brucella* species may require three or more weeks to grow in blood culture.[18] Serologic testing helps to confirm endocarditis caused by *Brucella,* fungi, rickettsiae or chlamydiae. Endocarditis from these organisms, with the exception of *Candida* species, are rarely diagnosed by blood culture.[81] Since these infections are often complicated by major artery embolism and progressive valvular destruction, surgery is often necessary; any operative specimens, including arterial emboli, should be examined and cultured for fungi and other unusual pathogens.

Guidelines to Antimicrobial Therapy

Susceptibility testing helps to determine the best drug(s) for a particular infection. Selection may be based on disc diffusion tests initially, but determination of the minimal inhibitory concentration (MIC) and the minimal lethal or bactericidal concentration (MLC or MBC) is preferable because of the need for bactericidal drugs. In brief, the MIC is that concentration of antibiotic which inhibits visible growth (i.e., no turbidity) in the test tube of a standard inoculum of bacteria (usually 10^5 colony-forming units per ml).[107] The MBC is that concentration which kills 99.9 per cent more of the original inoculum.[5] The MIC and MBC for a number of drugs should be determined in all cases. Even viridans streptococci, usually exquisitely sensitive to penicillin, should be tested because some strains require up to 4 μg per ml of penicillin for inhibition of growth, and may not be killed by even higher concentrations of penicillin.[12]

The next step is to document that peak concentrations in the patient's serum are sufficient to kill the organism. Two methods are commonly used and either is satisfactory. In one, serum is assayed for antimicrobial concentration to document that serum levels exceed by several-fold the MBC of the infecting organism. In the other, serum drawn from the patient during antimicrobial therapy is directly tested to determine the highest dilution that kills the organism. This serum bactericidal test (SBT), or Schlichter test,[90] is a tube-dilution test in which twofold serial dilutions of serum (usually obtained at a time when peak antibiotic levels are anticipated)

Table 12–2. THERAPEUTIC REGIMENS FOR ENDOCARDITIS OF KNOWN ETIOLOGY

Gram-Positive Organisms	Antibiotic Regimen*	Duration (Weeks)
Viridans streptococci	1. Penicillin G 2 mU q4h IV	4
	2. Procaine penicillin 1.2 mU q6h IM	2–4
	or Penicillin G 2mU q4h IV *plus*	2–4
	Streptomycin 500 mg q12h IM	2
	3. Vancomycin 500 mg q6h IV	4
	4. Cephalothin 2 gm q4h IV	4
Enterococcus§	1. Penicillin G 2.5 mU q4h IV	4–6
	or Ampicillin 1.5 gm q4h IV *plus either*	4–6
	Streptomycin 1 gm q12h IM	2
	then 500 mg q12h IM	2–4
	or Gentamicin 1 mg/kg q8h IV	4–6
	2. Vancomycin 500 mg q6h IV *plus either*	4–6
	Streptomycin 500 mg q12h IM	4–6
	or Gentamicin 1 mg/kg q8h IV *or* IM	4–6
Staphylococcus aureus†	1. Nafcillin 1.5 gm q4h IV	4
	2. Vancomycin 500 mg q6h IV	4
	3. Cephalothin 2 gm q4h IV	4
	4. Nafcillin 1.5 gm q4h IV *plus*	4
	Gentamicin 1 mg/kg IV *or* IM	1
Staphylococcus epidermidis	1. Vancomycin 500 mg q6h IV *plus*	6
	Gentamicin 1 mg/kg q8h IV *or* IM *plus*	2
	Rifampin 300 mg q12h PO	6
	2. Penicillin 2.5 mU q4h IV	6
	or Nafcillin 1.5 gm q4h IV	6
	or Cephalothin 2 gm q4h IV *plus*	6
	Gentamicin 1 mg/kg q8h IM *or* IV *plus*	2
	Rifampin 300 mg q12h PO	6
Streptococcus pneumoniae	1. Penicillin 2.5 mU q4h IV	4
	2. Cephalothin 2 gm q4h IV	4
	3. Vancomycin 500 mg q6h IV	4
Gram-Negative Organisms		
Pseudomonas	1. Ticarcillin 3 gm q4h IV	4–6
	or Piperacillin 3 gm q4h IV *plus*	4–6
	Tobramycin 2.5–3.0 mg/kg q8h IV	4–6
E. coli‡	1. Ampicillin 2 gm q4h IV	4–6
	2. Cephalothin 2 gm q4h IV	4–6
	3. Moxalactam 2 gm q6h IV	4–6
Serratia marcescens‡	1. Moxalactam 2 gm q6h IV	
	2. Ticarcillin 3 gm q6h IV *plus*	6
	Amikacin 3–5 mg/kg q8h IV *or* IM	6
Hemophilus spp.‡	1. Ampicillin 2 gm q4h IV	4
	2. Cefamandole 2 gm q4h IV	4
	3. Ampicillin 2 gm q4h IV	4
	or Cefamandole 2 gm q4h IV *plus*	4
	Gentamicin 1 mg/kg q8h IM *or* IV	2
	4. Moxalactam 2 gm q6h IV	4

*Antibiotic doses for 70-kg adult with normal renal function.
†If organism is sensitive to penicillin G, substitute penicillin G 2 mU q4h IV for nafcillin.
‡The recommendation for moxalactam is based only on in vitro sensitivity data.
§For enterococci highly resistant to streptomycin, use gentamicin.
Choices 1 to 4 throughout are in descending order of preference.

Table 12–3. CAUSES OF CULTURE-NEGATIVE ENDOCARDITIS

1. Antimicrobial therapy before cultures were obtained
2. Uremia
3. Fastidious organisms
   a. Anaerobic bacteria
   b. Nutritionally variant streptococci
   c. L-forms
   d. *Brucella*
   e. *Hemophilus* species
4. Nonbacterial or unusual bacterial causes
   a. Rickettsia (Q fever)
   b. *Chlamydia* (psittacosis)
   c. Fungi (especially *Aspergillus* species)
   d. Marantic endocarditis (nonbacterial thrombotic)
   e. Left atrial myxoma

are tested against a standard inoculum of the organism to document that a 1:8 dilution (i.e., SBT = 1:8) or greater of the patient's serum kills the organism.[5]

Justification for this 1:8 threshold is based mainly on treatment of endocarditis in rabbits with one of several doses of antibiotic.[19] Cure was associated with an SBT of 1:8 or more, and relapse with lesser dilutions. Although demonstration of the necessity of SBTs of 1:8 or more for cure in clinical studies has been more difficult, demonstration of this level of serum bactericidal activity is currently standard practice.[22, 42] Nevertheless, exceptions do occur. Occasionally, patients with an SBT of less than 1:8 may be cured; others with an SBT of 1:8 or more may relapse. Therefore, these and other in vitro susceptibility tests supply adjunctive information and should not be used as the sole basis of therapeutic decisions. Although favorable test results in patients who respond to antibiotics are encouraging, these tests in fact are clinically most useful for patients who continue to have fever and bacteremia while on therapy or who relapse after an appropriate course of treatment.

Persistent Bacteremia

In a patient with persistent or recurrent bacteremia, one of three causes are usually found: (1) the dose of antibiotic is too low; (2) the organism is not killed by the antibiotic even at high doses; or (3) a persistent focus of infection, cardiac or extracardiac, is responsible for continued sepsis (Table 12–4). The first and second causes should become evident after appropriate susceptibility testing. For example, the MIC and MBC given an indication of how susceptible the organism is in vitro to the chosen antibiotic. Determination of serum antibiotic concentration allows rational adjustment of the dose to give that concentration likely to exceed the MBC. The SBT substantiates how effectively the organism is killed by the patient's serum, and indirectly confirms the adequacy of antimicrobial selection and dosing.

Cases of persistent bacteremia have occurred despite seemingly appropriate therapy based on in vitro tests.[77] In some instances, organisms may be tolerant to bactericidial antibiotics (i.e., the MBC exceeds the MIC by a factor of 32 or more), and hence killing of bacteria within the vegetation occurs slowly or not at all.[82] In other instances, persistent bacteremia has been caused by organisms that, although not tolerant by in vitro tests, required addition of a second antibiotic for cure.[77] Whether tolerant strains are an important cause of persistent bacteremia and more complications is uncertain, but one study suggests that this is so.[75] Although routine administration of two antibiotics for patients infected by tolerant organisms cannot be recommended, those who have persistent bacteremia certainly should receive a second drug, such as rifampin or an aminoglycoside.

Occasionally the vegetation itself cannot be sterilized by antibiotics alone, and surgical intervention is necessary.[24] This is almost always the case for infections caused by fungi[81] and is often so for those caused by gram-negative organisms.[21, 60, 76]

Finally, an extracardiac site infected during the initial bacteremia may subsequently cause

Table 12–4. CAUSES OF PERSISTENT BACTEREMIA IN ENDOCARDITIS

1. Antibiotic dose too low or infrequent for therapeutic levels
2. Antibiotic not bactericidal for organism
   a. Resistant organism
   b. Tolerant organism
3. Persistent focus of infection
   a. Cardiac focus
      1. Valvular
      2. Myocardial or ring abscess
      3. Aneurysm
   b. Extracardiac focus
      1. Septic arthritis
      2. Pleural effusion
      3. Mycotic aneurysm
      4. Hepatic abscess
      5. Splenic abscess
      6. Osteomyelitis
      7. Epidural abscess

fever and, occasionally, positive blood cultures. Virulent organisms, particularly *S. aureus,* are most often responsible, but any organism can cause secondary infection. This secondary site is usually obvious after careful history-taking, physical examination, and laboratory studies; often it takes the form of focal abscesses large enough to require drainage.

Septic arthritis, pleural effusion, and osteomyelitis are frequently encountered as secondary sites of infection.[69] Septic arthritis can be managed by needle aspiration of infected joint fluid and systemic antibiotic therapy; drugs and doses adequate for endocarditis are also adequate for septic arthritis. Incision and open drainage is rarely necessary unless the infected joint (e.g., the hip joint) is relatively inaccessible to needle aspiration.[32]

Pleural effusions also can be drained by repeated needle aspiration, especially if the cultures are sterile. However, purulent pleural fluid, fluid with a pH <7.2, or fluid that grows bacteria upon culture often reaccumulates unless drained by a chest tube.[51, 52]

A treatment regimen effective for endocarditis usually cures an existing osteomyelitis. However, surgical drainage may be necessary for sequestration and contiguous abscesses (e.g., epidural or psoas muscle abscesses).[9]

Rarely, the cause of persistent bacteremia remains a mystery even after careful evaluation. In these instances, persistent valve infection should be strongly considered as the source, but it may also prove to be a clinically silent mycotic aneurysm, a hepatic abscess, or a splenic abscess.[36] Computerized tomography or liver-spleen scan may help detect these foci of infection, and surgical drainage of the abscess or excision of the aneurysm is then indicated.

Combination Chemotherapy

Combination therapy is often used before culture results are known, but definitive treatment with two or more antibiotics is indicated in only a few situations (Table 12–5).[88] Common to all these situations is a demonstrated need to achieve more rapid or effective killing of an organism or to shorten therapy. Since no single drug will kill the enterococcus in vitro at achievable serum concentrations, endocarditis caused by this organism must be treated with either penicillin, ampicillin, or vancomycin plus an aminoglycoside.[37, 108] Streptomycin is often used, but high-grade streptomycin resistance (MIC >2000 μg/ml) is now common. Routine susceptibility testing will detect this resistance. Gentamicin should be used in these cases because some enterococcal strains (e.g., *Streptococcus faecium*) are resistant to tobramycin.[63, 109]

Combination therapy with penicillin and streptomycin permits shorter courses of treatment (two weeks instead of four) for viridans streptococcal endocarditis,[114] but this combination is not essential for cure unless the organism has a high MIC against penicillin. Moreover, treatment with penicillin alone is preferred for those patients who are at risk of vestibular damage from streptomycin.

Prosthetic valve endocarditis caused by methicillin-resistant *Staphylococcus epidermidis* should probably be treated with vancomycin plus gentamicin, and possibly with the addition of rifampin. In vitro susceptibility tests indicate that this combination kills these organisms more rapidly, and one clinical study suggests that combination therapy may be more effective than a single drug.[44] If the organism is sensitive to beta-lactam antibiotics, these drugs can be used alone.

Since drug combinations may be more toxic than single drugs, particularly if an aminoglycoside is included, it is important to document that the combination selected is better than a single drug. In the case of persistent bacteremia, this is confirmed clinically by observation of the patient and microbiologically by serial blood cultures. Several in vitro methods are available for this

Table 12–5. INDICATIONS FOR COMBINATION CHEMOTHERAPY

1. Organism killed slowly or not at all by single antibiotic
   a. Enterococci
   b. Gram-negative rods
   c. Tolerant organisms
2. Persistent bacteremia for a valvular focus
3. Prosthetic valve endocarditis caused by methicillin-resistant *S. epidermidis*
4. Failure to achieve serum bactericidal test ≥1:8 with single drug
5. Two-week therapy of viridans streptococcal endocarditis

purpose also, and the SBT is probably the easiest to perform. In this instance, the addition of a new drug to the treatment regimen should increase the dilution of serum that kills the organism by at least fourfold.

MANAGEMENT OF CARDIAC COMPLICATIONS

Endocarditis interferes with cardiac function in three ways: (1) damage to valves from the infected vegetation; (2) impaired myocardial function from infarction, myocarditis, abscess, or purulent pericarditis; and (3) damage to the conduction system from local infection. Congestive heart failure, pericarditis and tamponade, arrhythmias, and sudden death are the clinical manifestations of these processes.

Heart Failure

The principal cardiac complication is heart failure, which occurs in 22 to 60 per cent of all cases and is now the leading cause of death from endocarditis.[49, 69, 103] Up to 90 per cent of all patients who die have congestive heart failure.[69] Similarly, patients with endocarditis who develop heart failure before or during medical therapy are more likely to die.[49, 61, 69]

Congestive heart failure may develop for several reasons (Table 12–6). Insufficiency from perforation of the aortic or mitral valve is the most common cause. Others include valvular prolapse or destruction due to weakening of the valve structure, often by virulent organisms; rupture of chordae tendineae; ventricular septal defect from destruction of the intraventricular septum; rupture of an infected sinus of Valsalva; myocarditis, pericarditis, or myocardial abscess; obstruction of the valve orifice by the vegetation; and intercurrent myocardial infarction.[110] Myocardial infarction due to embolism of a coronary artery occurs most often in aortic valve disease. Infarction probably arises more often than is suspected and is a relatively common cause of heart failure.[15, 72]

Certain clinical features are associated with a higher risk and increased severity of heart failure. Aortic valvular and mitral valvular infections cause significant heart failure in approximately 80 and 50 per cent of cases, respectively.[61] In contrast, infections of tricuspid valves or congenital defects cause heart failure in less than 20 per cent of cases. Endocarditis caused by *S. aureus*, pneumococci, and enterococci, particularly if the aortic valve is involved, increases the risk of heart failure.[61, 69, 103] Finally, patients in whom vegetations of the aortic or mitral valve are demonstrated by echocardiography are still more likely to develop heart failure.[23, 96, 97, 105]

To achieve the best results in the greatest number of patients, the clinician must differentiate those individuals likely to respond to antibiotics alone from those likely to need combined medical and surgical therapy. Patients who have endocarditis caused by streptococci and associated with mild or no heart failure, or who have infection of the tricuspid valve caused by *S. aureus*, can be expected to respond to antibiotics alone. In contrast, patients who develop heart failure, particularly in aortic valve infections, or who have left-sided endocarditis caused by virulent or rel-

Table 12–6. CAUSES OF HEART FAILURE IN ENDOCARDITIS

1. Valvular failure
   a. Insufficiency due to perforation
   b. Prolapse from valve ring damage
   c. Valvular stenosis from the vegetation
   d. Chordae tendineae rupture
   e. Papillary muscle rupture
2. Myocardial failure
   a. Myocardial infarction
   b. Myocarditis
   c. Myocardial abscess
3. Intracardiac shunt
   a. Fistula formation between aorta and cardiac chambers
   b. Ventricular septal defect
   c. Rupture of sinus of Valsalva
4. Cardiac tamponade
   a. Rupture of abscess into pericardium
   b. Purulent pericarditis from septicemia
   c. Rupture of vascular structure into pericardium

atively resistant organisms (*S. aureus,* possibly enterococci, gram-negative rods, fungi, rickettsiae and chlamydiae), are at risk of disastrous complications. In addition, persons who develop endocarditis of a prosthetic valve, especially within two months of implantation, are at great risk of severe heart failure and death. In fact, so ominous is endocarditis in this setting that unless the patient promptly responds to antibiotics and develops no complications, or unless there are strong contraindications, early valve replacement is advisable. Although patients with late-onset prosthetic valve endocarditis (i.e., more than two months after valve replacement) may respond to antibiotics alone, those who develop heart failure or a new regurgitant murmur, or have myocardial invasion (evidenced by persistent fever, atrioventricular conduction disturbances, or bacteriologic relapse), should be considered for early surgery.[45]

Evaluation of Heart Failure

Since clinical assessment alone is often unreliable or inaccurate, ways have been sought to improve the selection of patients with endocarditis who are most likely to benefit from early surgery. The findings of Wann and associates[105] have stimulated much interest in echocardiography as one way to improve patient selection. These authors noted in a retrospective study that, of 22 patients who had valvular vegetations detected by M-mode echocardiography, all 22 had heart failure and four had cerebral emboli. Furthermore, 20 of the 22 either died or required surgery within a mean period of 22 days from hospital admission. Of 43 patients without vegetations, 12 had heart failure, none had cerebral, emboli, and none died or required surgery. In a larger prospective study, Stewart and co-workers[96] confirmed that patients who had vegetations detectable by echocardiography also had a higher rate of complications; however, the prevalences of heart failure and emboli were considerably lower, both at 30 per cent. In addition, patients who did not have vegetations also developed complications, albeit at a lower rate.

The limitations of M-mode echocardiography, apart from the technical considerations, are those of resolution, time of examination, and field of view. The resolution of most equipment is such that vegetations smaller than 2 mm can be missed easily, especially if background signals associated with certain pre-existing valve abnormalities are present. Also, examination may be made too early in the course of the illness, before vegetations of sufficient size have formed. Finally, the field of view in M mode echocardiography is limited to the size of the beam of sound as it sweeps the heart. Two-dimensional echocardiography affords a wider field of view and may be superior to M mode. The former probably detects more vegetations and myocardial complications than M mode, although in some patients the two methods are complementary.[57,62] However, two-dimensional echocardiography does not have sufficient specificity to permit prediction of a patient's clinical course, and M-mode may be better in this regard.[55]

Echocardiography can detect other abnormalities besides vegetations, especially in aortic valve disease. Early closure of the mitral valve and increases in the left ventricular diameter correlate with the severity of aortic regurgitation.[105] Flail valve leaflets may be detected. Myocardial size and function can be assessed.

These encouraging developments notwithstanding, the role of echocardiography in the evaluation of patients with endocarditis for early surgery is still being defined. At present, the following conclusions seem valid: (1) patients in whom vegetations are detected by echocardiography are at increased risk of major cardiac and embolic events and should be closely monitored; (2) patients with aortic regurgitation and heart failure in whom vegetations are also detected by echocardiography constitute the highest risk category and generally require early surgery; (3) echocardiographic demonstration of valvular vegetation should not be regarded as a sole criterion for selection for surgery, and this finding must be assessed in light of the larger clinical picture.

Aside from echocardiography, the electrocardiogram may help in the selection of high-risk patients. Patients with aortic valve endocarditis who develop any degree of atrioventricular (AV) block, in the absence of any other identifiable cause, should be suspected of having extension of the infective process from the valve into the myocardium or of myocardial abscess formation. These patients are at great risk of sudden death. Therefore, any degree of AV block, including prolongation of the P-R interval, that develops without explanation is an indication for early aortic valve replacement.[8, 104] AV block in the setting of prosthetic endocarditis of the aortic valve is an extremely ominous sign and also is an indication for early surgery.

In the management of prosthetic valve endocarditis, cardiac fluoroscopy should be carried out to exclude the presence of abnormal rocking motions caused by valve dehiscence. The latter condition is often found in patients dying of prosthetic endocarditis and requires urgent surgery because of the progressive nature of the process.[98, 115]

Patients who have heart failure caused by endocarditis may not need preoperative cardiac catheterization. In particular, for those with active aortic valve infection, clinical examination and noninvasive tests are sufficiently accurate to determine whether compromise exists and to enable plans for surgery to be made if necessary. Moreover, cardiac catheterization, usually accomplished at relatively small risk in these patients, may be dangerous if heart failure is severe, because of the chance of dislodging infected emboli and the risk of serious complications during the procedure.[59, 98] On the other hand, in older patients, catheterization to define coronary artery anatomy may be useful. Also, catheterization can reveal other lesions not evident from clinical examination alone (e.g., aortic root abscess, sinus of Valsalve aneurysm, or fistulae).

Treatment of Heart Failure

Since cardiac complications, particularly heart failure, cause most of the deaths in infective endocarditis, emphasis has been on earlier diagnosis and more aggressive surgical management of these complications (Table 12–7). By far the most important factor determining outcome is the adequacy and preservation of myocardial function, whether one evaluates results of medical or of surgical therapy. Little is gained by temporizing measures in the patient who develops moderate or severe heart failure during the course of endocarditis.

Surgery is usually delayed in the mistaken belief that a more prolonged course of antibiotic provides a better chance of sterilzing the infection, and thus avoids the theoretical problem of sewing a prosthetic valve into friable tissue at a site of active infection. This approach is flawed. First, heart failure, not residual infection, is the principal cause of death in these patients, and antibiotics alone cannot arrest this process. Second, if heart failure is allowed to progress, the risk of death correspondingly increases, and surgery will become only a salvage maneuver in a moribund patient.[13] Finally, the fear that residual infection at the operative site will adversely affect the outcome is unfounded. Numerous studies confirm that valve replacement can be successfully performed during the early, active phase of endocarditis even while blood cultures are positive.[78, 112, 117] The risk of continuing infection is probably around 5 per cent.[98]

For these reasons, medical therapy for heart failure caused by endocarditis is adjunctive except in mild cases. Patients who develop mild heart failure, particularly if this is due to mitral valve infection, should be

Table 12–7. INDICATIONS FOR EARLY CARDIAC SURGERY IN ACTIVE ENDOCARDITIS

Definite	Possible
1. Moderate or severe heart failure, especially if progressive	1. Recurrent embolization
2. Prosthetic valve endocarditis with valve dehiscence or obstruction	2. Prosthetic valve endocarditis within two months of operation
3. New onset of heart block or bundle branch block presumed due to periaortic infection	**Adjunctive**
4. Fungal endocarditis	1. Echocardiographic abnormalities:
5. Persistent bacteremia from valve source despite appropriate antibiotic therapy according to laboratory tests	(a) Vegetations on mitral or aortic valves
	(b) Early mitral preclosure
	2. Endocarditis of aortic valve
	3. Endocarditis due to virulent organisms (e.g., *S. aureus)*
	4. Endocarditis due to gram-negative rods
	5. Prosthetic valve endocarditis
	(a) New regurgitant murmur
	(b) Persistent, unexplained fever

Definite = indication is sufficient justification for surgery.
Possible = indication may be sufficient reason for surgery.
Adjunctive = indication favors surgery if definite indication is not clearly present, or earlier surgery if definite indication is present.

given a trial of digitalis and diuretics. If the heart failure is easily controlled and does not progress, these patients may safely be treated medically. However, those who develop more severe heart failure, who have aortic valve endocarditis, or who require more aggressive medical therapy (e.g., afterload reducing drugs) are at serious risk of death from heart failure and should strongly be considered for early surgery.

When and if an operation is performed for active endocarditis, a full course of appropriate medical therapy is also given. If intraoperative cultures of tissue stains are positive, at least four more weeks of therapy is recommended; if negative, two weeks of postoperative antibiotics is a safe minimum. Anticoagulants are prescribed as needed according to the type of prosthetic valve. Postoperative embolic events and subsequent cerebral hemorrhage are infrequent occurrences in this setting,[117] probably because of excision of the vegetation and debridement of the infected site.

Conduction Disturbances

Serious disturbances of intracardiac conduction, although unusual, are potentially treatable complications of endocarditis. Conduction disturbances, which may be permanent or temporary, are caused by extension of the infection to the AV node or bundle of His. Because of its proximity to the AV node, the aortic valve is involved in almost all cases in which serious conduction disturbances occur.[8, 104] In patients with aortic prosthetic valves, conduction disturbances are common and usually signify the presence of a valve ring abscess.[8, 98] First- and second-degree heart block are the most common of these disturbances. Complete heart block has been reported in up to 4 per cent of cases and is frequently lethal.[104] Since digitalis, electrolyte disorders, and myocardial infarction can also cause abnormal conduction, these conditions must be excluded by appropriate evaluation.

Patients with endocarditis who develop any degree of heart block not attributable to other causes are at serious risk of death complications. They should be monitored in an intensive care unit and should undergo placement of a temporary transvenous pacemaker. Urgent surgery is advised for those with aortic valve infection. Patients in whom there might reasonably be another cause of heart block or who have only mitral valve infection may be observed, but surgery is advised if the heart block progresses or other complications (e.g., worsening heart failure, new murmurs) develop.

Endocarditis of Prosthetic Valves

Although not a complication in the strictest sense, endocarditis of prosthetic heart valves is different enough from that of native valves to merit special mention. Prosthetic valve endocarditis is classified as either early onset (within 60 days of surgery) or late onset (after 60 days), each type displaying particular clinical characteristics.[25] Early-onset prosthetic valve endocarditis usually occurs later than three weeks postoperatively, so that bacteremia (especially from gram-negative bacteria) that arises before then is more likely to be from a noncardiac source and not caused by endocarditis.[87] However, bacteremia occurring after the third week is more likely to be associated with changing murmurs and no obvious extracardiac focus of infection. *Staphylococcus aureus, S. epidermidis,* gram-negative rods, and fungi are the bacteria most commonly isolated from patients with early prosthetic valve endocarditis. Over 80 per cent of those developing this complication may die.[25, 46, 93, 115]

In contrast, late prosthetic valve endocarditis resembles native-valve infections in bacteriology and clinical course. Viridans streptococci are most commonly responsible and mortality rates average about 40 per cent.[25, 46, 115] As in native-valve endocarditis, cases of prosthetic endocarditis caused by streptococci are often cured by medical therapy alone and have a mortality rate correspondingly lower than infections caused by nonstreptococcal organisms.

With a few exceptions, the indications for early surgery in patients with prosthetic valve endocarditis are the same as for those with native-valve infections. Early prosthetic valve endocarditis is often due to virulent and resistant organisms that are present in the suture line and cause formation of local abscesses. So poor is the eventual outcome in these patients that early reoperation and replacement of the infected prosthesis is strongly advised. However, patients who have infections caused by streptococci and who have an uncomplicated clinical course otherwise may safely be treated medically and closely observed. As mentioned above, the diagnosis of valve dehiscence, whether in early or late endocarditis, is an indication for immediate operation.

Similarly, patients with late-onset prosthetic valve endocarditis caused by nonstreptococcal organisms are at increased risk of death. In fact, the triad of heart failure, a nonstreptococcal etiology, and a new regurgitant murmur has been associated with a 90 per cent mortality rate in these patients.[45] Therefore, if all these are present, early surgery should be considered.

Miscellaneous Cardiac Complications

Involvement of cardiac structures other than valves is common in endocarditis. The myocardium may be directly affected by spread of infection through a fistulous tract from a valve ring abscess, by focal abscess formation, or by a diffuse myocarditis. Infection extending to the intraventricular septum can cause necrosis and rupture of that structure and acute formation of ventricular septal defect. The conduction system is often damaged when the myocardium becomes involved.

Myocardial infarction may be caused by focal necrosis from the infection, but most commonly is due to embolization of debris from the vegetation to the coronary arteries. Medical management of this complication is recommended.

Extension of infection to the aortic root and contiguous structures can cause an aneurysm of the coronary artery or of the sinus of Valsalva. These may subsequently rupture or form a fistula into the pericardium or another cardiac chamber. Surgical therapy is indicated for these complications.

Pericarditis may be the result either of seeding during the bacteremia of endocarditis or of spread from a contiguous focus, such as a myocardial or aortic root abscess. This complication should be considered in patients with endocarditis who develop chest pain. Echocardiography is the most useful diagnostic test. Purulent pericarditis should be treated by immediate drainage and pericardiectomy, not only to remove the focus of infection but also to prevent the constrictive pericarditis that often develops later.

DIAGNOSIS AND MANAGEMENT OF NEUROLOGIC COMPLICATIONS

Neurologic complications occur in up to 50 per cent of patients and are the second most common cause of death in those with endocarditis.[41, 49, 74, 103, 119] Five syndromes are recognizable clinically: a diffuse neuropsychiatric disorder, meningoencephalitis, stroke, myelopathy, and neuropathy.[119] Neuropsychiatric manifestations include headache, seizures, confusion, personality changes, disorientation, hallucinations, and other findings characteristic of an acute organic brain syndrome. Coma is the most serious of these and is associated with a poor prognosis. These complications are more common in the elderly.

Meningoencephalitis, the most common of these syndromes, is characterized by headache, meningismus, and abnormal cerebrospinal fluid findings, which typically show a mild or moderate pleocytosis. CSF cultures are usually sterile, but acute purulent meningitis does occur, especially if *S. aureus* or the pneumococcus is the cause of the endocarditis.[47, 49, 74]

Stroke syndromes, which may be transient or permanent, are characterized by focal central neurologic deficits. Hemiplegia with or without aphasia is the usual findings, but any degree of paralysis or sensory deficit may occur. Half of all neurologic manifestations of endocarditis are strokes, and up to 3 per cent of strokes from all causes are secondary to endocarditis.[41, 119]

Myelopathy and cranial and peripheral neuropathy occur infrequently.[74, 119] Myelopathy due to spinal epidural abscess must be differentiated by appropriate tests from that caused by emboli to the spinal cord, because either may produce paraplegia, girdle pain, and incontinence.

Neuropathies affecting vision are the most common, causing double vision and blurring or loss of vision. Peripheral or central emboli to cranial nerves II, III, IV, and VI probably cause these disturbances, although emboli to cortical visual centers or the central retinal artery may produce similar signs and symptoms. Weakness or sensory disturbances in a peripheral nerve distrubiton are also probably due to microemboli.[119]

Evaluation of Neurologic Complications

Clinical findings in patients with central nervous system complications cannot be relied on to predict underlying pathologic processes. Those most commonly present are meningeal inflammation, cerebral infarction from major artery or microvascular occlusions, mycotic aneurysm formation, and microscopic brain abscesses.[74, 119] Meningeal inflammation is itself nonspecific and can be caused by any of the other pathologic lesions mentioned. Infarcted brain tissue can irritate or cause congestion of the meninges; a leaking mycotic aneurysm can provoke an inflammatory response; and brain abscess, especially if near the cortex, can inflame overlying meninges, or rupture and produce purulent meningitis.[14, 83]

Lumbar puncture is indicated in any patient with endocarditis who has altered mental status or focal neurologic signs, provided there is no increased intracranial pressure. If brain abscess or increased intracranial pressure is suspected, a computed tomographic brain scan should be obtained before the lumbar puncture. CT is an extremely accurate, noninvasive method of detecting brain abscess or intracranial bleeding.[1, 66] The lumbar puncture may reveal any of several abnormalities (Table 12–8). The most common findings is a pleocytosis of less than 500 white blood cells accompanied by normal protein and glucose—so-called aseptic meningitis. Since this abnormality is so common, endocarditis should be included in the differential diagnosis of aseptic meningitis. The presence of red blood cells suggests a leaking aneurysm, and patients with this finding should undergo cerebral angiography.[119] Likewise, patients who have focal neurologic signs, unilateral headache, and pleocytosis of the cerebrospinal fluid are more likely to have a mycotic aneurysm and should undergo angiography.[120]

The lumbar puncture is not otherwise predictive of the underlying pathologic process. Further evaluation by CT or angiography is indicated in those patients who develop focal neurologic deficits or who have progressive or significant alterations in mental status.

Meningoencephalitis and Meningitis

Meningoencephalitis responds to antimicrobial therapy alone. However, if cultures of cerebrospinal fluid grow the infecting organism (usually *Staphylococcus aureus* or *Streptococcus pneumoniae*), repeat lumbar puncture is indicated to document sterilization of the CSF. Depending on the organism, nafcillin or penicillin is preferred therapy for these infections because cephalosporins such as cephalothin, which are active against these organisms in vitro, do not achieve effective concentrations in the CSF.[54, 89]

Although vancomycin has been used occasionally to treat gram-positive meningitis, penetration of this drug into CSF is not well studied, and experience in treatment of meningitis is limited.[34] In penicillin-allergic patients who do not have anaphylaxis, desensitization and treatment with penicillin is strongly advised. Alternatively, rifampin (600 mg every 12 hr), which readily crosses the blood-brain barrier, can be added to vancomycin. Finally, intrathecal vancomycin may be tried in refractory cases.

Embolic Strokes

Cerebral infarction is caused by embolization from the cardiac vegetation to a major artery, usually the middle cerebral artery.

Table 12–8. TYPICAL CEREBROSPINAL FLUID CHANGES PRODUCED BY NEUROLOGIC COMPLICATIONS OF BACTERIAL ENDOCARDITIS

	Abnormalities Present				
	Cell Count (Cells/mm³)		*Protein*	*Glucose*	*Culture or*
Complication	*RBC*	*WBC*	*(mg%)*	*(mg%)*	*Gram Stain*
Meningoencephalitis	0	0–500	20–200	45–80	(−)
Meningitis	0	>1000, mostly PMNs	>60	<45	(+)
Septic embolism	0	100–1000	45–125	45–80	(−)
Mycotic aneurysm	0	<5	20–45	45–80	(−)
Leaking	>5–10	<50	20–45	45–80	(−)
Subarachnoid hemorrhage	Bloody	<50	20–1000	50–100	(−)
Intracerebral hemorrhage	200–50,000	<50	20–2000	50–100	(−)
Abscess	0	0–1000	45–200	45–80	(−)

RBC = red blood cells, WBC = white blood cells, PMN = polymorphonuclear leukocyte. Adapted from Ziment, I.: Nervous system complications in bacterial endocarditis. Am. J. Med. 47:593, 1969.

Multiple microinfarctions may occur alone or in combination with large-vessel embolism and may sometimes cause unexplained fluctuations in the level of consciousness in patients with endocarditis.[74] Most strokes occur early in the course of endocarditis when blood cultures are still positive, and usually require no specific therapy other than that for the underlying infection. However, evidence of repeated or ongoing cerebral or systemic embolization is an indication for valve replacement to remove the source of emboli.[24] Some authorities have suggested that demonstration of large valvular vegetations on echocardiography indicates a significant risk of cerebral embolism, and have advocated early valve replacement to prevent embolism in patients with this finding.[23, 97, 105] However, others have reported lower rates of embolism, and stress that management decisions should continue to be made from multiple clinical factors and not from echocardiographic findings alone.[96] Until more evidence becomes available, this latter course seems the more prudent.

The role of anticoagulation for embolic stroke caused by endocarditis is less controversial: this therapy is contraindicated in endocarditis of native valves. Evidence from both experimental and clinical studies supports this recommendation. Warfarin given to rabbits with streptococcal endocarditis caused an explosive infection characterized by high fevers and rapidly evolving bacteremia.[38, 100] In addition, mean survival was shorter in warfarin-treated rabbits than in those untreated. Similarly, Pruitt and coworkers found that 23 per cent of the intracranial hemorrhages in patients with embolic strokes and endocarditis occurred in the 3 per cent of individuals given anticoagulants.[74]

In contrast, anticoagulants should not be discontinued in patients with endocarditis of a prosthetic valve of a type (e.g., Starr-Edwards) requiring systemic anticoagulation to prevent emboli postoperatively. Discontinuation of anticoagulants in these patients has been associated with an increased incidence of central nervous system complications.[113] Prosthetic valve endocarditis is commonly caused by *Staphylococcus epidermidis,* and experimental evidence suggests that warfarin may have an inhibitory effect on the development of vegetations by this organism;[101] this may partly explain why anticoagulation causes fewer complications in prosthetic valve infections.

Evidence from Canada suggests that aspirin may benefit some patients who have transient ischemic attacks not caused by endocarditis.[17] Although platelets undoubtedly participate in the pathogenesis of endocarditis,[26] aspirin does not alter the course of experimental endocarditis in rabbits[50] and, although not harmful, probably offers little or no benefit.

Intracranial Mycotic Aneurysms

Mycotic aneurysms, a bacterial arteritis probably initiated by embolism to the vasa vasorum, reportedly occur in 2 to 10 per cent of patients with endocarditis[64, 74, 119] and are most commonly recognized in the central nervous system. The true prevalence is unknown because these may develop without symptoms and often are unsuspected unless bleeding occurs. Correspondingly, the cerebrospinal fluid may be normal, compatible with aseptic meningitis, or hemorrhagic. The presence of red cells in the CSF of a patient with endocarditis is very suggestive of mycotic aneurysm and merits further diagnostic studies.

Patients with intracranial mycotic aneurysms fall into one of three categories: (1) those who are asymptomatic; (2) those who are symptomatic because of meningeal irritation caused by a leaking aneurysm or because of associated focal neurologic deficits; and (3) those who develop massive, life-threatening hemorrhage. Asymptomatic patients should probably be observed clinically for evolution of neurologic or meningeal signs, and followed by repeat angiography during the course of therapy. Some cerebral aneurysms may resolve on antibiotic therapy alone, and surgery can be reserved for those that do not.[11, 65]

Symptomatic patients not manifesting life-threatening hemorrhage should probably undergo immediate surgery if possible. Single mycotic aneurysms of peripheral branches of the cerebral arteries may be easily approached and excised.[120] Multiple aneurysms or centrally located ones are more difficult to excise and should probably be observed over the course of therapy.[10]

Patients who have life-threatening hemorrhage should be evaluated to exclude the possibility of a mass effect from hematoma, which, if present, should be evacuated. Otherwise, these patients should be stabilized, followed by serial angiography, and explored surgically after inflammation has had time to subside in order to minimize the risk of repeat hemorrhage.[79]

Brain Abscess

Brain abscess is uncommon in patients with endocarditis, occurring with a frequency of 1 to 4 per cent;[41, 49, 74, 119] most are probably microabscesses discovered at atuopsy, which do not cause a mass effect and have uncertain importance. Similarly, of all patients with clinically significant, large brain abscess, bacterial endocarditis is the cause in less than 1 per cent.[14, 83] Acute endocarditis, characterized by a fulminant clinical course and often due to *S. aureus,* most commonly causes large abscesses when these do occur.[43, 74] Correspondingly, large abscesses are extremely rare in subacute cases caused by more indolent organisms.[49, 102, 119]

Since brain abscesses are often small and multiple, those caused by endocarditis rarely require (and often are not amenable to) surgical intervention.[74, 119] Furthermore, recent studies using computerized tomography to follow abscesses have documented resolution of even large abscesses with antibiotic therapy alone.[80] Nevertheless, patients who show clinical deterioration attributable to a mass lesion, or who have or develop evidence of compromised brain stem function, should have prompt neurosurgical consultation to consider drainage of the abscess.

MISCELLANEOUS COMPLICATIONS

Systemic Embolism

Embolic episodes occur in up to 50 per cent of patients and are second only to heart failure as complications of endocarditis.[69] Although embolism to the cerebral or coronary arteries is most serious, the spleen, kidney, lung, and mesenteric or major peripheral arteries are more common sites.

Emboli to major systemic vessels infrequently cause serious vascular compromise. When this does occur, however, embolectomy is advised if possible. Vascular compromise is more likely to happen from emboli in endocarditis caused by fungi or unusual organisms such as *Hemophilus parainfluenzae.*[20, 81] Emboli, especially those occurring during the course of culture-negative endocarditis, should be examined and cultured because the etiologic agent may be present.

Most embolic events occur early in the course of endocarditis when blood cultures are positive and specific antimicrobial therapy alone is usually adequate treatment. However, patients who experience recurrent systemic embolization while on therapy are at increased risk of a major central nervous system complication and should be considered candidates for early cardiac surgery. Patients with recurrent pulmonary embolism are at risk for development of significant pulmonary hypertension. Surgery should also be considered in these patients, although, if infection is limited to the right side of the heart only, a course of systemic anticoagulation may be cautiously tried first. Otherwise, and certainly in patients with systemic emboli, anticoagulation is absolutely contraindicated.

Extracranial Mycotic Aneurysm

In the pre-antibiotic era, infective endocarditis caused most cases of mycotic aneurysm.[95] Extracranial mycotic aneurysms now are rarely due to endocarditis and usually result from seeding of a damaged, atherosclerotic artery during bacteremia of any cause.[40]

When this complication does occur, the manifestations are hemorrhage; persistent bacteremia despite appropriate therapy; and signs and symptoms of either an expanding mass, vascular insufficiency, or both. Unless the aneurysm is large or peripherally located, a pulsatile mass is unusual. Any artery may be involved. Aneurysms of the sinus of Valsalva or proximal aorta are most common, but many of these are probably caused by direct extension of infection from the valve.[92] Elderly patients with pre-existent abdominal aortic aneurysms or severe atherosclerosis are more likely to seed this site.[118] Aneurysms of the mesenteric, hepatic, or splenic arteries are rare but should be suspected in patients who have abdominal pain, persistent fever or bacteremia, or gastrointestinal bleeding.

The diagnosis of extracranial mycotic aneurysm is confirmed by arteriography. Computed tomography and intravenous digital angiography may prove useful as experience increases. Since mycotic aneurysms are difficult to sterilize with antibiotics alone and may still enlarge and rupture, surgical drainage, excision, and repair or ligation of the infected arterial segment is necessary in nearly every case.[40, 68] Vascular surgical consultation should be sought as soon as the diagnosis is suspected. Antibiotics should be continued for four to six weeks postoperatively, depending on whether smears and cultures from the aneurysm are positive.

Renal Disease

Hematuria, pyuria, proteinuria, and azotemia are extremely common in infective endocarditis. Although abnormalities of urinary sediment are practically universal and renal infarction from emboli is present in over half of the cases at autopsy, clinically significant disturbance of renal function is uncommon. Rarely, glomerulonephritis, an immune-complex disease, does cause clinically important renal failure.[35] Low serum complement levels reflect the immune-complex nature of this complication. Since glomerulonephritis is usually benign and the diagnosis can be made if serum complement is depressed, renal biopsy is rarely indicated. The glomerulonephritis improves with appropriate antimicrobial therapy, and dialysis has largely eliminated uremia as a cause of death. Because antibiotics alone are adequate therapy in most cases, corticosteroids are not indicated. However, renal function abnormalities that progress during antibiotic therapy may be caused by the antibiotic itself. Consequently, antibiotics, other drugs, congestive heart failure, and volume depletion must be excluded as causes of renal failure before glomerulonephritis can be diagnosed confidently in the absence of biopsy. Renal biopsy may be indicated for patients who have progressive deterioration in renal function after these other causes have been reasonably excluded.

CONCLUSIONS

Infective endocarditis destroys valves, seeds distant sites with bacteria, disseminates embolic debris through the circulation, and initiates a host-immune response capable of tissue injury. Treatment of this disease is directed toward arresting growth of the infected cardiac vegetation. Since host defenses are ineffective in the milieu of the vegetation, antibiotics must be bactericidal and must be given in large doses for several weeks.

Despite modern antibiotic therapy, serious complications of the heart, central nervous system, and other vital organs often occur. Cardiac complications are the most serious and cause the most deaths. Clinical and laboratory findings can be used to assess risk for certain subsets of patients, and new noninvasive methods may help refine this estimate of risk. The presence and degree of heart failure correlate most strongly with poor outcome and all efforts should be directed toward preservation of myocardial function. Medical therapy alone is usually unsuccessful in patients with progressive heart failure. In addition, certain subsets of patients, free of complications early in the course of the illness, are destined to develop either heart failure or other serious complications. For these patients, close observation and aggressive, early surgical intervention are often needed to prevent further complications or death.

References

1. Abrams, H. L., and McNeil, B. J.: Medical implications of computed tomography ("Cat scanning"). N. Engl. J. Med. 298:255, 310, 1978.
2. Abrutyn, E., Lincoln, L., Gallagher, M., and Weinstein, A. J.: Cephalothin-gentamicin synergism in experimental enterococcal endocarditis. J. Antimicrob. Chemother. 4:153, 1978.
3. Abruzzo, J. L., and Christian, C. L.: The induction of a rheumatoid factor–like substance in rabbits. J. Exp. Med. 114:791, 1961.
4. Angrist, A. A., and Oka, M.: Pathogenesis of bacterial endocarditis. J.A.M.A. 183:249, 1963.
5. Anhalt, J. P., Sabath, L. D., and Barry, A. L.: Special tests: bactericidal activity, activity of antimicrobics in combination and detection of betalactamase production. *In* Lennette, E. H. (ed.): Manual of Clinical Microbiology, 3rd ed. Washington, DC, American Society for Microbiology, 1980, pp. 478–484.
6. Applefeld, M. M., and Woodward, T. E.: Infective endocarditis: a clinical overview. Curr. Probl. Cardiol. 2:1, 1977.
7. Archer, G. L.: Antimicrobial susceptibility and selection of resistance among *Staphylococcus epidermidis* isolates recovered from patients with infection of indwelling foreign devices. Antimicrob. Agents Chemother. 14:353, 1978.
8. Arnett, E. N., and Roberts, W. C.: Valve ring abscess in active infective endocarditis: frequency, location, and clues to clinical diagnosis from the

study of 95 necropsy patients. Circulation 54:140, 1976.
9. Baker, A. S., Ojemann, R. G., Swartz, M. N., and Richardson, E. P.: Spinal epidural abscess. N. Engl. J. Med. 293:463, 1975.
10. Bell, W. E., and Butler, C., II: Cerebral mycotic aneurysms in children. Two case reports. Neurology 18:81, 1968.
11. Bingham, W. F.: Treatment of mycotic intracranial aneurysms. J. Neurosurg. 46:428, 1977.
12. Bourgault, A., Wilson, W. R., and Washington, J. A., II: Antimicrobial susceptibilities of species of viridans streptococci. J. Infect. Dis. 140:316, 1979.
13. Boyd, A. D., Spencer, F. C., Isom, O. W., et al.: Infective endocarditis: an analysis of 54 surgically treated patients. J. Thorac. Cardiovasc. Surg. 73:23, 1977.
14. Brewer, N. S., MacCarty, C. S., and Wellman, W. E.: Brain abscess: a review of recent experience. Ann. Intern. Med. 82:571, 1975.
15. Brunson, J. G.: Coronary embolism in bacterial endocarditis. Am. J. Pathol. 29:689, 1953.
16. Burch, K. H., Quinn, E. L., Cox, F., et al.: Intramuscular clindamycin for therapy of infective endocarditis. Report of 23 cases and review of the literature. Am. J. Cardiol. 38:929, 1976.
17. Canadian Cooperative Study Group: A randomized trial of aspirin and sulfinpyrazone in threatened stroke. N. Engl. J. Med. 299:53, 1978.
18. Cannady, P. B., and Sanford, J. P.: Negative blood cultures in infective endocarditis: a review. South. Med. J. 69:1420, 1976.
19. Carrizosa, J., and Kaye, D.: Antibiotic concentrations in serum, serum bactericidal activity, and results of therapy of streptococcal endocarditis in rabbits. Antimicrob. Agents Chemother. 12:479, 1977.
20. Chunn, C. J., Jones, S. R., McCutchan, J. A., et al.: *Haemophilus parainfluenzae* infective endocarditis. Medicine 56:99, 1977.
21. Cohen, P. S., Maguire, J. H., and Weinstein, L.: Infective endocarditis caused by gram-negative bacteria: a review of the literature, 1945–1977. Prog. Cardiovasc. Dis. 22:205, 1980.
22. Coleman, D. L., Horwitz, R. I., and Andriole, V. T.: Association between serum inhibitory and bactericidal concentration and therapeutic outcome in bacterial endocarditis. Am. J. Med. 73:260, 1982.
23. Davis, R. S., Strom, J. A., Frishman, W., et al.: The demonstration of vegetations by echocardiography in bacterial endocarditis: an indication for early surgery. Am. J. Med. 69:57, 1980.
24. Dinuble, M. J.: Surgery in active endocarditis. Ann. Intern. Med. 96:650, 1982.
25. Dismukes, W. E., Karchmer, A. W., Buckley, M. J., et al.: Prosthetic valve endocarditis. Circulation 48:365, 1973.
26. Durack, D. T., and Beeson, P. B.: Experimental bacterial endocarditis. I: Colonization of a sterile vegetation. Br. J. Exp. Pathol. 53:44, 1972.
27. Durack, D. T., and Beeson, P. B.: Experimental bacterial endocarditis. II: Survival of bacteria in endocardial vegetations. Br. J. Exp. Pathol. 53:50, 1972.
28. Ellner, J. J., Rosenthal, M. S., Lerner, P. I., and McHenry, M. C.: Infective endocarditis caused by slow-growing, fastidious, gram-negative bacteria. Medicine 58:145, 1979.
29. Freedman, L. R., and Valone, J.: Experimental infective endocarditis. Prog. Cardiovasc. Dis. 22:169, 1979.
30. Garriques, I. L., and Duma, R. J.: Bacterial endocarditis: failure with clindamycin. Ann. Intern. Med. 79:756, 1973.
31. Garrison, P. K., and Freedman, L. R.: Experimental endocarditis. I: Staphylococcal endocarditis in rabbits resulting from placement of a polyethylene catheter in the right side of the heart. Yale J. Biol. Med. 42:394, 1970.
32. Goldenberg, D. L., Brandt, K. D., Cohen, A. S., and Cathcart, E. S.: Treatment of septic arthritis: comparison of needle aspiration and surgery as initial modes of joint drainage. Arthritis Rheum. 18:83, 1975.
33. Gregoratos, G., and Karliner, J. S.: Infective endocarditis: diagnosis and management. Med. Clin. North Am. 63:173, 1979.
34. Gump, D. W.: Vancomycin for treatment of bacterial meningitis. Rev. Infect. Dis. 3 (Suppl.): S289, 1981.
35. Gutman, R. A., Striker, G. E., Gilliland, B. C., and Cutler, R. E.: The immune complex glomerulonephritis of bacterial endocarditis. Medicine 51:1, 1972.
36. Healy, T. S.: Splenectomy in refractory subacute bacterial endocarditis. Northwest Med. 61:764, 1962.
37. Hook, E. W., Roberts, R. B., and Sande, M. A.: Antimicrobial therapy of experimental enterococcal endocarditis. Antimicrob. Agents Chemother. 8:564, 1975.
38. Hooke, W. E., and Sande, M. A.: Role of the vegetation in experimental *Streptococcus viridans* endocarditis. Infect. Immun. 10:1433, 1974.
39. Hopewell, P. C., and Murray, J. F.: The adult respiratory distress syndrome. Annu. Rev. Med. 27:343, 1976.
40. Jarrett, F., Darling, R. C., Mundth, E. D., and Austen, W. G.: The management of infected arterial aneurysms. J. Cardiovasc. Surg. 18:361, 1977.
41. Jones, H. R., Siekert, R. G., and Geraci, J. E.: Neurologic manifestations of bacterial endocarditis. Ann. Intern. Med. 71:21, 1973.
42. Jordan, G. W., and Kawachi, M. M.: Analysis of serum bactericidal activity in endocarditis osteomyelitis, and other bacterial infections. Medicine 60:49, 1981.
43. Kaplan, K.: Brain abscess. Infect. Dis. Pract. 4:1, 1981.
44. Karchmer, A. N., Archer, G. L., and Dismukes, W. E.: *Staphylococcus epidermidis* prosthetic valve endocarditis: microbiologic and clinical observations as guides to therapy. Ann. Intern. Med. 98:447, 1983.
45. Karchmer, A. N., Dismukes, W. E., Buckley, M. J., and Austen, W. G.: Late prosthetic valve endocarditis: clinical features influencing therapy. Am. J. Med. 64:199, 1978.
46. Kloster, F. E.: Infective prosthetic valve endocarditis. *In* Rahimtoola, S. H. (ed.): Infective Endocarditis. San Francisco, Grune & Stratton, 1978, pp. 291–305.
47. Kuegsegger, J. M.: Pneumococcal endocarditis. Am. Heart J. 56:867, 1958.
48. Lange, M., Salaki, J. S., Middleton, J. R., et al.: Infective endocarditis in heroin addicts: epide-

miological observations and some unusual cases. Am. Heart J. 96:144, 1978.
49. Lerner, P. I., and Weinstein, L.: Infective endocarditis in the antibiotic era. N. Engl. J. Med. 274:199, 259, 323, 388, 1966.
50. Levison, M. E., Carrizosa, J., Tanphaichitra, D., et al.: Effect of aspirin on thrombogenesis and on production of experimental aortic valvular *Streptococcus* viridans endocarditis in rabbits. Blood 49:645, 1977.
51. Light, R. W.: Pleural effusions. Med. Clin. North Am. 61:1339, 1977.
52. Light, R. W., MacGregor, M. I., Ball, W. C., Jr., and Luchsinger, P. C.: Diagnostic significance of pleural fluid pH and P_{CO_2}. Chest 64:591, 1973.
53. Lincoln, L. J., Weinstein, A. J., Gallagher, M., and Abrutyn, E.: Penicillinase-resistant pencillins plus gentamicin in experimental enterococcal endocarditis. Antimicrob. Agents Chemother., 12:484, 1977.
54. Mangi, R. J., Kundargi, R. S., Quintiliani, R., and Andriole, V. T.: Development of meningitis during cephalothin therapy. Ann. Intern. Med. 78:347, 1973.
55. Martin, R. P., Meltzer, R. S., Chia, B. L., et al.: Clinical utility of two-dimensional echocardiography in infective endocarditis. Am. J. Cardiol. 46:379, 1980.
56. McCarthy, L. R., and Bottone, E. J.: Bacteremia and endocarditis caused by satelliting streptococci. Am. J. Clin. Pathol. 61:585, 1974.
57. Melvin, E. T., Berger, M., Lutzker, L. G., et al.: Noninvasive methods for detection of valve vegetations in infective endocarditis. Am. J. Cardiol. 47:271, 1981.
58. Messner, R. P., Laxdal, T., Quie, P. G., and Williams, R. C., Jr.: Rheumatoid factors in subacute bacterial endocarditis—bacterium, duration of disease or genetic predisposition. Ann. Intern. Med. 68:746, 1968.
59. Mills, J., Abbott, J., Utley, J. R., and Ryan, C.: Role of cardiac catheterization in infective endocarditis. Chest 72:576, 1977.
60. Mills, J., and Drew, D.: *Serratia marcescens* endocarditis: a regional illness associated with intravenous drug abuse. Ann. Intern. Med. 84:29, 1976.
61. Mills, J., and Utley, J.: Heart failure in infective endocarditis: predisposing factors, course, and treatment. Chest 66:151, 1974.
62. Mintz, G. S., Kotler, M. N., Segal, B. L., and Parry, W. R.: Comparison of two-dimensional and M-mode echocardiography in the evaluation of patients with infective endocarditis. Am. J. Cardiol. 43:738, 1979.
63. Moellering, R. C., Jr., Wennersten, C., and Weinstein, A. J.: Penicillin-tobramycin synergism against enterococci: a comparison with penicillin and gentamicin. Antimicrob. Agents Chemother. 3:526, 1973.
64. Molinari, G. F.: Septic cerebral embolism. Stroke 3:117, 1972.
65. Moskowitz, M. A., Rosenbaum, A. E., and Tyler, H. R.: Angiographically monitored resolution of cerebral mycotic aneurysms. Neurology 24:1103, 1974.
66. New, P. F., Davis, K. R., and Ballantine, H. T.: Computed tomography in cerebral abscess. Radiology 121:641, 1976.
67. Nolan, C. M., and Beaty, H. N.: *Staphylococcus aureus* bacteremia: current clinical patterns. Am. J. Med. 60:495, 1976.
68. Patel, S., and Johnston, K. W.: Classification and management of mycotic aneurysms. Surg. Gynecol. Obstet. 144:691, 1977.
69. Pelletier, L. L., Jr., and Petersdorf, R. G.: Infective endocarditis: a review of 125 cases from the University of Washington Hospitals, 1963–1972. Medicine 56:287, 1977.
70. Perlman, B. B., and Freedman, L. R.: Experimental endocarditis. II: Staphylococcal infection of the aortic valve following placement of a polyethylene catheter in the left side of the heart. Yale J. Biol. Med. 44:206, 1971.
71. Perlman, B. B., and Freedman, L. R.: Experimental endocarditis. III: Natural history of catheter-induced staphylococcal endocarditis following catheter removal. Yale J. Biol. Med. 44:214, 1971.
72. Perry, E. L., Fleming, R. G., and Edwards, J. E.: Myocardial lesions in subacute bacterial endocarditis. Ann. Intern. Med. 36:126, 1952.
73. Pesanti, E. L., and Smith, I. M.: Infective endocarditis with negative blood cultures: an analysis of 52 cases. Am. J. Med. 66:43, 1979.
74. Pruitt, A. A., Rubin, R. H., Karchmer, A. W., and Duncan, G. W.: Neurologic complications of bacterial endocarditis. Medicine 57:329, 1978.
75. Rajashekaraiah, K. R., Rice, T., Rao, V. S., et al.: Clinical significance of tolerant strains of *Staphylococcus aureus* in patients with endocarditis. Ann. Intern. Med. 93:796, 1980.
76. Reyes, M. P., Palutke, W. A., Wylin, R. F., and Lerner, A. M.: *Pseudomonas* endocarditis in the Detroit Medical Center, 1969–1972. Medicine 52:173, 1973.
77. Reymann, M. T., Holley, H. P., and Cobbs, C. G.: Persistent bacteremia in staphylococcal endocarditis. Am. J. Med. 65:729, 1978.
78. Richardson, J. V., Karp, R. B., Kirklin, J. W., and Dismukes, W. E.: Treatment of infective endocarditis: a 10-year comparative analysis. Circulation 58:589, 1978.
79. Roach, M. R., and Drake, C. G.: Ruptured cerebral aneurysms caused by microorganisms. N. Engl. J. Med. 273:240, 1965.
80. Rosenblum, M. L., Hoff, J. T., Norman, D., et al.: Nonoperative treatment of brain abscesses in selected high-risk patients. J. Neurosurg. 52:217, 1980.
81. Rubinstein, E., Noriega, E. R., Simberkoff, M. S., et al.: Fungal endocarditis: analysis of 24 cases and review of the literature. Medicine 54:331, 1975.
82. Sabath, L. D., Laverdiere, M., Wheeler, N., et al.: A new type of penicillin resistance of *Staphylococcus aureus*. Lancet 1:443, 1977.
83. Samson, D. S., and Clark, K.: A current review of brain abscess. Am. J. Med. 54:201, 1973.
84. Sande, M. A.: Experimental endocarditis. *In* Kaye, D. (ed.): Infective Endocarditis. Baltimore, University Park Press, 1976, pp. 11–28.
85. Sande, M. A., and Courtney, K. B.: Nafcillin-gentamicin synergism in experimental staphylococcal endocarditis. J. Lab. Clin. Med. 88:118, 1976.
86. Sande, M. A., and Irvin, R. G.: Pencillin-aminoglycoside synergy in experimental *Streptococcus viridans* endocarditis. J. Infect. Dis. 129:572, 1974.
87. Sande, M. A., Johnson, W. D., Hook, W. E., and

Kaye, D.: Sustained bacteremia in patients with prosthetic cardiac valves. N. Engl. J. Med. 286:1076, 1972.

88. Sande, M. A., and Scheld, W. M.: Combination antibiotic therapy of bacterial endocarditis. Ann. Intern. Med. 92:390, 1980.
89. Sande, M. A., Sherertz, R. J., Zak, O., and Strausbaugh, L. J.: Cephalosporin antibiotics in therapy of experimental *Streptococcus pneumoniae* and *Haemophilus influenzae* meningtis in rabbits. J. Infect. Dis. 137 (Suppl.):S161, 1978.
90. Schlichter, J. G., and MacLean, H.: A method of determining the effective therapeutic level in the treatment of subacute bacterial endocarditis with penicillin. Am. Heart J. 34:209, 1947.
91. Shine, K. I., Kuhn, M., Young, L. S., and Tillisch, J. H.: Aspects of the management of shock. Ann. Intern. Med. 93:723, 1980.
92. Shnider, B. I., and Cotsonas, N. J.: Embolic mycotic aneurysms, a complication of bacterial endocarditis. Am. J. Med. 16:246, 1954.
93. Slaughter, L., Morris, J. E., and Starr, A.: Prosthetic valvular endocarditis: a 12-year review. Circulation 47:1319, 1973.
94. Staub, N. C.: Pulmonary edema due to increased microvascular permeability. Annu. Rev. Med. 32:291, 1981.
95. Stengel, A., and Wolferth, C. C.: Mycotic (bacterial) aneurysms of intravascular origin. Arch. Intern. Med. 31:527, 1923.
96. Stewart, J. A., Silimperi, D., Harris, P., et al.: Echocardiographic documentation of vegetative lesions in infective endocarditis: clinical implications. Circulation 61:374, 1980.
97. Stiles, G. L., and Friesinger, G. C.: Bacterial endocarditis with aortic regurgitation: implications of embolism. South. Med. J. 73:582, 1980.
98. Stinson, E. B.: Surgical treatment of infective endocarditis. Prog. Cardiovasc. Dis. 22:145, 1979.
99. Thadepalli, H., and Francis, C. K.: Diagnostic clues in metastatic lesions of endocarditis in addicts. West. J. Med. 128:1, 1978.
100. Thompson, J., Eulderink, F., Lemkes, H., and van Furth, R.: Effect of warfarin on the induction and course of experimental endocarditis. Infect. Immun. 14:1284, 1976.
101. Thorig, L., Thompson, J., and Eulderink, F.: Effect of warfarin on the induction and course of experimental *Staphylococcus epidermidis* endocarditis. Infect. Immun. 17:504, 1977.
102. Victor, M., and Banker, B. Q.: Brain abscess. Med. Clin. North Am. 47:1355, 1963.
103. Von Reyn, C. F., Levy, B. S., Arbeit, R. D., et al.: Infective endocarditis: an analysis based on strict case definitions. Ann. Intern. Med. 94:505, 1981.
104. Wang, K., Gobel, F., Gleason, D. F., and Edwards, J. E.: Complete heart block complicating bacterial endocarditis. Circulation 46:939, 1972.
105. Wann, L. S., Dillon, J. C., Weyman, A. E., and Feigenbaum, H.: Echocardiography in bacterial endocarditis. N. Engl. J. Med. 295:135, 1976.
106. Washington, J. A., II: Blood cultures: principles and techniques. Mayo Clin. Proc. 50:91, 1975.
107. Washington, J. A., II, and Sutter, V. L.: Dilution susceptibility test: agar and macro-broth dilution procedures. *In* Lennette, E. H. (ed.): Manual of Clinical Microbiology, 3rd ed. Washington, DC, American Society for Microbiology, 1980, pp. 453–458.
108. Watanakunakorn, C.: Penicillin combined with gentamicin or streptomycin: synergism against enterococci. J. Infect. Dis. 124:581, 1971.
109. Weinstein, A. J., and Moellering, R. C., Jr.: Penicillin and gentamicin therapy for enterococcal infections. J.A.M.A. 223:1030, 1973.
110. Weinstein, L., and Rubin, R. H.: Infective endocarditis—1973. Prog. Cardiovasc. Dis. 16:239, 1973.
111. Werner, A. S., Cobbs, C. G., Kaye, D., and Hook, E. W.: Studies on bacteremia of bacterial endocarditis. J.A.M.A. 202:199, 1967.
112. Wilson, W. R., Danielson, G. K., Giuliani, E. R., et al.: Valve replacement in patients with active infective endocarditis. Circulation 58:585, 1978.
113. Wilson, W. R., Geraci, J. E., Danielson, G. K., et al.: Anticoagulant therapy and central nervous system complications in patients with prosthetic valve endocarditis. Circulation 57:1004, 1977.
114. Wilson, W. R., Geraci, J. E., Wilkowski, C. J., and Washington, J. A., II: Short-term intramuscular therapy with procaine penicillin plus streptomycin for infective endocarditis due to viridans streptococci. Circulation 57:1158, 1978.
115. Wilson, W. R., Jaumin, P. M., Danielson, G. K., et al.: Prosthetic valve endocarditis. Ann. Intern. Med. 82:751, 1975.
116. Wofsy, D.: Culture-negative septic arthritis and bacterial endocarditis: diagnosis by synovial biopsy. Arthritis Rheum. 23:605, 1980.
117. Young, J. B., Welton, D. E., Raizner, A. E., et al.: Surgery in active infective endocarditis. Circulation (Suppl. I) 60:77, 1979.
118. Zak, F. G., Strauss, L., and Sapha, I.: Rupture of diseased large arteries in the course of enterobacterial *(Salmonella)* infections. N. Engl. J. Med. 258:824, 1958.
119. Ziment, I.: Nervous system complications in bacterial endocarditis. Am. J. Med. 47:593, 1969.
120. Ziment, I., and Johnson, B. L.: Angiography in the management of intracranial mycotic aneurysms. Arch. Intern. Med. 122:349, 1968.

13

Cardiac Tamponade

E. WILLIAM HANCOCK

Cardiac tamponade may be defined in general terms as "compression of the heart resulting from accumulation of fluid within the pericardial sac."[37] Since the term "compression" so used is somewhat vague, a more useful definition is that of Shabetai: "cardiac tamponade is the hemodynamic abnormality that results from accumulation of fluid in the pericardium with an increase in pressure of the pericardial fluid."[33] These definitions indicate that the essence of cardiac tamponade is the elevation of pressure within the pericardial space.

Spodick prefers the more restrictive wording: "cardiac tamponade is defined as the decompensated phase of cardiac compression resulting from an unchecked rise in intrapericardial fluid pressure."[35] He further points out that the term may also be used as a generalization to describe any degree of cardiac compression. This ambiguity in the use of the term "tamponade" is responsible for some confusion in discussions of the subject.

The principal effect of compression of the heart is an impairment of filling of the heart in diastole. Impaired filling of the heart, if not countered by compensatory mechanisms, would quickly result in impaired cardiac output and reduced systemic arterial pressure, a form of cardiogenic shock. A restricted use of the term "tamponade" for only such a syndrome certainly implies a true cardiac emergency. However, this is only the extreme end of the spectrum. In many circumstances there is severe compression of the heart, but because of the effects of compensatory mechanisms the systemic circulation is not severely impaired. This is the rule in medical, as opposed to surgical, patients with cardiac tamponade. In medical patients, in most circumstances, pericardial effusion and developing cardiac tamponade can be recognized at a stage well short of the crisis of cardiogenic shock. Thus, it is preferable to use the term "tamponade" for all degrees of compression of the heart, and to refer to the hypotensive shock–like condition as "decompensated" or "critical" tamponade.

PATHOPHYSIOLOGY

The pericardial space normally contains about 20 ml of fluid, or a layer less than 5 mm thick around most of the heart. The pressure in the pericardial space normally is essentially the same as that in the pleural space; i.e., negative in inspiration and slightly positive in expiration, with a mean pressure very close to zero, or atmospheric pressure. When fluid is added to the pericardial space, the pressure rises, slowly at first when the pericardial membrane is slack, and then steeply when the pericardium becomes tense. When the volume of fluid increases slowly, the pericardium stretches gradually; it may not reach its limit of distensibility until a very large effusion, such as 2000 ml or more, has developed. On the other hand, when fluid accumulates rapidly the pericardium has little opportunity to stretch; it reaches its limit of distensibility with effusions as small as 100 ml. Thus, the effect of increased pericardial fluid on the pericardial pressure depends not only on the amount of fluid, but also on the

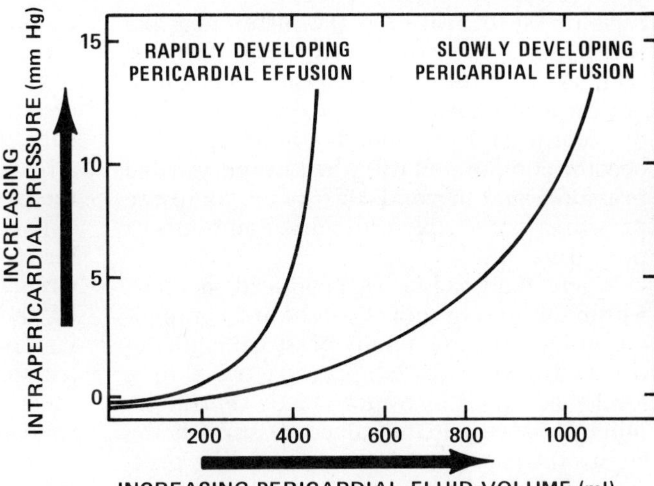

Figure 13–1. The effects of increasing amounts of pericardial effusion on intrapericardial pressure. In rapidly developing effusions, the pericardium has little opportunity to stretch and the pressure-volume curve is steep. In slowly developing effusions, the pericardium stretches and a very large effusion may develop before a steep rise in pressure occurs.

distensibility of the pericardium. The pericardium is composed primarily of dense connective tissue, mostly collagen. The collagen bundles have some waviness, particularly in younger people, which permits some stretch to occur.[17] However, the normal pericardium is extremely resistant to stretch that is applied acutely, and only after days and weeks of a persistent distending pressure does it stretch markedly. The pressure-volume characteristics of the pericardium for slowly and rapidly developing effusions are illustrated in Figure 13–1.

Central venous pressure is normally about 5 mm Hg higher than intrapericardial pressure; this differential maintains the right atrium and the central veins in an appropriate, slightly distended condition. Peripheral venous pressure, likewise, is up to 5 mm Hg higher than central venous pressure; this differential promotes continuous blood flow toward the heart from the periphery. When pericardial fluid begins to accumulate, raising intrapericardial pressure moderately, there is only a slight rise in central venous pressure and little or no initial rise in peripheral ve-

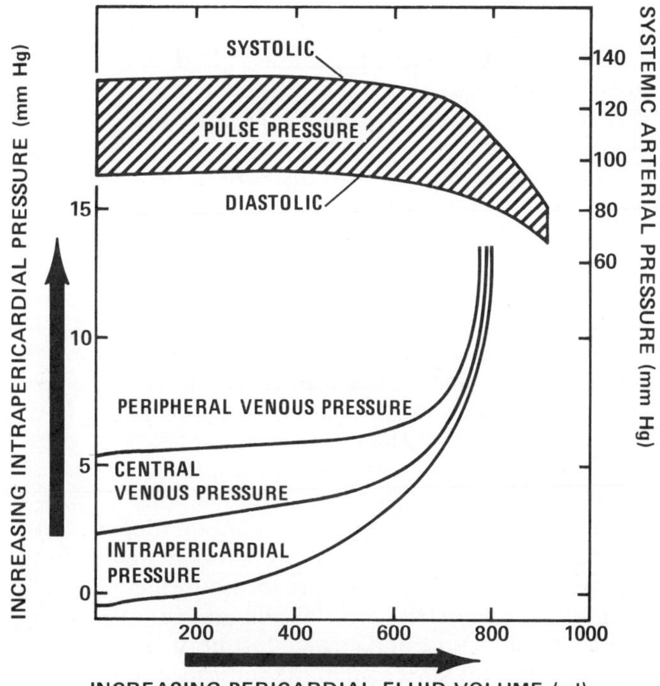

Figure 13–2. Diagram of the effects of cardiac tamponade on venous and arterial pressures. With moderate increase in intrapericardial pressure, the central and peripheral venous pressures rise slightly, but become more closely equilibrated than normal. After equilibration, they rise steeply with increasing tamponade. Reduction of arterial pulse pressure and a fall in mean arterial pressure occur only with severe tamponade.

nous pressure. However, the differences between these three pressure levels decrease (Fig. 13–2). With greater elevations of intrapericardial pressure, up to about 10 mm Hg, the central and peripheral venous pressures become equilibrated with the intrapericardial pressure, and beyond this point all three pressures rise steeply with added amounts of pericardial fluid.

When tamponade is produced acutely, within minutes or one to two hours, compensation by a rise in venous pressure is inadequate. Intrapericardial pressure rises to a level that equals or even exceeds central venous pressure and diastolic pressure in the right ventricle; the effective distending pressure of the right ventricle becomes critically reduced. In these circumstances, the circulation is maintained by the action of three more quickly acting compensatory mechanisms. First, the heart empties more completely with each contraction; the normal ejection fraction of about 0.50 increases to 0.70 to 0.80. Second, an increase in heart rate occurs, tending to maintain cardiac output even though the stroke volume is necessarily much diminished. Third, there is arteriolar vasoconstriction in the vascular bed of the skeletal muscles and the kidney, which tends to maintain systemic arterial pressure in the face of decreasing cardiac output, and thus to maintain perfusion of the heart and brain. These compensatory mechanisms are mediated by adrenergic stimulation. They could be attenuated by the administration of beta-adrenergic blocking agents, particularly the tachycardia and the increased ejection fraction.

Reduction in the effective distending pressure of the right ventricle leads to reduction in the volume of this chamber, i.e., to compression of the right ventricle. An important reduction in the volume of the left ventricle also occurs, not solely from direct compression as in the case of the right ventricle, but to some extent secondarily to the reduction in pulmonary blood flow and in the venous flow into the left side of the heart as a result of compression of the right ventricle. Ditchey and associates showed in experimental animals that cardiac tamponade, produced abruptly, caused an immediate compression of the right ventricle and reduction of pulmonary arterial blood flow, whereas the volume and stroke output of the left ventricle did not begin to fall until several beats later.[10] These events also lead to a reduction in pulmonary blood volume, which has the effect of displacing blood into the systemic veins, raising systemic venous pressure, and beginning, within the time span of a few beats, the circulatory compensation for the cardiac tamponade.

In cardiac tamponade, as in congestive heart failure, impairment of the systemic circulation leads to retention of salt and water by the kidney, increasing the intravascular volume. This volume increase is largely distributed to the systemic venous portion of the circulation. Together with a degree of venoconstriction, this leads to a further rise in venous pressure. The rise in venous pressure is the most important compensatory mechanism, which acts, largely after a period of hours or days, to maintain filling of the heart and adequacy of the systemic circulation in the face of cardiac tamponade. Typical measurements of the circulatory status in acute and in subacute or chronic cardiac tamponade are given in Table 13–1.

Abnormalities in the regional circulations are essentially the same in cardiac tamponade as in other forms of hypotension and circulatory failure. Diminished renal blood flow is the most striking and consistent alteration. The coronary circulation can be selectively impaired by compression of the epicardial coronary arteries when extremely severe cardiac tamponade is produced in experimental animals.[18] It is doubtful whether this occurs in humans, however.

A parasympathetic vasodepressor reflex, associated with vagally mediated bradycardia, may occur in cardiac tamponade.[13] This is seen in severe cases, particularly in the preterminal phase of electromechanical dissociation. Atropine may be effective in blocking this undesirable complication.

Restriction of filling of the heart by cardiac tamponade produces characteristic alterations of the pressure waveforms in the right ventricle, right atrium, and jugular veins. The right ventricle shows a narrow pulse pressure owing to an elevated diastolic pressure with a normal systolic pressure. The early diastolic pressure, as well as that in mid- and late diastole, is elevated; consequently, the "square root" or "dip-plateau" waveform seen in chronic constrictive pericarditis is not found in cardiac tamponade. The waveforms in the right atrium and jugular venous pulse show an exaggerated pressure drop in systole

Table 13–1. TYPICAL HEMODYNAMIC MEASUREMENTS IN ACUTE AND SUBACUTE CARDIAC TAMPONADE COMPARED WITH NORMAL, ILLUSTRATING THE COMPENSATORY MECHANISMS THAT MAINTAIN THE CIRCULATION IN SUBACUTE AND CHRONIC TAMPONADE

	Normal	Acute Tamponade	Subacute Tamponade
Pericardial pressure, mm Hg	0	10	18
Central venous pressure, mm Hg	4	10	20
Systemic venous pressure, mm Hg	8	10	20
Heart rate, per minute	70	100	75
Left ventricular end-diastolic volume, ml	142	40	110
Left ventricular ejection fraction	0.50	0.70	0.50
Stroke volume, ml	60	28	55
Cardiac output, l/min	4.2	2.8	4.1
Systemic vascular resistance, mm Hg/l/min	23.8	28.6	23.2
Mean arterial pressure, mm Hg	100	80	95

(X descent) and a reduced or absent drop in early diastole (Y descent); this also contrasts with constrictive pericarditis, in which both X and Y descents are prominent (Friedreich's sign). The central venous pressure waveform in cardiac tamponade reflects the waveform in the pericardial fluid pressure recording, which shows a systolic drop owing to the decompressive effect of the smaller heart size in systole. Forward flow from the veins to the right atrium occurs largely during systole, for the same reason.

Another difference between the venous pulse in tamponade and that in chronic constrictive pericarditis is Kussmaul's sign, which is defined as a rise in venous pressure with inspiration. This does occur in a minority of patients with constrictive pericarditis, but, contrary to frequent statements, is not found in patients in whom the compression of the heart is purely due to tamponade by fluid. In tamponade, the variation in venous pressure with respiration is normal; i.e., the venous pressure is constant or falls slightly with inspiration. It is not unusual to observe an increase in the amplitude of the venous waves with inspiration in cardiac tamponade, or indeed in many other circumstances; this should not be confused with Kussmaul's sign.

Paradoxical pulse, which is defined as an exaggerated fall in systemic arterial pressure with inspiration, occurs almost uniformly in cardiac tamponade. The long-time controversy about its mechanism is not entirely resolved, but several points have become established. The inspiratory fall in pressure is due to an inspiratory drop in the left ventricular stroke volume, and is accompanied by an inspiratory drop in left ventricular diastolic volume. At the same time that left-sided volume and output are decreasing, right-sided venous return and right ventricular volume are increasing.[32] In other words, the normal inspiratory augmentation of venous return is maintained in the presence of cardiac tamponade.

Two principal mechanisms are proposed to link these events to paradoxical pulse. First, the inspiratory augmentation of right ventricular volume, in the presence of a relatively restricted total cardiac volume, may shift the ventricular septum to the left and restrict the left ventricular volume, a kind of internal tamponade of the left ventricle by the right ventricle.[11] Second, the expansion of pulmonary blood volume by expansion of the lungs, the lungs being outside of the external compression that surrounds the heart, may impair the normal tendency for blood in the lungs and pulmonary veins to flow into the left atrium and left ventricle.[19] Probably both mechanisms are important, but their relative effect, quantitatively, is uncertain. The first mechanism is likely predominant in cardiac tamponade, whereas the second may play a more important role in constrictive pericarditis. Other mechanisms may also be important, including the effect of inspiration in increasing the left ventricular afterload and thus decreasing left ventricular stroke volume.[26] Any of these mechanisms may have an enhanced effect as a result of the reduced volume of all the cardiac chambers in cardiac tamponade. Phasic variations in filling of the cardiac chambers that may be qualitatively and quantitatively normal in absolute terms may have an exaggerated effect simply because they are large in proportion to the volume of the chambers.

HISTORY AND ETIOLOGY

Any of the causes of pericardial effusion may lead to cardiac tamponade, and the etiologies therefore range over a wide variety of medical and surgical conditions. The most frequent clinical circumstances, and some key considerations with regard to each etiology, are discussed below.

Acute hemopericardium, usually from trauma such as a knife or gunshot wound, or closed chest trauma such as a steering-wheel impact in an automobile accident, is the most frequent cause of acute cardiac tamponade. Perforation of the heart by intravascular catheters used for pacing or for diagnostic cardiac catheterization and angiography produces a similar syndrome. Textbook descriptions of cardiac tamponade, often presented along the lines of Beck's description of the triad of a small quiet heart, falling arterial pressure, and rising venous pressure, refer primarily to this very acute surgical type of cardiac tamponade.[3] This subject is discussed more fully in Chapter 14 on cardiac trauma.

Cardiac tamponade in medical patients can be classified into six groups of etiologies; neoplastic, uremic, rheumatic, hemorrhagic, infective, and idiopathic. Each of these has features worthy of individual discussion.

Patients with neoplastic disease are perhaps the largest group who present with cardiac tamponade in the usual practice of internal medicine and its subspecialities. Metastatic carcinoma from the lung or the breast is the most frequent type of neoplasm. Lymphoma and leukemia also produce tamponade relatively often, and a wide variety of other neoplasms may be responsible. There is a rare primary mesothelioma of the pericardium that behaves in a highly malignant fashion, similar to mesothelioma of the lung.

Neoplastic pericardial disease usually presents in patients in whom the neoplasm has been previously diagnosed, and generally when there is known active neoplastic disease elsewhere in the body. Occasionally this is not so, however, and the pericardial effusion and tamponade are the initial presenting features of neoplastic disease; carcinoma of the lung is the most likely primary source in such cases.

Cytologic examination of pericardial fluid is highly accurate for the diagnosis of carcinomatous invasion of the pericardium, particularly for lung and breast carcinoma. This is not true, however, for lymphoma and other miscellaneous neoplasms, in which the cytologic study is more likely to be falsely negative.

Radiation pericarditis causes all the clinical forms of pericardial disease, including acute pericarditis, subacute or chronic pericardial effusion, and chronic constrictive pericarditis.[4] Cardiac tamponade in these cases is most frequently seen in subacute pericarditis with effusion, and is often associated with constrictive pericarditis (effusive-constrictive pericarditis). In the past, radiation pericarditis has been seen in at least 5 per cent of patients who survived for a year or longer after doses of 4000 rads or more to the mediastinum. These most frequently were patients with Hodgkin's disease, less often breast carcinoma, and occasionally other neoplasms such as malignant thymoma. Radiation pericarditis has diminished considerably in incidence in the past ten years, owing to improved techniques of dosimetry, more complete shielding of the heart, recognition of the 4000-rad limit for cardiac tolerance, and a greater use of chemotherapy in Hodgkin's disease. New cases are still seen, however, sometimes occurring years after the radiotherapy has been completed. It is not unusual for radiation pericarditis to present as an important clinical problem for the first time more than five years, perhaps as long as 20 to 25 years, later.[2]

Uremic pericarditis causes cardiac tamponade occasionally, but this is relatively rare. Patients with uremic pericarditis who have circulatory congestion are often suffering more from volume overload and congestive heart failure than from tamponade. A more frequent condition than true uremic pericarditis is the pericarditis with effusion that occurs in patients who are on chronic dialysis. The factors responsible for dialysis pericarditis are not well understood. An impaired immune response to viral infection, for example, may play a role. Anticoagulation, often used systemically during hemodialysis, is probably an important factor in some cases.

Clinical assessment of cardiac tamponade is particularly difficult in dialysis patients, since elevated venous pressure, circulatory congestion, and peripheral edema can reflect various mechanisms in these individuals.

Tamponade is often first suspected when unusual hypotensive reactions occur during dialysis sessions. It is particularly critical to assess the role of congestive heart failure and intravascular volume excess or depletion accurately in dialysis patients who are suspected of having cardiac tamponade.

Bacterial or fungal infective pericarditis, producing purulent pericardial fluid, is a relatively rare condition in current medical practice, but an extremely important one because of its high mortality rate in the absence of timely diagnosis and treatment. Diagnosis is difficult, partly because such infections usually occur as a complication in already seriously ill patients. Postoperative thoracic and cardiovascular surgery patients, chest trauma, dialysis, neoplasm, and septicemia of any cause are some of the clinical settings in which purulent pericarditis occurs. Another important feature of this condition is the need for more complete drainage of the pericardial fluid than pericardiocentesis can accomplish in most instances, and the considerable tendency to progress rapidly to constrictive pericarditis. Tuberculous pericarditis shares these features with other types of bacterial and fungal infections involving the pericardium.

Connective tissue diseases, particularly rheumatoid arthritis and systemic lupus erythematosus, are associated with pericarditis and pericardial effusion rather frequently, but only occasionally lead to cardiac tamponade. This probably reflects the relatively chronic course of most patients with these conditions, and the effectiveness of corticosteroid therapy for control of the major visceral inflammatory crises. The postcardiotomy syndrome may be included with the rheumatic diseases as a form of pericarditis that occasionally leads to tamponade. Cardiac tamponade that develops days to weeks after cardiac surgery is likely to be related primarily to anticoagulant therapy, with an uncertain role for the postcardiotomy syndrome. However, patients not taking anticoagulants may develop severe tamponade, apparently due primarily to the postcardiotomy syndrome.[27]

Nontraumatic hemopericardium, although most frequently related to anticoagulant therapy, may also occur with slowly leaking aneurysms or dissections of the ascending aorta and in patients with acute myocardial infarction. Rupture of the heart in acute myocardial infarction is fatal because of massive acute hemopericardium and tamponade; this usually occurs so rapidly that diagnosis is retrospective and treatment impossible to apply.

CLINICAL DIAGNOSIS

The symptoms of cardiac tamponade are nonspecific and relate principally to the secondary circulatory embarrassment. The rise in venous pressure leads to fullness in the head, neck, and abdomen; abdominal pain and nausea due to hepatic and intestinal congestion is often the most prominent symptom in cardiac tamponade that follows a subacute course. Dyspnea is frequent and often severe, reflecting diminished cardiac output and also restriction of lung volume by pericardial and pleural effusions. Orthopnea is often present, but paroxysmal nocturnal dyspneic attacks do not occur in most instances. There is often a vague oppressive feeling in the chest, probably reflecting a combination of circulatory abnormality and a direct sensation of distention of the pericardial sac. Most patients with cardiac tamponade have additional symptoms that reflect the primary disorder, such as chest pain from trauma or pericarditis, chills and fever from infection, and so forth. Symptoms, therefore, are relatively nonspecific and are not likely to be the clue that leads to the diagnosis of cardiac tamponade.

Patients with the critical forms of cardiac tamponade are acutely ill and appear distressed and dyspneic, with rapid pulse and respiration. In the most severe decompensated cases they show the shocklike appearance of cold, pale moist skin; weak pulse; low blood pressure; and altered mental status. In most medical cases, however, shock is not present; the skin is warm and dry, and the pulse is reasonably full in volume. Blood pressure may be low, with a narrow pulse pressure, but this is not the rule; perfectly normal values of systolic and diastolic pressure and of pulse pressure are consistent with at least moderately severe cardiac tamponade. This is the picture seen in most patients in usual medical practice.[14]

Paradoxical pulse is virtually always present in cardiac tamponade. This physical sign has a key value, therefore, if it can be elicited and interpreted accurately. An inspiratory fall of 10 mm Hg is often said to be the upper limit of normal, with paradoxical pulse defined as a fall greater than 10 mm Hg.

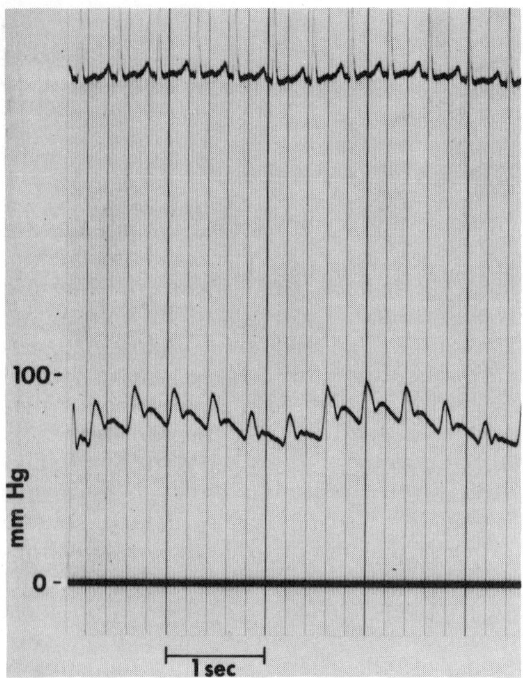

Figure 13–3. Direct intra-atrial pressure recording, showing paradoxical pulse in a 20-year-old woman with cardiac tamponade due to leukemic invasion. Arterial pressure is 93/74 on expiration, falling to 83/67 on inspiration. The inspiratory fall in systolic pressure is borderline in terms of absolute fall (10 mm Hg) but is large when expressed as a percentage of the pulse pressure (53 per cent).

This is a useful but arbitrary value, particularly when the measurement is made with a sphygmomanometer rather than a direct intra-arterial recording. Most patients with tamponade have a respiratory variation of 15 to 20 mm Hg or greater in arterial systolic pressure. When arterial pressure is low, however, a smaller degree of variation may be equally significant. Paradoxical pulse can also be defined in terms of the drop in systolic pressure as a percentage of pulse pressure; a drop of more than 50 per cent may be regarded as pathologic (Fig. 13–3).

Simple palpation of the radial pulse is an excellent method of assessing paradoxical pulse. Palpation probably detects pulse pressure more than it does the absolute systolic pressure levels. In a large majority of instances, a paradoxical pulse that is clinically important is palpable at the bedside and does not require a sphygmomanometer for its detection. Measurements with the sphygmomanometer are useful for confirmation in doubtful cases and for serial observations, but a value of 10 mm Hg shown by the sphygmomanometer should not be taken to rule out a paradoxical pulse if the variation can be detected by palpation.

Assessment of paradoxical pulse, whether by palpation or sphygmomanometry, should be carried out during quiet, uninstructed breathing, at least initially. Instructed deep breathing may then be used to bring out a doubtful abnormality. Many patients, when asked to take a deep inspiration, may actually perform Valsalva's maneuver, giving spurious results. If breathing is to be instructed, it should be in the form of continuous breathing in and out, without pauses.

Paradoxical pulse is difficult to assess when there is any cardiac arrhythmia, or when hypotension is severe. These situations are the principal exceptions to the rule that cardiac tamponade is always associated with a clinically detectable paradoxical pulse. On the other hand, paradoxical pulse does not necessarily reflect cardiac tamponade. The principal nonpericardial cause of paradoxical pulse is seen in the patient with dyspnea due to obstructive airway disease, either acute (asthma) or chronic obstructive pulmonary disease. Pulmonary embolism and shock have also been reported to cause paradoxical pulse. Paradoxical pulse in the presence of clearly normal central venous pressure should be assumed not to reflect cardiac tamponade.

Conversely, paradoxical pulse may be absent in certain circumstances of cardiac tamponade in which it would ordinarily be expected. The most important of these circumstances is left ventricular failure, when diastolic pressure in the left ventricle considerably exceeds intrapericardial fluid pressure. Here the right ventricle may be compressed, but not the left ventricle. This syndrome is most likely to be seen in dialysis patients.[29] Paradoxical pulse may also be absent in patients with atrial septal defect or with severe aortic regurgitation, even when cardiac tamponade is present.[22, 34]

Central venous pressure is always elevated in cardiac tamponade, with the exception of the first few minutes in some traumatic cases when central venous pressure has not yet risen, and the rare instances in which depletion of the circulating blood volume is severe enough to reduce central venous pressure to normal.[1] These circumstances are readily recognizable and it is therefore a good clinical rule that central venous pressure is always elevated in cardiac tamponade. It is vital to recognize, however, that "no jugular venous distention," the commonly used expression from the physical examination, may not reflect an examination that is sufficiently critical to rule out an elevated central venous pressure. If the external jugular veins are distended in the horizontal position and become nondistended in the upright position, it may be assumed that central venous pressure is normal. Failure to see distended external jugular veins in any position is nondecisive, however. It may be that the external jugular veins are very small or absent, that they are invisible beneath a layer of fat or other overlying tissue in the neck, or that along with other superficial veins in the body they are venoconstricted as part of the compensatory mechanisms that operate in the presence of circulatory impairment. This last circumstance is particularly frequent in cardiac tamponade of the more acute types, since the increase in blood volume and its redistribution to the venous system, producing widespread distention of the superficial veins, takes some time to occur. Furthermore, the expansion of venous blood volume may be opposed by diuretic therapy.

The critical examination needed to assess central venous pressure as normal, and thereby rule out cardiac tamponade in most instances, requires first of all that the external jugular veins be well seen, and that they be seen to be distended in the recumbent position and not distended in the upright position. If these observations are not clear-cut, there needs to be a careful observation of the internal jugular venous pulse. This is best done by first observing the patient in the sitting-up position, using a light to cast a shadow on the side of the neck. This should be followed by a similar observation with the patient in the recumbent position. If the internal jugular pulse is well seen in the recumbent position and is not seen in the sitting-up position, it may be presumed that central venous pressure is not elevated. On the other hand, any venous pulsation seen above the clavicles in the sitting-straight-up position should be presumed to be abnormal; this finding usually reflects elevated central venous mean pressure, although in some instances an abnormally prominent venous A wave (diastolic) or V wave (systolic) may be seen in the upright position in the presence of a normal mean central venous pressure. In some instances the venous pulsation seen in the neck may consist only of negative waves, one or two dips per cycle. This is particularly frequent in constrictive pericarditis, in which there is usually a systolic and a (more prominent) diastolic dip for each cardiac cycle. In cardiac tamponade only the systolic dip is prominent, and the dip is not so abrupt and visible as that in chronic constrictive pericarditis (Fig. 13–4). Most physicians should not expect to analyze the waveform of the venous pulse accurately in patients with cardiac tamponade, but the detection of elevated central venous pressure by accurate observation of the *level* of the internal jugular venous pulse is vital to the appropriate detection of this condition.

Kussmaul's sign, the rise in mean venous pressure with inspiration, does not occur in uncomplicated cardiac tamponade, despite being often quoted as one of the signs to look for. It is reasonable to seek this sign, as its presence should suggest constrictive pericarditis, or perhaps severe congestive heart failure, rather than uncomplicated tamponade. However, the *absence* of Kussmaul's sign should certainly not be quoted as evidence that cardiac tamponade is not present. Like paradoxical pulse, Kussmaul's sign should be first sought during quiet, uninstructed breathing; the patient should be in the position in which the external jugular venous distention or the internal jugular pulsation level is visible partway up the neck.

Apart from clues noted in the neck veins and arterial pulse, the physical examination gives little specific help in the diagnosis of cardiac tamponade. Hepatomegaly is often present and occasionally may be more readily elicited than the neck veins. Peripheral edema is not usually present, however, because of the rapidity of the development of elevated central venous pressure in most cases. Another factor in the frequent absence of peripheral edema in patients with cardiac tamponade is the relative youth of many of these with this condition; the frequency of peripheral edema in most types of congestive heart failure reflects the diminished tissue turgor and incompetent venous valves common to many elderly patients as much as it reflects the elevation of central venous pressure. Faint heart sounds and impalpable cardiac impulse are classic and understandable physical signs, but certainly are not necessar-

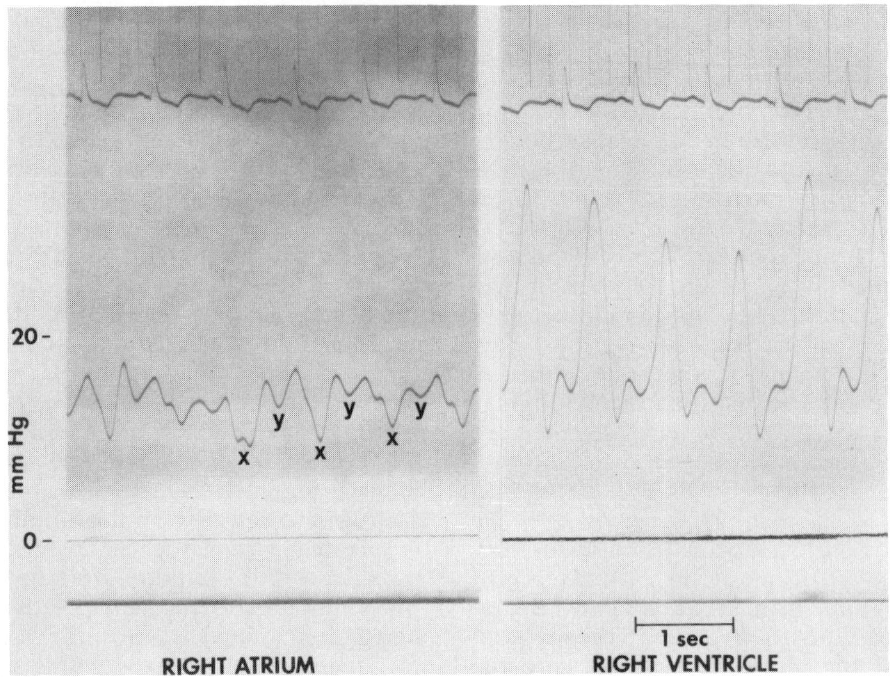

Figure 13–4. Right atrial *(left)* and right ventricular *(right)* pressure recordings in a 59-year-old woman with cardiac tamponade due to metastatic breast carcinoma. Right atrial pressure is elevated to a mean level of 12 mm Hg, with a predominant systolic *(X)* descent and a reduced diastolic *(Y)* descent. In the right ventricle there is a plateau of diastolic pressure elevated to 13 mm Hg. The early diastolic pressure is elevated as well as the mid- and late diastolic pressure, and the waveform does not have the "square root" appearance seen in chronic constrictive pericarditis.

ily present. Also, the presence of a pericardial friction rub does not weigh against the existence of a large pericardial effusion and cardiac tamponade; such rubs presumably are produced at the peripheral portion of the pericardial sac, where the parietal and visceral pericardial layers come together. The abnormal heart sounds in diastole, S3 and S4, are not ordinarily present in cardiac tamponade; their presence should raise the suspicion of congestive heart failure or, when only S3 is present, of constrictive pericarditis.

ELECTROCARDIOGRAPHY

The electrocardiogram in patients with cardiac tamponade usually shows sinus tachycardia, and often reveals low voltage and nonspecific ST- and T-wave abnormalities. These findings are not specific for cardiac tamponade, or even for pericardial disease. Low voltage in the limb leads only is particularly nonspecific, whereas generalized low voltage, with all complexes less than 0.5 mV in the limb leads and 1.0 mV in the precordial leads, can be a helpful clue to the diagnosis of pericardial effusion.

Cardiac tamponade due to acute pericarditis of various etiologies is often associated with ST-segment elevation diffusely in the ECG. In principle, all leads in which the positive electrode overlies the epicardial surface of the right or left ventricle show ST elevation. There is always ST depression in lead aVR in such cases, and leads III, aVL, and V1 may also show isoelectric or depressed ST segments, depending on the electrical axis of the heart. P-Q–segment depression also is often found in active pericarditis; this is virtually as frequent and specific as ST-segment elevation.[36]

Another electrocardiographic finding in pericardial effusion is electrical alternans. This does not necessarily imply the presence of tamponade, but in practice is usually associated with it. Neoplastic pericardial invasion is responsible for most instances of cardiac tamponade that are associated with electrical alternans. Electrical alternans is due to a swinging motion of the heart within a pericardial effusion, resulting in a beat-to-beat change in the electrical axis of the heart. The classical alternans pattern results when the heart swings from one position to another on alternate beats. Other patterns of swinging may occur, however, producing various patterns of changing electrical axis (seen as varying voltage in individual leads). Swinging motion of the degree that leads to electrical alternans implies a relatively large pericardial effusion, an absence of pericardial adhesions, and a relatively thin, serous type of pericardial fluid. The presence of these three factors in most cases of neoplastic pericardial effusion probably accounts for the association of electrical alternans with neoplastic effusions. Furthermore, the frequent occurrence of tamponade in neoplastic effusion is a likely explanation for the association of electrical alternans with tamponade, rather than simply a large pericardial effusion. There appears to be no direct reason why elevated intrapericardial fluid pressure per se should lead to more extensive swinging of the heart within the pericardial sac.

Electrical alternans may occur in situations other than cardiac tamponade, most notably during paroxysms of supraventricular tachycardia. Total electrical alternans, involving the P wave as well as the QRS complex, is a more specific indicator of pericardial effusion than is alternans of the QRS alone, but well developed examples of total alternans are rarely seen. There is also a form of pseudo-electrical alternans, in which a change in QRS axis occurs with respiration in a patient whose respiratory rate is about one half of the heart rate. This leads to alternation of the QRS voltage particularly in leads III and VI, which are usually the leads that best reflect changes in the electrical axis with respiration.

ROENTGENOGRAPHY

Most patients with cardiac tamponade have enlargement of the cardiac silhouette in the plain chest roentgenogram, as a result of the pericardial effusion. The small quiet heart referred to by Beck as part of the triad of findings in cardiac tamponade occurs primarily in acute hemopericardium of traumatic origin, and is not seen in medical patients, with rare exceptions.[3] Allegedly specific shapes of the heart shadow in the chest film, such as "water-bottle" or "globular" shapes, actually have little specificity for the presence of pericardial effusion. The chest films most suggestive of pericardial effusion are those with considerable enlargement of the heart shadow and a normal pulmonary vascular pattern, but often with pleural effusion.

Although the chest film often suggests the presence of pericardial effusion, it generally provides little or no evidence as to whether tamponade is present. Even though the pulmonary venous pressure is elevated in cardiac tamponade, the chest film does not usually show evidence of this in the form of redistribution of pulmonary blood flow or prominence of vascular or interstitial markings, because there is a redistribution of blood volume away from the lungs, rather than into the lungs as in ordinary congestive heart failure. One roentgenographic sign that may provide a clue to the diagnosis of cardiac tamponade in the presence of pericardial effusion is dilatation of the superior vena cava, reflecting elevated central venous pressure. It should also be pointed out that pleural effusion, although possibly due to various factors related to the primary disease, may also reflect tamponade, the pleural fluid forming as a transudate secondary to the elevated central venous pressure.

ECHOCARDIOGRAPHY

Echocardiography is the most reliable and convenient clinical method for detecting pericardial effusion, and for this purpose has essentially replaced other methods such as radioisotope scanning, intravenous carbon dioxide injection, and angiocardiography.[16] The M-mode echocardiogram, with a damping study of the left ventricle and a sweep study from aorta to left ventricle, is adequate to determine the presence or absence of pericardial effusion in a great majority of patients. Two-dimensional echocardiography is more definitive, since it displays the pericardial space around the entire circumference of the heart.[25] When the M-mode echocardiogram shows an echo-free space of 1.0 cm both anterior and posterior to the heart, the presence of a large pericardial effusion may be confidently inferred, and a pericardiocentesis may be expected to be successful. If only a posterior space is seen, the two-dimensional study is indicated in order to assess further the presence of pericardial fluid anteriorly or inferiorly, where it might be accessible to pericardiocentesis.

Echocardiography demonstrates the presence of pericardial fluid, but gives only indirect clues as to whether tamponade is present. One such clue is the presence of exaggerated swinging of the heart, as in electrical alternans.[38] Another is a conspicuous variation in the right ventricular and left ventricular dimensions with respiration;[31] associated with this may be a respiratory variation in the E to F slope and in the early diastolic opening excursion of the mitral valve, reflecting respiratory variation in filling of the left ventricle.[9] A third clue is a reduced diameter of the right ventricle, reflecting compression of the right ventricle by the increased intrapericardial fluid pressure.[30] This clue is usually recognized only in retrospect since the variability in the angle at which the ultrasonic beam crosses the right ventricular cavity makes this a variable measurement, and a comparable measurement before the advent of cardiac tamponade is usually unavailable.

HEMODYNAMIC STUDIES

Hemodynamic studies are not usually necessary to establish a diagnosis of cardiac tamponade, but they do provide characteristic findings that are useful in confirming the diagnosis, assessing possible associated abnormalities, and monitoring the clinical course and the results of treatment. The simplest study is a direct measurement of central venous pressure by means of an intravenous catheter, advanced to the superior vena cava or the right atrium. Central venous pressure is always elevated in cardiac tamponade, save for the highly unusual circumstance of volume depletion, mentioned above. The level of central venous pressure, referred to the midthoracic plane, is often in the moderate range of 10 to 20 mm Hg, but is likely to be 20 to 30 mm Hg or even higher in severe cases. Placement of the catheter in the right atrium, under fluoroscopic guidance, gives the additional information of the distance from the right lateral border of the right atrial cavity to the right lateral cardiac border, which is a fairly reliable indication of the extent of the pericardial fluid layer at that location.

A more complete catheterization of the right side of the heart, including measurement of pulmonary artery wedge pressure, provides a more complete assessment of cardiac tamponade than does central venous pressure determination alone. The balloon-tipped catheter is usually satsifactory for this purpose; fluoroscopic guidance is preferable, but not always essential. The right atrial and pulmonary artery wedge pressure levels should be equal, and should be equilibrated with the diastolic pressure levels in the right ventricle and pulmonary artery in cardiac tamponade. The right atrial pressure waveform shows a predominant systolic (X) descent, with a diminished or absent diastolic (Y) descent. The right ventricular pressure waveform shows elevation of the diastolic pressure to a level one third or more of the systolic pressure level; there is no early diastolic dip or "square root" pattern in cardiac tamponade, in contrast to the pattern seen in chronic constrictive pericarditis (Fig. 13–4).

Intra-arterial pressure monitoring is often useful in cardiac tamponade for following the course and treatment of a critically ill patient, for monitoring the results of pericardiocentesis, and for assessing the paradoxical pulse more accurately than can be done noninvasively. In addition, a phasic change in the arterial pressure waveform with inspiration may be seen, reflecting beat-to-beat changes in stroke volume, that provides additional evidence for the presence of a true paradoxical pulse (Fig. 13–5).

In more complex cases, catheterization of the left side of the heart may be useful and indicated in patients with cardiac tamponade. Left ventricular diastolic pressure should be equilibrated with that in the right ventricle. If the left ventricular diastolic pressure is substantially higher, the abnormality is more complex than that of cardiac tamponade alone and some type of left ventricular dysfunction is present. This circumstance is particularly frequent in dialysis patients, who are likely to have left ventricular abnormalities secondary to hypertension or coronary artery disease, and also intravascular fluid overload that precipitates disproportionate left ventricular failure.

Finally, measurement of intrapericardial fluid pressure, via a pericardiocentesis needle, provides the definitive diagnosis of cardiac tamponade. In cardiac tamponade, intrapericardial pressure is elevated to within

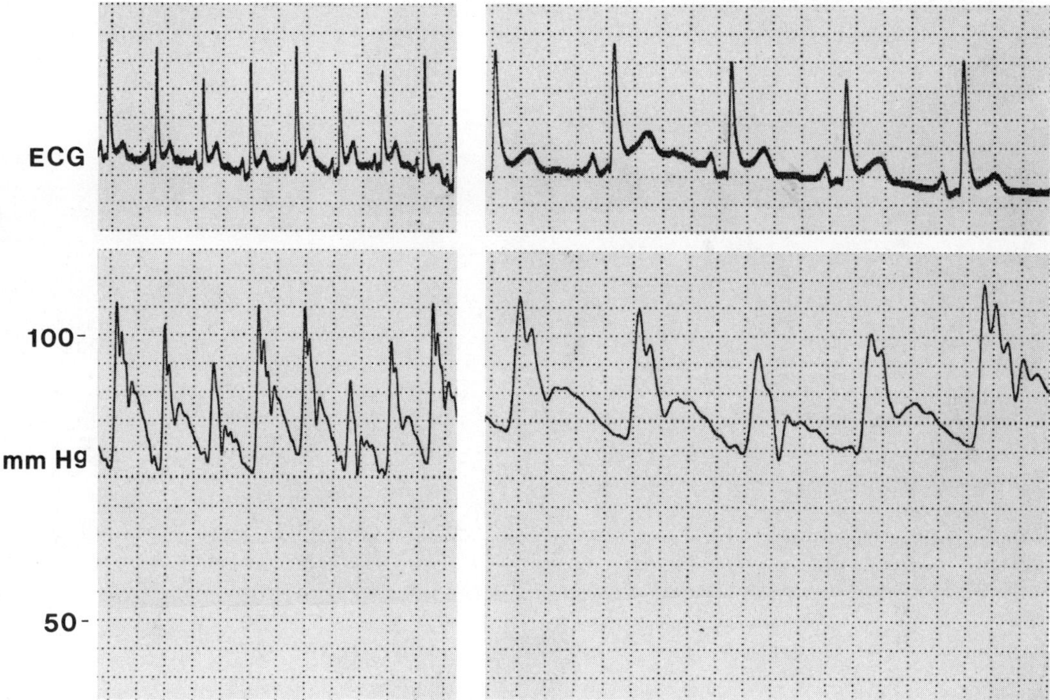

Figure 13–5. Recordings of central aortic pressure during respiration in a patient with paradoxical pulse due to dialysis-related pericardial effusion and tamponade. With inspiration there is a drop in systolic pressure and pulse pressure, owing to a drop in stroke volume. There is also a change in arterial pressure waveform, with a reduced pressure in late systole and a deeper incisura, again reflecting a drop in stroke volume.

3 to 4 mm Hg of right atrial or central venous pressure. Successful pericardiocentesis is documented by measurements of normal intrapericardial fluid pressure after removal of most of the fluid; i.e., a mean pressure level of less than 5 mm Hg with a transient fall below zero with inspiration. Hemodynamically successful relief of uncomplicated cardiac tamponade is documented by a fall in right atrial or central venous pressure to normal or nearly so, associated with reduction of intrapericardial pressure to normal (Fig. 13–6). Such measurements are particularly useful in patients who may have a combination of cardiac tamponade and constriction of the heart by the visceral pericardium (effusive-constrictive pericarditis).[15] This circumstance is particularly frequent in patients with relatively severe subacute pericarditis with effusion, especially those in whom the etiology is tuberculous, radiation-induced, or idiopathic.

MANAGEMENT

The essential step in management of cardiac tamponade is to relieve the compression of the heart by removing the fluid, either by pericardiocentesis or by surgical means. In extreme emergencies, pericardiocentesis should be done initially; however, surgery can also be accomplished very rapidly if necessary. There is usually a choice between pericardiocentesis and surgery; the factors involved are discussed later in this chapter.

In emergency circumstances, while preparations for removing the fluid are being made, certain types of supportive therapy may be helpful. Intravenous fluids may support the circulation in cardiac tamponade by further increasing central and pulmonary venous pressures, even when these pressure levels are already elevated and when there has been no loss of intravascular fluid. However, fluid replacement is most helpful in the management of acute traumatic hemopericardium, when there has been blood loss and when tamponade has developed too quickly for the renal adjustment of circulating blood volume to occur. Arterial pressure may be very responsive to volume infusion in such circumstances.

Intravenous isoproterenol is probably the most advantageous drug for support of the systemic circulation in cardiac tamponade.[12]

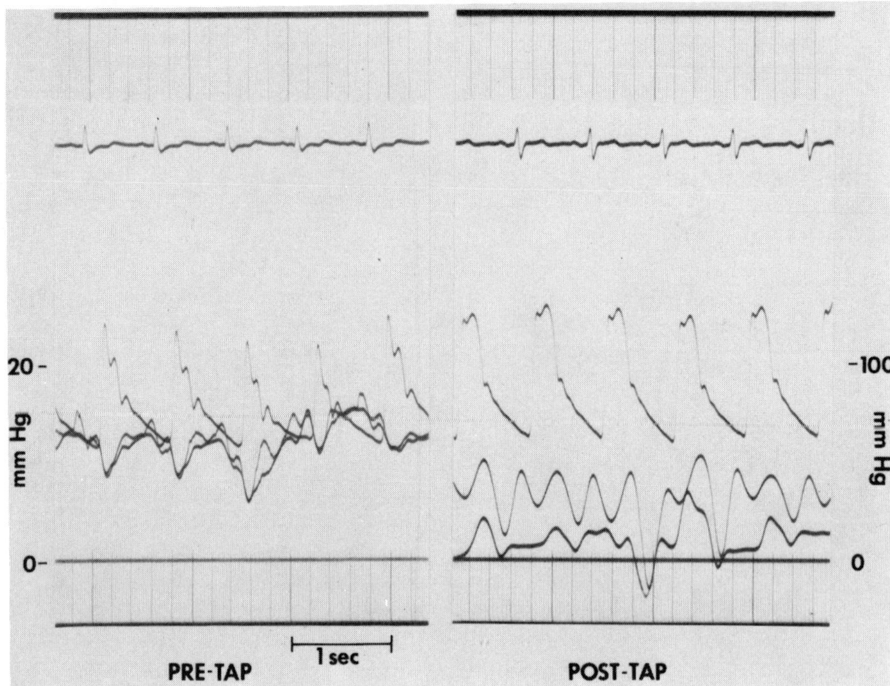

Figure 13–6. Pressure recordings before *(left)* and after *(right)* removal of fluid by pericardiocentesis in a 59-year-old woman with cardiac tamponade resulting from metastatic breast carcinoma. The three pressures recorded simultaneously are *(from above downward)*, aorta, right atrium, and pericardial space. Before removal of fluid *(left)*, the pericardial and right atrial pressures are elevated to 12 mm Hg and are essentially equilibrated; both show a predominant systolic dip. Aortic pressure is 120/70 with a prominent fall in inspiration. After removal of fluid *(right)*, pericardial pressure has fallen to near zero, documenting satisfactory relief of cardiac compression. Right atrial pressure has fallen to a normal level and aortic pressure has risen, with a reduced inspiratory drop. Pressure records of this type document the existence of tamponade as the cause of elevated central venous pressure, and its relief by pericardiocentesis.

It stimulates cardiac contractile force, dilates the resistance arterioles, and reduces the size of the heart, thus diminishing the effective degree of tamponade while increasing the cardiac output. A pressor drug that constricts the resistance arterioles, such as norepinephrine or methoxamine, may also be useful in patients who are hypotensive owing to critical tamponade. A combined infusion of isoproterenol and norepinephrine may be appropriate in these circumstances.

Vasodilator therapy alone, such as intravenous nitroprusside, should not be used in cardiac tamponade, since it is undesirable to reduce the cardiac filling pressure to the levels to which pure vasodilating drugs would be expected to reduce it.

Pericardiocentesis

Removal of pericardial fluid by percutaneous needle puncture of the pericardial sac is widely practiced as a method of diagnosis and management of pericardial effusion and tamponade. It is usually the quickest and most convenient procedure for these purposes. Controversy exists regarding its use as opposed to surgical methods, however, because of its risks and limited success rate.

Pericardiocentesis, or surgical pericardiostomy, is indicated as a rule when cardiac tamponade is believed to be present, i.e., when pericardial effusion is demonstrated and there are hemodynamic abnormalities suggesting tamponade. The procedure usually is relatively urgent, since even compensated tamponade can become decompensated quickly and without warning by the accumulation of a small amount of additional fluid in the pericardial space. The procedure is a true emergency when there is clinical shock, respiratory distress, or hypotension, e.g., arterial systolic pressure less than 100 mm Hg or arterial pulse pressure less than 30 mm Hg.

Ideally, pericardiocentesis should be performed in a cardiac catheterization laboratory, since it is an invasive cardiologic procedure with risks and technical requirements similar to those of cardiac catheterization and angiography. Correspondingly, the operator ideally should be a cardiologist who is skilled and experienced in invasive cardiologic procedures. Emergency circumstances may require that pericardiocentesis be done in other clinical settings and by other physicians, but this requires good clinical judgment as to whether such an acute emergency truly exists, whether supportive therapy may permit some delay in carrying out the procedure, and whether a surgical approach may be preferred.

Pericardiocentesis is best performed by a subxiphoid approach, although a left parasternal or an apical approach may be preferred in some instances. The subxiphoid approach is more likely to avoid injury to the coronary arteries on the surface of the heart than are the other two routes. In addition, it provides an approach that is more or less parallel to the anterior or inferior surface of the heart, whereas the intercostal and apical approaches are perpendicular to the surface of the heart and cross the pericardial space in a short dimension. It may be helpful to elevate the patient's upper body by 20° to 30°, but this is not essential since the heart does not consistently either sink or float within a pericardial effusion.

The subxiphoid puncture should be made about 5 cm below the xiphoid tip and about 1 cm to the left of the midline. The site must be far enough below the xiphoid to permit the needle to pass under the rib margin at a narrow angle with the skin surface, ideally about 20°. A frequent error is to select a puncture site too close to the rib margin, resulting in an excessively vertical position of the needle and in a needle track that will remain below the diaphragm.

It is useful to use atropine, 0.8 to 1.0 mg intravenously or intramuscularly, as premedication for pericardiocentesis, since vasodepressor ("vasovagal") reactions are not uncommon. These reactions may be due to pain or other nonspecific aspects of the procedure, but they are also likely if inadvertent puncture of the heart should occur, particularly if hemopericardium and aggravated cardiac tamponade should follow.

The local anesthetic should be instilled through a small-bore needle, such as a No. 20, which is long enough to reach the pericardial space, usually at least 10 cm. The local anesthetic needle should be advanced into the pericardial space, and a few milliliters of pericardial fluid aspirated; this maneuver clarifies the appropriate direction and distance for subsequent passage of the larger-bore needle. If the pericardial space cannot be reached by the local anesthetic needle, a different site of insertion should be chosen, usually further below the xiphoid than that selected initially.

Following the local anesthetic exploration, a needle of at least 16 gauge with a short bevel should be inserted. The short bevel is very important, since it provides greater tactile awareness by the operator of the structures encountered by the needle. Also, it is more likely to permit the needle tip to lie freely in the pericardial space, without touching the heart if inserted too far, and without requiring the needle tip to be just barely within the pericardial space if not inserted far enough. A small opening should be made in the skin with the tip of a scalpel blade, to facilitate insertion of the short-beveled pericardiocentesis needle. Either a trocar-type or a fluid-filled needle with a syringe attached may be used; however, the syringe offers the major advantage of signaling entrance into the pericardial space immediately, by the aspiration of fluid.

Connection of an electrocardiographic lead to the needle, using a unipolar V lead connection, is a useful monitoring device during pericardiocentesis.[5] When the tip of the needle touches the right ventricle, ST-segment elevation is recorded in this lead while little or none is seen in a surface ECG lead. Rarely, the needle contacts the right atrium, and P-R segment depression is recorded.[20] The experienced operator may make little or no use of this technique, however. Penetration of the pericardium is normally accompanied by a recognizable "plunk" or "give" sensation, particularly if an appropriately short-beveled needle is employed. This sensation signals entrance into the pericardial space, and there is no need to advance further or to contact the heart to obtain an ECG contact current. While the needle is in the pericardial space, contact of the tip with the heart is normally accompanied by a distinct grating or scratching sensation, due to movement of the heart against the needle tip during the cardiac cycle. This frequently occurs as fluid is removed and the pericardial space becomes smaller.

The initial measurement of the intrapericardial pressure level should be made before more than 3 to 5 ml of fluid are removed, since the pressure may fall considerably with removal of small amounts of fluid. Phasic electromanometric recordings, with simultaneous recordings of right atrial or central venous pressure, are preferable, but in a bedside or emergency room procedure a saline manometer may be used, just as in lumbar puncture.

If grossly bloody fluid is obtained, it must be questioned whether the needle tip may be within a cardiac chamber, with intracardiac blood being aspirated. There are several methods of making this distinction. ST-segment elevation should have been observed if the needle traversed the right ventricular wall. Intracardiac blood should clot rather quickly, while intrapericardial blood has usually been defibrinated by the action of the heart and does not clot. A pressure recording from the right ventricle should have a systolic peak of 20 to 30 mm Hg and be easily distinguished from the recording in the pericardial fluid, which has a fall in systole. A drop of intracardiac blood on a gauze pad should spread out as a homogeneous, deep red spot, while a drop of bloody pericardial fluid should separate into a central, deep red spot and a peripheral halo that is much less bloody. A small hand injection of radiographic contrast agent will disappear almost immediately from an intracardiac site, while remaining in a dependent site if injected into the pericardial sac. Echocardiography after saline injection into a questionable location usually permits a conclusion as to whether the needle is inside or outside the heart.[7] Finally, for confirmation, the packed cell volume or the blood gas levels of the fluid sample may be compared with similar determinations on a sample of circulating blood.

Pericardial fluid should be aspirated slowly with a syringe over 10 to 30 minutes. When little or no further fluid can be aspirated, intrapericardial and central venous pressure levels should be recorded again to assess the adequacy of the relief of tamponade. In a successful pericardiocentesis the intrapericardial pressure should be reduced to a normal level, even though there is always residual fluid within the pericardial space (Fig. 13–5). Central venous pressure may not fall to normal immediately, since there is an increased blood volume and venoconstriction that require time for reversal; it should fall substantially, however, and should not exceed 10 mm Hg at the end of the procedure. Paradoxical pulse should also be essentially eliminated by a successful pericardiocentesis for uncomplicated cardiac tamponade. Often there is a notable change in the arterial pulse waveform, consistent with an increase in stroke volume, in addition to a rise in systolic and pulse pressures (Fig. 13–6).

As a rule, an indwelling catheter should be placed in the pericardial space at the end of the procedure, to allow further slow drainage of fluid and to prevent rapid recurrence of tamponade from reaccumulated fluid. The catheter is best placed by the Seldinger flexible guidewire technique. It may be placed earlier in the procedure, before aspiration of the fluid, but there is sometimes difficulty with kinking of the catheter and occlusion of its tip when fluid is aspirated under negative pressure. Such catheters should not be left indwelling in the pericardial space for longer than about 48 hours because of the risk of infection.

Instillation of air or carbon dioxide into the pericardial space at the end of a pericardiocentesis is a frequent procedure to permit air-contrast roentgenograms to be made. Such films, in the upright position, show an air-fluid level and permit assessment of the amount of residual fluid and the size of the heart. These two points can be well assessed by echocardiography, however, and since the instillation of air obscures the echocardiogram for the next 24 to 48 hours, the air instillation has a lesser role than in the past. Nonetheless, it may still be useful in certain cases to assess the thickness of the parietal pericardium and to determine whether the entire pericardial sac is a single open space or whether the tap was done in a loculated area of effusion.

Surgery

Surgical treatment of cardiac tamponade may be divided into three types of procedures. The first is subxiphoid pericardiostomy.[6] This is usually done under local anesthesia, and involves resection of the xiphoid process and the creation of a small opening

PROFESSIONAL BOOK STORE

MEDICAL BOOKS FROM ALL PUBLISHERS

PHONE 955-1620

1122 EAST 53rd ST. CHICAGO, ILL. 60615

Customer's Order No.	Date 4/25 19 84
Sold to	
Address	
City	

Sold by	Cash	C.O.D.	Charge	On Acct.	Mdse. Ret.	Paid Out	
	X						

Quantity	Description	Price	Amount
1	Schwiman		40 00
		tax	2 80
			42 80
		Tax	
Thank You In case of claims or returned goods please present this bill.		Total	

RS 510-8

No. A10439

Uarco Business Forms

Received by ____________

into the inferior aspect of the pericardial space. Through such an opening the fluid is easily drained, and a limited manual exploration of the pericardial space may be carried out. Light pericardial adhesions may be broken up. A pericardial biopsy can also be obtained. A drainage tube may be left in place for several days. This approach is most useful in reversible nonconstrictive forms of tamponade, such as that in most patients with dialysis-related or idiopathic pericarditis. Most patients who are suitable for subxiphoid pericardiostomy are also suitable for pericardiocentesis, so that this approach is used the most frequently in those centers in which pericardiocentesis is rarely performed.

The second surgical approach is the parietal pericardiectomy through a left intercostal thoracotomy. This is a more extensive procedure, usually done under general anesthesia. It permits a more definitive relief of tamponade by removing a considerable amount of the anterolateral parietal pericardium, usually as far as the phrenic nerve on the left side. It is often referred to as a "window procedure," but the term partial parietal paricardiectomy is preferable in order to emphasize that a considerable amount of pericardium should be removed, not merely a small opening. This approach is particularly useful in purulent pericarditis, in which adequate drainage of often loculated effusion is essential.

The third method is pericardiectomy through a vertical or transverse sternotomy. This is the most extensive and definitive approach to pericardiectomy, and permits stripping of a constricting visceral pericardium if necessary, as well as extensive parietal pericardiectomy. This method is particularly useful in patients in whom visceral constriction is likely, e.g., those with radiation-induced or tuberculous pericarditis. In some of these operations cardiopulmonary bypass may even be employed, to permit a difficult visceral pericardiectomy to be performed on the quiet heart, with less risk of perforating the atrial and ventricular chamber walls.[8]

Surgery vs. Pericardiocentesis

The choice between pericardiocentesis and surgery for the management of cardiac tamponade is a controversial one. Pericardiocentesis is practiced frequently in many medical centers.[21, 23] In other centers, however, it is rarely performed and surgery is favored as the initial approach.[24, 28] In the smaller hospital, because a thoracic surgeon is more likely to be available than is a cardiologist experienced in pericardiocentesis and a suitably equipped cardiac catheterization laboratory, surgery is often preferred.

Pericardiocentesis has probably become safer in recent years, particularly because of the development of echocardiography, which permits the procedure to be restricted to those patients known to have large pericardial effusions that are distributed at least partially in the anterior and apical region of the pericardial space. Probably many of the complications of the procedure in the past have occurred with the "blind tap," done on suspicion only, often in a critically ill or terminal patient who actually had no pericardial effusion. On the other hand, there has been a greater recognition of the inherent risks of the procedure and of the fact that it probably should be practiced routinely only by experienced invasive cardiologists. A further consideration is that the subxiphoid surgical procedure has become widely known and practiced only in recent years, and may be considered the most conservative and inherently safe of the several procedures available for cardiac tamponade.

Some of the advantages and disadvantages of pericardiocentesis, relative to a surgical approach, are listed in Table 13–2. Apart from these general points, and apart from local experience and tradition, each method has specific advantages in particular types of pericardial disease. In traumatic hemopericardium, for example, surgery is usually preferable, because the clotted blood cannot be aspirated and because a source of continuing bleeding often needs surgical correction. Surgery is also preferred in purulent pericarditis, because thorough drainage is required to control the infection. In most other forms of pericardial disease, including those associated with dialysis, neoplasm, radiation, rheumatic disease, and idiopathic pericarditis, pericardiocentesis is a feasible alternative that enables surgery to be avoided in most instances.[21]

When cardiac tamponade is managed successfully by pericardiocentesis, it must always be recognized that recurrence of tamponade and the need for repeat pericardiocentesis is likely. There should be a readiness to pro-

Table 13–2. ADVANTAGES AND DISADVANTAGES OF PERICARDIOCENTESIS COMPARED WITH SURGICAL METHODS IN MANAGEMENT OF CARDIAC TAMPONADE

Advantages	Disadvantages
Quickly applicable in varying clinical settings	Requires good-quality echocardiography, skilled invasive cardiologist, and cardiac catheterization facilities for best results
Readily combined with hemodynamic studies	Occasionally misses diagnoses (tuberculosis, lymphoma) that could be made by pericardial biopsy
Diagnostic study of fluid provides nearly all diagnoses that could be made by pericardial biopsy	Fails to relieve tamponade in one third of cases
Effectively relieves tamponade in two thirds of cases, with no subsequent need for surgery	May delay necessary surgery because of temporary or illusory relief of tamponade
	Risk of hemopericardium from puncture of heart

ceed to surgery if two or three pericardiocenteses are required, or if relatively severe tamponade recurs quite soon after pericardiocentesis.

References

1. Antman, E. M., Cargill, V., and Grossman, W.: Low-pressure cardiac tamponade. Ann. Intern. Med. 91:403, 1979.
2. Applefeld, M. M., Cole, J. F., Pollock, S. H., et al.: The late appearance of chronic pericardial disease in patients treated by radiotherapy for Hodgkin's disease. Ann. Intern. Med. 94:338, 1981.
3. Beck, C. S.: Two cardiac compression triads. J.A.M.A. 104:714, 1935.
4. Cohn, K. E., Stewart, J. R., Fajardo, L. F., and Hancock, E. W.: Heart disease following radiation. Medicine 46:281, 1967.
5. Bishop, L. H., Jr., Estes, E. H., Jr., and McIntosh, H. D.: Electrocardiogram as a safeguard in pericardiocentesis. J.A.M.A. 162:264, 1956.
6. Cassel, P., and Cullum, P.: The management of cardiac tamponade. Drainage of pericardial effusions. Br. J. Surg. 54:620, 1967.
7. Chandraratna, P. A. N., First, J. Langeuin, E., et al.: Echocardiographic contrast studies during pericardiocentesis (brief report). Ann. Intern. Med. 87:199, 1977.
8. Copeland, J. G., Stinson, E. B., Griepp, R. B., et al.: Surgical treatment of chronic constrictive pericarditis using cardiopulmonary bypass. J. Thorac. Cardiovasc. Surg. 69:236, 1975.
9. D'Cruz, I. A., Cohen, H. C., Prabhu, R., et al.: Diagnosis of cardiac tamponade by echocardiography. Circulation 52:460, 1975.
10. Ditchey, R., Engler, R., LeWinter, M., et al.: The role of the right heart in acute cardiac tamponade in dogs. Circ. Res. 48:701, 1981.
11. Dornhorst, A. C., Howard, P., and Leathart, G. L.: Pulsus paradoxus. Lancet 1:746, 1952.
12. Fowler, N. O., and Holmes, J. C.: Hemodynamic effects of isoproterenol and norepinephrine in acute tamponade. J. Clin. Invest. 48:502, 1969.
13. Friedman, H. S., Lajam, F., Gomes, J. A., et al.: Demonstration of a depressor reflex in acute cardiac tamponade. J. Thorac. Cardiovasc. Surg. 73:278, 1977.
14. Guberman, B. A., Fowler, N. O., Engel, P. J., et al.: Cardiac tamponade in medical patients. Circulation 64:633, 1981.
15. Hancock, E. W.: Subacute effusive-constrictive pericarditis. Circulation 43:183, 1971.
16. Horowitz, M. S., Schultz, C. S., Stinson, E. B., et al.: Sensitivity and specificity of echocardiographic diagnosis of pericardial effusion. Circulation 50:239, 1974.
17. Ishihara, T., Ferrans, V. J., Jones, M., et al.: Histologic and ultrastructural features of normal human parietal pericardium. Am. J. Cardiol. 46:744, 1980.
18. Jarmakani, J. M. M., McHale, P. A., and Greenfield, J. C., Jr.: The effect of cardiac tamponade on coronary haemodynamics in the awake dog. Cardiovasc. Res. 9:112, 1975.
19. Katz, L. N., and Gauchat, H. W.: Observations on pulsus paradoxus (with special reference to pericardial effusions). Arch. Intern. Med. 33:371, 1924.
20. Kerber, R. G., Ridges, J. D., and Harrison, D. C.: Electrocardiographic indications of atrial puncture during pericardiocentesis. N. Engl. J Med. 282:1142, 1970.
21. Krikorian, J. G., and Hancock, E. W.: Pericardiocentesis. Am. J. Med. 65:808, 1978.
22. Kronzon, I., and Winer, H. E.: Absence of paradoxical pulse in patients with atrial septal defect and cardiac tamponade. Am. J. Cardiol. 41:446, 1978 (Abstr.).
23. Kuhn, L. A.: Acute and chronic cardiac tamponade. Cardiovasc. Clin. 7:177, 1976.
24. Lajos, T. Z., Black, H. E., Cooper, R. G., et al.: Pericardial decompression. Ann. Thorac. Surg. 19:47, 1975.
25. Martin, R. P., Rakowski, H., French, J., and Popp, R. L.: Localization of pericardial effusion with wide angle phased array echocardiography. Am. J. Cardiol. 42:904, 1978.
26. McGregor, M.: Pulsus paradoxus. N. Engl. J. Med. 301:480, 1979.
27. Ofori-Krakye, S. K., Tyberg, T. I., Geha, A. S., et al.: Late cardiac tamponade in open heart surgery: incidence, role of anticoagulants in its pathogenesis and its relationship to the postcardiotomy syndrome. Circulation 63:1323, 1981.
28. Pradhan, D. J., and Ikins, P. M.: The role of pericardiotomy in treatment of pericarditis with effusion. Am. Surg. 42:257, 1976.
29. Reddy, P. S., Curtiss, E. I., O'Toole, J. D., and Shaver, J. A.: Cardiac tamponade: hemodynamic observations in man. Circulation 58:265, 1978.

30. Schiller, N. B., and Botvinick, E. H.: Right ventricular compression as a sign of cardiac tamponade. Circulation 56:774, 1977.
31. Settle, H. P., Adolph, R. J., Fowler, N. O., et al.: Echocardiographic study of cardiac tamponade. Circulation 56:951, 1977.
32. Shabetai, R.: The pathophysiology of cardiac tamponade and constriction. Cardiovasc. Clin. 7:67, 1976.
33. Shabetai, R.: The Pericardium. New York, Grune & Stratton, 1981.
34. Shabetai, R., Fowler, N. O., Braunstein, J. R., and Gueron, M.: Transmural ventricular pressures and pulsus paradoxus in experimental cardiac tamponade. Dis. Chest 39:557, 1961.
35. Spodick, D. H.: Acute cardiac tamponade. Pathologic physiology, diagnosis, and management. Prog. Cardiovasc. Dis. 10:64, 1967.
36. Spodick, D. H.: Diagnostic electrocardiographic sequences in acute pericarditis: significance of PR segment and PR vector changes. Circulation 48:575, 1973.
37. Stedman's Medical Dictionary, 23rd ed. Baltimore, Williams & Wilkins Co., 1976.
38. Usher, B. W., and Popp, R. L.: Electrical alternans: mechanism in pericardial effusion. Am. Heart J. 83:459, 1972.

14

The Internist's Role in the Recognition and Management of Cardiovascular Trauma

MELVIN D. CHEITLIN

and JOSEPH A. ABBOTT

Cardiovascular trauma is initially the province and responsibility of the surgeon. However, the internist and cardiologist become involved in both the acute and later phases of this acquired condition, usually because of the development of new and abnormal physical or laboratory findings, or late complications. The role of the internist in the management of the patient who has sustained cardiovascular trauma is reviewed in this chapter.

Until this century, trauma to the heart was considered to be fatal and thus a pathologic curiosity rather than a clinical problem. In the modern era, several circumstances have conspired to increase the significance to both surgeon and internist of cardiovascular trauma. First, the increase in population, the stresses of modern life, and technologic advances such as high-speed transportation have resulted in a marked rise in both military and civilian violence. The number of trauma patients therefore has also increased and with it the number of individuals with cardiovascular injury. Second, the development of trained ambulance crews, police, and firemen who are rapidly responding and capable of first-echelon resuscitation and rapid transport of injured patients to a sophisticated care facility has made possible prompt recognition and treatment of cardiovascular trauma. Patients with cardiovascular trauma who would have died rapidly from hemorrhage, asphyxia, or pericardial tamponade are being kept alive long enough to reach the hospital. Third, there have been marked advances in diagnostic and surgical techniques that enable the physician to recognize and treat the patient with cardiovascular trauma. Physicians today are more aware of the possibility of cardiovascular trauma, and specifically search for evidence that it has occurred. Patients who have had cardiac trauma in the past, with problems missed at the time of acute injury when head and abdominal injury or multiple fractures masked the relatively asymptomatic trauma to the cardiovascular system, are now being recognized by abnormal findings on electrocardiograms, chest roentgenograms, enzyme studies, and radioisotopic examinations.

Most authorities divide cardiovascular trauma into two groups: penetrating and nonpenetrating. Any structure in the cardiovascular system can be injured, and, in general, all types of injuries have been described in patients with penetrating or nonpenetrating trauma. Table 14–1 presents a classifica-

Table 14–1. CLASSIFICATION OF CARDIOVASCULAR TRAUMA

I. Pericardial contusion and laceration
   A. Pericardial tamponade
   B. Pericarditis: (1) immediate, (2) purulent, (3) posttraumatic
   C. Laceration of pericardium with subluxation of heart
II. Myocardial contusion and laceration
   A. Myocardial failure
   B. Arrhythmias and atrioventricular conduction defects
   C. Myocardial rupture
   D. Left ventricular aneurysm: (1) true, (2) false
   E. Rupture of interventricular septum and interatrial septum
   F. Mural thrombosis and distal embolization
III. Valvular insufficiency
   A. Mitral, aortic, tricuspid, and pulmonary insufficiency
IV. Coronary artery injury
   A. Thrombosis and laceration
   B. Coronary arteriovenous fistulae; coronary arteriocameral fistulae
V. Arterial and venous injury
   A. Arterial laceration and thrombosis
   B. Arteriovenous fistulae
   C. Venous laceration, thrombosis, and pulmonary embolism
   D. Arterial false aneurysm including aortic traumatic aneurysm
VI. Retained intracardiac and intraluminal foreign bodies
VII. Iatrogenic trauma

tion of cardiovascular trauma. The forces involved in injury to the cardiovascular system can be categorized as follows:

1. Penetrating
   a. Low-velocity missles
   b. High-velocity missles
2. Nonpenetrating
   a. Unidirectional force to thoracoabdominal region
   b. Direct compression of thorax
   c. Blast
   d. Rapid deceleration
   e. Indirect forces to abdomen or extremities
   f. Physical agents: electric shock, heat, cold

The tissue damage caused by penetrating missiles and objects is related to the mass and shape of the penetrating object as well as to the tumbling characteristics of the object at the time of impact. A major determinant of tissue injury is the velocity of the missile as it strikes the body. Passage of the missile through the body transfers energy to the tissues and produces a temporary cavitation along the penetrating tract, the size of which is proportional to the velocity of the missile.[5] This cylinder of cavitation alternately expands and collapses, oscillating for several cycles and causing tissue necrosis at a distance from the actual path of the missile. For this reason, the mass of necrotic tissue that must be debrided at the time of surgery is much larger than would be suspected by the size of the entrance and exit wounds.

The path of the missile, once it strikes the body, can be deflected by bone or even by tissue planes when the velocity of the missile is low, resulting in an unpredictable path that injures tissue and organs in areas unsuspected on the basis of the location of the entrance wound. We have seen gunshot victims with apparent abdominal wounds in whom the missile deflected into the thorax and produced cardiac injury; even gunshot wounds in the shoulder or neck have caused cardiac trauma.[96]

Although people of any age can be victims of cardiovascular trauma, the most frequent victims involved in violent trauma tend to be male, young, and (for the most part) previously healthy. For this reason, if the patient survives the initial trauma, recovery from the acute damage is usually quite good and residual ventricular cardiac function is often well preserved.

Cardiac injury occurs in 3 to 5 per cent of all patients with initial thoracoabdominal trauma.[32,78] The mortality rate for penetrating cardiac wounds varies with the type of injury, but overall is about 65 to 80 per cent. Gunshot wounds are the most lethal,[93] and appear to be increasing in frequency compared with knife wounds.[65] Once the patient arrives at the hospital alive, the mortality rate varies from 5 to 30 per cent.[18,62,102] There is evidence that alcohol can affect marked reductions in ventricular performance and exacerbate arrhythmias in the presence of minor degrees of myocardial trauma. This may enhance mortality after cardiovascular trauma. Since so many accidents occur in intoxicated patients, mortality may be increased beyond what would be expected from the myocardial injury incurred.

THE ACUTELY INJURED PATIENT

The acutely injured patient is usually first seen and evaluated by a surgeon.[24,103,109] A rapid history of the traumatic event must be obtained either from the patient or from persons accompanying him while his physical condition is rapidly evaluated. Airway patency must be established immediately, and rapid measurements made of pulse, respiration, and blood pressure. Pneumothorax, especially "sucking" pneumothorax, must be identified and treated with chest tubes. Signs of shock must be sought, such as "thready" pulse, peripheral vasoconstriction, and cold, clammy skin. Sites of obvious external injury should be looked for and external bleeding controlled. The height of central venous pressure should be assessed rapidly; if the deep cervical venous pulsations cannot be seen, an intravenous catheter should be placed for measurement of central venous pressure as well as for delivery of intravenous fluids. Blood should be drawn for type and crossmatch, although Type O blood can be given in an acute emergency. In the presence of hemodynamic compromise, two large intravenous catheters should be placed either by cutdown or percutaneously.

Rapid death from cardiovascular trauma results from four conditions: (1) hemorrhage and shock; (2) pericardial tamponade occurring from laceration of a cardiac chamber or a great vessel within the pericardial sac; (3) myocardial contusion with heart failure; and (4) arrhythmia. Usually, with pericardial tamponade, there is a rise in central venous pressure. Thus, the classic Beck's triad of a small quiet heart, shock, and elevated central venous pressure is often present in patients with pericardial tamponade. However, there frequently is associated blood loss in patients with cardiac trauma, and the resultant decreased intravascular volume, even in the presence of pericardial tamponade, may prevent elevation of central venous pressure.[49, 99] In this situation, restriction of filling of the right and left ventricle causes an even greater decrease in stroke volume and profound shock.

Since the pericardium is relatively noncompliant, rapid accumulation of a small amount (150–200 ml) of blood is all that is necessary to produce fatal pericardial tamponade. If bleeding occurs slowly enough and there is little or no external blood loss, then, as the ventricular filling is restricted by the increasing pericardial pressure, with decreasing stroke volume there is reflex sympathetic vasoconstriction involving both arterioles and peripheral veins. This increases venous tone and venous pressure, and thus supports the filling of both ventricles and the maintenance of stroke volume.

In the presence of external bleeding, volume replacement with colloid fluid followed by blood must be started immediately. Central venous pressure is a good measure of the adequacy of blood volume in a previously healthy patient. Fluid and blood should be transfused rapidly until central venous pressure is in the range of 5 to 10 cm H_2O. In a patient with a thoracoabdominal wound, if the blood pressure does not return after apparently adequate volume replacement, especially if central venous pressure rises rapidly, pericardial tamponade should be suspected and immediate pericardiocentesis carried out preparatory to opening the chest surgically. In cases of tamponade, when cardiac output is seriously compromised, induction of anesthesia can cause blunting of autonomic nervous system reflexes with resultant cardiovascular collapse and cardiac arrest. The patient should be prepared for surgery and the surgeon should be ready to operate before induction of anesthesia is begun. At San Francisco General Hospital Medical Center, approximately half of the patients with traumatic pericardial tamponade who are without pulse or pressure have been successfully resuscitated by this aggressive approach.

Pericardial tamponade associated with gunshot and knife wounds requires direct suture of the cardiac laceration to stop the bleeding.[88, 99] Pericardiocentesis by needle can be effective in low-velocity penetrating injuries such as knife wounds. In about one fourth of the patients, however, pericardiocentesis is unsuccessful primarily because there is clotted blood in the pericardium that cannot be removed through the needle.[93, 111] Recurrent or delayed bleeding frequently occurs and causes repeated pericardial tamponade; therefore, pericardiotomy to examine the heart directly is necessary in all such patients. For this reason, if a patient with pericardial tamponade is maintaining adequate blood pressure, we attempt pericardiocentesis in the emergency room while the operating room is being readied for thoracotomy. If the patient has marked hemodynamic compromise with barely palpable pulse and low blood pressure, the chest should be opened at once, even in the emergency room.[64] Laceration of the cardiac chambers, usually the right ventricle but frequently the left, or even the atria, can be successfully sutured. Coronary arterial injury and injury to the root of the aorta and pulmonary artery, both of which are intrapericardial, should be sought. Occasionally, if a lacerated coronary artery is overlooked and the patient is in shock and vasoconstricted, the artery may not be bleeding at the time of exploration. With resuscitation and return of blood pressure to normal levels, the lacerated retracted artery can begin to bleed anew and again cause tamponade.

If the bleeding is venous as a result of a small laceration of the vena cava or atrium, relatively slow accumulation of blood can occur and, after some stretching of the pericardium, late pericardial tamponade can arise hours or even several days after the injury. In these situations, the triad of a small quiet heart, elevated venous pressure, and falling systolic pressure usually occurs. The clue in such cases is elevation of central venous pressure. If the patient has a thick neck or an injury that prevents visualization of the neck veins, a catheter must be placed intravenously for measurement of central venous pressure.

During physical examination, a pericardial friction rub frequently can be heard, and signs of pericardial tamponade are present in addition to elevated central venous pressure. Such signs include a sudden, sharp dip in the elevated venous pressure (the X descent) as cardiac contraction occurs, causing the base of the ventricle to descend and the size of the atria to increase, with lesser dips at the time of the opening of the tricuspid valve (the Y descent). Other signs of pericardial tamponade are paradoxical pulse, or a drop in blood pressure of 10 mm Hg or greater with quiet inspiration; Kussmaul's sign, or increasing central venous pressure with quiet inspiration instead of the usual drop; and electrical alternans on the electrocardiogram. The patient develops tachycardia, and when decompensation occurs finally, blood pressure is low with narrow pulse pressure.

The chest roentgenogram may show signs of chest trauma such as fractured ribs or pleural effusion. Fracture of the first or second rib and sternal fracture is an especially common association with cardiovascular trauma.[81,110] Slight cardiomegaly may be present but frequently may not be obvious on roentgenograms taken quickly by a portable machine. If air-containing organs, such as the esophagus, trachea, or bronchi, are ruptured, there may be pneumomediastinum, pneumopericardium, or pneumothorax.

An echocardiogram can be helpful by showing pericardial effusion and possibly other signs of cardiac tamponade, such as pseudoprolapse of the mitral valve and collapse of the right ventricular outflow tract in expiration. Since the patient's chest is frequently covered with surgical dressings, echocardiography may be impractical during the acute management stage. Caution must be observed in evaluating the echocardiogram. In one of our patients the echocardiogram was negative for pericardial fluid, but obvious pericardial tamponade resulting from a large posteriorly placed clot and unclotted blood in the pericardium was found during surgery. There is some evidence that clots may have an echo reflectance similar to that of the myocardium, and thus may not be detectable as fluid by echocardiography.[52]

With penetrating injury, contaminated foreign material can be deposited in the pericardium, together with fragments of cloth, metal, wood, and other materials, that can cause infection and purulent pericarditis. If this occurs, the patient usually has a septic course with high fever. For purulent pericarditis, appropriate antibiotic therapy after culture of the microorganism, and often open drainage, are necessary.

Up to this point in management, the internist rarely is primarily involved. Once the patient's condition is stabilized, and abnormalities observed during physical examination and on the ECG and chest roentgenogram are evaluated more carefully, the internist or cardiologist is consulted. The problems of cardiovascular trauma that the internist subsequently faces are discussed separately below.

POSTTRAUMATIC CHEST PAIN

After trauma, the patient frequently may complain of chest pain.[84] Most often, this can be related to trauma to the chest wall, especially if there are signs of external injury, pinpoint localization of the pain as occurs with fractured ribs, and increased sharp somatic pain with respiration or muscle movement. On occasion, the pain is visceral in nature, not well localized, and even compressive or squeezing. If pericardial injury is involved, a pleuritic component to the pain may be present. In older patients, the question of acute myocardial infarction frequently arises, as a result of either the trauma or coronary disease precipitated by the stress of the trauma.

Myocardial Contusion, Laceration, and Infarction

Myocardial contusion can result from penetrating trauma or nonpenetrating trauma, owing to the heart striking the spine or sternum sharply during sudden deceleration or to direct compression between the sternum and the spine by impact of a steering wheel. There is hemorrhage into the cardiac muscle and muscle necrosis, and the pain can be quite similar to the discomfort of myocardial infarction.

In cases of penetrating injury, such as a knife or gunshot wound, laceration of the coronary artery can occur and is most often fatal. The myocardial injury results from either direct trauma or indirect involvement by the cylinder of cavitation. An ECG in such a patient may reveal an acute myocardial infarction. Although the coronary artery can be lacerated without showing the acute ECG changes that indicate an infarction, ECG changes of acute infarction are usually apparent after the bleeding artery is found and ligated. More frequently, subendocardial myocardial infarction may occur because of a prolonged period of hypotension. The diagnosis of infarction can easily be missed because the ST elevations of the acute infarction are often mistaken for the changes of pericarditis, and the importance of pathologic Q waves is often unappreciated. Preinjury ECGs are rarely available.

When the ECG shows acute myocardial infarction in a patient who has suffered nonpenetrating thoracic injury, the cause is almost always myocardial contusion or a myocardial infarction precipitated by the stress of trauma in an individual with coronary artery disease.[105] Although coronary thrombosis can result directly from nonpenetrating trauma, it is rare.[4, 72]

Myocardial contusion can be present without effecting significant changes in the ECG, but its presence can be suspected by ST-segment and T-wave changes, prolonged Q-T intervals, Q waves consistent with an acute myocardial infarction, or development of tachyarrhythmias.[50] Unfortunately, ST-segment and T-wave changes and arrhythmias after trauma can be associated with increased vagal or sympathetic tone, increased catecholamines, and electrolyte and blood gas abnormalities; they therefore are nonspecific.[66] On physical examination, contusion can be suspected when a pericardial friction rub is heard or when an older patient has an S3 gallop or other signs of congestive heart failure.

Experimental evidence indicates that the degree of ventricular functional impairment is related to the amount of cardiac muscle damaged.[105] After myocardial contusion, depression of cardiac output can be demonstrated.[74] Sutherland and colleagues noted significant right ventricular contusion by radioisotopic angiography after nonpenetrating chest trauma.[95]

In addition to congestive heart failure, all the complications of acute myocardial infarction resulting from coronary artery disease can occur with infarction due to myocardial contusion. These include arrhythmias, both ventricular and atrial; atrioventricular (AV) block; cardiac arrest due to ventricular fibrillation; pericarditis; and even late cardiac rupture and ventricular aneurysm.[71] For these reasons, when cardiac contusion is suspected, the patient should be managed in a coronary or intensive care unit with constant ECG monitoring and treatment, including direct cardioversion of ventricular tachycardia or fibrillation, as in any case of myocardial infarction.

The common enzymes measured (serum glutamic oxaloacetic transaminase [SGOT], lactic dehydrogenase [LDH], and creatine kinase [CK]) are all elevated in patients with muscular, hepatic, or renal injury and after hemorrhage and metabolic acidosis, even without myocardial infarction. Injury to the myocardium with necrosis should be suspected if the MB fraction of the CK or the cardiac "fast" fraction of LDH is elevated.[60] The value of pyrophosphate radioactive scanning is not yet established,[54] but there are reports suggesting that it may be helpful in more objective diagnosis of patients with myocardial contusion.[12, 41] Potkin and coworkers[76] reported 100 consecutive patients with severe, nonpenetrating chest trauma.

Noninvasive tests performed were serial ECGs, CPK-MB enzymes, continuous ECG monitoring for arrhythmias, and technetium Tc-99m pyrophosphate scintigraphy. Elevations of CPK-MB enzyme occurred in 72 patients, ECG abnormalities in 70 patients, and Lown Grades III–V dysrhythmias in 27 patients. Clinically important cardiac damage did not occur in these patients. Fifteen patients died, none from cardiac injury, and at postmortem five had myocardial contusion. None of the noninvasive tests were abnormal more often in these five than in the ten patients without cardiac contusion.

The treatment of the patient with suspected myocardial contusion depends on the clinical condition. Most often, cardiac contusion is an incidental finding suspected by ECG or CPK-MB enzyme rise, and not the primary problem. If the patient has an arrhythmia, this should be treated as if there were myocardial necrosis just as for an acute myocardial infarction. If congestive heart failure is present, the patient should be treated with diuretics or inotropic agents such as dopamine and dobutamine;[61] even balloon counterpulsation has been employed.[40, 85] In severely injured patients, pulmonary wedge pressure and cardiac output should be monitored, and care should be taken to avoid hypervolemia and the precipitation of congestive heart failure. If the myocardial contusion is manifest by ECG changes alone, observation and rest for several days is all that is necessary, since almost all these patients do very well. Late complications of myocardial necrosis should be looked for on follow-up examination.

Posttraumatic Pericarditis

The problem of chest pain occurring at a time remote from the acute injury will now be discussed. In a subgroup of patients, chest pain may develop a week to several months after the direct trauma. Fever may also accompany the chest pain, which frequently has a pleuritic component and may be accompanied by pericardial friction rub. Such posttraumatic pericarditis is currently considered to have an etiology similar to that of the postmyocardial infarction and postpericardiotomy syndromes.[34] The mechanism may be associated with the development of autologous antibodies, with the damage related to antigen-antibody-complement complexes.[100] The problem can be accompanied by pericardial effusion, and even occasionally by pericardial tamponade that requires pericardiocentesis.

The syndrome is most often self-limited and can be treated with reassurance; analgesics; anti-inflammatory agents such as aspirin and acetaminophen; and even a short-term course of corticosteroids, which should be tapered as rapidly as possible. It is our impression that precordial pain often returns after cessation of the steroids, and for this reason they should be used infrequently and for as short a time as possible. At times, only removal of a retained foreign body in the pericardium will stop recurrent pericarditis.[112] Unfortunately, postinjury pericarditis has a tendency to recur, sometimes two or more times. Pericardiectomy has occasionally been necessary in patients with multiple episodes of recurrent posttraumatic pericarditis.

Late constrictive pericarditis has been reported after myocardial trauma.[42] There is experimental evidence that hemopericardium alone will resolve without constriction, but hemopericardium accompanied by myocardial injury can result in chronic constrictive pericarditis.[86] Since this is a late phenomenon, the patient must have late follow-up for this to be discovered and surgically treated.

ARRHYTHMIAS AND ABNORMAL ELECTROCARDIOGRAPHIC FINDINGS

After myocardial contusion, the major trauma can be injury of the conduction system. At times, the only manifestation of myocardial injury may be the onset of a ventricular or atrial arrhythmia. These arrhythmias have been observed after penetrating and nonpenetrating trauma as well as after electric shock. The usual arrhythmias are ventricular ectopy; atrial ectopy occurs less frequently. Atrial tachyarrhythmias (including tachycardia, fibrillation and flutter) and ventricular arrhythmias (including ectopy, tachycardia, and fibrillation) may also occur. These arrhythmias have been reported after nonpenetrating chest injury, and may be related to contusion of the myocardium. They may also be related to severe stimulation of the autonomic nervous system;[58] and also to increased catecholamines and electrolyte and blood gas abnormalities in the absence of myocardial contusion.

Bradyarrhythmias including sinus bradycardia, sinus pauses, and sinoatrial arrest have also been described. All degrees of AV block as well as bundle branch block have been observed, including right bundle branch block with left anterior or left posterior hemiblock, and even complete heart block with junctional or lower ventricular escape rhythms.[30]

Fatal arrhythmias can occur with nonpenetrating chest trauma, which results in low energy transfer to the myocardium, causing depolarization and repolarization changes that produce ventricular tachyarrhythmias and even ventricular fibrillation.[31] At postmortem examination, there is no gross or histologic evidence of myocardial damage. These arrhythmias are said to be the result of myocardial concussion and have been called "commotio cordis."[31]

The clinical effect of brady- and tachyarrhythmias depends on the extent of other cardiovascular damage. Since patients with cardiovascular trauma are usually young and of previous good health, they tend to tolerate supraventricular arrhythmias fairly well. Ventricular tachycardia and fibrillation demand prompt therapy. These arrhythmias are similar clinically and electrocardiographically to those of a nontraumatic etiology. Because most of these arrhythmias are transient, treatment usually depends on their hemodynamic effects. If the patient is tolerating the rhythm well, close observation may be all that is necessary. In cases of multiple ventricular ectopy and tachyarrhythmias, antiarrhythmic drugs are useful, and at times even cardioversion must be carried out to convert malignant tachyarrhythmias. Obviously, in patients with arrhythmias and hemodynamic compromise, rapid slowing of the ventricular response is required by administration of digitalis, propranolol, or verapamil, or even by cardioversion. In the case of changing and progressively developing AV block, a temporary pacemaker may have to be implanted. In cases of complete heart block, especially with a wide idioventricular pacemaker, insertion of a temporary pacemaker is indicated. Most often, these are transient arrhythmias that disappear without complication.

Electrocardiographic abnormalities including ST-segment and T-wave changes and Q-T interval prolongation tend to support the diagnosis of myocardial contusion, but most patients with ST-segment and T-wave changes as their only abnormality do very well without complications.[76] Elevation of ST segments later followed by T-wave inversion has been seen in patients with either early or late pericarditis. It has already been noted that typical Q waves with ST-segment elevation and T-wave inversion can occur in patients with acute myocardial damage resulting from contusion, as well as in patients with acute myocardial infarction; unless diligently sought, these changes are not infrequently misdiagnosed as indicating pericarditis.

With pericardial effusions, electrical alternans of QRS or, more specifically, total electrical alternans may be the clue pointing to pericardial tamponade.

DEVELOPMENT OF A HEART MURMUR

Any intracardiac structure can be damaged during penetrating and nonpenetrating cardiac injury.

Valvular Insufficiency

Mitral and Tricuspid Insufficiency

Rupture of an atrioventricular valve is more uncommon than rupture of the chordae tendineae cordis or papillary muscle tip as a cause of AV valvular insufficiency.[39, 72] Both mitral and tricuspid valve insufficiency produce a pansystolic murmur located characteristically at the apex for the mitral valve and at the left sternal border for the tricuspid valve. Carvallo's sign is frequently heard in patients with tricuspid insufficiency with an increased loudness of the murmur on inspiration. The hemodynamic effect of these lesions depends on the severity of the insufficiency. We have seen cases of traumatically induced tricuspid insufficiency in which a murmur is present without central venous pressure changes.[53] If the volume load is severe, S3 and S4 gallop sounds can be heard, as well as a short diastolic flow rumble due to the marked increase in the diastolic flow across the valve.

The hemodynamic effect of these lesions depends on the magnitude of the regurgitant volume of blood and the compliance of the chambers receiving the regurgitant blood. Valvular insufficiency compromises myocardial function by sudden development of a volume overload that affects the right ventricle when the tricuspid valve is damaged and the left ventricle when the mitral valve is damaged. This volume load occurs in an unprepared ventricle inside a relatively noncompliant pericardial sac. With sudden valvular insufficiency, the diastolic volume of the ventricle increases and usually results in a marked increase in the filling pressure of the ventricle. The atrium and venous beds are unprepared for the increased volume resulting from regurgitant blood in systole, and so a V wave of varying magnitude occurs. In this way, the mean atrial pressure is increased. On the right side of the heart, this causes systemic venous hypertension and right heart failure. Because of the low-resistance regurgitant run-off into the right atrium, the forward effective right ventricular output may drop, thus decreasing flow through the lungs to the left side of the heart. This may cause a drop in the systemic cardiac output, especially if there is increased resistance to right ventricular ejection because of pulmonary vascular or left heart disease.

With sudden mitral insufficiency, pulmonary edema results.[45] Frequently, there is also severe pulmonary arterial hypertension, and therefore afterload problems for the right ventricle with resultant right ventricular failure. Undoubtedly, some of the elevation in right ventricular filling pressure results from the sudden increase in left ventricular diastolic volume and change of right ventricular compliance through the restrictive effects of the noncompliant pericardium and the effect of increasing left ventricular volume on the commonly shared interventicular septum.

In cases of severe tricuspid insufficiency, the chest roentgenogram often shows no abnormality; later, superior vena caval and right atrial and right ventricular shadows may become enlarged. In cases of severe mitral insufficiency, the heart size, including the left atrium, may not be abnormally enlarged.[48] Pulmonary vascular redistribution, Kerley B lines, and frank pulmonary edema may be present. Later, enlargement of the left atrium, left ventricle, pulmonary artery, and right ventricle may occur.

The ECG also is of little help in the early stages, frequently showing no abnormalities or only ST-segment and T-wave changes. Later, in cases of tricuspid insufficiency, an rSR′ commonly occurs in lead V1, representing incomplete right bundle branch block or mild right ventricular hypertrophy. Although the ECG can be normal early in the course of mitral insufficiency, left ventricular hypertrophy and even biventricular hypertrophy can develop rapidly.

Aortic Insufficiency

Aortic insufficiency can result from penetrating as well as nonpenetrating trauma.[70] In cases of sudden chest or abdominal compression, systemic vascular resistance and blood pressure may increase markedly and may rupture an aortic cusp. Moffat and colleagues showed that intra-aortic pressure of 400 mm Hg could be generated in dogs struck on the sternum.[68] This occurs most frequently in patients who suffered chest compression during an automobile accident. The murmur of severe traumatic aortic insufficiency is frequently shorter and lower pitched than the usual murmur of chronic aortic insufficiency, because there is a rapidly decreasing gradient due to equalization of pressure in the aorta and the left ventricle in mild- and late diastole. The left ventricle resists the sudden volume overload for the same reasons as those described above for mitral insufficiency. The left ventricular filling pressure, therefore, is quite high; at times, it exceeds the left atrial pressure in mid- and late diastole, and thus closes the mitral valve and results in a soft, almost inaudible first heart sound. Frequently, S4 and S3 gallops are heard together with a short systolic ejection murmur due to the increased stroke volume. High left atrial pressure occurs, and pulmonary edema and even severe pulmonary hypertension develop rapidly. The initial chest roentgenogram may show no abnormalities or only a slightly increased heart size, but severe pulmonary congestion and even pulmonary edema are often evident. Concomitant injuries to the ascending aorta and the aortic valve are not uncommon as well as, in penetrating injuries, aortic valvular insufficiency and ventricular septal defects.[23, 28] These associated injuries should be recognized and repaired at the time of valve replacement.

Pulmonary Insufficiency

Valvular pulmonary insufficiency is the rarest of all the trauma-induced valvular lesions. Pulmonary insufficiency can result from penetrating injury; when this occurs, a short, low-pitched, diastolic, diamond-shaped murmur is heard along the left sternal border, starting distinctly after the aortic component of the second sound and ending in mid-diastole. A systolic ejection murmur may also be heard along the left sternal border. Usually no immediate clinical problem results from right ventricular volume overload. Eventually, the pulmonary artery and right ventricle may become enlarged.

The Echocardiogram in Valvular Insufficiency. The echocardiogram in each of these types of valvular insufficiency can be of great help in that there is a dilatation of the appropriate volume-overloaded chambers and, in the case of tricuspid insufficiency and pulmonary insufficiency, paradoxic motion of the interventricular septum. With aortic insufficiency, diastolic fluttering of the anterior leaflet of the mitral valve is apparent. With mitral insufficiency, diastolic and even systolic fluttering of the anterior leaflet of the mitral valve can be seen, with transient echoes appearing in the left atrium in systole if there is chordal rupture.

Management of Valvular Insufficiency. The prognosis of valvular insufficiency is good if the valves of the right side of the heart are involved, but poor if there is severe insufficiency of the mitral or aortic valve. Massive mitral insufficiency is better tolerated than massive aortic insufficiency, because of the favorable effect on wall tension development gained in mitral insufficiency by ejecting blood with the onset of contraction into the low-resistance left atrium. In this way, by the time the left ventricle develops sufficiently high pressure to eject blood through the aortic valve, the left ventricular volume is small, compared with a comparable degree of aortic insufficiency in which all the blood must be ejected out of the aorta. As a result, patients with comparable degrees of volume overload from mitral insufficiency have lesser developed wall tension (wall tension $\propto$ systolic pressure $\times$ ventricular radius) for a given volume overload than patients with aortic insufficiency. Because it takes time for hypertrophy to develop, the strain in the left ventricular wall is markedly increased early in the course, so that there is some heart failure and the patient's condition is frequently poor soon after injury. If survival is prolonged, hypertrophy can occur with thickening of the ventricle and normalization of the wall stress. In this way, these patients may well become compensated and develop the clinical picture of severe chronic mitral or aortic insufficiency, with dilatation of the appropriate chambers.[104]

Treatment consists of recognition of the condition, which is facilitated by Swan-Ganz catheterization and the finding of large V waves in the right atrium in patients who have tricuspid insufficiency, or in the pulmonary capillary wedge in patients who have mitral insufficiency without evidence of a left-to-right shunt. The usual doses of digitalis and diuretics should be administered to support cardiac output and decrease pulmonary congestion. Nitroprusside, as a combination preload-and-afterload–reducing agent, has been most beneficial in acute mitral and aortic insufficiency.[46] This drug acts by increasing venous capacitance, thereby reducing ventricular filling pressure, and, as an afterload-reducing agent, thereby increasing the effective stroke volume and cardiac output and decreasing regurgitant volume. With lower V waves, there is further reduction in left atrial and pulmonary capillary wedge pressures. If hemodynamic effects of the valvular insufficiency result in continued poor ventricular function after stabilization, the patient will require valve replacement.

Ventricular Septal Rupture

Rupture of the ventricular septum can result from penetrating as well as nonpenetrating trauma.[83, 90] About half of the cases reported in the literature have resulted from nonpenetrating injury.[10] Unlike the congenital ventricular septal defect, the rupture can occur anywhere in the muscular septum, and so the systolic murmur may be located either at the left sternal border or at the apex. Usually, the murmur is loud and accompanied by a systolic thrill. With a large left-to-right shunt at the ventricular level, the volume load is on the left ventricle even though pulmonary blood flow is increased. The left ventricle ejects blood through the ventricular septal defect during systole when the right ventricle is contracting, and thereby ejects blood directly out of the right ventricle outflow tract into the pulmonary artery. There is therefore no volume overload of the right ventricle. If the ventricular septal defect is large enough, there is equilibration of pressure in the left and right ventricles, and the size of the shunt will depend solely on the relative pulmonary-to-systemic vascular resistance. In this instance, there is both a volume load on the left ventricle and a pressure load or afterload on the right ventricle.

Usually, there is pulmonary congestion with left ventricular failure and frequently an increase in the pulmonic component of the second heart sound consistent with pulmonary hypertension. In the acute stage, the ECG findings and the heart size on the chest roentgenogram may remain within normal limits.[10] Roentgenographically, pulmonary vascular congestion with an increase in pulmonary arterial and venous markings may be seen. The echocardiogram will show dilatation of the left ventricle and probably the left atrium, with good left ventricular wall motion. Definitive diagnosis depends on proving an oxygen step-up in the right ventricle by cardiac catheterization, which can be carried out in the intesive care unit with a Swan-Ganz catheter. Additional intracardiac injuries are common: e.g., aortic and mitral insufficiency, coronary artery laceration, and especially aortic and right heart fistulae. For this reason, full cardiac catheterization and angiocardiography should be performed before surgery.[7, 10, 28, 94, 101] If the shunt is large enough and the patient is having hemodynamic difficulty, surgical correction can be performed. If the patient is hemodynamically stable, medical management should be pursued because spontaneous closure of these defects has been reported.[108] Afterload reduction may be helpful in these patients by reducing the systemic vascular resistance and increasing the effective forward cardiac output.

Atrial Septal Rupture

Rupture of the atrial septum is both less common and less readily detected than that of the ventricular septum. First, atrial septum is better protected by the sternum from penetration by knife wounds. Second, perforation of the atrial septum is less easily detected clinically, because the atria are low-pressure chambers and the only murmur associated with left-to-right shunt at the atrial level is the systolic ejection murmur of increased right ventricular stroke volume across the pulmonary valve. If the shunt is large, a short, low-pitched, diastolic rumbling murmur reflecting increased tricuspid flow may be present along the left sternal border. These are not impressive murmurs and may be overlooked.

The pathophysiologic problem of atrial septal rupture is right ventricular overload, which eventually manifests as right ventricular and pulmonary arterial enlargement. The ECG eventually shows as rSR′ in lead V_1 of right ventricular overload. When discovered, the defect can be closed surgically if the shunt is large; the surgical mortality is low.

ARTERIOVENOUS AND CORONARY-CAMERAL FISTULAE

Arteriovenous and coronary-cameral fistulae usually result from penetrating injuries, although occasionally they have been reported to occur with nonpenetrating trauma.[37] Any vessel can be involved, but in cases of cardiac trauma the coronary arterial vessels are most often affected. This can result in a coronary arteriovenous or coronary-cameral fistula where the blood empties directly into the cardiac chamber, usually the right atrium or right ventricle, occasionally the left ventricle, and rarely the left atrium.[57, 79] Coronary arteriovenous and cameral fistulae result in continuous murmurs, usually along the left sternal border or at the apex, that are commonly accentuated in diastole. The fistulae tend to enlarge and may result in a low-resistance shunt that reduces distal myocardial perfusion, causing myocardial ischemia, the "coronary steal" syndrome.[51] Angina pectoris has also occurred in these patients. Because of progressive enlargement of the fistula and the probability of myocardial ischemia, surgical closure has been recommended when such fistulae are detected. Occasionally, however, such fistulae exist for many years without changing in size[21]; when they are thus small and asymptomatic, medical follow-up may be preferable to surgical repair.[11]

A relatively frequent intracardiac fistula can be caused by aortic injury with resulting fistulous formation with the right atrium, right ventricle, pulmonary artery, and rarely the left atrium.[94] In this situation the size of the defect determines the size of the left-to-right shunt since fistulae entering the right heart are connecting the aorta with a low pressure system emptying into the low-resistance pulmonary vascular bed. Large fistulae cause massive left-to-right shunts, right and left ventricular volume overload, and congestive heart failure. Findings usually consist of a continuous murmur over the precordium, wide pulse pressure, and signs of left and right ventricular volume overload and failure if the shunts are large. Most often, these shunts require surgical repair.

Occasionally, fistulae between a systemic artery and a heart chamber can result from a penetrating injury, or rarely from a nonpenetrating injury.[27] We have seen internal mammary-to-right-ventricular fistulas in patients with knife wounds. The major manifestation of this lesion is a continuous murmur.

Arteriovenous fistulae involving systemic arteries are not unusual after penetrating trauma. These lesions tend to enlarge and are associated with a loud, continuous murmur that is accentuated in systole, maximal over the site of the fistula, and usually accompanied by a thrill. If the vessel involved is large (as large as or larger than the femoral artery), the arteriovenous fistula can result in a big enough increase in cardiac output and volume overload of the left ventricle to cause congestive heart failure.[80] The organ or limb distal to the fistula may show the effects of ischemia. Because such fistulas tend to enlarge, it is recommended that they be repaired when discovered, even if they are asymptomatic.

A special type of arteriovenous fistula is that between the pulmonary artery and the aorta. This causes volume overload of the left ventricle and the hemodynamic effects that occur in patients with a patent ductus arteriosus. The murmur is continuous, usually can be heard at the left base, and is accentuated during late systole.

ABNORMAL CHEST ROENTGENOGRAPHIC FINDINGS

Occasionally, the clue to cardiac trauma is an abnormality on the chest roentgenogram. There may be no history of cardiovascular trauma per se and the damage to the cardiovascular system may not be recognized at the time of injury, the abnormality often being discovered accidentally years later on the chest roentgenogram.[48]

Pericardial Injury

At the time of injury, pericardial hemorrhagic effusion can cause enlargement of the cardiac silhouette. If the accumulation of fluid is slow and the clinical picture is dominated by trauma to other systems, the only evidence that the heart has been damaged may be the large cardiac silhouette on the chest roentgenogram.

Rupture of the pericardium has been described with herniation of the heart or part of it, for instance the left atrial appendage, through the tear; if the tear is small enough, strangulation of the atrium or even the entire heart can occur, with disastrous consequences.[63] If the tear is large, the heart can be displaced into the left side of the chest and appear moved to the left more than is normal. Lung containing air may thus appear to be inferior to the heart.[6]

Rupture of the diaphragmatic portion of the pericardium also occurs, producing continuity between pericardial and abdominal cavities. In these cases, abdominal content can herniate into the pericardial cavity.[54]

Cardiac Contusion or Laceration and Ventricular Aneurysm

With cardiac contusion and extensive necrosis, generalized cardiomegaly with resultant congestive heart failure can occur as in cases of cardiomyopathy. If there has been localized myocardial necrosis, either with contusion or laceration, a true or false left ventricular aneurysm can develop.[89] The consequences are similar to those of a left ventricular aneurysm developing in a patient with coronary artery disease. In general, these patients have less trouble with a true left ventricular aneurysm than patients with coronary disease, because the former individuals tend to be young and have normal coronary arteries, and thus the remaining normal cardiac muscle is capable of compensating for the damaged myocardium.[47] However, mural thrombus with systemic embolization can develop; congestive heart failure and arrhythmias can also occur. Indications for aneurysmectomy are similar to those in patients with arteriosclerotic heart disease.[9]

False aneurysms are those in which there has been a rupture of the myocardium contained by the epicardium and pericardium. Unlike true ventricular aneurysms, these have a tendency to rupture even at a time remote from their formation.[107] Differentiation of a false from a true aneurysm is not always possible, even with angiocardiography. False aneurysms frequently show a small neck on the angiocardiogram and tend to be spherical. Spherical aneurysms tend to increase in size with increasing wall tension, resulting in eventual rupture. When found, false aneurysms should be repaired. Since posttraumatic ventricular aneurysms can be associated with other intracardiac defects, full catheterization and angiography should be carried out prior to surgical repair.

Aortic Injury

After trauma, either penetrating or nonpenetrating, damage to the aorta with formation of a false aneurysm is not uncommon. In deceleration and steering-wheel injuries, a sudden shearing force is applied to the aorta that causes tearing of the intima and media; frequently, complete separation occurs in the aorta at the locations of greatest stress, just beyond the point of origin of the left subclavian artery and in the ascending aorta just above the coronary arteries.[73] If the adventitia of the ascending aorta also ruptures, pericardial tamponade quickly results and the patient usually dies immediately. In the descending aorta, if the adventitia does not rupture, the pleura and mediastinal tissues can tamponade the hemorrhage and allow a false aneurysm to develop. This occurs in about 15 per cent of patients with aortic rupture. In a study by the United States Armed Forces Institute of Pathology, about one third of the patients with aortic rupture had minimal or no external signs of chest trauma.[73]

A clue to the possibility of aortic injury is the finding on the chest roentgenogram of a widened mediastinum, which is caused by mediastinal hemorrhage.[48, 73, 97] Obviously, bleeding and widening of the mediastinum can result from venous injury and from tearing of small arteries. In these instances, resolution of the widening occurs with time, leaving a perfectly normal mediastinal shadow. When widening of the mediastinum is seen in an individual with chest trauma, aortography should be performed when the patient is stable to rule out the possibility of rupture of the aorta or another large artery.

Occasionally, dissection of the adventitia occurs with rupture, compromising vessels that arise from the aorta such as the left subclavian artery, and producing a decrease in distal pulses and blood pressure or even compression of the descending aorta, with a decrease in femoral pulses.[44, 97] In these instances, systolic bruits can be heard, especially in the interscapular region to the left of the spine. Aortic rupture is thought especially likely to occur in patients who have had a fracture of the first rib, and should be specifically sought in such patients.[110]

If the aortic injury is overlooked during the acute episode, it is not unusual to discover the abnormal mediastinal shadow on a chest roentgenogram some time later. This follow-up film is often taken for reasons unrelated to the previous chest trauma. Occasionally, the aneurysm is discovered five to ten years after the traumatic episode, and has a thin layer of calcium deposited in the wall of the thrombus.

When the aortic rupture is diagnosed at the time of the traumatic event, it is recommended that surgery be performed in a medical center where this type of surgery is done frequently; otherwise, the operative mortality rate is extremely high. As in the emergency treatment of dissection of the aorta, the force of left ventricular contraction and blood pressure can be decreased by administering propranolol and lowering the blood pressure to minimally tolerated levels with trimethaphan camsylate, nitroprusside, or other afterload-reducing drugs. This therapy decreases the forces that tend to rupture the aorta further and can sustain the patient until surgery can be performed.[8]

If the aneurysm is chronic and has been there for a long time, the question arises of whether or not to repair it.[67] Bennett and Cherry[14] reported in a review of the literature that about half of the chronic aneurysms eventually enlarge, become symptomatic, or rupture. For these reasons, they recommend elective repair when such aneurysms are discovered. Fleming and Green,[35] in a study from Walter Reed General Hospital, reported 43 cases of chronic aortic aneurysm in which 39 per cent eventually enlarged or became symptomatic; the authors came to the same conclusions as did Bennett and Cherry.

Intracardiac Foreign Bodies

Metallic foreign bodies are the only ones visible on the roentgenogram. In general, if the foreign bodies are free in the lumen they can migrate.[55, 87] If they are present in veins, migration occurs centrally and the objects end up in the right side of the heart or the pulmonary arteries. If they are present in the left side of the heart or in the pulmonary veins, migration occurs distally, causing embolization to distal arteries.[22, 69] The diagnosis of embolized foreign body should be suspected when there is no exit wound and the object is not found in the suspected area by roentgenography.[98] Intraluminal foreign bodies in the left side of the heart should be removed because of the possibility of embolization or embolization from fibrin deposited on the foreign body.

Intracardiac, but not intraluminal, foreign bodies that do not cause hemodynamic embarrassment or interference with valves have been evaluated in long-term follow-up studies. Bland and Beebe[15] described 40 patients with retained intracardiac foreign bodies; only two had any major complications. One patient had moderate aortic insufficiency, and in one individual the object eroded through the pulmonary artery into the bronchus and required pneumonectomy. However, a substantial number of patients had extreme psychosomatic problems due to their knowledge of the presence of the intracardiac foreign body, and five were incapacitated by this anxiety. For this reason, Bland and Beebe recommended removal of any object greater than 1 cm in size. Another problem consists of repeated precipitation of recurrent pericarditis by an intrapericardial object that will not abate until the object is removed. If such objects are free-floating within the pericardial sac, their removal presents a real challenge to the surgeon.

TRAUMA TO ARTERIES AND VEINS

Systemic arteries and veins can be traumatized by either laceration or thrombus resulting from direct injury to the wall that is caused by the vessel being in the cylinder of cavitation around the path of the high-velocity missile.[80] Vascular injury can also occur from blunt trauma. Arterial thrombosis presents as sudden ischemia of the limb or organ supplied by the artery. There is pain, numbness, pallor, and pulselessness of the extremity caused by the sudden marked drop in blood flow to the limb. Since the obstruction is sudden, there is no time for collateral vessels to develop, and vasoconstriction of the other arterial vessels in the extremity arises. If the injury is not treated, such involvement of a large vessel results in gangrene of the extremity. The longer the ischemia lasts, the more likely is there to be localized edema upon relief of the ischemia. In this case, fasciotomy to relieve the local tissue pressure is very important.[77] In penetrating injuries due to low-velocity missiles, e.g., knife wounds, there is little tissue damage, and primary repair of the vessel is possible. In these cases angiography is often unnecessary before repair.[77] In cases in which vascular injury results from high-velocity missiles, e.g., gunshot wounds, or in which there is blunt trauma, large areas of tissue damage may occur, extensive debridement may be necessary, and grafting may be needed in repair. Angiography before surgery is very useful in these patients.

Laceration of the artery results in hemorrhage. If there is no free access to the exterior, a large hematoma can develop and, if contained, can result in a false aneurysm. This aneurysm has a tendency to expand, and distal flow to the extremity or organ is often diminished, causing ischemia. Pulsatile masses in the extremity, with or without bruits, should be considered false aneurysms and studied by angiography. If present, they must be repaired.

If there has been laceration of the artery and the accompanying vein, a traumatic arteriovenous fistula can develop. The low-resistance pathway into the vein increases flow from the artery to the vein and enlarges both vessels. This increased proximal run-off can rob the distal circulation of flow and result in distal ischemia. If the vessels involved are large enough (the size of the femoral artery or larger), congestive heart failure results.[38] In the case of an aorta–inferior vena cava fistula, massive increase in cardiac output and severe congestive heart failure occur and death ensues rapidly. Auscultation over such a fistula reveals a loud continuous murmur that is pathognomonic of an arteriovenous fistula.

Venous injury can result in laceration or thrombosis. With laceration, unless the vessel is quite large (for instance, the size of the inferior vena cava or the portal vein) or the bleeding is into a low–resistance area such as the peritoneal cavity or the pericardium, enough tissue turgor has usually developed to slow and finally stop the hemorrhage. If bleeding continues and blood volume cannot be kept normal by transfusion, primary repair of the vein is indicated.

If thrombosis occurs, the consequences of chronic venous obstruction may result in edema and dependent turgor of the extremity. More dangerous is the possibility of the development of pulmonary embolism. For this reason, any patient who has had trauma to a large vein and in whom there is no contraindication should receive anticoagulant therapy.

As mentioned above, injury to the heart can result in a contusion causing formation of a mural thrombus that can subsequently embolize to the lungs if it is on the right side of the heart, or produce systemic embolization if it is on the left side.

In cases of whiplash injuries to the neck, there can be laceration involving the intima that lifts a flap in the common carotid or internal carotid arteries, occasionally resulting in late obstruction of the vessel and late development of stroke. These intimal flaps can be discovered by careful angiography with multiple views.[25]

FOLLOW-UP OF THE POSTCARDIAC TRAUMA PATIENT

Many of the patients who survive cardiac trauma continue to be symptomatic. As mentioned previously, postpericardiotomy pericarditis is not uncommon and may be recurrent. However, many resuscitated victims of otherwise lethal cardiac trauma continue to have symptoms that often are not explainable on the basis of the hemodynamic impairment that they continue to manifest.

At San Francisco General Hospital Medical Center, we have studied 20 long-term survivors who were successfully resuscitated by emergency surgery after traumatic cardiac wounds. Before injury, 18 were gainfully employed. After successful resuscitation and for a mean follow-up time of two years, all 20 were still symptomatic with chest pain, fatigue, and/or shortness of breath. However, careful examination revealed that only six had major residual cardiovascular defects. Tested by graded treadmill exercise, 18 had a normal functional capacity. Only eight of the 20 patients resumed employment. Sixteen had a traumatic neurosis documented by psychologic testing.[1] The problem of secondary gain influencing the symptoms is difficult to assess, of course, but no victim had received compensation from the "Victim of Violent Crimes Program" of the State of California. In addition, we suspected that the persistent chest pain, fatigability, and breathlessness, which were unrelated to the objective physical response to exercise, also constituted evidence of a deep-seated psychosomatic problem related to the serious cardiovascular trauma. We proposed that early rehabilitation and reassurance as to the capability of ultimate recovery, with return to normal activity and work, must be an explicit goal of medical therapy, initiated by the internist, if there is to be a decrease in the incidence of major psychosomatic residual problems.

IATROGENIC INJURY

With the increasing use of invasive diagnostic and therapeutic techniques, a growing number of iatrogenic cardiovascular complications have arisen. Cardiac catheterization in the diagnostic laboratory, in which needles and catheters are introduced into arteries and veins and directed into the heart, involves a relatively low incidence of complications.[20, 92] However, with long-term hemodynamic monitoring as in the intensive care unit and the coronary care unit areas, cases have been observed of septicemia with nosocomial infections, fatal ventricular arrhythmias, venous occlusion and phlebitis, arterial thrombus and embolization, and pulmonary infarction due to prolonged wedging of a Swan-Ganz catheter or repeated catheter injections.[36, 43] Traumatic and, at times, expanding false aneurysms and arteriovenous fistulae have been reported even after short-term arterial cannulation. Traumatic injury of the brachial nerve has been noted. With jugular and subclavian intravenous approaches to the placement of large-bore venous catheters, pneumothorax and hemothorax have occurred. False aneurysms and traumatic arteriovenous fistulae have also arisen after needle biopsy of the kidney.[56] Lumbar disc surgery has occasionally resulted in the formation of traumatic arteriovenous fistulae between the iliac artery and vein, with consequent congestive heart failure.[91]

With the increasing use of intravenous catheters, there is an appreciable incidence of lost catheters that migrate centrally and come to rest in the right atrium, right ventricle, or pulmonary artery.[29] Fortunately, these can sometimes be retrieved with catheter snares passed fluoroscopically, thus avoiding the necessity of thoracotomy and direct surgical removal.[16, 82] The passage of catheters into the heart also can result in cardiac perforation, which if untreated has led to tamponade and death in some cases. Catheters that gradually perforate the right ventricular wall, such as pacemaker catheters, rarely cause such a major complication as cardiac tamponade; the reason for this is not clear. Cardiac catheterization and angiography have also caused cardiac perforation. This is a special risk in transseptal catheterization of the left side of the heart in which a needle is passed through a catheter and the intra-atrial septum is deliberately perforated. Perforation of the atrium out into the pericardium or the ascending aorta has occurred and resulted in death.[33]

Angiography has also caused cardiac tamponade by perforation of the left ventricular wall as a result of entrapment of the catheter tip between trabeculae carneae cordis, or through recoil of the angiographic catheter bringing the high-velocity angiographic jets into apposition with the ventricular surface during the injection.[2] There is a long overdue and mandatory need to standardize angiocardiographic procedures, including injection flow rates and the types of catheters used since the advent of modern pump injectors. Rarely, the high-density contrast material is inadvertently introduced into the pericardial sac, and osmotic action drawing more body fluid into the pericardium results in late tamponade.[75]

Finally, cardiopulmonary resuscitation has resulted in rupture of cardiac structures or the aorta, tearing of the venae cavae, and laceration of the heart with rupture.[3, 17] Laceration of the venae cavae has also been reported in cases of traumatic delivery of a baby.

CONCLUSION

In our society and environment in which speed and violence are prevalent, there is an increasing incidence of cardiovascular trauma. As awareness of the possibility of salvage from cardiac trauma is heightened following better organization of emergency units and trauma centers to receive and care for such patients, there will be increasing involvement of the internists in the care of those who survive cardiac trauma. More patients will present with the residuals of this trauma and attendant neurosis, challenging internists not only to recognize but also to treat these complications effectively. Although this acquired disease is first managed by surgeons, internists and cardiologists will play a definite role in the diagnosis of late complications and of subtle signs of cardiac involvement, which are often overlooked during the dramatic phase of the patient's initial presentation. Indications are that the incidence of cardiac trauma will increase and thus present a continuing and accelerating challenge.

References

1. Abbott, J. A., Cousineau, M., Cheitlin, M.D., et al.: Late sequelae of penetrating cardiac wounds. J. Thorac. Cardiovasc. Surg. 75:510, 1978.
2. Abbott, J. A., Lipton, M. J., Kosek, J., et al.: Cardiac trauma from angiographic injections; a quantitative study. Circulation 57:91, 1978.
3. Agdal, N., and Jorgensen, T. G.: Penetrating laceration of the pericardium and myocardium and myocardial rupture following closed-chest cardiac massage. Acta Med. Scand. 194:477, 1973.
4. Allen, R. P., and Liedtke, A. J.: The role of coronary artery injury and perfusion in the development of cardiac contusion secondary to nonpenetrating chest trauma. J. Trauma 19:153, 1979.
5. Amato, J. J., and Rich, N. M.: Temporary cavity effects in blood vessel injury by high velocity missiles. J. Cardiovasc. Surg. 13:147, 1972.
6. Anderson, M., Fredens, M., and Olesen, K. H.: Traumatic rupture of the pericardium. Am. J. Cardiol. 27:566, 1971.
7. Anyanwu, C. H.: Mitral incompetence and ventricular septal defects following nonpenetrating injury. Thorax 31:113, 1976.
8. Aronstam, E. M., Gomez, A. C., O'Connell, T. J.,

et al.: Recent surgical and pharmacologic experience with acute dissecting and traumatic aneurysms. J. Thorac. Cardiovasc. Surg. 59:231, 1970.

9. Aronstam, E. M., Strader, L. D., Geiger, J. P., et al.: Traumatic left ventricular aneurysms. J. Thorac. Cardiovasc. Surg. 59:239, 1970.
10. Asfaw, I., Thoms, N. W., and Arbulu, A.: Interventricular septal defects from penetrating injuries of the heart: a report of 12 cases and review of the literature. J. Thorac. Cardiovasc. Surg. 69:450, 1975.
11. Austin, S. M., Applefeld, M. M., Turney, S. Z., and Mech, K. F., Jr.: Traumatic left anterior descending coronary artery to right ventricle fistula: report of two cases. South. Med. J. 70:581, 1977.
12. Bayer, M. J., and Burdick, D.: Diagnosis of myocardial contusion in blunt chest trauma. J.A.C.E.P. 6:238, 1977.
13. Beall, A. C., Jr.: Discussion. *In* Rea, W. J., Sugg, W. L., Wilson, L. C., et al.: Coronary artery lacerations. An analysis of 22 patients. Ann. Thorac. Surg. 7:518, 1969.
14. Bennett, D. E., and Cherry, J. K.: The natural history of traumatic aneurysms of the aorta. Surgery 61:516, 1967.
15. Bland, E. F., and Beebe, G. W.: Missiles in the heart. A twenty-year follow-up report of World War II cases. N. Engl. J. Med. 274:1039, 1966.
16. Bloomfield, D. A.: The nonsurgical retrieval of intracardiac foreign bodies—an international survey. Cathet. Cardiovasc. Diagn. 4:1, 1978.
17. Bodily, K., and Fisher, R. P.: Aortic rupture and right ventricular rupture induced by closed chest cardiac massage. Minn. Med. 62:225, 1979.
18. Borja, A. R., Lansing, A. M., and Ransdell, H. T., Jr.: Immediate operative treatment for stab wounds of the heart. Experience with fifty-four consecutive cases. J. Thorac. Cardiovasc. Surg. 59:662, 1970.
19. Brantigan, C. O., Burdick, D., Hopeman, A. R., and Eiseman, B.: Evaluation of technetium scanning for myocardial contusion. J. Trauma 18:460, 1978.
20. Braunwald, E., and Swan, H. J. C. (eds.): Cooperative study on cardiac catheterization. Circulation 37 (Suppl. III): III-1, 1968.
21. Bravo, A. J., Glancy, D. L., Epstein, S. E., et al.: Traumatic coronary arteriovenous fistula. A 20 year follow up with serial hemodynamic and angiographic studies. Am. J. Cardiol. 27:673, 1971.
22. Buriham, E., Pepe, E. V. A., and Miranda, F., Jr.: Bullet embolism following gunshot wounds of the chest: case report and review of the literature. J. Cardiovasc. Surg. 21:711, 1980.
23. Charles, K. P., Davidson, K. G., Miller, H., and Caves, P. K.: Traumatic rupture of the ascending aorta and aortic valve following blunt chest trauma. J. Thorac. Cardiovasc. Surg. 73:208, 1977.
24. Corso, P. J.: Chest trauma. Primary Care 5:543, 1978.
25. Crissey, M. M., and Bernstein, E. F.: Delayed presentation of carotid intimal tear following blunt craniocervical trauma. Surgery 75:543, 1974.
26. Defalque, R. J., and Campbell, C.: Cardiac tamponade from central venous catheters. Anesthesiology 50:249, 1979.
27. DeSa'Neto, A., Padnick, M. B., Desser, K. B., and Steinhoff, N. G.: Right sinus of Valsalva–right atrial fistula secondary to nonpenetrating chest trauma. Circulation 60:205, 1979.
28. Desser, K. B., Benchimol, A., Cornell, W. P., and Nelson, A. R.: Traumatic ventricular septal defect, aortic insufficiency, and sinus aneurysm. J. Thorac. Cardiovasc. Surg. 62:830, 1971.
29. Doering, R. B., Stemmer, E. A., and Connolly, J. E.: Complications of indwelling venous catheters, with particular reference to catheter embolus. Am. J. Surg. 114:259, 1967.
30. Dolara, A., and Pozzi, L.: Atrioventricular and intraventricular conduction defects after nonpenetrating trauma. Am. Heart J. 72:138, 1966.
31. Doty, D. B., Anderson, A. E., Rose, E. F., et al.: Cardiac trauma. Clinical and experimental correlation of myocardial contusion. Am. Surg. 180:452, 1974.
32. Dougall, A. M., Paul, M. E., Finely, R. J., et al.: Chest trauma—current morbidity and mortality. J. Trauma 17:547, 1977.
33. Enghoff, E., and Cullhed, I.: Experiences with transseptal left heart catheterization. A review of 454 studies. Am. Heart J. 81:398, 1971.
34. Engle, M. A., Klein, A. A., Hepner, S., and Ehlers, K. H.: The postpericardiotomy and similar syndromes. Cardiovasc. Clin. 7:211, 1976.
35. Fleming, A. W., and Green, D. C.: Traumatic aneurysms of the thoracic aorta. Report of 43 patients. Ann. Thorac. Surg. 18:91, 1974.
36. Foote, G. A., Schabel, S. I., and Hodges, M.: Pulmonary complications of the flow-directed balloon-tipped catheter. N. Engl. J. Med. 290:927, 1974.
37. Forker, A. D., and Morgan, J. R.: Acquired coronary artery fistula from nonpenetrating chest injury. J.A.M.A. 215:289, 1971.
38. Frishman, W., Epstein, A. M., Kulick, S., and Killip, J.: Heart failure 63 years after traumatic arteriovenous fistula. Am. J. Cardiol. 34:733, 1974.
39. Gerry, J. L., Bulkley, B. H., and Hutchins, G. M.: Rupture of the papillary muscle of the tricuspid valve. Am. J. Cardiol. 40:825, 1977.
40. Gewertz, B., O'Brien, C., and Kirsh, M. M.: Used intra-aortic balloon support for refractory low cardiac output in myocardial contusion. J. Trauma 17:325, 1977.
41. Go, R. T., Doty, D. B., Chiu, C. L., et al.: A new method of diagnosing myocardial contusion in man by radionuclide imaging. Radiology 116:107, 1975.
42. Goldstein, S., and Yu, P. N.: Constructive pericarditis after blunt chest trauma. Am. Heart J. 69:544, 1963.
43. Greene, J. F., and Cummings, K. C.: Aseptic thrombotic endocardial vegetation. J.A.M.A. 225:1525, 1973.
44. Griffin, J. S., Ochsner, J. L., and Bower, P. J.: Posttraumatic coarctation of the aorta. Diagnostic clues. Am. J. Cardiol. 31:391, 1973.
45. Harada, J., Osawa, M., Kosukegawa, K., et al.: Isolated mitral valve injury from nonpenetrating cardiac trauma. J. Cardiovasc. Surg. 18:459, 1977.
46. Harshaw, C. W., Grossman, W., Munro, A. B., et al.: Reduced systemic vascular resistance as therapy for severe mitral regurgitation of valvular origin. Ann. Intern. Med. 83:312, 1975.
47. Hellman, R. M., and Rufty, A. J.: Left ventricular aneurysms caused by blunt chest trauma. South. Med. J. 71:652, 1978.

48. Hipona, F. A., and Paredes, S.: The radiologic evaluation of patients with chest trauma. Med. Clin. North Am. 59:65, 1975.
49. Jones, E. W., and Helmsworth, J.: Penetrating wounds of the heart: thirty years experience. Arch. Surg. 96:671, 1968.
50. Jones, J. W., Hewitt, R. L., and Drapanas, T.: Cardiac contusion: capricious syndrome. Ann. Surg. 181:567, 1975.
51. Jones, R. C., and Jahnke, E. J.: Coronary artery–atrioventricular fistula and ventricular septal defect due to penetrating wound of the heart. Circulation 32:995, 1965.
52. Kerber, R. E., and Payvandi, M. N.: Echocardiography in acute hemopericardium: production of false-negative echocardiograms by pericardial clots. Circulation 55–56 (Suppl. III): III-24, 1977 (abstr.).
53. Kessler, K. M., Foianni, J. E., Davia, J. E., et al.: Tricuspid insufficiency due to nonpenetrating trauma. Am. J. Cardiol. 37:442, 1976.
54. Larrieu, A. J., Wiener, I., Alexander, R., and Wolma, F. J.: Pericardiodiaphragmatic hernia. Am. J. Surg, 139:436, 1980.
55. Ledgerwood, A. M.: The wandering bullet. Surg Clin. North Am. 57:97, 1977.
56. Leiter, E., Gribetz, D., and Cohen, S.: Arteriovenous fistula after percutaneous needle biopsy—surgical repair with preservation of renal function. N. Engl. J. Med. 287:971, 1972.
57. Liberthson, R. R., Barron, K., Harthorne, J. W., et al.: Traumatic coronary arterial fistula. A case report and review of the literature. Am. Heart J. 86:817, 1973.
58. Liedtke, A. J., and DeMuth, W. E., Jr.: Nonpenetrating cardiac injuries: a collective review. Am. Heart J. 86:687, 1973.
59. Liedtke, A. J., and DeMuth, W. E.: Effects of alcohol on cardiovascular performance after experimental nonpenetrating chest trauma. Am. J. Cardiol. 35:243, 1975.
60. Lindsey, D., Navin, T. R., and Finley, P. R.: Transient elevation of serum activity of MB isoenzymes of creatine phosphokinase in drivers involved in automobile accidents. Chest 74:15, 1978.
61. Macdonald, R. C., Hanning, C. D., and Ledingham, I. McA.: The use of inotropic drugs in myocardial contusion: 2 case reports. Intensive Care Med. 6:19, 1980.
62. Mandal, A. K., Awariefe, S. O., and Dparah, S. S.: Experience in the management of 50 consecutive penetrating wounds of the heart. Br. J. Surg. 66:565, 1979.
63. Mattilla, S., Silvola, H., and Ketonen, P.: Traumatic rupture of the pericardium with luxation of the heart. Case report and review of the literature. J. Thorac. Cardiovasc. Surg. 70:495, 1975.
64. Mattox, K. L., Beall, A. C., Jr., Jordan, G. L., and DeBakey, M. E.: Cardiorrhaphy in the Emergency Center. J. Thorac. Cardiovasc. Surg. 68:886, 1974.
65. Mattox, K. L., Koch, V., Beall, A. C., Jr., and DeBakey, M. E.: Logistic and technical considerations in the treatment of the wounded heart. Circulation (Suppl. 51–52):I-210, 1975.
66. Menzies, R. C.: Cardiac contusion. A review. Med. Sci. Law 18:3, 1978.
67. Midley, F., and Behrendt, D. M.: Surgical repair of chronic post-traumatic aneurysm of the aortic arch. J. Thorac. Cardiovasc. Surg. 67:229, 1974.
68. Moffat, R. C., Robert, V. L., and Berkas, E. M.: Blunt trauma to the thorax: development of pseudoaneurysms in the dog. J. Trauma 6:666, 1966.
69. Moncada, R., Matuga, T., Unger, E., et al.: Migrating traumatic cardiovascular foreign bodies. Circulation 57:186, 1978.
70. Najafi, H., Dye, W. S., Javid, H., et al.: Rupture of an otherwise normal aortic valve. Report of two cases and review of the literature. J. Thorac. Cardiovasc. Surg. 56:57, 1968.
71. Parmley, L. F., and Cheitlin, M. D.: Traumatic heart disease. *In* Fowler, N. O., (ed.): Cardiac Diagnosis and Treatment. Hagerstown, Maryland, Harper & Row, 1976, pp. 1095–1122.
72. Parmley, L. F., Manion, W. C., and Mattingly, T. W.: Nonpenetrating traumatic injury of the heart. Circulation 18:371, 1958.
73. Parmley, L. F., Mattingly, T. W., Manion, W. C., et al.: Nonpenetrating traumatic injury of the aorta. Circulation 17:1086, 1958.
74. Pomerantz, M., Delgado, F., and Eiseman, B.: Unsuspected depressed cardiac output following blunt thoracic or abdominal trauma. Surgery 70:865, 1971.
75. Popper, R. W., Schumacher, D., and Quinn, C. H.: Cardiac tamponade due to hypertonic contrast medium in the pericardial sac following cineangiography. Clinical observation and experimental study. Circulation 35:933, 1967.
76. Potkin, R. T., Werner, J. A., Trobaugh, B. G., et al.: Cardiac contusion. Evaluation of noninvasive tests of cardiac damage in suspected cadiac contusion. Circulation 66:627, 1982.
77. Reichle, F. A., and Golsorkhi, M.: Diagnosis and management of penetrating arterial and venous injuries in the extremities. Am. J. Surg. 140:365, 1980.
78. Reul, G. J., Jr., Mattox, K. L., Beall, A. C., Jr., et al.: Recent advances in the operative management of massive chest trauma. Ann. Thorac. Surg. 16:52, 1973.
79. Reyes, L. H., Mattox, K. L. Gaasch, W. H., et al.: Traumatic coronary artery in right heart fistula. Report of a case and review of the literature. J. Thorac. Cardiovasc. Surg. 70:52, 1975.
80. Rich, N. M.: Vascular trauma. Surg. Clin. North Am. 53:1367, 1973.
81. Richardson, J. D., McElvein, R. B., and Trinkle, J. K.: First rib fracture: a hallmark of severe trauma. Ann. Surg. 181:251, 1975.
82. Rossi, P.: "Hook catheter," technique for transfemoral removal of foreign body from right side of the heart. Am. J. Roentgenol. 109:101, 1970.
83. Rotman, M., Peter, R. H., Sealy, W. C., et al.: Traumatic ventricular septal defect secondary to nonpenetrating chest trauma. Am. J. Med. 48:127, 1970.
84. Saunders, C. R., and Doty, D. B.: Myocardial contusion. Surg. Gynecol. Obstet. 144:595, 1977.
85. Saunders, C. R., and Doty, D. B.: Myocardial contusion: effect of intraaortic balloon counterpulsation on cardiac output. J. Trauma 18:706, 1978.
86. Sbokos, C. G., Karayannacos, P. E., Kontaxis, A., et al.: Traumatic hemopericardium and chronic

constrictive pericarditis. Ann. Thorac. Surg. 23:225, 1977.

87. Schechter, D. C., and Gilbert, L.: Injuries of the heart and great vessels due to pins and needles. Thorax 24:246, 1969.
88. Sherman, M. M., Saini, V. K., Yarnoz, M. D., et al.: Management of penetrating heart wounds. Am. J. Surg. 135:553, 1978.
89. Singh, R., Nolan, S. P., and Schrank, J. P.: Traumatic left ventricular aneurysm. J.A.M.A. 234:412, 1975.
90. Sinha, S. N., Bhattacharya, S. K., Mymin, D., et al.: Ventricular septal defects due to penetrating injuries of the heart. Can. Med. Assoc. J. 107:1182, 1972.
91. Spittel, J. A., Jr., Palumbo, P. J., Love, J. G., et al.: Arteriovenous fistula complicating lumbar-disk surgery. N. Engl. J. Med. 268:1162, 1963.
92. Stanger, P., Heymann, M. A., Tarnoff, H., et al.: Complications of cardiac catheterization of neonates, infants, and children. Circulation 50:595, 1974.
93. Sugg, W. L., Rea, W. J., Ecker, R. R., et al.: Penetrating wounds of the heart. An analysis of 459 cases. J. Thorac. Cardiovasc. Surg. 56:531, 1968.
94. Summerall, C. P., Lee, W. H., Jr., and Boone, J. A.: Intracardiac shunts after penetrating wounds of the heart. N. Engl. J. Med. 272:240, 1965.
95. Sutherland, G. R., Calvin, J. E., Driedger, A. A., et al.: Anatomic and cardiopulmonary responses to trauma with associated blunt chest injury. J. Trauma 21:1, 1981.
96. Symbas, P. N.: Cardiac trauma. Am. Heart J. 92:387, 1976.
97. Symbas, P. N.: Great vessels injury. Am. Heart J. 93:518, 1977.
98. Symbas, P. N., and Harlaftis, N.: Bullet emboli in the pulmonary and systemic arteries. Ann. Surg. 185:318, 1977.
99. Szentpetery, S., and Lower, R. R.: Changing concepts in the treatment of penetrating cardiac injuries. J. Trauma 17:459, 1977.
100. Tabatznik, B., and Isaacs, J. P.: Postpericardiotomy syndrome following traumatic hemopericardium. Am. J. Cardiol. 7:83, 1961.
101. Thandroyen, F. T., and Matisonn, R. E.: Penetrating thoracic trauma producing cardiac shunts. J. Thorac. Cardiovasc. Surg. 81:569, 1981.
102. Triukle, J. K., Toons, R. S., Franz, J. L., et al.: Affairs of the wounded heart: penetrating cardiac wounds. J. Trauma 19:467, 1979.
103. Trunkey, D. D., and Lewis, F. R.: Chest trauma. Surg. Clin. North Am. 60:1541, 1980.
104. Urschel, C. W., Covell, J. W., Sonnenblick, E. H., et al.: Myocardial mechanics in aortic and mitral valvular regurgitation: the concept of instantaneous impedance as a determinant of the performance of the intact heart. J. Clin. Invest. 47:867, 1968.
105. Utley, J. R., Doty, D. B., Coklins, J. C., et al.: Cardiac output, coronary flow, ventricular fibrillation and survival following varying degrees of myocardial contusion. J. Surg. Res. 20:539, 1976.
106. Vlay, S. C., Blumenthal, D. S., Shoback, D., et al.: Delayed acute myocardial infarction after blunt chest trauma in a young woman. Am. Heart J. 100:907, 1980.
107. Vlodaver, Z., Coe, J. I., and Edwards, J. E.: True and false left ventricular aneurysms. Propensity for the latter to rupture. Circulation 51:567, 1975.
108. Walker, W. J.: Spontaneous closure of traumatic ventricular septal defect. Am. J. Cardiol. 15:263, 1965.
109. Ward, R. E.: Study and management of blunt trauma in the immediate post-impact period. Radiol. Clin. North Am. 19:3, 1981.
110. Wilson, J. M., Thomas, A. N., Goodman, P. C., and Lewis, F. R.: Severe chest trauma. Morbidity implication of first and second rib fracture in 120 patients. Arch. Surg. 113:846, 1978.
111. Yao, S. T., Carey, J. S., Shoemaker, W. C., et al.: Hemodynamics and therapy of acute hemopericardium from stab wounds of the heart. J. Trauma 7:783, 1967.
112. Zeft, H. J., and McIntosh, H. D.: Postpericardiotomy syndrome in a patient with a retained foreign body. Am. J. Cardiol. 16:593, 1965.

15

Drug Therapy for Cardiac Emergencies: Pharmacokinetic Considerations

PAUL PENTEL

and NEAL L. BENOWITZ

Drug therapy for cardiac emergencies is characterized by several unique considerations.

1. Because of the urgency of the patient's condition, therapeutic drug concentrations must be achieved rapidly, often within minutes. To accomplish this, a route of drug administration must be chosen that allows prompt drug absorption and delivery to target organs.
2. Most cardiac emergencies are associated with some degree of circulatory dysfunction that in turn may alter the pharmacokinetics of therapeutic agents. Drug dosage regimens must be tailored to accommodate these changes.
3. The clinical status of the acutely compromised patient often changes rapidly, requiring adjustment of drug dosing.
4. The acutely ill patient can be expected to tolerate drug toxicity poorly, so that the avoidance of excessive drug dosage is of critical importance.

In addition to these factors, time usually does not permit the measurement of drug concentrations in blood for use as a guide for dosing. Decisions about drug doses must often be made entirely on the basis of a knowledge of a particular drug's pharmacokinetic characteristics, the patient's underlying circulatory disorder, and an appreciation of how the two will interact. In this chapter the effects of acute cardiac dysfunction on drug pharmacokinetics, and the principles underlying the use of drugs in emergent situations, are considered. These principles are illustrated by a discussion of several frequently used drugs. Attention is focused on the first few hours of management. The influence of chronic cardiac failure on pharmacokinetics has been reviewed elsewhere.[10]

EFFECTS OF CIRCULATORY FAILURE ON PHARMACOKINETICS

Pathophysiology of Circulatory Dysfunction in Cardiac Emergencies

Circulatory Failure. Circulatory failure, or the inability of the heart to provide sufficient cardiac output to satisfy tissue metabolic requirements, is the most important and most common cause of altered pharmacokinetics during cardiac emergencies. Circulatory failure may result from decreased myocardial contractility, arrhythmias that allow insufficient time for diastolic filling or impair atrioventricular synchrony, circulatory stresses such as increased afterload or hypovolemia, valvular dysfunction, tamponade, or a variety of less common insults. Regardless of etiology, circulatory failure elicits characteristic compensatory hemodynamic adjustments

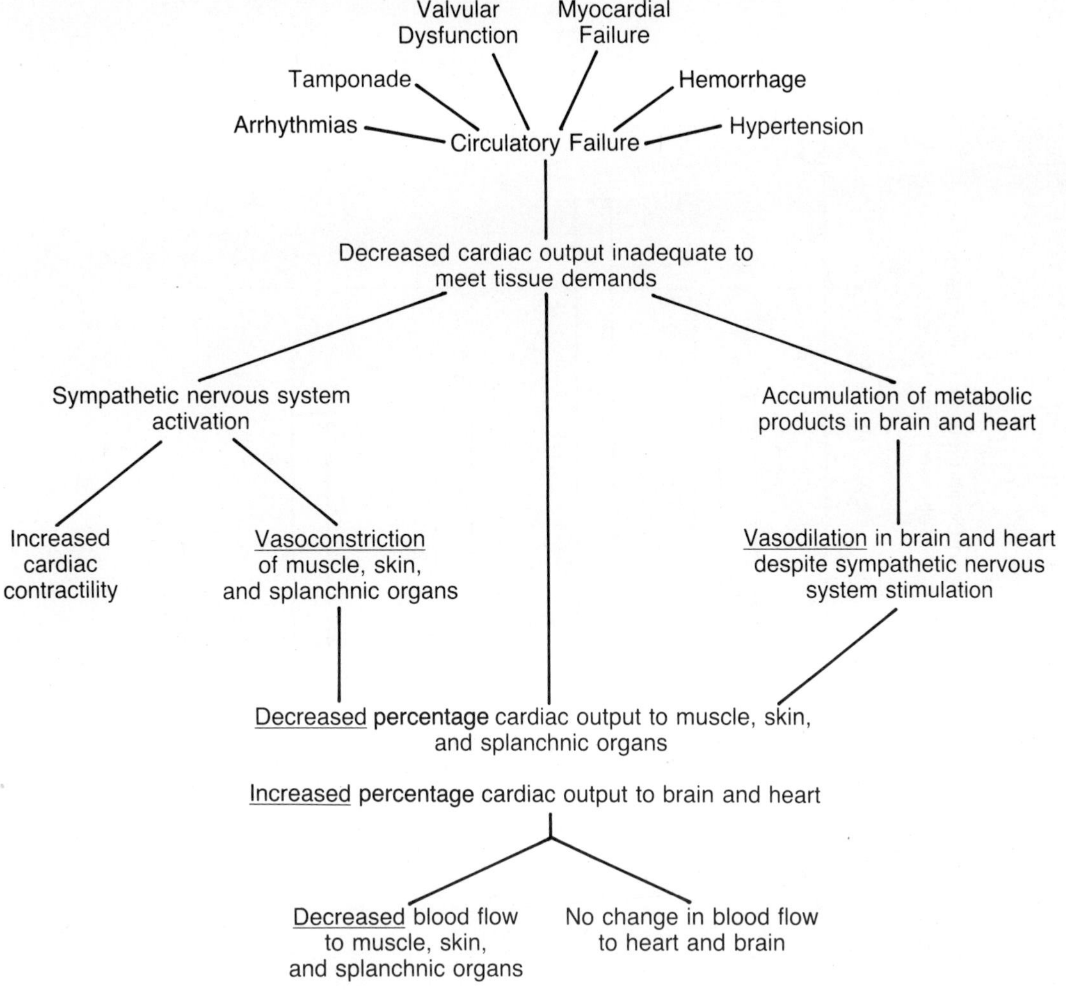

Figure 15–1. Effects of circulatory failure on blood flow distribution.

mediated in large part by activation of the sympathetic nervous system (Fig. 15–1).[8, 12, 48, 49, 106, 107] Enhanced sympathetic tone increases cardiac contractility and peripheral vascular resistance, both of which serve to maintain arterial blood pressure. The increase in peripheral vascular resistance, however, is not uniform among different vascular beds. Organs with high metabolic requirements such as heart and brain exhibit autoregulation; their vessels remain relatively vasodilated despite sympathetic stimulation due to the effects of hypoxia, lactic acid, or other products of anaerobic metabolism that accumulate when organ perfusion is reduced. Blood flow to heart and brain tends to be preserved while vasoconstriction decreases blood flow in other locations such as skin, muscle and splanchnic organs. Thus, a disproportionate fraction of the available cardiac output is delivered to heart and brain (Fig. 15–2).

Cardiopulmonary Resuscitation (CPR). Cardiac output during CPR is severely compromised; in humans the mean arterial pressure is less than 50 per cent of normal,[15, 70] and in dogs cardiac output is less than 30 per cent of normal.[102] Hemodynamic measurements are difficult to obtain in patients during CPR, but animal data suggest that changes in blood flow distribution are qualitatively similar to those observed with circulatory failure and spontaneous circulation. Blood flow during CPR in anesthetized, electrically fibrillated dogs is reduced to all organs, but least so to brain and next least to heart (Fig. 15–3).[102] It is important to note, however, that these studies differ from those

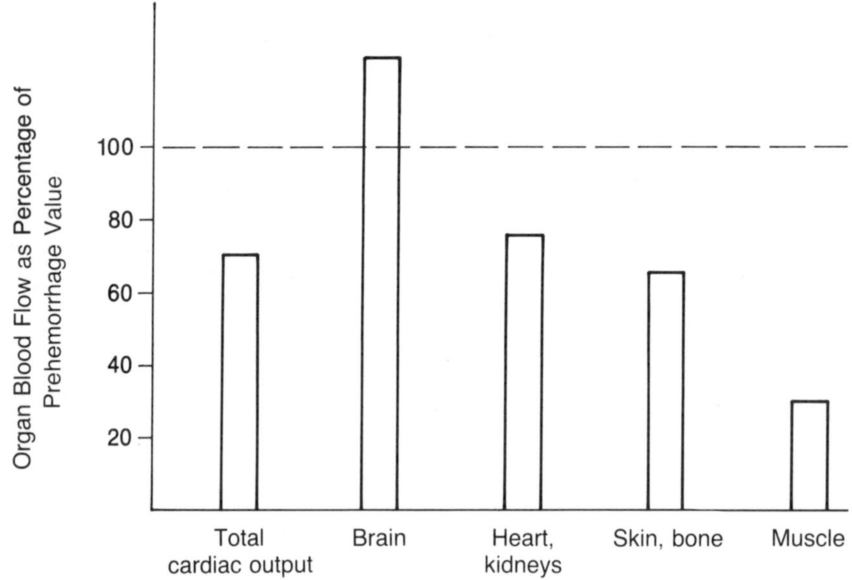

Figure 15–2. Effects of 30 per cent hemorrhage on organ blood flow in monkeys. Blood flow to heart and kidneys is relatively well preserved, and blood flow to brain is actually greater than before hemorrhage. The marked decrease in flow to skeletal muscle is particularly important since muscle represents 30 to 40 per cent of body weight and is a major organ of drug uptake. (Adapted from Benowitz et al.: Lidocaine disposition kinetics in monkeys and man. II. Effects of hemorrhage and sympathomimetic drug administration. Clin. Pharmacol. Ther. 16:99, 1974.)

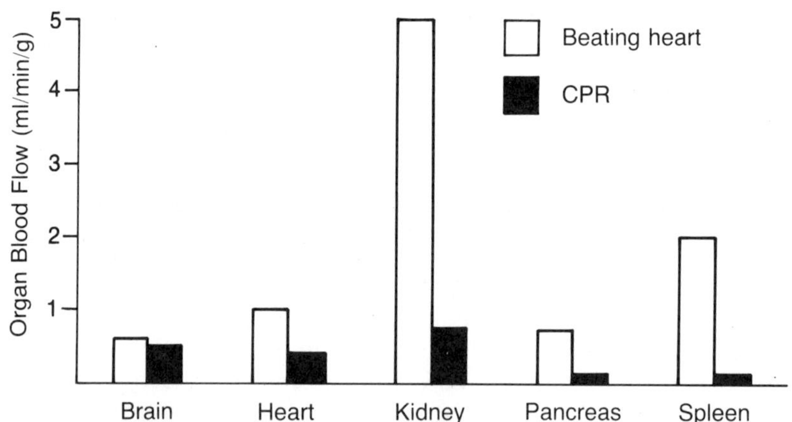

Figure 15–3. Organ blood flow in anesthetized dogs with normally beating hearts and during CPR in animals with electrically induced ventricular fibrillation. Blood flow is well preserved to brain, reduced to heart and kidneys, and lowest to pancreas and spleen. (Adapted from Voorhees et al.: Regional blood flow during cardiopulmonary resuscitation in dogs. Crit. Care Med. 8:134, 1980.)

of cardiac arrest in humans in that CPR is initiated in the animals without delay, whereas patients are often without effective circulation for a period before initiation of CPR. In dogs subjected to 20 minutes of complete circulatory arrest, cerebral blood flow during subsequent resuscitation decreases from 45 per cent of the prearrest value at the start of resuscitation to less than 10 per cent one hour later despite a constant cardiac output.[34] The reason for this decrease is not clear, but this observation demonstrates that the control of organ blood flow during CPR is a complex process. For the purpose of pharmacokinetic considerations, CPR and circulatory failure with spontaneous circulation may be considered to be similar in that total cardiac output is reduced and the pattern of blood flow redistribution during promptly initiated CPR resembles that seen in circulatory failure.

Pneumatic Trousers (Military Anti-Shock Trousers, MAST Suit). The MAST suit consists of inflatable trousers that compress the lower extremities and abdomen. It has been employed widely in the initial management of hypotension secondary to blood loss.[50] There is current interest in the use of the MAST suit in cardiogenic shock and as an adjunct to CPR. When the MAST suit is applied to supine normotensive subjects, mean arterial pressure increases by 10 to 20 mm Hg. This is due to an increase in total peripheral resistance produced by compression of lower extremity arterioles, and is accompanied by a decrease in cardiac output. During 60° upright tilt, the MAST suit produces a small increase in cardiac output despite increased peripheral vascular resistance, suggesting that there is also a reduction of venous pooling in the lower limbs.[35] Since lower extremity venous pooling is not expected during circulatory failure, it is likely that the beneficial hemodynamic effect of the MAST suit in this situation is primarily due to increased peripheral resistance. The expected redistribution of blood flow would be similar in many respects to the sympathetic vasoconstriction seen in cardiac failure, the major difference being preservation of upper limb blood flow (as well as preservation of splanchnic blood flow if the abdominal portion of the suit is not inflated). Although it is difficult to extrapolate data from normotensive subjects to patients in shock or undergoing CPR, it is likely that the MAST suit exaggerates the redistribution of blood flow already present.

Drug Absorption

Absorption of drugs from sites with impaired blood flow is slow, possibly incomplete, and subject to changes in circulatory status. Thus, the oral, subcutaneous, and intramuscular routes may not be reliable in acute cardiac emergencies, and an intravascular route is preferred. When intravascular access cannot be established rapidly, however, intratracheal or intramuscular drug administration may be useful. The pulmonary tree provides an extensive surface for drug absorption, and pulmonary venous blood empties directly into the heart. Consequently, some drugs (epinephrine, lidocaine)[29, 44, 80, 81] appear to be well absorbed from this site even when cardiac output is markedly decreased. The intramuscular route has been used to administer lidocaine to patients suspected of having acute myocardial infarction.[6, 18, 93, 108] Therapeutic blood concentrations of lidocaine can be readily achieved, and this route has been suggested for prehospital prophylaxis of ventricular arrhythmias. It should be noted, however, that intramuscular administration of lidocaine has been studied primarily in patients without circulatory failure, and the adequacy of lidocaine absorption in patients with moderate or severe circulatory failure is not known. Absorption of lidocaine is more rapid from deltoid muscle than from gluteus maximus or vastus lateralis (Fig. 15–4).[18] Injection of drugs into the base of the tongue has also been suggested when intravascular access cannot be established because of the area's prominent vascularity. This location appears to have no advantage over other intramuscular sites.[78]

Drug Distribution

Relationship of Blood Concentration of Drug to Drug Effect. For most drugs, the magnitude of therapeutic or toxic effect is determined by their concentration at the target organ. At steady state, when the concentration of drug in blood is in equilibrium with the concentration of drug in tissues, blood concentration of drug is proportional to tis-

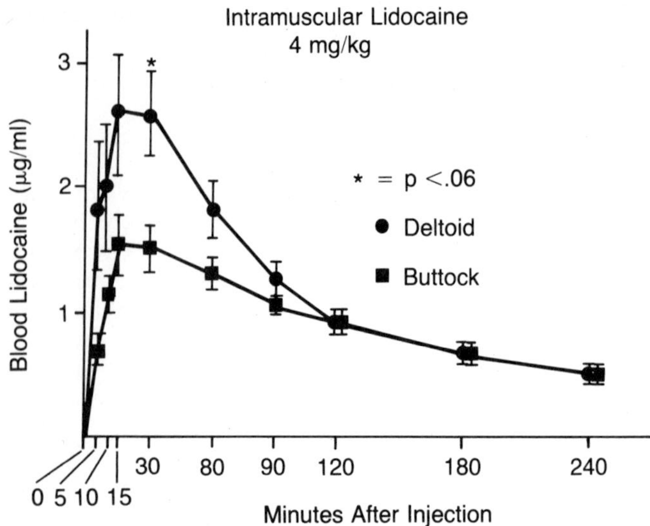

Figure 15–4. Blood lidocaine concentrations after 4 mg/kg of 10 per cent lidocaine injected into the deltoid or gluteal muscles of patients with suspected myocardial infarction but without overt cardiac failure. (From Zener et al.: Blood lidocaine levels and kinetics following high-dose intramuscular administration. Circulation 47:984, 1973. Reproduced by permission of The American Heart Association, Inc.)

sue concentration of drug. For most cardioactive drugs, the blood concentration of drug at steady state correlates with the magnitude of effect of the drug, and can be used as a predictor of therapeutic effect or toxicity. Since all drugs take time to distribute from blood to tissues, the blood concentration of drug may not correlate with the tissue concentration of drug immediately after administration. It is important to consider this relationship in order to design and monitor drug dosage in acute situations.

Drugs That Distribute Rapidly. A computer simulation of lidocaine kinetics after a one-minute infusion illustrates the time course of distribution of lidocaine from blood into various organs: a well-perfused tissue (heart) and two poorly perfused tissues (muscle and adipose) (Fig. 15–5).[9] Blood concentration of lidocaine falls rapidly after infusion, owing to tissue uptake of drug. During this phase, blood concentrations are quite high while tissue concentrations are still low. Distribution of lidocaine to the heart, because of its relatively high rate of perfusion, is rapid, and lidocaine concentration in the heart is proportional to that in blood within four minutes of infusion. Therapeutic or toxic concentrations (and effects) of lidocaine are achieved in the heart within minutes of lidocaine administration. Distribution of lidocaine to muscle and adipose tissue is, by comparison, much slower, but these tissues represent a storage reservoir of greater magnitude. The consequence of uptake into these tissues is that the blood concentration of

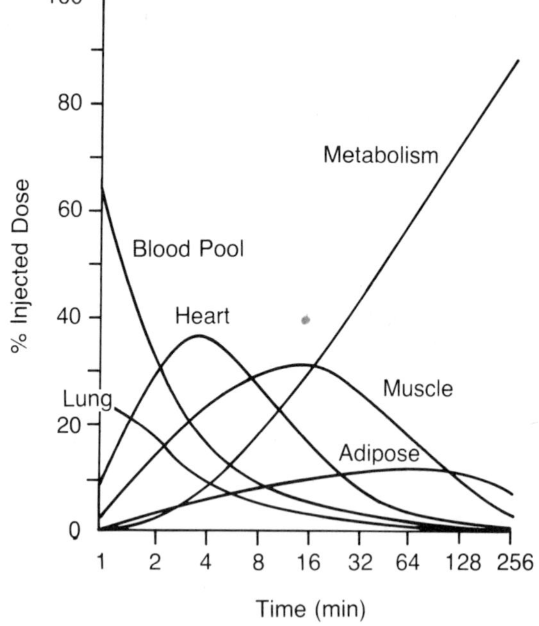

Figure 15–5. Computer simulation based on a perfusion model of the distribution of lidocaine to various tissues in man after a 1-min intravenous infusion (note log time scale). The initial rapid decline in blood concentration is primarily due to drug distribution to tissues. Myocardial lidocaine concentration peaks at 4 min, and blood lidocaine concentration from this time on parallels myocardial concentration. Distribution of lidocaine to other tissues is slower, and blood lidocaine concentration continues to decline rapidly for 20 to 30 min owing to tissue uptake. The subsequent slower decline in blood lidocaine concentration is primarily due to metabolism. (From Benowitz et al.: Lidocaine disposition kinetics in monkey and man. I. Prediction by a perfusion model. Clin. Pharmacol. Ther. 16:87, 1974. Reproduced with permission.)

lidocaine continues to decline at a rate faster than can be explained by metabolism for 20 to 30 minutes after administration. Thereafter, blood concentration of lidocaine declines much more slowly, the rate being determined by the rate of hepatic metabolism and rate of distribution out of tissues. Thus, although the overall distribution of lidocaine to body tissues takes about 30 minutes, the high initial blood concentrations of lidocaine seen after intravenous injection are reflected within a few minutes by high concentrations in well-perfused organs such as heart and brain.

Drugs That Distribute Slowly. Although many cardiac drugs such as lidocaine are distributed rapidly to the heart, others such as digoxin are distributed more slowly. The distribution half-life for lidocaine is five to ten minutes,[11] consistent with the observation that distribution is essentially complete within 30 minutes.[9] In contrast, the distribution half-life of digoxin is much longer (range 20–90 min),[25, 59, 79] and peak cardiac digoxin effect is not achieved until 30 minutes to five hours after an intravenous dose.[79, 90, 94] Serum digoxin concentration before this time does not correlate well with the effect on the myocardium. The use of a single large dose of digoxin for initiating digoxin therapy does not cause early myocardial toxicity, and the full loading (digitalizing) dose can be administered at once. The common and preferable practice of dividing the digitalizing dose into two or three boluses administered at three- to six-hour intervals serves the purpose of incrementally determining a dose that yields the desired myocardial effect for a given patient. It should be noted, however, that whereas the myocardial effects of intravenous digoxin are delayed, vascular effects occur rapidly and seem to be related to high plasma concentrations.[19, 87] Thus, an increase in systemic vascular resistance of up to 50 per cent occurs within minutes of a rapid intravenous injection. This may be due to more rapid distribution of digoxin to peripheral vessels than to myocardium. Because the increase in systemic vascular resistance precedes the increase in cardiac contractility, rapid intravenous administration of digoxin may have adverse hemodynamic consequences such as a decrease in cardiac output.[87] It has been demonstrated that slower administration of an intravenous loading dose of the related cardiac glycoside ouabain (over 15 min) prevents the increase in systemic vascular resistance seen with administration over ten seconds,[23] and this probably is also true of digoxin.[66] Thus, large doses of intravenous digoxin can be administered without causing early myocardial toxicity, but should be infused slowly to prevent a rapid increase in systemic vascular resistance.

Circulatory Influences on Drug Distribution. In response to impaired cardiac output, sympathetically mediated vasoconstriction results in redistribution of blood flow. A relatively large fraction of the available cardiac output is delivered to heart and brain, and less to muscle, skin, splanchnic organs, and kidney. Thus, blood flow and distribution of drugs to locations other than heart and brain is delayed. In addition, the initial drug concentration in blood minutes after administration of the drug is higher in patients with circulatory failure than in those with normal circulatory states. This point is illustrated by a computer simulation of the effects of hypovolemic shock on lidocaine distribution (Fig. 15–6).[8] Hypovolemia resembles other causes of reduced cardiac output in that the pattern of sympathetic stimulation and blood flow redistribution is similar. Blood lidocaine

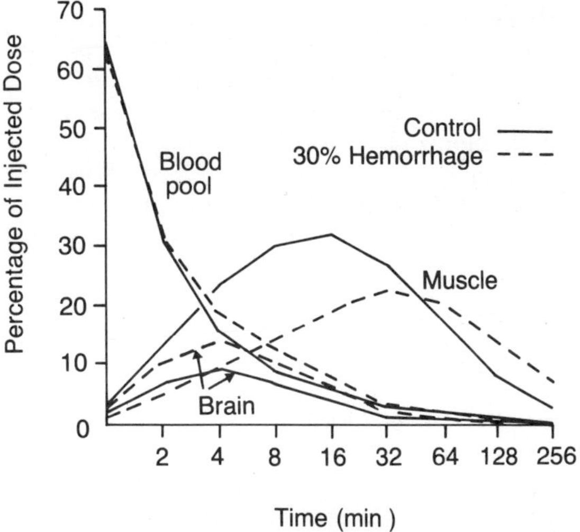

Figure 15–6. Computer simulation based on a perfusion model of the distribution of lidocaine to various tissues after a 1-min intravenous infusion of 100 mg in a 70-kg person. During hemorrhage, vasoconstriction in muscle decreases muscle blood flow and the rate and extent of drug uptake. As a result, blood lidocaine concentration is higher and brain (as well as heart, which is not shown), with preserved blood flow, achieves a higher lidocaine concentration. (From Benowitz et al.: Lidocaine disposition kinetics in monkey and man. II. Effects of hemorrhage and sympathomimetic drug administration. Clin. Pharmacol. Ther. 16:99, 1974. Reproduced with permission.)

concentration is higher than normal minutes after drug administration during hemorrhage owing to reduced tissue perfusion. Lidocaine concentrations are also initially higher in well-perfused tissues such as brain than in other tissues. This explains why cardiac or central nervous system toxicity may result when standard lidocaine doses are administered to patients with circulatory failure. Individuals with myocardial infarction and circulatory failure can convulse after a single rapid injection of 75 or 100 mg of lidocaine despite subtherapeutic blood concentrations of lidocaine measured shortly after the event.[11]

Drug Metabolism

The rate of hepatic drug metabolism is determined by both the intrinsic metabolic capacity and the rate of drug delivery to the liver (hepatic blood flow).[85] Drugs for which intrinsic hepatic metabolizing capacity is high are rapidly and extensively cleared from hepatic blood, and their rate of metabolism is dependent primarily on hepatic blood flow. Lidocaine is such a drug, and hepatic lidocaine clearance has been correlated with hepatic blood flow as estimated by indocyanine green clearance (Fig. 15–7).[109] In circulatory failure, decreased cardiac output is associated with a roughly proportional decrease in hepatic blood flow, and metabolic clearance of lidocaine is therefore diminished. This may have substantial therapeutic implications. The elimination half-life of lidocaine has been shown to be prolonged up to threefold in patients with myocardial infarction without overt cardiac failure, and up to sixfold in those with overt cardiac failure.[77] Just as circulatory failure may decrease hepatic blood flow and impair the clearance of highly extracted drugs by the liver, drugs that impair hepatic blood flow may have the same effect. Propranolol decreases hepatic blood flow by lowering cardiac output, and the administration of therapeutic doses of propranolol to normal subjects during lidocaine infusion increases the steady state plasma lidocaine concentration by 30 per cent.[75] Similarly, cimetidine impairs hepatic blood flow by blocking H_2 receptors in mesenteric, gastric, and hepatic arteries, and administration of therapeutic doses of cimetidine in normal subjects has been shown to decrease lidocaine clearance by 25 per cent.[31] Catecholamines and inotropic agents can also alter hepatic blood flow. Although the effects in humans have not been studied, norepinephrine decreases and isoproterenol increases hepatic blood flow and lidocaine clearance in monkeys.[8]

Drugs such as digoxin and quinidine, for which intrinsic hepatic metabolizing capacity is low, are, by contrast, slowly and incompletely cleared from hepatic blood. Their rates of metabolism are relatively independent of hepatic blood flow and are determined instead primarily by the intrinsic metabolic capacity of the liver. Injury to hepatocytes due to reduced perfusion, arterial hypox-

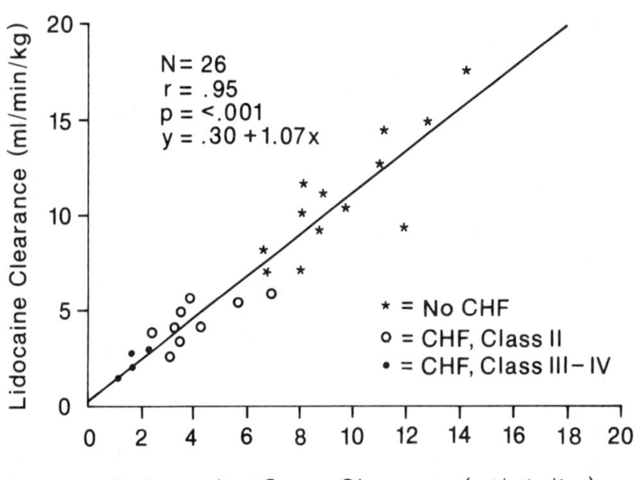

Figure 15–7. Lidocaine clearance is markedly impaired in patients with congestive heart failure, and correlates with hepatic blood flow as measured by indocyanine green clearance. (From Zito, R. A., and Reid, P. R.: Lidocaine kinetics predicted by indocyanine green clearance. N. Engl. J. Med. 298:1160, 1078. Reprinted by permission, from The New England Journal of Medicine.)

emia, or passive congestion can impair intrinsic metabolic capacity and slow the metabolic clearance of drugs. For example, antipyrine clearance, which is independent of hepatic blood flow, is reduced in patients with congestive heart failure.[77]

Drug Excretion

Circulatory failure, with the resulting decrease in renal blood flow, may have several important effects on the renal excretion of drugs. The kidney does have a modest capacity for autoregulation, and when renal blood flow is moderately reduced (10 to 20%), the glomerular filtration rate (GFR) does not fall. However, further reductions in renal blood flow lower the GFR and consequently slow the excretion of drugs cleared by filtration, such as procainamide and digoxin.[27] The tubular reabsorption of drugs may be increased as a consequence of decreased urine flow accompanying a decrease in GFR, as well as by sympathetically mediated shunting of blood from cortical to juxtamedullary nephrons, but documentation of clinically important decreases in drug excretion due to these mechanisms is lacking. Reduced renal blood flow might also be expected to slow the elimination of drugs that are actively secreted by reducing their rate of delivery to secretion sites. Digoxin is excreted by both filtration and secretion, and impaired digoxin secretion due to hypovolemia has been postulated in a report of two patients in whom renal digoxin clearance was impaired to a greater extent than creatinine clearance.[7] Thus, renal hemodynamic changes induced by circulatory failure all serve to decrease drug excretion by the kidney and may necessitate reductions in the maintenance dose of drugs that depend on renal elimination (Fig. 15–8).

Other Factors Associated With Cardiac Disease

Many, if not most, patients who present with acute cardiac emergencies have other manifestations of chronic cardiac disease that may further influence drug kinetics. For example, fluid retention may increase the volume of distribution of water-soluble drugs. Hypoproteinemia may increase the volume of distribution of highly protein-bound drugs or reduce the hepatic clearance of highly extracted drugs. Coexisting drug therapy may produce hemodynamic effects that alter drug disposition. These factors will be considered below only as they relate to acute hemodynamic compromise; the review of Benowitz and Meister provides further discussion of this topic.[10]

DRUG ADMINISTRATION DURING CIRCULATORY FAILURE

Routes of Drug Administration*

Intravenous. Although the peripheral intravenous route is the most commonly employed, it is often difficult to establish a peripheral intravenous line in the presence of shock because of intense peripheral vasoconstriction. A central venous catheter, introduced via the subclavian or internal jugular vein, is often used to administer fluids and drugs in this situation. Administration of drugs through a central venous catheter results in higher initial cardiac concentrations than administration via peripheral intravenous catheter, because (1) there is less dilution of drug with venous blood when it is administered centrally, and (2) sluggish blood flow in a vasoconstricted extremity can reduce the rate of delivery of drug to the central circulation from this site. This has been shown experimentally in dogs undergoing CPR: the appearance of the indicator dye Cardio-Green in central arterial blood is delayed and the concentration lower after peripheral, as opposed to central, intravenous administration.[60] Although use of the central intravenous route during CPR therefore has a potential advantage, drug administration by this route has also been associated with serious toxicity. In a review of 132 cases of cardiac arrest occurring in critically ill hospitalized patients, 17 arrests were believed to result from administration of drugs through a central intravenous catheter. The majority[12] were due to aminophylline; epinephrine and digoxin were implicated in the remainder.[14] The central intravenous route, therefore, should be used cautiously for administration of potentially cardiotoxic drugs: other routes, if available, are preferable. If the central

*See Table 15–1.

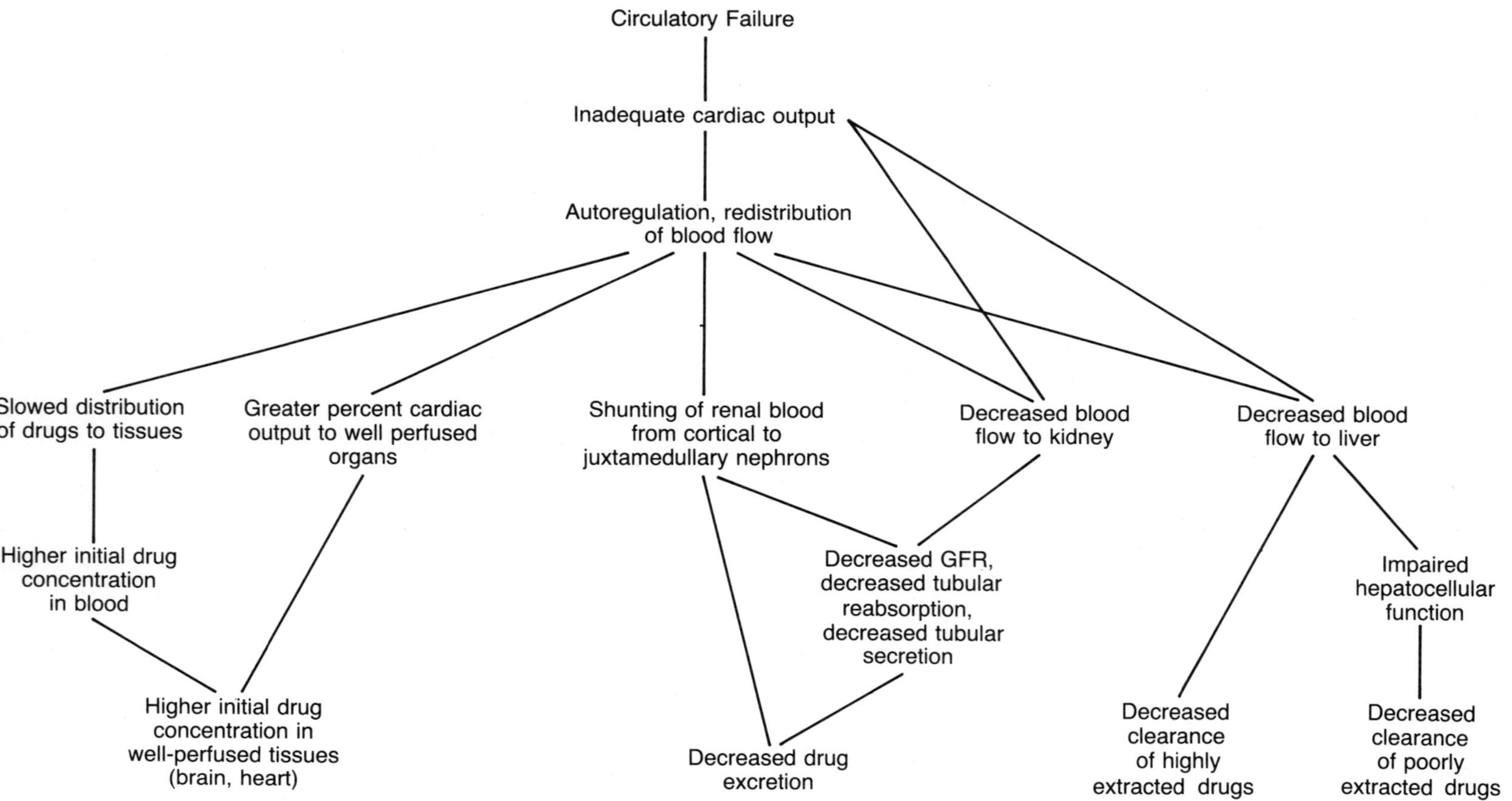

Figure 15–8. Pharmacokinetic consequences of circulatory failure. GFR = glomerular filtration rate.

Table 15–1. ROUTES OF DRUG ADMINISTRATION USED IN CARDIAC EMERGENCIES.

Route	Advantages	Disadvantages	Drugs Administered Via This Route	Principal Clinical Use	Precautions
Intramuscular, subcutaneous	Always available	Absorption may be slow, erratic	Lidocaine (intramuscular)	Prehospital arrhythmia prophylaxis for suspected myocardial infarction when intravenous route not available	Deltoid muscle best; absorption may be poor in vasoconstricted patients; intravascular route always preferred
			Epinephrine (subcutaneous)	Anaphylaxis in normotensive patients, or in hypotensive patients when intravenous route not available	
Peripheral Intravenous	Safe procedure; data regarding most drugs pertain to this route	Difficult to obtain when cardiac output low and patient severely vasoconstricted; distribution to heart possibly slowed during CPR with poor peripheral perfusion	Most		
Central intravenous (subclavian, internal jugular)	Catheter can be placed even in severely hypotensive patients	Risks of procedure (pneumothorax, hemothorax); drugs reach heart at very high concentration	Many	When peripheral intravenous route not available	Cardiac arrest associated with administration of aminophylline and other potentially cardiotoxic drugs via this route; administer all drugs slowly (over a minimum of 2–3 min)
Intratracheal	Available in intubated patients	New technique, few kinetic data available	Epinephrine	During cardiac arrest when intramuscular route not available	Drug doses not well established; some drug solutions (bicarbonate) can injure lungs
Intracardiac	Always available	Risks of procedure (pneumothorax, coronary artery laceration, intramyocardial injection, CPR must be interrupted, very high initial drug concentration in heart)	Epinephrine, Calcium	When no other route available	All other intravascular routes and intratracheal administration preferred

CPR = cardiopulmonary resuscitation.

route is used, drugs should be given slowly, ideally by controlled infusion to allow maximal drug dilution. It remains to be determined whether central intravenous drug administration during CPR offers any clinical advantage to patients who have not responded to drugs given via a peripheral vein.

Intracardiac. The intracardiac route has been used for administration of epinephrine in cases of cardiac arrest when an intravenous catheter is not available, or in the hope that direct cardiac administration may achieve a therapeutic cardiac concentration when the peripheral intravenous route has not. Intracardiac injection into the right ventricle offers no pharmacokinetic advantage over central intravenous administration. Left ventricular injection could potentially produce a higher arterial concentration of drug by preventing drug uptake by the lung, but an advantage of the intracardiac route over other intravascular routes has not been demonstrated. Transthoracic intracardiac injection may result in pneumothorax, laceration of a coronary artery, intramyocardial injection, or pericardial tamponade.[40, 54] The subxiphoid approach is safer than transthoracic injection, but both require interruption of CPR.[22] The intracardiac route of drug administration is considered by many to be an alternative for use only when both the intravenous and intratracheal routes are not available.[71]

Intratracheal. The intratracheal route has been evaluated as a means of drug administration when intravenous access cannot be established, primarily during CPR. Intratracheal administration of drug is accomplished by injecting drug into the tracheobronchial tree at the level of the carina, using a flexible catheter introduced through the lumen of an endotracheal tube. This is immediately followed by five to ten bag ventilations, which are believed to distribute drug to more distal airways. Intratracheal administration of epinephrine, lidocaine, or atropine in 10 ml of water to dogs does not appear to have adverse pulmonary effects as judged by serial arterial blood gases. However, sodium bicarbonate solutions, perhaps because of hypertonicity, do cause pulmonary injury and illustrate a potential limitation of this route.[29] The intratracheal route was compared with the intravenous route during cardiopulmonary arrest in dogs: epinephrine diluted in 10 ml of water administered intratracheally resulted in a resuscitation rate equal to that obtained with femoral intravenous administration.[78] It is of note that undiluted 1:1000 epinephrine (volume of 1 ml) was ineffective in resuscitating dogs from hypoxic arrest, perhaps because of drug remaining in the endotracheal tube.

Intratracheal and intravenous administration of lidocaine, epinephrine, and atropine during hypoxic arrest have also been compared in dogs: time to onset of drug effect as judged by the cardiac rhythm was shorter via the intratracheal route for all drugs.[29] Response to peripheral intravenous dosing may be delayed in this circumstance owing to sluggish return of femoral venous blood, or more extensive dilution of femoral than of pulmonary venous blood. However, when epinephrine was used to treat histamine-induced hypotension in dogs that still had spontaneous circulation and did not require CPR, the onset of therapeutic effect was slower after intratracheal administration than after administration via a peripheral leg vein.[44] Thus, the initial rate of delivery of drug to the heart via the intratracheal and intravenous routes may depend on the adequacy of the existing circulation, and the intratracheal route may provide more rapid drug distribution to the central circulation when cardiac output is severely compromised.

The duration of drug action may also be longer with intratracheal than with intravenous administration. Electrocardiographic effects of epinephrine, lidocaine, and atropine persist longer with intratracheal than with intravenous administration in dogs in hypoxic arrest.[29] A slower decline in plasma epinephrine concentration has been observed in anesthetized normotensive dogs after intratracheal than after intravenous administration.[81] This suggests a pulmonary depot of epinephrine after intratracheal dosing, resulting in a relatively sustained drug action. No pharmacokinetic data regarding the use of the intratracheal route in humans have been obtained. One adult given 10 ml of epinephrine intratracheally during resuscitation from cardiac arrest regained a palpable pulse and sinus rhythm one minute later, but the blood pressure then increased to 230/130 mm Hg, illustrating that further study is necessary to establish appropriate dosing regimens.[80] At present, the use of epinephrine 1:10,000 via the intratracheal route in the same dose as is indicated for intravenous injection appears warranted if intravenous access cannot be established. Use of the intratracheal route for other drugs, such as lidocaine, appears feasible but requires further study.

Principles of Intravenous Dosing

A variety of dosing regimens have been proposed for the rapid achievement and maintenance of therapeutic blood concentrations of drug. Intravenous infusion at a constant rate is sufficient for some drugs. The rate at which a drug achieves a steady state plasma concentration is determined by the drug's elimination half-life; 90 per cent of the steady state concentration is reached after about 3.5 half-lives. For a rapidly eliminated drug such as epinephrine (half-life 2 min), this would take only seven minutes. For lidocaine (half-life 1.5 hr) the corresponding time would be 5.2 hours, so that a more rapid method of initially achieving a therapeutic blood concentration of drug is required (Fig. 15–9). A single intravenous bolus injection (loading dose) can produce a therapeutic concentration almost immediately, but this is maintained only briefly because of lidocaine's rapid and extensive tissue distribution (Fig. 15–10). A larger bolus would prolong the

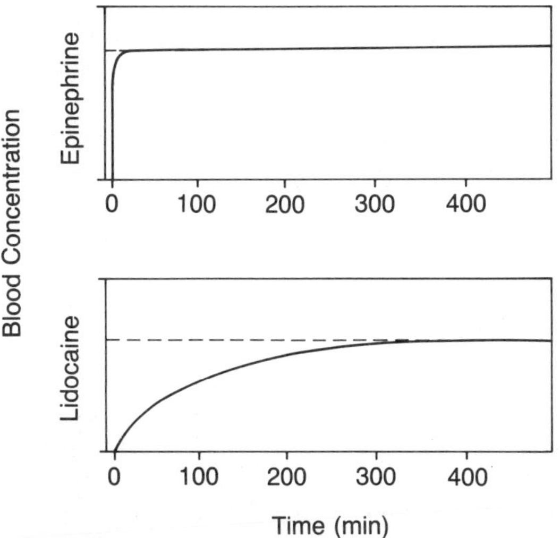

Figure 15–9. A constant-rate intravenous infusion of norepinephrine (half-life 2 min) achieves 90 per cent of the steady state plasma concentration in 3.5 half-lives, or 7 min. The corresponding interval after starting a lidocaine infusion (half-life 90 min) is almost 5.2 hr.

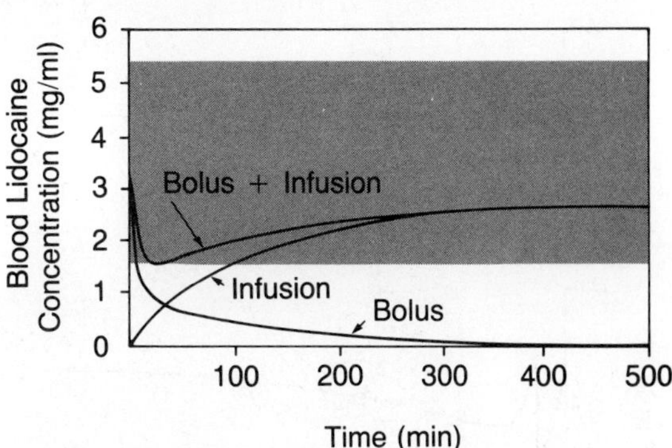

Figure 15–10. A single 100-mg bolus injection of lidocaine administered to a 70-kg person produces blood concentrations that rapidly fall below the therapeutic range (*shaded area*). The combination of a bolus and continuous intravenous infusion (2 mg/min) rapidly achieves and maintains a therapeutic concentration. (Adapted from Harrison, D. C.: Practical guidelines for the use of lidocaine. Prevention and treatment of cardiac arrhythmias. J.A.M.A. 233:1202, 1975.)

therapeutic effect somewhat, but the concentration would be in the toxic range initially. Combination of a bolus dose and a constant rate infusion is often sufficient to achieve and maintain an effective drug concentration.[47] Even with this method, however, some patients have a dip in blood concentration of drug to subtherapeutic levels 20 to 30 minutes after the initial bolus injection. Other loading regimens have been used to overcome this problem: two or three boluses plus infusion, rapid infusion followed by slow infusion, and bolus plus rapid and slow infusions (Fig. 15–11).[86, 105] All these methods offer advantages over the single bolus plus infusion, but they also require increasing amounts of attention and patient monitoring. The choice of an appropriate loading regimen is considered further in the discussions on individual drugs below.

After a desired steady state drug concentration has been achieved, it may become necessary to increase or decrease the blood concentration of drug because of inadequate or excessive drug effect. If this is accomplished by increasing or decreasing the drug infusion rate, the time required to reach 90 per cent of the new steady state concentration will again be about 3.5 half-lives (Fig. 15–12). For drugs with long half-lives, a small bolus dose (e.g., 25–50 mg lidocaine) can be used to approach a new higher steady state concentration more rapidly.[11] Similarly, achievement of a lower steady state concen-

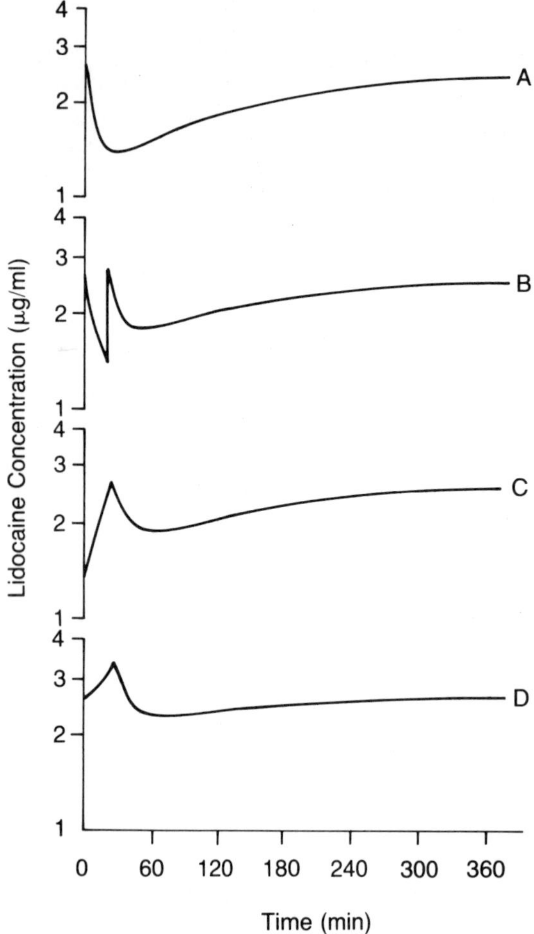

Figure 15–11. Computer simulation of four regimens of lidocaine administration in a 70-kg person. *A*, 100-mg bolus plus 2 mg/min infusion; *B*, 100-mg bolus plus 2 mg/min infusions supplemented by a 50-mg bolus at 20 min; *C*, two infusions, 8 mg/min for 25 min followed by 2 mg/min; and *D*, 100-mg bolus plus two infusions, 8 mg/min for 25 min followed by 2 mg/min. (From Salzer et al: A comparison of methods of lidocaine administration in patients. Clin. Pharmacol. Ther. 29:617, 1981. Reproduced with permission.)

tration can be hastened by discontinuing the drug infusion entirely until an appropriate plasma concentration is obtained, and then resuming the infusion at a slower rate. For example, if an infusion of lidocaine is stopped, assuming an elimination half-life of 100 minutes, the blood lidocaine concentration will fall by 25 per cent in 41 minutes, 50 per cent in 100 minutes, and 75 per cent in 200 minutes.

PHARMACOKINETIC CONSIDERATIONS FOR INDIVIDUAL DRUGS

Several drugs frequently used in the management of cardiac emergencies and representative of a wide variety of pharmacokinetic characteristics are discussed below. Each drug illustrates in some way how the pharmacokinetic principles referred to above may be applied to the selection of appropriate dosing regimens.

Lidocaine

Lidocaine is administered intramuscularly or intravenously for acute control of ventricular arrhythmias and for arrhythmia prophylaxis in patients with proved or suspected myocardial infarction.

The intramuscular route, as discussed previously, has been studied primarily in patients without circulatory failure. In such patients, 4 to 5 mg per kg body weight injected into the deltoid muscle produces therapeutic plasma lidocaine concentrations within five to ten minutes that are sustained for 60 to 90 minutes (Fig. 15–4).[6, 18, 93, 108] Since intramuscular injection does not allow titration of dose, the intravenous route is preferred, when possible, even in patients without circulatory failure.

Pharmacokinetics. The therapeutic plasma concentration range for lidocaine is 1.5 to 5.5 µg/ml.[11] Serious toxicity is uncommon at these concentrations. Intravenous administration of lidocaine (Fig. 15–10) is followed by a rapid decline in plasma concentration due to tissue distribution (half-life of 10 min) and a subsequent slower decline due primarily to lidocaine elimination (half-life of 100 min).[47] Lidocaine is metabolized by the liver to monoethylglycinexylidide (MEGX), which has antiarrhythmic activity and toxicity similar to that of lidocaine.[11] Although plasma concentrations of MEGX are usually quite low, some patients receiving lidocaine infusions, particularly those with circulatory failure, may achieve MEGX concentrations as high as the concurrent lidocaine concentration. A case has been described in which toxicity developed despite a therapeutic plasma concentration of lidocaine, probably owing to a high plasma concentration of MEGX.[46] MEGX is further metabolized to glycinexylidide, which is only 10 to 15 per cent as potent an antiarrhythmic agent. Lidocaine is highly extracted from blood by the liver, and the metabolic capacity of the liver for lidocaine is high. Lidocaine clearance has been shown to be proportional to hepatic blood flow as estimated by indocyanine green clearance (Fig. 15–7),[109] although a 1980 study demonstrating no correlation should be noted.[5]

Effects of Circulatory Failure. Since hepatic blood flow is rate limiting, lidocaine clearance would be expected to be independent of the intrinsic metabolic capacity of the liver. In the hemorrhaged monkey, however, and probably also in patients with severe cardiac disease, lidocaine clearance is decreased beyond that which can be accounted for by diminished blood flow to the liver.[8] Thus, hepatocellular dysfunction with reduced intrinsic metabolic capacity of the liver may contribute to decreased lidocaine clearance in patients with congestive heart failure. In support of this possibility, patients with myocardial infarction and congestive heart failure have been shown to have slowed clearance of antipyrine, a drug that is believed to be eliminated independently of hepatic blood flow.[77]

A second important effect of circulatory failure on lidocaine kinetics is reduction of the rate of drug distribution to tissues. In patients with circulatory failure, the initial plasma concentration of lidocaine produced by a bolus dose is increased by 50 to 100 per cent, and it is frequently recommended that the initial bolus dose of lidocaine be reduced by half in the presence of circulatory failure.[11]

Plasma lidocaine concentration has been shown to increase progressively during constant infusion of the drug for more than 24 hours in patients with myocardial infarction. At the same time there is an increase in the plasma concentration of α_1-acid glycoprotein (AGP), an acute-phase reactant to myocardial necrosis, and a protein to which lidocaine binds.[84] The close correlation of plasma lidocaine and AGP concentrations suggests that the increased plasma concentration of lidocaine could be due to increased protein binding. However, the plasma clearance and steady state concentration of a highly extracted drug such as lidocaine would not be expected to change with alterations in protein binding,[85] and the role of AGP in lidocaine cumulation is speculative. The plasma concentration of lidocaine has also been shown to increase during prolonged infusion in normal subjects (in whom AGP concentration remains constant), perhaps because of decreased hepatic extraction.[4] To avoid toxicity, the rate of lidocaine infusion may therefore need to be reduced with prolonged infusions in patients with and without myocardial infarction. Specific guidelines regarding the magnitude of reduction required are not currently available.

Dosing. Since most studies have not shown a close correlation between body weight and lidocaine concentrations, some investigators adjust lidocaine dose for body weight and others do not. Loading regimens have been discussed and illustrated previously (Fig. 15–11). A single bolus dose of 100 mg with

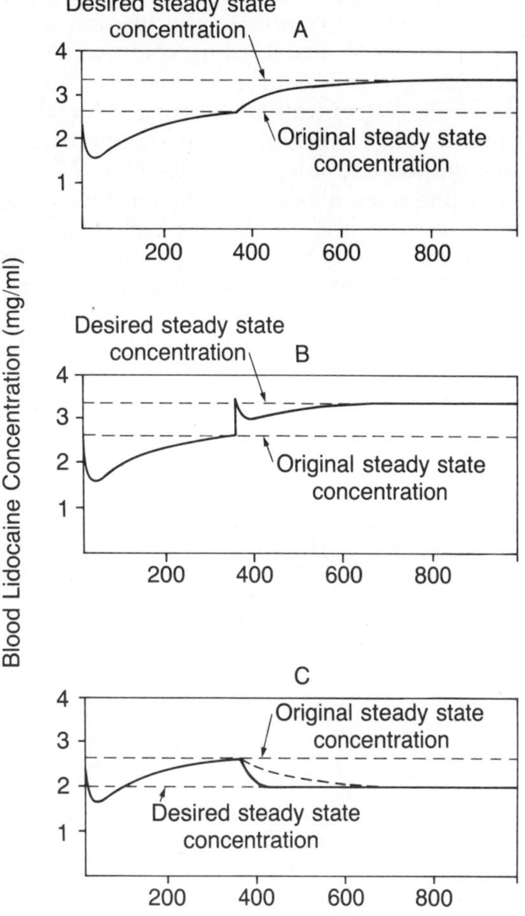

Figure 15–12. Methods of changing the steady state concentration of lidocaine in a 70-kg person. An initial 100-mg bolus followed by an infusion of 2 mg/min has been administered to achieve the original steady state concentration. *A,* The lidocaine infusion rate is increased to 2.5 mg/min. The new steady state concentration is achieved slowly, requiring 350 min (3.5 half-lives of lidocaine). *B,* The new steady state can be achieved more rapidly by administering a small (25-mg) bolus dose of lidocaine along with the higher infusion rate. *C,* When a lower blood lidocaine concentration is desired, this can be achieved most rapidly by discontinuing the infusion until the lower concentration is reached and then resuming the infusion at a lower rate (*solid line*) rather than immediately starting the slower infusion (*dashed line*). (Adapted from Winkle et al.: Pharmacologic therapy of ventricular arrhythmias. 36:629, 1975.)

normal circulatory function or 50 mg in the presence of circulatory failure, followed by a constant infusion of 2 mg/min without or 1 mg/min with circulatory failure, is often adequate for treating ventricular arrhythmias. Additional bolus doses of 25 to 50 mg can be given if arrhythmias reappear during the expected dip in the plasma lidocaine concentration.[11]

When lidocaine is administered for arrhythmia prophylaxis, there is no clinical end point to allow titration of the loading dose, and a multiple dose-loading regimen would provide greater assurance that the plasma lidocaine concentration remains in the therapeutic range. Multiple bolus regimens have in common administration of 200 to 225 mg lidocaine over about 20 minutes. One regimen uses an initial bolus dose (1-min infusion) of 75 mg intravenously followed by three 50-mg bolus doses at five-minute intervals.[105] The mean plasma lidocaine concentrations measured in 23 patients receiving this regimen (Fig. 15–13) were within the therapeutic range at all times except at five minutes after the initial dose, and serious toxicity did not develop in any patient. In patients with arrhythmias, the loading regimen can be stopped after one, two, or three doses if the arrhythmia is suppressed. A maintenance infusion is then initiated. This dosing schedule has the advantage of being simple enough for prehospital use. In agreement with other studies, plasma lidocaine concentration one minute after the first bolus dose of the regimen was twice as high in patients with classes II or III cardiac failure as in patients without failure. This difference became smaller with successive doses, however, and all patients achieved therapeutic plasma concentrations of lidocaine regardless of the presence or absence of moderate cardiac failure. It did not appear to be necessary to adjust the dose for a moderate degree of circulatory failure with this loading regimen. For patients with severe failure or cardiogenic shock, one half the loading dose should be used until more data regarding dosing requirements for this group are available.[11]

To maintain a therapeutic plasma concentration, a loading dose of lidocaine must be followed by an infusion. The desired infusion rate in patients with arrhythmias is often determined by titration. When lidocaine is administered for arrhythmia prophylaxis, titration is impossible and the selection of an appropriate infusion rate is more difficult. In one study demonstrating the efficacy of prophylactic lidocaine, patients with myocardial infarction and no circulatory failure received a 100-mg loading dose followed by a 3-mg-

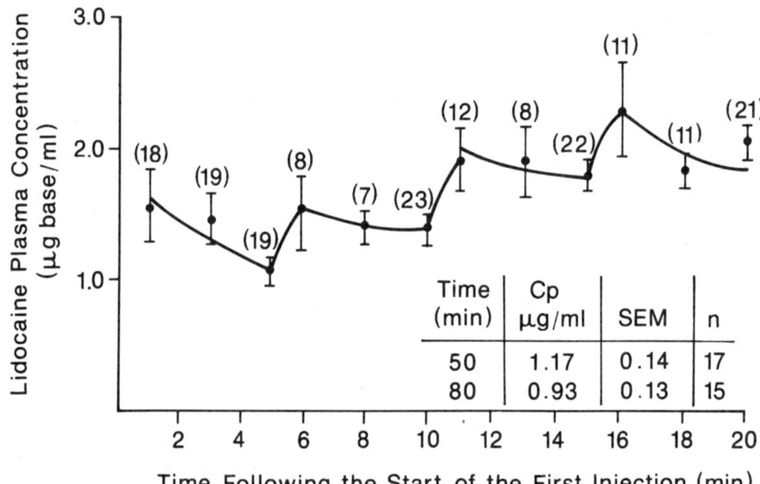

Time (min)	Cp µg/ml	SEM	n
50	1.17	0.14	17
80	0.93	0.13	15

Figure 15–13. Plasma lidocaine concentrations after administration of 75 mg lidocaine (t = 0) followed by 50 mg at 5, 10, and 15 min. Figures in parentheses are numbers of plasma determinations at the times indicated. Data include patients both with and without congestive heart failure. The mean plasma lidocaine concentrations are, with the single exception of 5 min, all within the therapeutic range (defined in this study as 1.2–6.0 µ/ml). (From Wyman et al.: Multiple bolus technique for lidocaine administration during the first hours of acute myocardial infarction. Am. J. Cardiol. 41:313, 1978. Reproduced with permission.)

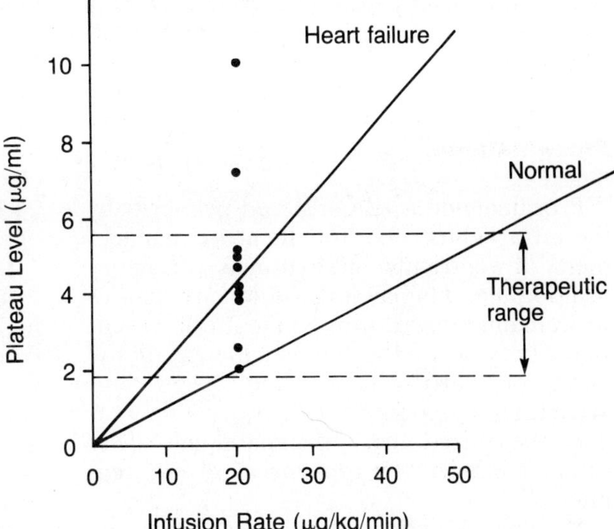

Figure 15–14. Relation between the steady state plasma concentration of lidocaine and the rate of lidocaine infusion for persons with normal cardiac output and those with heart failure. The solid lines represent mean data; the solid dots are the predicted plateau concentrations for the heart failure patients, calculated from their individual lidocaine clearance values. (From Thomson et al.: Lidocaine pharmacokinetics in advanced heart failure, liver disease, and renal failure in humans. Ann. Intern. Med. 78:499, 1973. Reproduced with permission.)

per-min infusion.[101] The mean plasma lidocaine concentration was 3.5 μg/ml (range 1.5–6.4 μg/ml). Other studies using lower infusion rates have failed to demonstrate a beneficial effect of lidocaine in preventing ventricular arrhythmias.[74] Comparable data are not available regarding effective doses in patients with circulatory failure.

Assuming that comparable plasma lidocaine concentrations also provide arrhythmia prophylaxis in patients with circulatory failure, a method of relating lidocaine infusion rate to the plasma concentration produced would be useful. Figure 15–14 shows an attempt to relate the steady state plasma lidocaine concentration to the infusion rate in patients with congestive heart failure.[100] There is considerable variability in this relationship because of marked individual variability in lidocaine clearance even in normal persons,[11] and possibly also because of variation in the severity of circulatory failure. These considerations limit the accuracy of any attempt to predict plasma concentrations of lidocaine during an infusion. One approach is to use average values for lidocaine clearance of 700 ml/min with normal circulation and 440 ml/min with circulatory failure to estimate the steady state plasma concentration of lidocaine:

$$\text{concentration } (\mu\text{g/ml}) = \frac{\text{infusion rate } (\mu\text{g/min})}{\text{clearance } (\text{ml/min})}$$

A nomogram has also been proposed that takes into account the severity of circulatory failure (Fig. 15–15).[100] This nomogram has

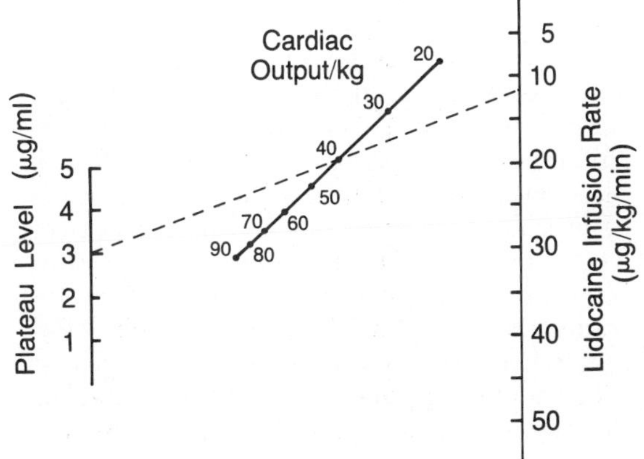

Figure 15–15. Nomogram for determining the infusion rate of lidocaine necessary to attain the desired steady state plasma concentration when cardiac output per kg body weight is known. This nomogram is based on patients' data but has not been tested in a clinical setting. (From Thomson et al.: Lidocaine pharmacokinetics in advanced heart failure, liver disease, and renal failure in humans. Ann. Intern. Med. 78:499, 1973. Reproduced with permission.)

not been explicitly tested but may provide a useful first approximation when cardiac output is known.

Procainamide

Procainamide is administered primarily by the intravenous route for the acute management of ventricular arrhythmias refractory to lidocaine. The clinical use of intravenous procainamide was unpopular until recent years because of the high incidence of hypotension, cardiac conduction delays, and arrhythmias associated with this route. It is now recognized that procainamide toxicity can be minimized by appropriate dosing regimens.

Pharmacokinetics. The commonly accepted therapeutic plasma concentration range for procainamide is 4 to 10 μg/ml.[13] However, one study showed that plasma procainamide concentrations as high as 33 μg/ml may be required to suppress recurrent ventricular tachycardia in some patients, and are usually tolerated well.[45] The loading dose of procainamide in this study was administered during close hemodynamic monitoring (usually during cardiac catheterization) on an elective basis. Whether such high plasma concentrations of procainamide are also safe in acutely ill patients, and whether these high concentrations are useful for suppressing arrhythmias other than recurrent ventricular tachycardia, is not certain.

Distribution of procainamide to tissues is extensive and rapid. Its elimination half-life averages three hours, and a loading dose is required when initiating therapy in patients with life-threatening arrhythmias.[57] Elimination of procainamide is approximately 50 per cent by renal excretion and 50 per cent by hepatic metabolism. The plasma half-life of procainamide is prolonged to eight hours in patients with end-stage renal failure. Procainamide is metabolized in part to *N*-acetyl procainamide (NAPA), which also has antiarrhythmic activity. Accumulation of NAPA in plasma is negligible during the first few hours of procainamide infusion, but increases over 24 to 48 hours. In patients who are slow acetylators of procainamide, plasma concentrations of NAPA at 24 hours are well below antiarrhythmic levels. Rapid acetylators achieve plasma concentrations that may be therapeutic within 24 hours, but these patients also have lower plasma concentrations of procainamide.[63] The contribution of NAPA to the therapeutic effect of a given dose of procainamide is therefore varied and difficult to quantitate.[13] There are no data, to our knowledge, demonstrating that a change in procainamide dose during the first 24 hours of therapy is required on the basis of a patient's acetylator status.

Dosing and Effects of Circulatory Failure. Procainamide toxicity is usually related to high plasma concentrations and often results from excessively rapid drug administration. For example, the intravenous infusion of 1 gm of procainamide at a rate of 100 mg/min is associated with initial plasma concentrations well above the therapeutic range, and infusions exceeding this rate have produced vascular collapse.[57] In contrast, infusion of the same dose of procainamide at a rate of 20 mg/min results in therapeutic plasma concentrations and does not produce significant hypotension.[38] Toxic plasma concentrations of procainamide may also result from administration of an excessive total dose. It is difficult to predict the loading dose a patient will require because of individual variability in both effective and toxic concentrations.[57] The risk of procainamide administration can therefore be minimized by giving the loading dose incrementally until antiarrhythmic effect or toxicity is noted.

Several loading regimens have been reported that appear both safe and effective. Giardina et al.[38] administered 100 mg of procainamide intravenously over one minute to patients with arrhythmias of various etiologies, and repeated this dose every five minutes until the arrhythmia was suppressed, toxicity supervened, or 1 gm had been given. The arrhythmia was suppressed or abolished in 19 of 20 patients, and the resulting plasma concentrations of procainamide correlated with the doses administered (Fig. 15–16).

Although a higher initial concentration would be expected in patients with circulatory failure because of slowed distribution of procainamide to tissues, no effect of circulatory failure on the relationship between dose and plasma concentration was observed. This somewhat surprising result could be due to the five-minute interval between doses, which may have been long enough to allow extensive tissue distribution even in the patients with circulatory failure. A similar loading regimen consisting of a constant intravenous

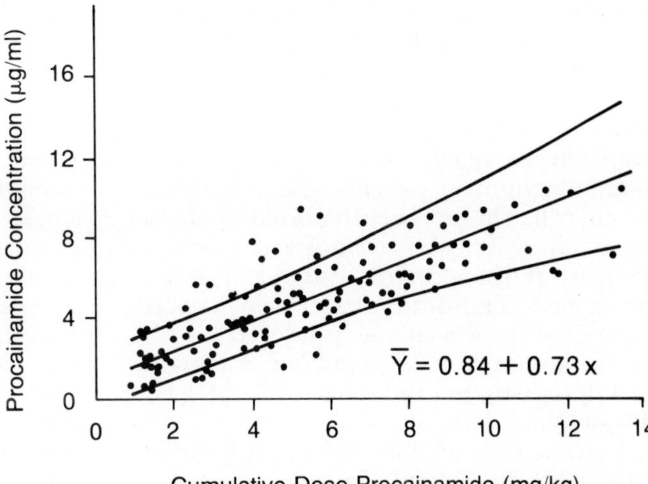

Figure 15–16. Plasma procainamide concentration (Y: µg/ml) is plotted as a function of cumulative dose (mg/kg body weight) for 20 patients who received 100 mg procainamide intravenously every 5 min. Plasma samples for study of drug concentration were obtained 4½ min after each dose. The black dots represent individual values in these patients. There is a gradual linear increase in plasma level as the cumulative dose increases for each patient. The middle line drawn through the points is the average regression line calculated from each individual's data. The two black lines above and below the overall regression line represent the 68 per cent confidence interval. (From Giardina et al.: Intermittent intravenous procaine amide to treat ventricular arrhythmias. Correlation of plasma concentration with effect on arrhythmia, electrocardiogram, and blood pressure. Ann. Intern. Med. 78:183, 1973. Reproduced with permission.)

infusion of 17 mg/kg body weight administered over one hour has also been used,[64] and the choice between a constant infusion and intermittent one-minute infusions appears to be one of convenience.

A maintenance infusion of procainamide is required after a loading dose because of the drug's relatively rapid elimination. Procainamide clearance is proportional to body weight in patients with normal renal and hepatic function,[104] and this relationship can be used to estimate the infusion rate needed to maintain a given plasma concentration of procainamide (Table 15–2). Thus, one can estimate a patient's plasma concentration of procainamide after a loading dose and then calculate the approximate infusion rate required to maintain this concentration, using Table 15–2. This infusion rate should be reduced in patients with renal insufficiency; one half the calculated infusion rate has been used for patients with a serum creatinine concentration of ≥ 1.5 mg/dl.[64] It should be cautioned that this method of determining the required procainamide infusion rate has not been tested and that the clinical advan-

Table 15–2. AN APPROACH TO PROCAINAMIDE DOSING, USING PATIENT RESPONSE TO A PROCAINAMIDE LOADING DOSE TO PREDICT THE REQUIRED MAINTENANCE INFUSION RATE

The estimated plasma procainamide concentration produced by a loading dose administered according to the method of Giardina et al.[38] (see text) was calculated using data from Figure 15–16. The infusion rate required to maintain this concentration was then calculated using the relationship:

$$\text{Infusion rate (mg/min)} = \text{Total body clearance (ml/min)} \times \text{Desired Plasma Concentration (mg/ml)}.$$

Total body clearance was calculated as (6.27 × body weight) − 40 (from Wyman et al.[104]). Because of individual variability in pharmacokinetic parameters and clinical response, these values should be viewed as first approximations only.

	Procainamide Infusion Rate (mg/min) Required to Maintain a Steady State Plasma Concentration of		
Body Weight (kg)	*4 µg/ml**	*6 µg/ml**	*8 µg/ml**
50	1.1	1.6	2.2
60	1.3	2.0	2.7
70	1.6	2.4	3.2
80	1.8	2.8	3.7
90	2.1	3.1	4.2
100	2.4	3.5	4.7

*Plasma procainamide concentrations of 4, 6, and 8 µg/ml correspond to loading doses of 4.3, 7.1, and 9.8 mg/kg, respectively.

tage of individualizing the steady state plasma concentration of procainamide rather than a fixed-dose regimen, although likely, has not been established. The use of fixed infusion rates of 2.8 mg/kg body weight/hr in patients with normal renal function, and 1.4 mg/kg body weight/hr in patients with renal insufficiency, has in fact been reported to abolish ventricular arrhythmias in 74 per cent of patients resistant to conventional doses of lidocaine.[64] The steady state plasma concentration of procainamide produced by this regimen was 6.9 ± 3.7 μg/ml (mean ± standard deviation), but the range was wide (1.7–17 μg/ml.).

Congestive heart failure did not influence procainamide clearance in the study used to generate Table 15–2, but higher steady state plasma concentrations of procainamide in patients with severe (classes III and IV) failure have been noted by others.[64] A 50 per cent reduction in maintenance infusion rate has been suggested for such patients.

Verapamil

Verapamil is an antiarrhythmic agent that blocks the slow inward calcium current. Because of its ability to slow atrioventricular conduction, verapamil is useful in the conversion of paroxysmal supraventricular tachycardia to sinus rhythm and in the slowing of ventricular rates associated with atrial fibrillation or flutter.[98] Verapamil can also decrease cardiac contractility, and it is contraindicated in patients with severe circulatory failure unless the failure is due to the arrhythmia for which verapamil is intended.[92] Most patients receiving verapamil have either normal baseline myocardial function or at most mild-to-moderate cardiac failure. Although the kinetics of verapamil has been studied in both normal and cardiac failure groups, direct comparison of studies is difficult because of differences in verapamil dose or rate of administration.

Pharmacokinetics. In both normal subjects and patients with congestive heart failure, there is an initial rapid decline in serum concentration of verapamil after an intravenous bolus dose.[55, 88] Peak effect, judged by slowing of ventricular rate, is achieved in one to 15 minutes, suggesting that verapamil distributes to myocardium rapidly.[43] Elimination is primarily by hepatic metabolism, and verapamil is highly extracted from blood by the liver.[28] The elimination half-life averages four to six hours, but is variable (range 2.8–15 hr) and increases with long-term administration.[55, 88] The active metabolite norverapamil accumulates with oral verapamil administration but is not detectable after a single intravenous dose.[55] The contribution of norverapamil to the antiarrhythmic activity of oral verapamil is uncertain.

Dosing and Effects of Circulatory Failure. Duration of effect from a single intravenous dose is variable but may be up to three hours.[3] In dogs the steady state serum concentration of verapamil correlates well with clinical effect (prolongation of the A-H interval),[65] but the correlation in humans following a single intravenous dose is less precise. In a study of patients with atrial fibrillation or flutter who received 0.075 to 0.225 mg of verapamil per kg of body weight intravenously, plasma concentration of drug did not correlate with the maximal decrease in ventricular rate.[26] The best predictor of response proved to be the presence or absence of circulatory failure: in all patients without failure, heart rate decreased to less than 100 beats per minute after a single dose of 0.075 mg/kg/body weight, whereas patients with circulatory failure required an additional dose of 0.15 mg/kg body weight and still had mean heart rates greater than those of patients without failure. The reason for this decreased response to verapamil in patients with circulatory failure is not clear, but it may be due to an antagonism of verapamil effect by increased sympathetic nervous system tone. The effects of circulatory failure on serum concentration of verapamil were not directly addressed in this study, but the myocardial concentration of verapamil would be expected, if anything, to be higher with circulatory failure because of slowed distribution to other tissues. Thus, the effects of cardiac failure on verapamil kinetics may be of less importance than other physiologic consequences of circulatory failure in determining cardiac response to verapamil.

Although the correlation of serum concentration of verapamil to clinical effect in a population of patients is poor, increases in serum concentration of drug in individual patients are associated with increased effect. A satisfactory clinical response to verapamil (slowing of ventricular rate or conversion to sinus rhythm) is often achieved with an intravenous dose of 0.075 mg/kg body weight, although the percentage of patients responding increases when a second dose of 0.15 mg/kg body weight is administered.[3] It is commonly recommended, therefore, that the lower dose be used initially for patients with circulatory failure to minimize the chance of further impairing cardiac function. It is advisable to wait at least 15 minutes before administering a second dose to ensure that the maximal effect of the first dose has been achieved. Patients without cardiac failure tolerate 0.15 mg/kg body weight well, obviating the need to start with the lower dose.[28, 88] A maximal total dose of 0.15 mg/kg body weight has been suggested because this is the largest dose used in most clinical studies. Infusion of verapamil over one minute is well tolerated. Faster infusion rates, at least in the dog, may cause high-degree AV block.[68] Maintenance therapy is usually accomplished with the oral form of verapamil, 80 to 120 mg every eight hours.[43] Considering the drug's relatively long half-life of four to six hours, periodic intravenous infusions should also suffice for maintenance therapy.

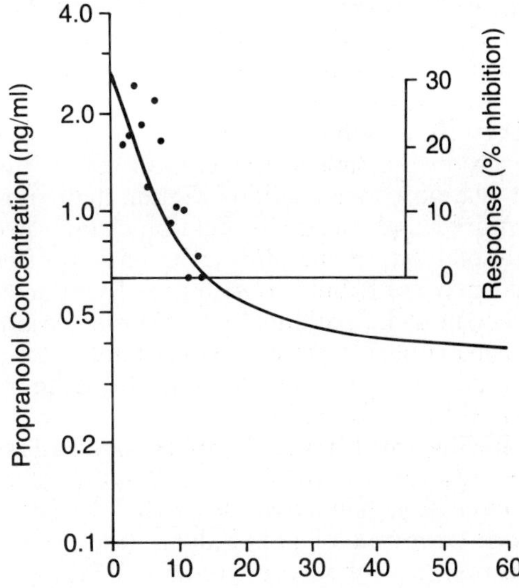

Figure 15–17. Percentage inhibition of isoproterenol-induced tachycardia (●) produced by 0.1 mg intravenous propranolol in normal persons, in relation to the plasma propranolol concentration (——). Percentage inhibition is maximal within 4 min and thereafter correlates well with propranolol concentration, implying rapid distribution of propranolol to the heart. (From McDevitt, D. G., and Shand, D. G.: Plasma concentrations and the time-course of beta blockade due to propranolol. Clin. Pharmacol. Ther. 18:708, 1975. Reproduced with permission.)

Propranolol

Intravenous propranolol is used in the acute management of supraventricular tachycardia, atrial fibrillation, ventricular tachycardia, and ventricular fibrillation, particularly when these rhythms occur in the setting of excessive sympathetic nervous stimulation. Since patients with circulatory failure are often dependent on stimulation of the sympathetic nervous system to maintain cardiac output, propranolol is generally reserved for persons with normal or only mildly impaired cardiac function. Most kinetic studies of propranolol have been performed on normal subjects.

Pharmacokinetics. The plasma concentration of propranolol falls rapidly after an intravenous bolus dose owing to distribution to tissues, and thereafter declines as a result of hepatic metabolism with a half-life of two to three hours (Fig. 15–17).[42, 89] Like lidocaine, propranolol is highly extracted from blood by the liver. Maximal beta-blockade resulting from intravenous propranolol measured by inhibition of exercise-induced tachycardia occurs at a plasma concentration of 100 ng/ml (comparable beta-blockade is seen at lower concentrations after oral dosing owing to the presence of a pharmacologically active metabolite, 4-hydroxy-propranolol). The intravenous dose required to achieve this plasma concentration in normal subjects is 0.15 to 0.3 mg/kg body weight infused over two minutes.[20] Peak effect occurs within four minutes of an intravenous dose, implying rapid distribution of drug to the myocardium.[69] Plasma propranolol concentration correlates well with its cardiac effects in the experimental setting (Fig. 15–17). However, in clinical use the response to a given dose, or plasma concentration, is considerably more variable for several reasons: (1) Propranolol is a competitive beta-antagonist, and the dose required to produce a given effect depends on the magnitude of the agonist stimulus. In humans, for example, increasing doses of propranolol are needed to antagonize tachycardia produced by increasing doses of the beta-agonist isoproterenol.[20] (2) Patients with normal circulatory function tolerate high plasma concentrations of propranolol well, and doses much larger than those needed to produce maximal beta-blockade can be administered to prolong the duration of therapeutic effect.[69] (3) It is not always necessary to achieve complete beta-blockade to produce a satisfactory clinical result.[76] (4) At plasma concentrations higher than those required for maximal beta-blockade, propranolol has a membrane-stabilizing effect that may contribute to its antiarrhythmic efficacy in some patients.[103] For these reasons, plasma concentrations of propranolol are of limited value in determining the dose required by an individual patient.

Dosing and Effects of Circulatory Failure. We are aware of no data regarding the effects of circulatory failure on propranolol kinetics. Since propranolol generally is not used in the presence of severe circulatory failure, it is probable that any such changes would be less important than the other determinants of clinical effect discussed above.

In view of the risk of precipitating circulatory failure in patients with underlying cardiac disease, intravenous propranolol is usually administered by titrating small-dose increments against clinical response and toxicity. Although rapid infusion rates are well tolerated in normal subjects, and even in patients with acute myocardial infarction without circulatory failure,[53] a rate of 1 mg infused over one to five minutes is more commonly recommended for acutely compromised patients. Doses should be no more frequent than every five minutes to allow development of maximal effect before the next dose is administered. A maximal total dose of 3 to 5 mg has been recommended.[71] Although this relatively low dose should minimize toxicity and be adequate for many patients, it may provide insufficient beta-blockade in others. Doses as high as 7.5 to 15 mg administered to patients with acute myocardial infarction and no overt circulatory failure have resulted in a low incidence of serious toxicity.[53] It is reasonable, then, to exceed a total dose of 5 mg, when necessary, in a patient without circulatory failure if the rate of administration is slow and the patient is observed for toxicity. Propranolol administration after an intravenous bolus dose is most often continued using oral dosing or intermittent intravenous bolus injections. A single oral dose of 40 to 120 mg propranolol provides about the same maximal inhibition of exercise-induced tachycardia as 0.3 mg/kg intravenous propranolol infused over two minutes in normal subjects.[20]

Maintenance therapy may also be provided by continuous intravenous infusion of propranolol with the infusion rate calculated using the equation on page 303. Assuming a clearance of 12 ml/min/kg,[58] a steady state plasma propranolol concentration of 100 ng/ml would be expected from an infusion rate of 1.2 μg/min/kg (5.0 mg/hr for a 70-kg person). Somewhat slower infusions were used in one study of postoperative patients, with a mean rate of 3 mg/hr irrespective of body weight that resulted in a mean plasma concentration of 80 ng/ml.[95] It is possible that this low maintenance requirement was due to impaired propranolol clearance in these patients, but it is not clear whether true steady state concentrations were achieved. Because of the large individual variability in propranolol clearance, careful monitoring of clinical end points is advisable when using a propranolol infusion.

Bretylium

Bretylium is useful in the management of recurrent or refractory ventricular tachycardia and fibrillation.

Pharmacokinetics. Bretyium is concentrated in adrenergic neurons and is extensively bound to tissues, including the heart.[56, 73] Its distribution is slow, and peak myocardial bretylium concentrations in the dog are delayed three to six hours after an intravenous dose (Fig. 15–18). Maximal antifibrillatory activity in the dog is also delayed three to six hours and correlates with the myocardial concentration rather than the serum concentration.[1] In humans, maximal suppression of premature ventricular depolarizations has been reported to occur eight hours after intramuscular administration of bretylium, even though the peak serum concentration occurs within one hour.[83] When bretylium is administered as an intravenous bolus injection to treat ventricular tachycardia or fibrillation, however, onset of action is usually within 20 minutes and may be as soon as one to two minutes.[24, 99] The reason for this apparent discrepancy is not clear, but it is possible that, in the doses used to treat ventricular tachycardia and fibrillation, bretylium concentrations in the heart rapidly rise to therapeutic levels even though peak

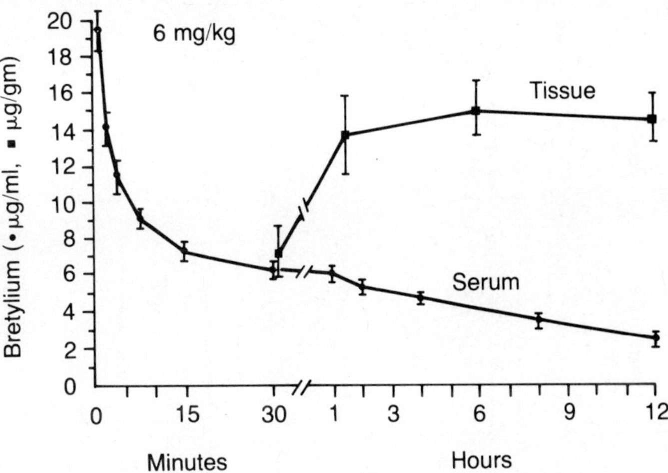

Figure 15–18. Concentration of bretylium in serum and myocardium after intravenous injection of 6 mg/kg over 60 sec to anesthetized, open-chest dogs. The tissue/serum bretylium ratio increases up to 12 hr, after which (*data not shown*) the concentrations in tissue and serum fall in parallel. (From Anderson et al.: Kinetics of antifibrillatory effects of bretylium: correlation with myocardial drug concentrations. Am. J. Cardiol. 46:583, 1980. Reproduced with permission.)

concentrations occur much later. Hypotension, the most common side effect of bretylium, usually appears within one hour;[83] it is possible that distribution of bretylium to sympathetic neurons is more rapid than distribution to the heart. It is not clear whether hypotension is more severe with bolus dosing than with slower administration. Bretylium is eliminated by renal excretion, with reported half-lives of 7.8 to 13.6 hours.[2, 73]

Dosing and Effects of Circulatory Failure. Serum bretylium concentration does not correlate with therapeutic effect, and dosing regimens have been developed using clinical end points such as arrhythmia termination. Since these end points are frequently difficult to assess in acutely ill patients who may be receiving multiple simultaneous therapies, current dosing recommendations for bretylium are not precise. For the treatment of ventricular fibrillation or life-threatening ventricular tachycardia, bretylium is usually administered as an intravenous bolus of 5 mg/kg/body weight. If this is not effective after five to ten minutes, additional boluses may be given and repeated to a maximal dose of 30 mg/kg body weight.[17, 56] Slower administration is recommended in conscious patients, to minimize nausea and vomiting.

Owing to bretylium's relatively long half-life and slow distribution to the myocardium, maintenance doses may be given every six to eight hours as a 10- to 20-minute intravenous infusion or intramuscular injection. A maintenance dose of 5 mg/kg body weight administered according to this schedule has been reported to be effective and well tolerated for up to one week.[24] Constant intravenous infusion of 1 to 2 mg/min has also been used for maintenance therapy, with the rate adjusted as necessary to achieve the desired clinical effect;[56] however, with a very long half-life and slow equilibration with myocardium, this approach does not seem necessary. Data are not available regarding the effects of circulatory failure on bretylium kinetics.

Catecholamines

Unlike the antiarrhythmic drugs (Table 15–3), catecholamines are rapidly removed

Table 15–3. REPRESENTATIVE PHARMACOKINETIC PARAMETERS FOR ANTIARRHYTHMIC DRUGS IN HEALTHY SUBJECTS

Drug	Distribution Half-Life (hr)	Elimination Half-Life (hr)	Volume of Distribution (l/kg)	Clearance ml/min/kg
Lidocaine[11]	0.08 – 0.17	1.3 to 1.8	0.7 to 2.2	6 to 14
Procainamide[36]	0.09 ± 0.02	2.9 ± 1.1	2.6 ± 1.0	11.8 ± 6.1
Verapamil[28, 55]	0.3 ± 0.58	3.7 – 6.3	3.5 ± 1.2	19.7 ± 3.2
Propranolol[42, 58]	0.09	3.8 ± 1.1	4.8 ± 0.9	12.9 ± 1.0
Bretylium[2, 73]	0.42 ± 0.15	7.8 to 13.6	3.4 to 5.9	4.3 to 12.1
Digoxin[59]	0.35 ± 0.06	43.2 ± 7.1	8.1 ± 2.0	2.7 ± 0.8

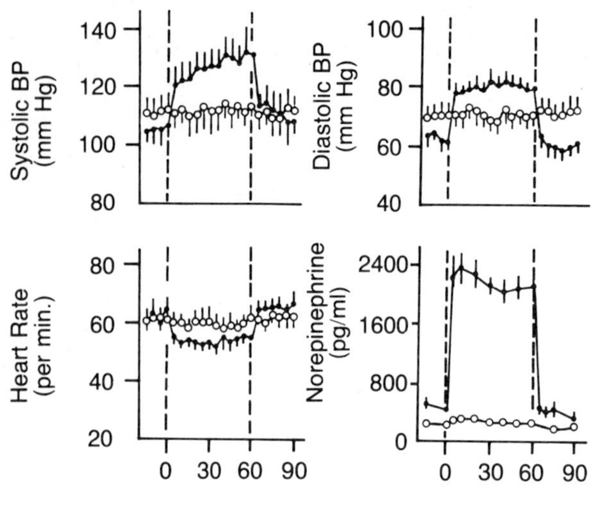

Figure 15–19. Mean (± SE) systolic blood pressures, diastolic blood pressures, heart rates, and plasma norepinephrine concentrations in five normal men during intravenous infusion of norepinephrine in doses of 5.0 (●) and 0.1 μg/min (○). (From Cryer, P.E.: Am. J. Physiol. 234:E252, 1978. Reproduced with permission.)

from the circulation by neuronal uptake or metabolism. All have short half-lives of only several minutes and can therefore be administered by intravenous infusion without requiring a loading dose.

Norepinephrine. Endogenous norepinephrine functions locally as a neurotransmitter in the brain and peripheral nervous system. Norepinephrine found in plasma is primarily due to spillover or leakage from neuronal synaptic clefts. In the usual circulating plasma concentrations (150–250 pg/ml at rest), norepinephrine is not pharmacologically active. When infused in normal subjects, a plasma concentration of greater than 1800 pg/ml is required to produce hemodynamic and metabolic effects (Fig. 15–19). This concentration is produced on the average by an infusion rate of 5 μg/min in normal subjects.[91]

After an intravenous bolus dose, the plasma concentration of norepinephrine initially declines rapidly, with a half-life of two minutes followed by a slower decline with a longer half-life (Fig. 15–20).[30, 33] The time course of accumulation of norepinephrine in plasma is determined by the kinetics of the initial rapid decline in plasma concentration because most of an administered dose of norepinephrine leaves the circulation during this time. In view of this short half-life, steady state plasma concentrations of norepinephrine are reached rapidly and a loading dose is not required (Fig. 15–19).[91] Neuronal reuptake is a major route of removal of norepinephrine from the circulation, and conditions that inhibit neuronal reuptake are associated with slowed elimination. For example, a 50 per cent increase in half-life is seen in patients taking therapeutic doses of

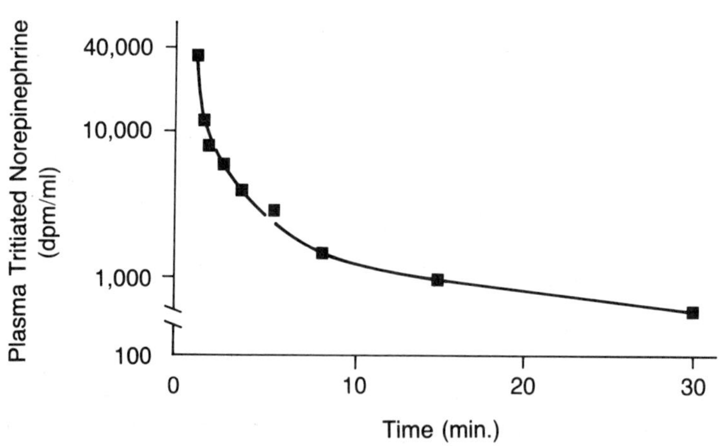

Figure 15–20. Plasma ^{3}H-norepinephrine concentration in normal persons after an intravenous bolus injection, demonstrating an initial half-life of 2 min. (Adapted from Esler et al.: Effect of norepinephrine uptake blockers on norepinephrine kinetics. Clin. Pharmacol. Ther. 29:12, 1981.)

the tricyclic antidepressant desipramine, an inhibitor of neuronal reuptake.[30] This could increase the resulting steady state plasma concentration of norepinephrine. Norepinephrine kinetics during cardiac emergencies or in patients with circulatory failure has not been well studied. An initial infusion rate of 4 to 8 μg/min is usually recommended, with the dose subsequently increased as needed.

Epinephrine. Epinephrine is commonly used during CPR for the treatment of nonperfusing rhythms such as fine ventricular fibrillation, asystole, or slow idioventricular rhythm. Its use in these situations as an intravenous bolus or an intratracheal or intracardiac injection is discussed earlier in the chapter. The plasma epinephrine half-life is about two minutes and steady state is approached rapidly.[32] Hemodynamic and metabolic effects of epinephrine are seen in normal subjects with intravenous infusion rates of greater than 1 μg/min (that produce a plasma concentration of epinephrine of 100–150 pg/ml).[16, 37]

Doses of epinephrine recommended to treat nonperfusing rhythms are greatly in excess of those needed to produce hemodynamic effects in normal subjects. Intravenous infusion of 10 ml of 1:10,000 epinephrine (1 mg) over one minute would be expected to produce a peak plasma concentration of epinephrine approximately 100 times greater than the steady state concentration from a 5 μg/min infusion. Although such high epinephrine doses may be indicated for nonperfusing rhythms, it is likely that lower doses would be effective and less toxic in other circumstances. In the treatment of hypotension due to anaphylaxis, for example, an intravenous infusion starting at 5.0 μg/min could be increased incrementally, allowing titration of the dosing rate according to the patient's clinical status.

For patients in whom intravenous access is not immediately available, as is the case in many patients with anaphylaxis, an initial subcutaneous dose of 0.3 mg can be administered. Although the absorption of drug from subcutaneous sites is unreliable in hypotensive patients, subcutaneous epinephrine has proved effective in anaphylaxis when administered early, and it is clearly preferable to an interval in which the patient receives no drug at all.

Dopamine. Dopamine is a catecholamine with complex, dose-dependent cardiovascular effects. Few data are available regarding plasma concentrations of dopamine, and dosing regimens are based on infusion rates and clinical end points. At low infusion rates (1–5 μg/kg body weight/min), dopamine increases cardiac contractility because of its beta-adrenergic agonist activity, and increases renal and mesenteric blood flow because of its dopaminergic-vasodilator activity. At higher infusion rates (5–10 μg/kg body weight/min), alpha-adrenergic agonist activity also becomes apparent, resulting in an increase in systemic vascular resistance.[41] There is considerable variation in response to dopamine. One study of patients with congestive heart failure reported that infusion rates of dopamine of 2 to 16 μg/kg body weight/min were required to increase mean arterial pressure 15 mm Hg.[51] The maximal infusion rate is often limited by the development of tachycardia and arrhythmias due to excessive beta-stimulation or by increased systemic vascular resistance as evidenced by decreasing cardiac output.[61, 72] In cardiogenic shock, for example, continued improvement in mean arterial pressure and cardiac index has been reported with infusion rates up to a mean of 17 μg/kg body weight/min, but at this level hemodynamic improvement was accompanied by deterioration in myocardial metabolism, with increased myocardial lactate production and oxygen consumption.[72] The optimal dopamine infusion rate for cardiogenic shock is probably ≤ 10 μg/kg body weight/min, although infusion rates of up to 53 μg/kg body weight/min have been reported to be of benefit in some patients with circulatory failure after surgery, as well as some with circulatory failure due to myocardial infarction.[52, 82]

When time permits, the initial infusion rate of dopamine should be 0.5 to 1.0 μg/kg body weight/min and should be increased at no less than 10-minute intervals to allow steady state to be approximated. In patients with life-threatening hypotension or during CPR, an initial infusion rate of 5 μg/kg body weight/min is often used. Dosing requirements during CPR have not been established, and infusion rates of greater than 10 μg/kg body weight/min may be needed to establish an adequate blood pressure.

Dobutamine. Dobutamine is a synthetic catecholamine with relatively selective inotropic action. It is most commonly administered to patients with chronic heart failure, and its kinetics have been studied in this population. Plasma dobutamine half-life in

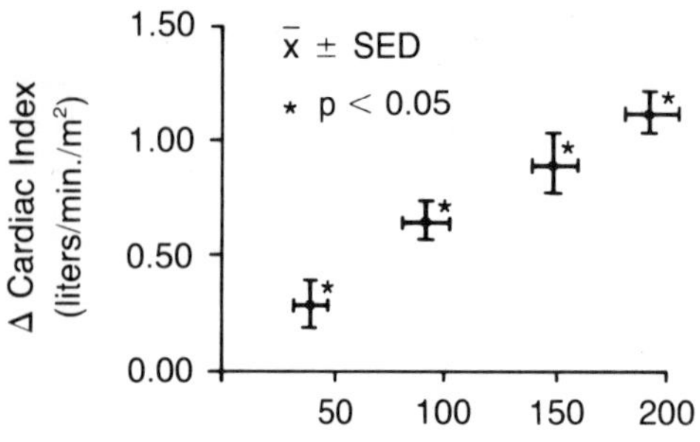

Figure 15–21. Increase in cardiac index is linearly related to plasma dobutamine concentration in patients with NYHA class IV congestive heart failure. Dobutamine infusion rates were 2.5, 5.0, 7.5, and 10 μg/kg/min. (From Leier et al.: The relationship between plasma dobutamine concentrations and cardiovascular responses in cardiac failure. Am. J. Med. 66:238, 1979. Reproduced with permission.)

patients with severe congestive heart failure is 2.4 minutes. Both the plasma concentration and the clinical effects of dobutamine are proportional to the rate of infusion (Fig. 15–21).[62] The therapeutic range for plasma dobutamine concentration is 50 to 200 ng/ml.[62] The minimal effective infusion rate is about 2.5 μg/kg body weight/min, and the usual maximal rate is 10 to 15 μg/kg body weight/min.[96] The use of higher infusion rates is limited in many patients by the development of sinus tachycardia or arrhythmias, although rates as high as 40 μg/kg body weight/min have been used in some patients with acute myocardial infarction without having serious toxic effects.[39] Because of dobutamine's short half-life, a loading dose is not required.

SUMMARY

In drug therapy for cardiac emergencies, it is necessary to (1) achieve therapeutic drug concentrations rapidly, (2) allow for the effects of cardiac dysfunction on drug pharmacokinetics, and (3) adjust drug dose as the patient's clinical status changes. Circulatory failure causes sympathetically mediated vasoconstriction of most tissues, with relative sparing of brain and heart due to autoregulation. Blood flow to vasoconstricted tissues is reduced, and the available cardiac output is redistributed so that heart and brain receive a greater fraction. Drug distribution to tissues is slowed, and the initial concentration of drug in blood is higher when circulatory failure is present than when it is absent. This higher blood concentration is reflected by higher concentrations of drug in the brain and heart, which are relatively well perfused. Initial doses of many drugs need to be reduced in patients with circulatory failure to prevent cardiac or central nervous system toxicity.

Drug metabolism in circulatory failure may be impaired by reduced hepatic blood flow resulting in decreased clearance of highly extracted drugs, or hepatocellular dysfunction resulting in decreased clearance of poorly extracted drugs. Drug excretion may be impaired by reduced renal blood flow, resulting in decreased filtration or secretion. The maintenance dose of many drugs must therefore be reduced in the presence of circulatory failure.

Intravenous drug administration is preferred in patients with circulatory failure. The central intravenous route is often convenient but must be used cautiously when potentially cardiotoxic drugs are being administered. Intratracheal administration appears to be a promising alternative for some drugs, such as epinephrine. Intracardiac injections are hazardous and offer no demonstrated advantage over other routes.

Most antiarrhythmic drugs have half-lives of at least several hours and require many hours to reach a steady state blood concentration when administered as a constant-rate intravenous infusion. Therapeutic blood concentrations of drug can be achieved more rapidly by administering a loading dose consisting of one or more intravenous bolus doses or rapid infusions. Catecholamines have half-lives of several minutes, and a loading dose is not required. Several representative drugs have been discussed to illustrate the application of pharmacokinetic principles to drug dosing in cardiac emergencies.

References

1. Anderson, J. L., Patterson, E., Conlon, M., et al.: Kinetics of antifibrillatory effects of bretylium: correlation with myocardial drug concentrations. Am. J. Cardiol. 46:583, 1980.
2. Anderson, J. L., Patterson, E., Wagner, J. G., et al.: Oral and intravenous bretylium disposition. Clin. Pharmacol. Ther. 28:468, 1980.
3. Aronow, W. S., Landa, D., Plasencia, G., et al.: Verapamil in atrial fibrillation and atrial flutter. Clin. Pharmacol. Ther. 26:578, 1979.

4. Bauer, L. A., Brown, T., Gibaldi, M., et al.: Influence of long-term infusions on lidocaine kinetics. Clin. Pharmacol. Ther. 31:433, 1982.
5. Bax, N. D. S., Tucker, G. T., and Woods, H. F.: Lignocaine and indocyanine green kinetics in patients following myocardial infarction. Br. J. Clin. Pharmacol. 10:353, 1980.
6. Bellet, S., Roman, L., Kistis, J. B., and Fleischmann, D.: Intramuscular lidocaine in the therapy of ventricular arrhythmias. Am. J. Cardiol. 27:291, 1971.
7. Benowitz, N.: Effect of cardiac disease on pharmacokinetics: pathophysiologic considerations. *In* Benet, L. Z., Massoud, N., and Gaubertoglio, J. (eds.): The Pharmacokinetic Basis of Drug Treatment. (in press.)
8. Benowitz, N., Forsyth, R. P., Melmon, K. L., and Rowland, M.: Lidocaine disposition kinetics in monkey and man. II. Effects of hemorrhage and sympathomimetic drug administration. Clin. Pharmacol. Ther. 16:99, 1974.
9. Benowitz, N., Forsyth, R. P., Melmon, K. L., and Rowland, M.: Lidocaine disposition kinetics in monkey and man. I. Prediction by a perfusion model. Clin. Pharmacol. Ther. 16:87, 1974.
10. Benowitz, N. L., and Meister, W.: Pharmacokinetics in patients with cardiac failure. Clin Pharmacokinet. 1:389, 1976.
11. Benowitz, N. L., and Meister, W.: Clinical pharmacokinetics of lignocaine. Clin. Pharmacokinet. 3:177, 1978.
12. Braunwald, E.: Heart Disease: A Textbook of Cardiovascular Medicine. Philadelphia, W. B. Saunders Co., 1980, p. 453.
13. Brown, J. E., and Shand, D. G.: Therapeutic drug monitoring of antiarrhythmic agents. Clin. Pharmacokinet. 7:125, 1982.
14. Camarata, S. J., Weill, M. H., Hanashiro, P. K., and Shubin, H.: Cardiac arrest in the critically ill. I. A study of predisposing causes in 132 patients. Circulation 44:688, 1971.
15. Chandra, N., Snyder, L. D., and Weisfeldt, M. L.: Abdominal binding during cardiopulmonary resuscitation in man. J.A.M.A. 246:351, 1981.
16. Clutter, W. E., Bier, D. M., Shah, S. D., and Cryer, P. E.: Epinephrine plasma metabolic clearance rates and physiologic thresholds for metabolic and hemodynamic actions in man. J. Clin. Invest. 66:94, 1980.
17. Cohen, H. C., Gozo, E. G., Jr., Langendorf, R., et al.: Response of resistant ventricular tachycardia to bretylium. Relation to site of ectopic focus and location of myocardial disease. Circulation 47:331, 1973.
18. Cohen, L. S., Rosenthal, J. E., Horner, D. W., Jr., et al.: Plasma levels of lidocaine after intramuscular administration. Am. J. Cardiol. 29:520, 1972.
19. Cohn, J. N., Tristani, F. E., and Khatri, I. M.: Cardiac and peripheral vascular effects of digitalis in clinical cardiogenic shock. Am. Heart J. 78:318, 1969.
20. Coltart, D. J., and Shand, D. G.: Plasma propranolol levels in the quantitative assessment of β-adrenergic blockade in man. Br. Med. J. 3:731, 1970.
21. Crawford, M. H., Ludden, T. M., Kennedy, G. T., et al.: Hemodynamic effects of *N*-acetylprocainamide in heart disease. Clin. Pharmacol. Ther. 31:459, 1982.
22. Davison, R., Barresi, V., Parker, M., et al.: Intracardiac injections during cardiopulmonary resuscitation. J.A.M.A. 244:1110, 1980.
23. DeMots, H., Rahmitoola, S. H., McAnulty, J. H., and Porter, G. A.: Effects of ouabain on coronary and systemic vascular resistance and myocardial oxygen consumption in patients without heart failure. Am. J. Cardiol. 41:88, 1978.
24. Dhurandhar, R. W., Teasdale, S. J., and Mahon, W. A.: Bretylium tosylate in the management of refractory ventricular fibrillation. Can. Med. Assoc. J. 105:161, 1971.
25. Doherty, J. E., and Perkins, W. H.: Studies with tritiated digoxin in human subjects after intravenous administration. Am. Heart J. 63:582, 1962.
26. Dominic, J., McAllister, R. G., Jr., Kuo, C. S., et al.: Verapamil plasma levels and ventricular rate response in patients with atrial fibrillation and flutter. Clin. Pharmacol. Ther. 26:710, 1979.
27. Duchin, K. L., and Schrier, R. W.: Interrelationship between renal hemodynamics, drug kinetics and drug action. Clin. Pharmacokinet. 3:58, 1978.
28. Eichelbaum, M., Somogyi, A., von Unruh, G. E., and Dengler, H. J.: Simultaneous determination of the intravenous and oral pharmacokinetic parameters of *D,L*-verapamil using stable isotope-labelled verapamil. Eur. J. Clin. Pharmacol. 19:133, 1981.
29. Elam, J. O.: The intrapulmonary route for CPR drugs. *In* Safar, P. (ed.): Advances in Cardiopulmonary Resuscitation. New York, Springer, 1977, p. 132.
30. Esler, M., Jackman, G., Leonard, P., et al.: Effect of norepinephrine uptake blockers on norepinephrine kinetics. Clin. Pharmacol. Ther. 29:12, 1981.
31. Feely, J., Wilkinson, G. R., McAllister, C. B., and Wood, J. J.: Increased toxicity and reduced clearance of lidocaine by cimetidine. Ann. Intern. Med. 96:592, 1982.
32. FitzGerald, G. A., Barnes, P., Hamilton, C. A., and Dollery, C. T.: Circulating adrenaline and blood pressure: the metabolic effects and kinetics of infused adrenaline in man. Eur. J. Clin. Invest. 10:401, 1980.
33. FitzGerald, G. A., Hossmann, V., Hamilton, C. A., et al.: Interindividual variation in kinetics of infused norepinephrine. Clin. Pharmacol. Ther. 26:669, 1979.
34. Gadzinski, D. S., White, B. C., Hoehner, P. J., et al.: Canine cerebral cortical blood flow and vascular resistance post cardiac arrest. Ann. Emerg. Med. 11:58, 1982.
35. Gaffney, F. A., Thal, E. R., Taylor, W. F., et al.: Hemodynamic effects of medical anti-shock trousers (MAST garment). J. Trauma 21:931, 1981.
36. Galeazzi, R. L., Benet, L. Z., and Sheiner, L. B.: Relationship between the pharmacokinetics and pharmacodynamics of procainamide. Clin. Pharmacol. Ther. 20:278, 1976.
37. Galster, A. D., Clutter, W. E., Cryer, P. E., et al.: Epinephrine plasma thresholds for lipolytic effects in man. J. Clin. Invest. 67:1729, 1981.
38. Giardina, E. G. V., Heissenbuttel, R. H., and Bigger, J. T.: Intermittent intravenous procaine amide to treat ventricular arrhythmias. Correlation of plasma concentration with effect on arrhythmia, electrocardiogram, and blood pressure. Ann. Intern. Med. 78:183, 1973.
39. Gillespie, T. A., Ambos, H. D., Sobel, B. E., and Roberts, R.: Effects of dobutamine in patients with

acute myocardial infarction. Am. J. Cardiol. 39:588, 1977.
40. Goldberg, A. H.: Cardiopulmonary arrest. N. Engl. J. Med. 290:381, 1974.
41. Goldberg, L. I. Hsieh, Y. Y., and Resnekov, L.: Newer catecholamines for treatment of heart failure and shock: an update on dopamine and first look at dobutamine. Prog. Cardiovasc. Dis. 19:327, 1977.
42. Gomeni, R., Bianchetti, G., Sega, R., and Morselli, P. L.: Pharmacokinetics of propranolol in normal healthy volunteers. J. Pharmacokinet. Biopharm. 5:183, 1977.
43. Gonzales, R., and Scheinman, M. M.: Treatment of supraventricular arrhythmias with intravenous and oral verapamil. Chest 80:465, 1981.
44. Greenberg, M. I., Roberts, J. R., Krusz, J. C., and Baskin, S. I.: Endotracheal epinephrine in a canine anaphylactic shock model. J.A.C.E.P. 8:500, 1979.
45. Greenspan, A. M., Horowitz, L. N., Spielman, S. R., and Josephson, M. E.: Large dose procainamide therapy for ventricular tachyarrhythmia. Am. J. Cardiol. 46:453, 1980.
46. Halkin, H., Meffin, P., Melmon, K. L., and Rowland, M.: Influence of congestive heart failure on blood levels of lidocaine and its active monodeethylated metabolite. Clin. Pharmacol. Ther. 17:669, 1975.
47. Harrison, D. C.: Practical guidelines for the use of lidocaine. Prevention and treatment of cardiac arrhtymias. J.A.M.A. 233:1202, 1975.
48. Higgins, C. B., Vatner, S. F., Franklin, D., and Braunwald, E.: Effects of experimentally produced heart failure on the peripheral vascular response to severe exercise in conscious dogs. Circ. Res. 31:186, 1972.
49. Higgins, C. B., Vatner, S. F., Millard, R. W., et al.: Alterations in regional hemodynamics in experimental heart failure in conscious dogs. Trans. Assoc. Am. Physicians 85:267, 1972.
50. Hoffman, J. R.: External counterpressure and the MAST suit: current and future roles. Ann. Emerg. Med. 9:419, 1980.
51. Holloway, E. L., Polumbo, R. A., and Harrison, D. C.: Acute circulatory effects of dopamine in patients with pulmonary hypertension. Br. Heart J. 37:482, 1975.
52. Holzer, J., Karliner, J. S., O'Rourke, R. A., et al.: Effectiveness of dopamine in patients with cardiogenic shock. Am. J. Cardiol. 32:79, 1973.
53. Jugdutt, B. I., and Lee, S. J. K.: Intravenous therapy with propranolol in acute myocardial infarction. Effects on changes in the S-T segment and hemodynamics. Chest 74:514, 1978.
54. Kaplan, B. M., and Knott, A. P., Jr.: Closed-chest cardiac massage for circulatory arrest. Arch. Intern. Med. 114:5, 1964.
55. Kates, R. E., Keefe, D. L. D., Schwartz, J., et al.: Verapamil disposition kinetics in chronic atrial fibrillation. Clin. Pharmacol. Ther. 30:44, 1981.
56. Koch-Weser, J.: Bretylium. N. Engl. J. Med. 300:473, 1979.
57. Koch-Weser, J., and Klein, S. W.: Procainamide dosage schedules, plasma concentrations, and clinical effects. J.A.M.A. 215:1454, 1971.
58. Kornhauser, D. M., Wood, A. J. J., Vestal, R. E., et al.: Biological determinants of propranolol disposition in man. Clin. Pharmacol. Ther. 23:165, 1978.
59. Koup, J. R., Greenblatt, D. J., Jusko, W. J., et al.: Pharmacokinetics of digoxin in normal subjects after intravenous bolus and infusion doses. J. Pharmacokinet. Biopharm. 3:181, 1975.
60. Kuhn, G. J., White, B. C., Swetnam, R. E., et al.: Peripheral vs central circulation times during CPR: a pilot study. Ann. Emerg. Med. 10:417, 1981.
61. Leier, C. V., Heban, P. T., Huss, P., et al.: Comparative systemic and regional hemodynamic effects of dopamine and dobutamine in patients with cardiomyopathic heart failure. Circulation 58:466, 1978.
62. Leier, C. V., Unverferth, D. V., and Kates, R. E.: The relationship between plasma dobutamine concentrations and cardiovascular responses in cardiac failure. Am. J. Med. 66:238, 1979.
63. Lima, J. J., Conti, D. R., Goldfarb, A. L., et al.: Pharmacokinetic approach to intravenous procainamide therapy. Eur. J. Clin. Pharmacol. 13:303, 1978.
64. Lima, J. J., Goldfarb, A. L., Conti, D. R., et al.: Safety and efficacy of procainamide infusions. Am. J. Cardiol. 43:98, 1979.
65. Mangiardi, L. M., Hariman, R. J., McAllister, R. G., Jr., et al.: Electrophysiologic and hemodynamic effects of verapamil. Circulation 57:366, 1978.
66. Marcus, F. I.: Use of digitalis in acute myocardial infarction. Circulation 62:17, 1980.
67. McAllister, R. G., Jr.: Intravenous propranolol administration: a method for rapidly achieving and sustaining desired plasma levels. Clin. Pharmacol. Ther. 20:517, 1976.
68. McAllister, R. G., Jr., Bourne, D. W. A., and Dittert, L. W.: The pharmacology of verapamil. I. Elimination kinetics in dogs and correlation of plasma levels with effect on the electrocardiogram. J. Pharmacol. Exp. Ther. 202:38, 1977.
69. McDevitt, D. G., and Shand, D. G.: Plasma concentrations and the time-course of beta blockade due to propranolol. Clin. Pharmacol. Ther. 18:708, 1975.
70. McDonald, J. L.: Systolic and mean arterial pressures during manual and mechanical CPR in humans. Crit. Care Med. 9:382, 1981.
71. McIntyre, K. M.: Cardiovascular pharmacology: Part II. *In* McIntyre, K. M., and Lewis, A. J. (eds.): Textbook of Advanced Cardiac Life Support. American Heart Assocation, 1981, p. IX-6.
72. Mueller, H. S., Evans, R., and Ayres, S. M.: Effect of dopamine on hemodynamics and myocardial metabolism in shock following acute myocardial infarction in man. Circulation 57:361, 1978.
73. Narang, P. K., Adir, J., Josselson, J., et al.: Pharmacokinetics of bretylium in man after intravenous administration. J. Pharmacokinet. Biopharm. 8:363, 1980.
74. Noneman, J. W., and Rogers, J. F.: Lidocaine prophylaxis in acute myocardial infarction. Medicine 57:501, 1978.
75. Ochs, H. R., Carstens, C., and Greenblatt, D. J.: Reduction in lidocaine clearance during continuous infusion and by coadministration of propranolol. N. Engl. J. Med. 303:373, 1980.
76. Pine, M., Favrot, L., Smith, S., et al.: Correlation of plasma propranolol concentration with therapeutic response in patients with angina pectoris. Circulation 52:886, 1975.
77. Prescott, L. F., Adjepon-Yamoah, K. K., and Talbot, R. G.: Impaired lignocaine metabolism in

patients with myocardial infarction and cardiac failure. Br. Med. J. 1:939, 1976.
78. Redding, J. S., Asuncion, J. S., and Pearson, J. W.: Effective routes of drug administration during cardiac arrest. Anesth. Analg. 46:253, 1967.
79. Reuning, R. H., Sams, R. A., and Notari, R. E.: Role of pharmacokinetics in drug dosage adjustment. I. Pharmacologic effect kinetics and apparent volume of distribution of digoxin. J. Clin. Pharmacol. 13:127, 1973.
80. Roberts, J. R., Greenberg, M. I., and Baskin, S. I.: Endotracheal epinephrine in cardiorespiratory collapse. J.A.C.E.P. 8:515, 1979.
81. Roberts, J. R., Greenberg, M. I., Knaub, M. A., et al.: Blood levels following intravenous and endotracheal epinephrine administration. J.A.C.E.P. 8:53, 1979.
82. Rosenblum, R., and Frieden, J.: Intravenous dopamine in the treatment of myocardial dysfunction after open-heart surgery. Am. Heart J. 83:743, 1972.
83. Romhilt, D. W., Bloomfield, S. S., Lipicky, R. J., et al.: Evaluation of bretylium tosylate for the treatment of premature ventricular contractions. Circulation 45:800, 1972.
84. Routledge, P. A., Shand, D. G., Barchowsky, A., et al.: Relationship between α_1-acid glycoprotein and lidocaine disposition in myocardial infarction. Clin. Pharmacol. Ther. 30:154, 1981.
85. Rowland, M., and Tozer, T. N.: Clinical Pharmacokinetics: Concepts and Applications. Philadelphia, Lea & Febiger, 1980, p. 138.
86. Salzer, L. B., Weinrib, A. B., Marina, R. J., and Lima, J. J.: A comparison of methods of lidocaine administration in patients. Clin. Pharmacol. Ther. 29:617, 1981.
87. Schinz, A., Schnelle, K., Klein, G., and Blömer, H.: Time sequence of direct vascular and inotropic effects following intravenous administration of digoxin in normal man. Int. J. Clin. Pharmacol. 15:189, 1977.
88. Schomerus, M., Spiegelhalder, B., Stieren, B., and Eichelbaum, M.: Physiological disposition of verapamil in man. Cardiovasc. Res. 10:605, 1976.
89. Shand, D. G., Nuckolls, E. M., and Oates, J. A.: Plasma propranolol levels in adults with observations in four children. Clin. Pharmacol. Ther. 11:112, 1969.
90. Shapiro, W., Narahara, K., and Traubert, K.: Relationship of plasma digitoxin and digoxin to cardiac response following intravenous digitalization in man. Circulation 42:1065, 1970.
91. Silverberg, A. B., Shah, S. D., Haymond, M. W., and Cryer, P. E.: Norepinephrine: hormone and neurotransmitter in man. Am. J. Physiol. 234:252, 1978.
92. Singh, B. N., Ellrodt, G., and Peter, C. T.: Verapamil: a review of its pharmacological properties and therapeutic use. Drugs 15:169, 1978.
93. Singh, J. B., and Kocot, S. L.: A controlled trial of intramuscular lidocaine in the prevention of premature ventricular contractions associated with acute myocardial infarction. Am. Heart J. 91:430, 1976.
94. Smith, T. W.: Drug therapy. Digitalis glycosides. N. Engl. J. Med. 288:719, 1973.
95. Smulyan, H., Weinberg, S. E., and Howanitz, P. J.: Continuous propranolol infusion following abdominal surgery. J.A.M.A. 247:2539, 1982.
96. Sonnenblick, E. H., Frishman, W. H., and LeJemtel, T. H.: Dobutamine: a new synthetic cardioactive sympathetic amine. N. Engl. J. Med. 300:17, 1979.
97. Stenson, R. E., Constantino, R. T., and Harrison, D. C.: Interrelationships of hepatic blood flow, cardiac output, and blood levels of lidocaine in man. Circulation 43:205, 1971.
98. Stone, P. H., Antman, E. M., Muller, J. E., and Braunwald, E.: Calcium channel blocking agents in the treatment of cardiovascular disorders. Part II: Hemodynamic effects and clinical applications. Ann. Intern. Med. 93:886, 1980.
99. Terry, G., Vellani, C. W., Higgins, M. R., and Doig, A.: Bretylium tosylate in treatment of refractory ventricular arrhythmias complicating myocardial infarction. Br. Heart J. 32:21, 1970.
100. Thomson, P. D., Melmon, K. L., Richardson, J. A., et al.: Lidocaine pharmacokinetics in advanced heart failure, liver disease, and renal failure in humans. Ann. Intern. Med. 78:499, 1973.
101. Valentine, P. A., Frew, J. L., Mashford, M. L., and Sloman, J. G.: Lidocaine in the prevention of sudden death in the pre-hospital phase of acute infarction. A double-blind study. N. Engl. J. Med. 291:1327, 1974.
102. Voorhees, W. D., Babbs, C. F., and Tacker, W. A.: Regional blood flow during cardiopulmonary resuscitation in dogs. Crit. Care Med. 8:134, 1980.
103. Woosley, R. I., Shand, D., Kornhauser, D., et al.: Relation of plasma concentration and dose of propranolol to its effect on resistant ventricular arrhythmias. Clin. Res. 25:262A, 1977 (abstr.).
104. Wyman, M. G., Goldreyer, B. N., Cannom, D. S., et al.: Factors influencing procainamide total body clearance in the immediate postmyocardial infarction period. J. Clin. Pharmacol. 21:20, 1981.
105. Wyman, M. G., Lalka, D., Hammersmith, L., et al.: Multiple bolus technique for lidocaine administration during the first hours of an acute myocardial infarction. Am. J. Cardiol. 41:313, 1978.
106. Zelis, R., and Mason, D. T.: Compensatory mechanisms in congestive heart failure—the role of the peripheral resistance vessels. N. Engl. J. Med. 282:962, 1970.
107. Zelis, R., Mason, D. T., and Braunwald, E.: Partition of blood flow to the cutaneous and muscular beds of the forearm at rest and during leg exercise in normal subjects and in patients with heart failure. Circ. Res. 24:799, 1969.
108. Zener, J. C., Kerber, R. E., Spivack, A. P., and Harrison, D. C.: Blood lidocaine levels and kinetics following high-dose intramuscular administration. Circulation 47:984, 1973.
109. Zito, R. A., and Reid, P. R.: Lidocaine kinetics predicted by indocyanine green clearance. N. Engl. J. Med. 298:1160, 1978.

16

Cardiopulmonary Catastrophes in Drug-Overdosed Patients

NEAL L. BENOWITZ,

JON ROSENBERG,

and CHARLES E. BECKER

Cardiopulmonary complications of drug overdose are frequent and include circulatory shock or hypertension, arrhythmias, and pulmonary edema. The objectives of this review are to discuss selected aspects of general management of drug overdose, to review the pathophysiology and management of drug-induced cardiovascular syndromes, to review the literature on cardiovascular complications of specific drug overdose, to attempt to relate pharmacology of the drugs to the pathophysiology of the overdose, and to make recommendations for management. Drugs have been selected for review that are most commonly taken in cases of overdose and have major cardiovascular manifestations. The list by no means includes all drugs involved in cases of overdose, but the principles of management are applicable to other drugs. A broader review of the spectrum of drugs and toxins that cause cardiac disturbances and a more comprehensive review of drug-induced arrhythmogenesis in particular are provided by Benowitz and Goldschlager.[23]

It should be emphasized that the literature on drug overdose consists largely of case reports or series of cases. Identification of the involved drug or drugs is often inadequate. Most cases of overdose involve more than one drug. Furthermore, data on which to base therapeutic recommendations are few. It is likely also that many reported cases represent the end of the extreme of the effects of drug overdose, ranging from mildly intoxicated patients who responded well but would have improved without specific treatment to severely overdosed patients who did not respond well to treatment. It is difficult to compare different series of cases of overdose with respect to morbidity and mortality because of different criteria chosen for the inclusion of patients.

GENERAL PRINCIPLES

General Clinical Management after Drug Overdose

A number of reviews discuss general principles of management of drug overdose.[19, 74] We wish to emphasize a few particularly relevant points. Patient's history of the drug taken is notoriously unreliable; often they do not know what drug they took. Medication containers or samples of the particular drug or substance are most helpful in diagnosis. Gastric contents, urine, and blood should be collected as early as possible for toxicologic examination. Toxicologic evaluation is reviewed briefly in the discussion of individual drugs.

Removal of unabsorbed drug is an important step in treatment because it can potentially modify the clinical course. Emesis is the most effective means of emptying the stomach. Syrup of ipecac is usually successful in inducing emesis in alert patients. In comatose patients, gastric lavage is indicated. Endotracheal intubation to prevent aspiration is mandatory before lavage. The drowsy patient who is too awake to be intubated, but who may aspirate if emesis is induced, presents a particularly difficult problem; it is advisable to wait until the patient becomes either more alert or more depressed before removal of the drug is attempted by emesis or lavage, respectively. Many drugs, especially those with anticholinergic activity, delay gastric emptying, so emesis or lavage may be of value and should be attempted regardless of the time interval since ingestion. Induction of emesis is contraindicated if corrosive substances have been ingested, which should be suspected if there is evidence of ulceration of the lips or pharynx. Whether to induce emesis after ingestion of petroleum distillates is still controversial. Animal studies indicate that pneumonitis due to petroleum distillates is related to aspiration and not systemic absorption.[49] Depression of the central nervous system resulting from systemic absorption of petroleum distillates is uncommon. Therefore, unless the petroleum distillate contains other toxins, such as pesticides, we do not recommend emesis.

Activated charcoal can potentially bind and prevent absorption of drug that was not removed by emesis or lavage, and in addition may remove a drug that undergoes enterohepatic or enteroenteric recirculation. In the latter instances, repeated doses of activated charcoal may substantially accelerate elimination of drug from the body. Drugs for which repeated doses of charcoal have been shown to be effective include phenobarbital,[137] carbamazepine,[137] dapsone,[138] and digitoxin.[148] Repeated administration of activated charcoal, Fuller's earth, or bentonite clay–based (adsorbing) substances improve survival after paraquat ingestion in animals and are recommended for use in humans.[169] Adequate amounts of charcoal must be given to compete with other drug-binding contents of the gastrointestinal tract. Doses of 50 to 100 gm should be administered as soon as possible. However, because charcoal binds ipecac, charcoal must be given after completion of ipecac-induced vomiting. For administration of repeated doses of charcoal, doses of 50 gm every four to six hours are recommended.

Monitoring of comatose patients after they have left the emergency room is best carried out in an intensive care setting. Patients with arrhythmias or abnormal electrocardiographic findings should be monitored electrocardiographically until the ECG shows no abnormalities. The lethargic patient in the emergency room presents a problem because delayed drug absorption, again most commonly after anticholinergic drug overdose, or progression of the pathophysiologic process, such as sometimes occurs in later phases of salicylate poisoning, can result in sudden deterioration. Intensive care monitoring, if available, is recommended until there is a clear trend toward improvement.

A number of techniques have been proposed for accelerating the removal of the offending drug from the body. These are discussed briefly later in the sections on specific drugs.

Drug-Induced Cardiopulmonary Syndromes

Hypotension and Circulatory Shock

Mechanisms. Hypotension occurs after overdosage with many different types of drugs. The mechanisms of hypotension are multiple, and hemodynamic patterns differ with different drugs in different stages of overdose and according to the presence and nature of underlying medical illness. Cardiac output may be reduced owing to drug-induced myocardial depression, relative hypovolemia resulting from venous pooling, or true hypovolemia resulting from vascular injury and fluid loss from the vascular space. Peripheral vascular resistance may be reduced because of drug-induced vascular relaxation, adrenergic-receptor blockade, or depression of central vasomotor tone. Myocardial and vascular dysfunction resulting from hypoxia, acidosis, and hypotension may complicate the picture.

The major importance of hypotension is that it warns the physician of possible circulatory insufficiency; blood pressure is also one of several indicators of response to treatment. The diagnosis of circulatory shock depends on evidence of tissue hypoperfusion. In previously healthy persons, urine output is usually the most sensitive indicator of hypoperfusion. Lactic acidosis is biochemical evidence that a substantial amount of tissue is hypoperfused. In patients with underlying coronary artery or cerebrovascular disease, cardiac or cerebral dysfunction may limit the tolerable extent of hypotension.

Management. Hypotensive patients should be placed in an intensive care unit where vital signs, fluid intake and output, body weight, and other parameters of circulatory function can be monitored continuously. Since indirect measurements of arterial blood pressure are difficult to obtain and often do not reflect true intra-arterial pressure in hypotensive states, direct measurement of intra-arterial blood pressure is preferred.

If hypotension is present without signs of tissue hypoperfusion, fluids should be administered at sufficient rates to maintain urine output and to compensate for insensible losses; fluids should be of appropriate composition to provide electrolyte needs. In many patients with signs of hypoperfusion of tissues, correction of acid-base and electrolyte disturbances and modest fluid therapy are sufficient to increase perfusion to adequate levels. However, increased pulmonary vascular permeability complicates many cases of drug overdose, and fluid therapy may cause pulmonary edema. For this reason, fluids must be administered cautiously. A reasonably safe method is by short infusions of small volumes (100–200 ml) of normal saline solution. If the clinical response is inadequate and if there is no evidence of pulmonary edema, the short infusions should be repeated but should not exceed a total of 1000 to 2000 ml over one to two hours. Evidence of pulmonary edema includes worsening hypoxia, decreasing lung compliance (manifested by increasing pressure necessary to ventilate a patient with a given tidal volume), and the appearance of pulmonary rales.

If shock persists despite fluid challenge, catheterization of the pulmonary artery and measurement of pulmonary capillary wedge (PCW) pressure, cardiac output, and/or venous oxygen saturation are recommended to monitor subsequent fluid therapy and to optimize drug treatment. The goal of fluid therapy is to re-establish adequate tissue perfusion with as little effect on PCW pressure as possible. As long as PCW pressure remains low, further fluid can be administered. Although there are no published data in this regard, an end point of a mean PCW pressure of 8 to 12 mm Hg in a person with previously normal cardiac function appears to be reasonable in light of the possibility of increased pulmonary vascular permeability. (In these patients, fluid therapy is based on clinical assessment of pulmonary edema rather than the measured PCW pressure.) This is in contrast to treatment of hemorrhagic or cardiogenic shock in which a PCW pressure of 15 to 18 mm Hg is often the end point. If evidence of tissue hypoperfusion persists when PCW pressures have been restored to "normal" or pulmonary edema is evident, pressor or inotropic agents should be administered to restore adequate perfusion. It should be noted that in persons with chronic cardiac failure, higher pressures (up to 20 mm Hg) may be necessary to maintain an adequate cardiac output.

Hemodynamic monitoring aids in the selection of pressor or inotropic drugs. For example, if circulatory failure is associated with low or low-normal peripheral vascular resistance, pressor drugs with substantial direct vasoconstricting activity, such as norepinephrine and dopamine, should be selected. Normalization of vascular resistance is a useful end point for titration of infusion rate.

If vascular resistance is normal or high, and depressed cardiac output is the determining factor in circulatory failure, drugs or interventions that increase cardiac output should be selected. Isoproterenol is particularly useful when myocardial depression is associated with bradyarrhythmias, although it may be arrhythmogenic; dobutamine, a dopamine analogue with relatively selective inotropic activity and less arrhythmogenic potential, is useful when the heart rate is already adequate. When both myocardial depression and low vascular resistance are present, epinephrine or combinations of norepinephrine or dopamine and isoproterenol may be useful. Drug-overdosed patients with severe myocardial depression are usually severely hypotensive, making vasodilator therapy difficult. Also, high vascular resistance is unusual because most myocardial poisons are also vascular poisons.

Dopamine has now become the pressor agent of choice in most cases of drug overdose, primarily because of its renal vasodilating effect. An exception is overdose with drugs that have alpha-adrenergic receptor–blocking effects, such as phenothiazines or tricyclic antidepressants, in which case more selective alpha-adrenergic agonists, such as norepinephrine or phenylephrine, may be required.

Pressor therapy has potential risks: pressor-induced venoconstriction can increase venous return and worsen pulmonary edema, and arteriolar constriction can further reduce tissue perfusion. However, in studies of the effects of infusion of norepinephrine into patients who overdosed with sedative drugs, the positive effects of norepinephrine on cardiac output outweighed the vasoconstrictor effects, and blood pressure increased without an increase in vascular resistance.[165]

Hypertension

Hypertension is relatively uncommon, usually following overdose of sympathomimetic or anticholinergic drugs. Severe hypertension has also been observed after therapeutic doses of over-the-counter cold preparations, and is likely to be observed with increasing frequency in view of the widespread use of amphetamine "look-alikes."

Unlike the development of hypertension in patients with chronic essential hypertension, in whom blood vessels have had time to adapt to high perfusion pressures, drug-induced hypertension can occur rapidly and be potentially more injurious to blood vessels. Thus, cerebrovascular accidents or malignant hypertension might occur at lower blood pressure in patients with drug-induced hypertension than in those with essential hypertension. Since sympathetic nervous excitation, resulting from locally or systemically released catecholamines, plays a major role in drug-induced hypertension, treatment is similar to that for pheochromocytoma. Use of sympathetic blocking drugs such as phentolamine (Regitine) (alpha-adrenergic blocker) and propranolol (Inderal) (beta-adrenergic blocker), as well as direct arteriolar dilators such as sodium nitroprusside (Nipride) and diazoxide (Hyperstat), may be helpful.

Arrhythmias

Drug-induced arrhythmias may be produced by general metabolic disturbances including hypotension, hypoxia, and acid-base and electrolyte disturbances, or may relate specifically to the pharmacologic effect of the overdose drug. Mechanisms of drug-induced arrhythmogenesis include direct or indirect sympathomemetic effects, anticholinergic effects, effects of altered central nervous system regulation of peripheral autonomic activity, and direct myocardial cell membrane effects. Mechanisms of arrhythmogenesis in poisoned patients are discussed in detail in a recent review.[23]

Supraventricular Tachyarrhythmias. Sinus tachycardia and other supraventricular tachyarrhythmias commonly occur after overdoses, and may also be a complication of any severe illness. Such arrhythmias often respond to general medical management and require no specific treatment. Propranolol and physostigmine may be indicated for sympathomimetic and anticholinergic drug ingestions, respectively. However, if there is concomitant evidence of cardiac membrane depression, as occurs with overdose of tricyclic antidepressants, such an approach may itself be hazardous (see below). Digitalis, propranolol, or verapamil may be useful in slowing a rapid ventricular response to atrial fibrillation or flutter, although these arrhythmias may be only transient. Electrical conversion is an acceptable alternative when supraventricular arrhythmias are life threatening and fail to respond to pharmacologic treatment.

Ventricular Tachyarrhythmias. Pharmacologic therapy for drug-induced ventricular irritability is similar to that employed in the setting of acute myocardial ischemia. There is an important exception in cases of overdose of membrane-depressant drugs such as quinidine or tricyclic antidepressants; in these instances, similar agents such as procainamide and disopyramide are contraindicated, and lidocaine or phenytoin are the drugs of choice. Selection of secondary drugs depends on the particular overdose; thus, propranolol might be indicated for sympathomimetic drug overdose, phenytoin for digitalis overdose, and isoproterenol for polymorphous ventricular tachycardia with a long Q-T interval due to quinidine-like drug overdose. Cardiac pacing usually proves very effective treatment for the latter group of patients. Bretylium tosylate has been useful in the treatment of intractable ventricular arrhythmias, especially fibrillation that is unresponsive to cardioversion and occurs in the setting of acute ischemic heart disease, and might be tried for similar arrhythmias arising during drug overdose. Its use has the potential disadvantage of causing or worsening hypotension. It should be recalled that bretylium is a unique antiarrhythmic agent, being actually an antifibrillatory drug. As such, it might prevent ventricular fibrillation while failing to suppress ventricular ectopy. Sustained ventricular tachycardia and fibrillation require electrical conversion.

Bradyarrhythmias. Bradyarrhythmias, particularly atrioventricular (AV) block, may occur unpredictably and require temporary transvenous cardiac pacing. Before pacemaker insertion, pharmacologic therapy may be necessary in an attempt to maintain heart rate, blood pressure, and cardiac output. Intravenous administration of atropine should be tried to treat sinus or junctional bradycardia; intravenous administration of isoproterenol may be used for unresponsive sinus, junctional, or ventricular bradycardias. These agents should be used with caution, however, because both may cause significant sinus or junctional tachycardia, and isoproterenol may cause ventricular extrasystolic activity including ventricular tachycardia. Low doses of atropine (< 0.5 mg) may cause parodoxical bradycardia.

Antiarrhythmic treatment strategies for particular drug-induced arrhythmias are discussed in sections on individual drugs.

Unusual Vascular Complications: Bowel Infarction and Pulmonary Embolism

Peripheral vascular complications of drug overdose are infrequently described in the medical literature. However, two patients recently treated at our hospital suggest that these may be more common and serious problems than previously recognized. One case occurred after a phenobarbital overdose in a young man in whom the abdomen became distended and hypotension worsened 12 hours after admission. He had multiple areas of infarction in the terminal ileum and ascending colon, presumably resulting from mesenteric arterial hypoperfusion. At surgery, the mesenteric vessels were patent and appeared free of disease. The patient recovered after hemicolectomy. Thus, there is a potential for ischemic bowel disease after drug-induced hypotension even in the absence of underlying arterial disease. Ischemic bowel complications are more likely to occur in older patients with underlying arterial disease.

The other case involved a middle-aged woman who was admitted to the hospital because of seizures, hypotension, and a low output state after overdose with tricyclic antidepressants. She was treated with fluids and pressors, and eventually awakened and regained apparently normal cardiovascular function. Four days later, she died suddenly. Initially, this was thought to be a case of late arrhythmic death due to tricyclic antidepressant overdose (see the discussion on tricyclic overdose below), but at autopsy the patient was found to have massive pulmonary embolism. It is likely that venous thrombosis resulted from a prolonged course of low-output circulatory failure secondary to the drug overdose. Pulmonary embolism should be considered a complication of drug overdose and a potential cause of late death. During prolonged periods of hypotension, anticoagulation, such as with low doses of heparin, might even be considered.

Pulmonary Edema

Pulmonary edema frequently complicates overdose with agents such as narcotics, sedative-hypnotic drugs, salicylates, and sympathomimetic drugs.[175] It may also occur as part of a cholinergic syndrome due to cholinesterase inhibition, particularly after ingestion of organophosphate pesticides.[29] Drug- or toxin-induced pulmonary edema may be the result or combination of different pathophysiologic processes (Fig. 16–1). Most commonly, edema is due to increased pulmonary vascular permeability indicated by normal or low PCW pressures and pulmonary edema fluid containing a protein concentration similar to that of plasma.[60, 175]

In a series of 24 patients with pulmonary edema, those with drug-induced and other noncardiogenic pulmonary edema had PCW pressures of < 20 mm Hg and edema fluid protein concentration:plasma protein concentration ratios of > 0.6.[60] Patients with hydrostatic or cardiogenic pulmonary edema had PCW pressures of > 20 mm Hg and edema fluid protein concentration:plasma protein concentration ratios of < 0.56.

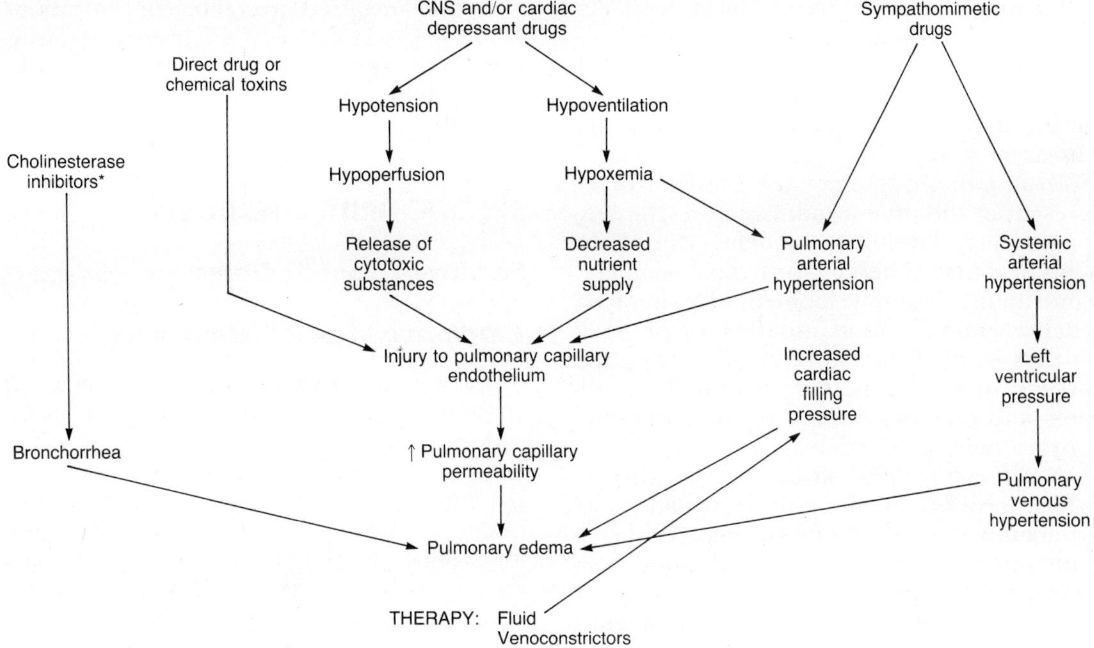

Figure 16–1. Mechanisms of drug-induced pulmonary edema.

The mechanisms by which sedative-hypnotic drugs produce capillary endothelial damage are still unknown. Pulmonary vascular injury may be a complication of systemic hypotension or hypoxemia. Resultant tissue injury may release vasoactive substances and inflammatory mediators and activate complement, contributing to endothelial injury.[97, 175]

Depression of respiration may lead to hypoxemia, precapillary pulmonary hypertension, increased vascular permeability, and finally extravasation of fluid. An analogy has been made to cases of pulmonary edema at high altitude in which hypoxia produces a similar picture, which is rapidly reversed by oxygen therapy. Ethchlorvynol, when injected intravenously, is an example of a drug that directly injures the alveolocapillary membrane.[70] Infused salicylate, possibly by means of its effects on prostaglandin synthesis, increases microvascular premeability.[175] Pulsatile lymphatic activity is reduced and lymphatic drainage is retarded during barbiturate anesthesia.[83] This might also contribute to the net accumulation of fluid in the lung after drug overdose.

Neurogenic pulmonary edema occurs after a variety of central nervous system events in humans and experimental animals, and may be mediated through the hypothalamus and the alpha-adrenergic sympathetic nervous system.[181] This may be analogous to the pulmonary edema produced by large infusions of catecholamines, and observed with increasing frequency in women treated with adrenergic agents for premature labor.[108] An analogy has also been made to drugs that injure the central nervous system, either indirectly by hypoxia or directly as has been postulated for salicylates.

Stimulant drugs increase sympathetic nervous systemic activity by both central and peripheral mechanisms. These agents may contribute to pulmonary edema by causing pulmonary arterial hypertension with injury to the endothelium; by increasing systemic vascular resistance, thereby causing severe hypertension and left ventricular overload; or by venoconstriction, thereby increasing cardiac filling and PCW pressure. Pulmonary edema due to stimulant drugs occurs most commonly after intravenous administration. By the time the patient is evaluated by the physician, blood pressure may be normal or even low, with evidence of hypovolemia resulting from sequestration of fluid into the lung and other extravascular sites.

Cardiogenic pulmonary edema with elevated PCW pressure may occur after poisoning with cardiac depressant drugs, often in the context of fluid therapy for hypotension or in the presence of pre-existing myocardial disease.

Drug-induced pulmonary edema can be present at the time of admission to the hospital or may develop subsequently during the clinical course. Therapy for hypotension may contribute to the development of pulmonary edema. Fluid filtration into the lung depends in part on PCW pressure. Fluid therapy and pressor drugs can increase central blood volume and pulmonary capillary pressure, and worsen pulmonary edema.

A difficult clinical situation may arise in which intracardiac filling pressures adequate to maintain cardiac output may result in pulmonary transudation. Suggestions concerning fluid therapy and the use of PCW pressures have been discussed. In anemic patients, transfusion of red blood cells may be useful in increasing blood pressure and improving oxygen delivery to tissues. Reduction of fluid intake and diuretics may limit pulmonary transudation by decreasing hydrostatic pressures, but may also be hazardous in potentiating hypotension. Animal studies of oleic acid–induced vascular permeability pulmonary edema suggest that infusion of nitroprusside may decrease lung water by decreasing cardiac filling and PCW pressures (via venodilation), while increasing cardiac output by arteriolar vasodilation.[150] Such therapy may prove useful in treating certain forms of drug-induced pulmonary edema, although studies to support its benefit in such patients have not yet been reported.

Atropine is the treatment of choice for pulmonary hypersecretion syndromes due to cholinesterase inhibition. Enormous doses of atropine are often required, and the dosing must be guided by clinical response, such as diminished bronchorrhea or excessive tachycardia.

The use of mechanical ventilation improves blood-air gas exchange and is an important adjunct to treatment of pulmonary edema. Adding positive end-expiratory pressure increases functional residual capacity, reduces intrapulmonary shunting, increases pulmonary compliance, and improves oxygenation. Positive end-expiratory pressure is useful in maintaining adequate arterial oxygen tensions while the lung is ventilated with nontoxic inspired oxygen concentrations. However, positive end-expiratory pressure does not reduce lung water in vascular permeability pulmonary edema in experimental animals.[150]

SPECIFIC DRUG OVERDOSES

Sedative-Hypnotic Drugs

*Cardiopulmonary Disturbances**

The sedative-hypnotic drugs are the major contributors to morbidity from drug intoxication. Coma, respiratory failure, and circulatory shock are commonly present when the patient is first seen at the hospital. Subsequent management problems include prolonged coma, pneumonia, and pulmonary edema. In one series of 52 critically ill patients, the prognosis for survival was best correlated with systolic blood pressure, arterial pH, and mean central venous pressure on admission.[3] These are indicators of the overall severity of drug overdose, but if the patient dies they do not indicate a cardiovascular cause of death. In most cases respiratory complications are responsible for fatalities.[101]

Hypotension is common in cases of sedative-hypnotic overdose. In the majority of patients reported in two series, cardiac output was reduced while systemic vascular resistance was either normal or increased.[165, 182] However, systemic vascular resistance was less than anticipated from the extent of hypotension if sympathetic reflexes were intact.

The major action of sedative-hypnotic drugs is on the central nervous system, and results in reduced sympathetic and increased parasympathetic peripheral autonomic tone. Barbiturates have been shown to depress myocardial function in animals, but severe myocardial depression is uncommon in humans.[9, 166] Cardiac output is commonly reduced because of relative hypovolemia due to increased venous capacitance and absolute hypovolemia due to fluid loss into tissues, the latter a consequence of increased vascular permeability.[164] Cardiac output and heart rate may be lower than normal owing to hypothermia and reduced metabolic demands. As a consequence of inhibition of

*See Table 16–1.

Table 16–1. MANIFESTATIONS, MECHANISMS, AND TREATMENT OF COMPLICATIONS OF SEDATIVE-HYPNOTIC DRUG OVERDOSE

Manifestations	Mechanisms	Treatment
a. Respiratory depression, coma	Depression of CNS (medullary) respiratory center, other CNS functions	Assisted ventilation
b. Hypotension	Venodilation, depression of CNS vasomotor centers, impairment of vascular reflexes, loss of intravascular volume	Fluids (cautiously), pressors (dopamine)
c. Pulmonary edema	Increase in pulmonary vascular permeability	Positive end-expiratory pressure, assisted ventilation if necessary, oxygen (to maintain P_{O_2} 60–70 mm Hg)
d. Hypothermia	Lowering of metabolic rate, ? alteration of temperature regulation	None
e. Sudden apnea, papilledema, convulsions (glutethimide)	Cerebral edema	Assisted ventilation, hyperventilation, anticonvulsant drugs
f. Ventricular arrhythmias (chloral hydrate)	Sensitization of myocardium to effects of catecholamines	Propranolol, lidocaine, phenytoin, hemodialysis

sympathetic function, the heart rate is frequently less than expected for the degree of hypotension.

In spite of hypotension and relative bradycardia, cardiac output is often sufficient to meet tissue metabolic demands. This is because sedative-hypnotic drugs cause hypothermia and reduce tissue metabolism and oxygen consumption. The reduction in cardiac output may be in part a response to reduced tissue oxygen requirements.

An important complication of sedative-hypnotic drug overdose is pulmonary edema, which results from increased pulmonary vascular permeability as discussed above. As a consequence, hypoxia and metabolic acidosis develop, which may worsen myocardial performance and potentiate arrhythmias.

Pulmonary edema is rarely manifest on initial presentation; it occurs more frequently with administration of fluid.[75] Noncardiac pulmonary edema is claimed to be more common with some of the nonbarbiturate sedative-hypnotic drugs,[9] but the relative incidence is related to how the patients were managed and is impossible to quantitate.

General Management

Management of hypotension and shock due to sedative-hypnotic overdose includes judicious use of fluids and pressor drugs. Since venous pooling contributes to reduced cardiac output, the head-down legs-up (Trendelenburg) position may substantially increase venous return, cardiac output, and blood pressure. Infusion of modest amounts of colloid or crystalloid fluids is sufficient to correct hypovolemia and to increase cardiac output and tissue perfusion to adequate levels in many patients. Failure to achieve adequate tissue perfusion despite increased cardiac filling pressure or evidence of pulmonary edema is an indication for the use of pressor drugs, as discussed previously.

There are specific data relating to the use of pressor drugs in cases of sedative-hypnotic overdose. In healthy, nonintoxicated persons, infusion of norepinephrine increases blood pressure by increasing vascular resistance, and results in a reflex decrease in cardiac output and heart rate. In contrast, infusion of norepinephrine in hypotensive, drug-overdosed patients increases blood pressure, owing to an increase in stroke volume and cardiac output, while systemic vascular resistance remains unchanged or even decreases.[93, 165] The cardiac-stimulating and peripheral-venoconstricting effects of norepinephrine are presumably responsible for the increased cardiac output. Increased cardiac output increases blood pressure, activates the baroreceptor reflex, and reduces sympathetic nervous vascular tone, presumably counteracting any direct arteriolar constricting effect of norepinephrine. With high infusion rates of norepinephrine, however, vasoconstriction and increased systemic vascular resistance can occur, with consequent adverse effects on tissue perfusion. Like norepinephrine, dopamine has alpha-adrenergic agonist effects, but it also has a direct renal vasodilating effect. For this reason, dopamine is the drug of choice in cases of sedative overdose. Norepinephrine is reserved as a second-line drug. Digoxin has been shown to reverse the myocardial depressive effects of barbiturates in animals,[166] but myocardial failure is a rare complication of sedative-hypnotic overdose and digoxin therefore is rarely indicated.

Specific Sedative-Hypnotic Drugs

The major differences between different sedative-hypnotic drugs and management of the overdose situation are the pharmacokinetics, routes of elimination, and methods used to facilitate drug removal from the body. These differences are summarized below.

Barbiturates. Barbiturates are divided into two groups: intermediate-acting (secobarbital [Seconal], pentobarbital [Nembutal], amobarbital [Amytal]) and long-acting (phenobarbital). Ingestion of shorter acting barbiturates results in faster progression and a higher incidence of deep coma and hypotension at the time of admission to the hospital than that caused by phenobarbital.[162] For barbiturates in general, hypoventilation and apnea generally precede hypotension.

Benzodiazepines. Benzodiazepines, which include diazepam (Valium), flurazepam (Dalmane), oxazepam (Serax), clorazepate (Tranxene), chloridiazepoxide (Librium), and a number of other recently released drugs, are now the most commonly used drugs for intoxication in this country. Extremely large oral doses produce minimal respiratory or cardiovascular depression, although such doses may have a significant synergistic effect with other drugs. A review of 12 cases of overdoses with benzodiazepines alone revealed no significant complications.[76] There are few documented cases in which benzodiazepine overdose resulted in death. Cardiac arrest was reported in a child after oral ingestion of diazepam, and sinus arrest persisted during early recovery.[25]

Intravenous administration of diazepam, for treatment of seizures or as preparation for elective cardioversion or endoscopy, has been associated with apnea and hypotension.[77] This complication seems to occur only after rapid injection (< 30 sec), and extremely high blood concentrations of diazepam are probably required to affect the brain and circulatory system. The cardiovascular effects of intravenous diazepam might be contributed to by the propylene glycol solvent. Acute pulmonary edema has also been reported after injection of dissolved chlordiazepoxide capsules.[153]

Recent reports indicate that physostigmine[13, 50] or naloxone[20] may be useful in reversing diazepam-induced narcosis, although there is no evidence that respiratory depression is ameliorated. Since physostigmine may have serious adverse effects, including bradyarrhythmias and convulsions, and since narcosis per se is rarely a severe clinical problem, there appears to be little overall benefit in the use of physostigmine in benzodiazepine intoxication.

Methaqualone. Methaqualone (Quaalude) is now one of the most widely abused street drugs; intoxication from it is common and may be fatal.[15, 130] The most common cardiovascular effect is tachycardia. Hypotension is relatively uncommon. Muscular hyperactivity, myoclonus, or generalized seizures with the associated metabolic derangements (see the discussion of sympathomimetic drugs later in this chapter) may complicate the overdose.[1]

Glutethimide. Glutethimide (Doriden) overdose cases are reported to be associated with greater morbidity and mortality in some (but not all) series than in barbiturate overdose cases.[11, 42, 125, 192] A greater degree of accompanying ventilatory depression has been reported. Cerebral edema, sudden apnea, and convulsions further contribute to toxicity. Fluctuating levels of consciousness, due either to erratic absorption or accumulation of a toxic metabolite, are common.[84]

Ethchlorvynol. Ethchlorvynol (Placidyl) overdose cases are not infrequent. The clinical presentation differs from that of barbiturates in that the average duration of coma is extremely long (102 hours compared with an average of 40 hours for barbiturates) and bradycardia is more marked.[179] Pulmonary edema may occur after either ingestion or intravenous injection of ethchlorvynol.[70, 189]

Meprobamate. Meprobamate usage, and consequent intoxication, has markedly decreased since the introduction of benzodiazepines. The pharmacologic effects are similar to those of the short-acting barbiturates.[61, 124] The duration of coma tends to be short.[120] Hypotension may be severe. In one patient studied hemodynamically, systemic vascular resistance was decreased and cardiac output was depressed. Hypotension in this patient responded to infusion of isoproterenol. Pulmonary edema during fluid therapy for meprobamate-induced hypotension has been reported.[14]

Chloral Hydrate. Chloral hydrate is historically the oldest hypnotic drug. It is rapidly metabolized to trichloroethanol, which is the major hypnotic chemical. Trichloroethanol and a second metabolite of chloral hydrate, trichloroacetic acid, are believed to be responsible for the cardiac toxicity that occurs after overdose. For the most part, intoxication resembles that of barbiturates, and treatment is the same. Nausea and vomiting characteristically result from gastric irritation, and gastric necrosis occurs.[191] Additional features of chloral hydrate overdose are supraventricular and ventricular tachyarrhythmias, including ventricular fibrillation.[80, 127] The ventricular tachycardia may be paroxysmal and polymorphous. There is usually no evidence of atrioventricular or intraventricular conduction block. It has been proposed that, like hydrocarbon anesthetics, chloral hydrate or its metabolites sensitize the myocardium to circulating catecholamines, resulting in myocardial irritability. Lidocaine is most often used in treating ventricular arrhythmias, but in several cases it has been ineffective, whereas intravenous beta-blockers abolished the ectopy. Since the actions of catecholamines on the heart are thought to cause arrhythmias, beta-blockers are the logical first choice of antiarrhythmic drug so long as myocardial depression due to other drugs or intrinsic disease is not evident. Noncardiogenic pulmonary edema has also been reported in cases of chloral hydrate overdose.[32]

Methyprylon. Methyprylon (Noludar) overdose is relatively uncommon;[126, 198] to our knowledge only one death has been reported.[151] There are no clear clinical features that distinguish this type of overdose from that of barbiturates.

Anticholinergic and Antihistaminic Drugs.* Many over-the-counter sleep preparations (e.g., Sominex, Nytol, and Sleepeze) contain anticholinergic (e.g., scopolamine) and/or antihistaminic (e.g., methapyrilene or doxylamine) drugs. Frequently, antihistamines such as diphenhydramine hydrochloride (Benadryl) are prescribed for sleep. In addition to coma, anticholinergic features commonly occur including sinus tachycardia with mild hypertension, dilated pupils, flushed and dry skin, bowel hypomotility, hallucinations, and convulsions.[90] Serious arrhythmias resulting from purely anticholinergic compounds are uncommon unless there is underlying ischemic heart disease. For example, in patients after myocardial infarction, atropine has caused ventricular tachycardia and fibrillation, presumably as a result of tachycardia-related imbalance between myocardial oxygen demand and supply.[129] In cases of massive overdose with diphenhydramine, myocardial function may be depressed and cardiac condition (wide QRS, AV block, slow junctional or idioventricular rhythm) may be impaired.[113]

If treatment is necessary because of hypotension, organ ischemia, or severe hypertension due to anticholinergic drugs, the most specific therapy is administration of a cholinesterase inhibitor. Physostigmine is most commonly used because it enters the brain and antagonizes both the central nervous system and peripheral autonomic effects. Alternatively, since anticholinergic drugs result in an imbalance between sympathetic and parasympathetic activity with a predominance of the former, propranolol may be effective in treating supraventricular tachyarrhythmias. Both physostigmine and propranolol may be hazardous and should be avoided in persons with depressed cardiac conduction or myocardial contractility (see the discussion of physostigmine in the section on tricyclic antidepressant drug poisoning later in this chapter).

Toxicology

Blood levels of drug correlate poorly with the clinical course in cases of sedative-hypnotic drug overdose. The reasons for this include different degrees of tolerance among casual and chronic users, the combined effects of several drugs in cases of mixed drug overdose, the presence of active metabolites not reflected by blood levels of the parent drug, and extensive tissue distribution of the drug.[156] Sequential determinations of blood level of drug are helpful in following the course of drug elimination, especially when coma is prolonged and there is a question of drug intoxication versus irreversible neurologic damage. Absence of electroencephalo-

*See Table 16–2.

Table 16–2. MANIFESTATIONS, MECHANISMS, AND TREATMENT OF COMPLICATIONS OF ANTICHOLINERGIC AND ANTIHISTAMINIC DRUG OVERDOSE

Drug	Manifestations	Mechanisms	Treatment
Atropine Belladonna Scopolamine Antihistamines (most over-the-counter hypnotics) Propantheline Plants (such as jimsonweed)	a. Sedation, delirium, coma, dry skin and mucous membranes, dilated pupils, reduced gastrointestinal motility, fever	Anticholinergic effects	None, physostigmine (for diagnosis, with caution)
	b. Myoclonus, convulsions*	Possibly antihistaminic action	Diazepam, phenytoin
	c. Sinus or atrial tachycardia	Anticholinergic effects	None (if hemodynamically stable), propranolol, physostigmine (if hypotensive or evidence of rate-related ischemia)
	d. Ventricular arrhythmias (usually with underlying ischemic heart disease)	Rate-related ischemia	Slow rate as above, lidocaine
	e. Conduction disturbances* (AV block, ↑ QRS)	Myocardial depression	None, pacing
	f. Bradyarrhythmias*		Isoproterenol (temporarily), pacing
	g. Hypotension*		Fluids, correct bradyarrhythmias, pressors

*Reported with diphenhydramine.

graphic activity followed by return of normal brain function has been reported after barbiturate intoxication.[82, 103]

Accelerated Drug Removal

A critical discussion of techniques for accelerating removal of sedative-hypnotic drugs from the body is beyond the scope of this chapter. A summary of these techniques is presented below, but the reader is referred elsewhere for more in-depth discussion.[149, 178] Repeated doses of charcoal by mouth or nasogastric tube and forced alkaline diuresis are useful in cases of phenobarbital overdose.[72, 131] As discussed earlier, the use of diuresis must be weighed against the substantial risks of pulmonary edema. Aqueous hemodialysis, lipid hemodialysis, and hemoperfusion with charcoal or adsorbent resins have all been proposed for cases of overdose with various sedative-hypnotic drugs. Hemoperfusion is a relatively new technique in which the patient's blood (usually obtained from the inferior vena cava via a femoral vein catheter) is pumped through a column (actually a cartridge) containing charcoal or a resin that adsorbs drugs from the blood, which is then returned to the patient via another venous catheter. In many cases it has been reported that substantial amounts of drug are removed from the body, but no controlled studies have been undertaken to demonstrate the effects of these procedures on the duration of coma or overall morbidity. Hemodialysis is especially efficacious for removal of water-soluble drugs such as methanol, ethylene glycol, salicylates, and chloral hydrate.[178] Hemoperfusion appears to be more effective in removal of lipid-soluble drugs; drugs with low intrinsic clearance and a relatively small volume of distribution, such as phenobarbital, are the best candidates.[149] Other sedative-hypnotic drugs with high intrinsic clearance and large distribution spaces are less effectively removed.

Sympathomimetic Drugs*

General Considerations

Sympathomimetic drugs include (1) stimulants such as amphetamine, methylphenidate (Ritalin), and cocaine, (2) hallucinogenic drugs such as phencyclidine, (3) anorectic agents such as phenylpropanolamine, and (4) the methylxanthine drugs caffeine and theophylline. Intoxication with these results in sinus or atrial tachycardia, hypertension (except from methylxanthines), generalized seizures, and (after massive ingestions) cardiovascular collapse and respiratory arrest. Ventricular arrhythmias occasionally occur.

Major causes of serious morbidity or death from stimulant drugs include the following: (1) Cerebrovascular accidents, which occur most likely as a result of hypertension.[43, 105] Patients with pre-existing vascular disease and persons taking monoamine oxidase–inhibiting drugs or large doses of amphetamines account for most of this category of deaths. (2) Cardiovascular complications, including arrhythmic deaths, which most likely arise as a result of ventricular fibrillation, and pulmonary edema.[7, 105] (3) Hyperpyrexia, with rhabdomyolysis, disseminated intravascular coagulation, and acute renal failure, which accounts for a significant number of late deaths.[69, 109, 167]

Hyperpyrexia usually occurs in patients with evidence of muscular hyperactivity (fasciculations, myoclonus, convulsions). Studies of amphetamine and cocaine toxicity in conscious dogs indicate that hyperpyrexia contributes significantly to death.[41] Pretreatment with pancuronium, which paralyzes the muscles that are the source of heat generation; diazepam, which prevents convulsions; chlorpromazine, which sedates the animal, lessens the severity of the seizures, and possibly also facilitates heat dissipation via peripheral alpha-adrenergic blockade and environmental cooling; all substantially improve survival. In contrast, propranolol, which effectively blocks cardiovascular responses to ampheta-

*See Table 16–3.

Table 16–3. MANIFESTATIONS, MECHANISMS, AND TREATMENT OF COMPLICATIONS OF SYMPATHOMIMETIC DRUG OVERDOSE

Drug	Manifestations	Mechanisms	Treatment
Sympathomimetic drugs (amphetamines, cocaine, phencyclidine, phenylpropanolamine, theophylline, and others)	a. Agitation, psychosis, convulsions, coma, cerebellar dysfunction*	All: release of catecholamines, direct stimulation of sympathetic nervous system	Minimize stimulation, diazepam, anticonvulsants
	b. Tachyarrhythmias		
	1. Sinus or atrial		None, propranolol, verapamil
	2. Ventricular		Propranolol, lidocaine, electrical cardioversion
	c. Hypertension		Phentolamine, sodium nitroprusside, beta-blocker (preferably β-1-selective) if associated with tachycardia
	d. Hyperthermia	Catecholamine excess, muscular hyperactivity	Stop seizures; paralysis (pancuronium) if seizures are uncontrollable, external cooling, oxygen, chlorpromazine or haloperidol†
	e. Hypotension, cardiovascular collapse		Fluids (may require large volume in presence of hyperthermia), pressors (unpredictable sensitivity)
	f. Rhabdomyolysis	Muscle hyperactivity	Fluids, mannitol, bicarbonate

*Especially phencyclidine.
†Experience is primarily in children with amphetamine intoxication.

mines, or bicarbonate infusion, which reverses metabolic acidosis, have not been reported to improve survival.[41]

Amphetamine-Like Drugs

Amphetamine (Benzedrine, Dexedrine), methamphetamine (Desoxyn), and many other amphetamine-like drugs (e.g., phenmetrazine [Preludin], diethylpropion [Tenuate], and fenfluramine [Pondimin]) are marketed as anorectic agents or, as for propylhexedrine (Benzedrex), nasal inhalers. The use of these, as well as illicitly manufactured amphetamines and their derivatives, has dramatically increased in recent years, as has that of cocaine. Stimulants are used for their euphoric effects, which are associated with central nervous system and adrenomedullary sympathetic activation, producing typical sympathomimetic syndromes and complications, as discussed earlier.

An opportunity for careful observation of massive cocaine overdose (presumably similar to massive amphetamine overdose) was afforded when a cocaine-filled condom ruptured in a patient's stomach during esophagoscopy.[177] Four hours after the balloon ruptured, extreme hypotension, tachycardia, apnea, and dilated nonreactive pupils occurred. Generalized seizures followed and required muscle paralysis by administration of pancuronium after anticonvulsants failed to control seizure activity. With respiratory support, fluids, and dopamine therapy, vital signs returned to normal in three hours although the patient remained comatose for many hours afterward. Gastrotomy was eventually performed to extract the remaining bag of cocaine. The picture of sudden onset of generalized seizures, followed by respiratory arrest, typically preceded death in one large series.[196]

Another type of overdose occurs with repeated use of amphetamine or cocaine over many hours or days.[21, 112] The duration of the euphoric effects of amphetamine and cocaine is usually much shorter than that of the actual presence of the drug in the blood. With repeat injections to maintain a "high," dangerous blood and tissue levels of the drugs can accumulate and produce increasing effects on the peripheral nervous system. For example, the speed or cocaine "freak" after a sustained period of drug use may appear flushed, diaphoretic, tachycardiac, and hypertensive and have cardiac arrhythmias at a time when he is no longer euphoric or is even depressed.

Recreational use of cocaine has been associated with myocardial ischemia and infarction.[44] Case reports of patients with cardiomyopathy suggest the possibility that chronic amphetamine abuse may result in myocarditis.[63, 168]

Amphetamines displace and release catecholamines stored in neurons, directly stimulate postsynaptic adrenergic receptors, and may inhibit monoamine oxidase, the enzyme responsible for intraneuronal degradation of catecholamines. Cocaine in particular is a potent inhibitor of neuronal catecholamine uptake, which is a major route of detoxification for norepinephrine released from nerve endings or the adrenal medulla, or administered exogenously.

Management of amphetamine and cocaine drug toxicity depends on the specific manifestations. Hypertension and tachycardia can be managed by alpha- and beta-adrenergic blocking agents or vasodilators such as sodium nitroprusside. Because arrhythmias result primarily from beta-adrenergic stimulation, a beta-blocking agent is the drug of choice. Theoretically, a relatively specific beta-1-blocker such as metoprolol is preferable in order not to antagonize the beta-2-mediated arteriolar dilation that may be opposing alpha-mediated constriction. Thus, beta-2-blockade could result in unopposed alpha-adrenergic effects and worsen hypertension.

Hyperpyrexia is potentially life threatening. Chlorpromazine or haloperidol may reverse hyperthermia by central nervous or peripheral vascular actions, as discussed previously.[41, 58] Although these drugs are known to lower seizure threshold in some experimental seizure models, chlorpromazine seems to lessen the severity of seizures due to sympathomimetic drugs. Seizures should be treated as rapidly and effectively as possible: intravenous administration of diazepam is usually effective in terminating them, but loading with phenytoin and, if necessary, phenobarbital should also be carried out.

If hyperthermia or severe metabolic acidosis complicates seizures or other evidence of muscular hyperactivity, external or internal cooling and paralysis with pancuronium or curare are indicated. Even when muscular hyperactivity is prevented by paralysis, persistent seizure activity may cause brain injury.[132] Therefore, electroencephalographic monitoring should be performed in paralyzed patients, and seizures should be controlled with anticonvulsant drugs or general anesthesia (thiopental or halothane) if necessary. Increased ventilation with high oxygen concentrations is indicated for all hyperthermic patients to meet the extreme metabolic demands of muscular hyperactivity and the effects of hyperthermia on metabolism in other body organs. Acute renal failure may result from hypovolemia, hypotension, and rhabdomyolysis with myoglobinuria, and may be prevented by vigorous fluid replacement and the use of mannitol and diuretics to increase urine flow, and by bicarbonate administration to alkalinize the urine.

In view of the catastrophic nature of adverse effects, tests of urinary and blood levels of amphetamine and cocaine are not usually helpful except to provide retrospective diagnostic information.

Renal elimination of amphetamine can be markedly accelerated by acidifying the urine.[79] However, the hazards of worsening systemic acidosis and of precipitating myoglobin in the kidney may outweigh possible benefits. When there is evidence of cocaine intoxication in a person who has swallowed bags or balloons of cocaine as a means of illicit drug transport (the "body packer" syndrome), surgical removal of unruptured packets of cocaine is recommended.[177]

Phencyclidine

Phencyclidine (PCP) has many of the stimulant actions of amphetamines, especially on the cardiovascular system, but also has prominent sedative and psychotomimetic actions. Use of PCP has increased tremendously in the past few years; it is smoked (sometimes in marijuana cigarettes), sniffed, injected intravenously, and ingested. Phencyclidine is sold as tetrahydrocannabinol (THC), lysergide (LSD), mescaline, or other drugs, and overdosed patients often do not know that they have taken PCP. The toxicity of PCP is significant and often leads to emergency room visits or hospitalization. Numerous deaths have been reported resulting from both pharmacologic toxicity and behavioral consequences of drug use.[38]

Most frequently, patients overdosed with PCP arrive at the emergency room with altered mental status ranging from an alcohol-like intoxication to agitated or catatonic psychosis and coma. Bizarre behavioral and neurologic signs are common and distinguish the PCP overdose from most other drug overdoses. The general signs and symptoms of PCP overdose on admission have been reviewed.[38, 107] Cerebellar dysfunction is almost always present and includes ataxia, spontaneous coarse horizontal and vertical nystagmus, and dysarthria. Convulsions may occur, and death due to status epilepticus with subsequent hypoxic neuronal degeneration has been reported. The cardiovascular complications of PCP resemble those of amphetamines. In most cases, hypertension and tachycardia are present.[38, 56] A case has been reported of severe hypertension in a 13-year-old boy after PCP overdose; intracerebral hemorrhage and death occurred.[56] Following large doses, hypotension and respiratory arrest develop.[186]

The mechanism of the pressor effect of PCP is believed to involve potentiation of the effects of endogenous catecholamines and possibly direct vasoconstrictor effects.[87, 95] There is some evidence suggesting that neuronal uptake of norepinephrine is blocked by PCP as it is by cocaine. Myocardial depression has been observed in isolated cardiac muscle preparations.[95] The pressor effects of PCP in animals are not blocked by ganglionic-blocking drugs or by adrenalectomy, but *are* blocked by alpha-adrenergic blockers, which suggests a direct alpha-adrenergic agonist effect.[95] With high doses of PCP in animals and humans, both hypotension and respiratory depression occur.[51, 186] A fascinating aspect of the pharmacology of PCP is that environmental stimulation aggravates the toxic state. Commonly, patients appear sedated and withdrawn when alone, but after external stimulation become extremely agitated. In our experience, blood pressure and heart rate are also extremely labile and increase markedly in association with behavioral agitation. This might again reflect increased sensitivity to endogenously released catecholamines.

Therapy for the cardiovascular complications caused by PCP consists of the use of alpha- and beta-adrenergic blocking drugs and vasodilators, as for amphetamines. Both nitroprusside and diazoxide have been used to treat PCP-induced hypertension. Because PCP enhances sensitivity to catecholamines, increased sensitivity to pressor drugs may be observed when these are used to treat hypertensive patients. Reduction of environmental stimulation is helpful in minimizing toxicity. Diazepam is often administered for sedation, and haloperidol to control extreme agitation.

Methods are available for measuring blood and urinary concentrations of PCP, and positive results confirm the diagnosis.[16] Since PCP is a weak base and partitions into acid, concentrations are higher in acidic than in neutral urine, and highest in acidic gastric juice. Acidification of urine has been shown to increase renal excretion of PCP.[52] PCP is eliminated from the body primarily by hepatic metabolism rather than renal excretion.[46] It is doubtful whether urinary acidification would increase renal clearance enough to have a significant effect on the course of the overdose, and (as discussed for amphetamines) acidification of the urine may aggravate kidney damage related to rhabdomyolysis.

Phenylpropanolamine and Other Over-the-Counter Sympathomimetic Drugs

Phenylpropanolamine, ephedrine, and many other over-the-counter decongestants and appetite-suppressant drugs have both direct and indirect (catecholamine-releasing) sympathomimetic effects. In most cases of overdose with cold or decongestant preparations, mild hypertension occurs but requires no specific therapy. Heart rate may be slow, owing to reflex slowing after ingestion of predominantly vasoconstrictor drugs such as phenylpropanolamine, or rapid, owing to coingested caffeine or anticholinergic antihistamines. After overdose and occasionally after therapeutic doses, severe hypertension may occur.[26,144,146] This may be associated with ventricular arrhythmias or SI-segment and T-wave changes on the ECG and abnormally elevated myocardial creatine kinase concentrations, suggesting myocardial injury.[44] Unusual responsiveness to catecholamines may explain some of the exaggerated blood pressure response in some patients. In one such patient, pressor hypersensitivity to infused norepinephrine related to a previously unrecognized autonomic insufficiency state was documented (Pentel, P., personal communication, 1982). Similar hypersensitivity to sympathomimetic drugs is expected in persons taking a tricyclic antidepressant and the antihypertensive drug guanethidine, which blocks uptake and increases pressor sensitivity to released catecholamines, respectively.[30,142]

Antihistamines found in common cold preparations may contribute to sympathomimetic-induced hypertension by inhibiting vagally mediated cardiac deceleration, which normally serves to compensate for vasoconstrictor-mediated hypertension.

Amphetamine "look-alikes," containing phenylpropanolamine, ephedrine, and/or caffeine, are available without prescription and are becoming increasingly popular. Several sudden deaths in the context of overdosage, presumably from arrhythmias, have been reported to the Food and Drug Administration.[128]

Management of overdose with phenylpropanolamine and related drugs includes careful monitoring of blood pressure and ECG monitoring. Management of hypertension, tachycardia, and arrhythmias is as discussed for amphetamines.

Theophylline and Caffeine

Cardiac toxicity of theophylline occurs in a different context from that of stimulant drugs. The most common circumstance is overdosage during therapy for obstructive airway disease, often as a result of hepatic dysfunction that reduces the rate of theophylline metabolism. Accidental or suicidal overdosage often occurs in persons with underlying medical illnesses. The nature and severity of these medical conditions impacts strongly on the course and severity of cardiac toxicity. Slow-release theophylline preparations are now widely prescribed. The physician should be alert to the possibility that a patient without much toxicity a few hours after an overdose may still be at risk of severe toxicity 12 or more hours after ingestion. Serial monitoring of blood theophylline concentrations is necessary to ensure that absorption is complete and that levels will not continue to rise.

The typical cardiovascular manifestations of theophylline overdose result from beta-adrenergic stimulation, and include tachycardia and arrhythmias.[57,98,159] Hypotension occurs more frequently than hypertension. Like amphetamines, theophylline causes systemic and local vascular catecholamine release and also (in high doses) may inhibit phosphodiesterase, an enzyme that degrades cyclic adenosine monophosphate, which in turn mediates beta-adrenergic actions. Theophylline also directly relaxes vascular smooth muscle. Convulsions typically occur with an overdose; cardiac and respiratory arrest are usual causes of death.[199] Administration of theophylline by means of central venous catheters has been found to be particularly hazardous, resulting in several cases of cardiac arrest.[40]

Management of cardiac toxicity due to theophylline in persons with chronic pulmonary disease may be difficult. Beta-adrenergic blocking agents are the most logical treatment for supraventricular and ventricular arrhythmias, but beta-blockers also worsen airway obstruction. Relatively cardiospecific beta-blockers such as metoprolol might be tried and the antiarrhythmic effects closely titrated against evidence of worsening airway obstruction.

Hypotension due to theophylline usually results from peripheral vasodilation, at least early in the course of overdose. However, in animals with prolonged beta-sympathetic stimulation due to theophylline, myocardial necrosis has been observed;[176] a similar event may contribute to hypertension late in the course of theophylline overdose in humans. In addition, many older patients with chronic pulmonary disease have ischemic heart disease. In the context of tachycardia and hypotension, myocardial perfusion may be inadequate and myocardial function impaired on that basis. Hypoxia due to underlying lung disease, hypokalemia due to sustained beta-adrenergic stimulation,[155] or acidosis due to pulmonary disease or convulsions may also contribute to hypotension.

Management of theophylline-induced hypotension includes correction of metabolic disturbances and arrhythmias, and administration of fluids and pressor agents. In cases of severe overdose, patients should be monitored with pulmonary arterial catheters. If pressor drugs are to be used, it is also useful to know the cardiac output and to be able to compute the systemic vascular resistance. If cardiac output is high and systemic vascular resistance low, as it is in many patients after theophylline overdose, administration of vasoconstrictors such as norepinephrine and beta-adrenergic antagonists is indicated. If cardiac output is low despite adequate cardiac filling pressures, and systemic vascular resistance is normal or high, as occurs sometimes late in the course of theophylline overdose and in persons with pre-existing myocardial disease, inotropic agents such as dobutamine might be selected.

In the presence of severe toxicity, particularly in a patient with serious underlying medical disease, the persistence of theophylline in the body and the time course of toxicity are quite prolonged; drug removal should be accelerated by institution of hemoperfusion.[57, 159]

Caffeine is widely consumed in beverages such as coffee and colas, in over-the-counter stimulants, and various other combination analgesic and cold medications. Caffeine has pharmacologic actions similar to those of theophylline. Caffeine potentiates the effects of sympathomimetic drugs and might contribute to adverse cardiac events, including sudden death from amphetamine "look-alikes" as discussed earlier. It is thought that caffeine alone causes severe cardiac toxicity only rarely, although cases of supraventricular tachycardias have been described.[24, 104] There are reports of severe caffeine intoxication with bradyarrhythmias followed by cardiovascular collapse in neonates.[18] We recently treated an adult for a massive ingestion of caffeine (No-Doz) tablets who had sinus tachycardia at a rate of 190 beats per minute, metabolic acidosis, hypokalemia, hyperglycemia, and extremely high levels of circulating catecholamines, particularly epinephrine.[24]

Narcotics*

Acute narcotic poisoning occurs in a variety of settings. Intravenous heroin overdose in the addict or casual user is most common. Overdoses with oral methadone and propoxyphene (Darvon) are less frequent but not uncommon. Morphine and meperidine (Demerol) overdose occasionally occurs during therapeutic administration. Death resulting from narcotic overdose, notably heroin, is well known and in most cases occurs before the patient can receive medical care. The mortality rate for narcotic overdose is low once treatment is initiated, and morbidity is low compared with that of sedative-hypnotic drug overdose, primarily because of the short

*See Table 16–4.

Table 16–4. MANIFESTATIONS, MECHANISMS, AND TREATMENT OF COMPLICATIONS OF NARCOTIC OVERDOSE

Manifestations	Mechanisms	Treatment
a. Respiratory depression, coma	Depression of CNS (medullary) respiratory center, other CNS functions	Naloxone, assisted ventilation
b. Hypothermia	Depression of CNS	None
c. Bradycardia	CNS-mediated increase in vagal, and decrease in sympathetic, tone	Naloxone
d. Atrial fibrillation		If rate is rapid, verapamil, propranolol, digitalis
e. Hypotension	Dilation of arteriolar and venous blood vessels	Naloxone, fluids
f. Pulmonary edema	Increase in pulmonary vascular permeability	Naloxone*, positive end-expiratory pressure, assisted ventilation if necessary
g. Seizures (propoxyphene, meperidine)	? Epileptogenic effect of toxic metabolite	Naloxone (large doses required), anticonvulsants

*May in some cases aggravate pulmonary edema (see text).

duration of action of narcotics and the availability of pharmacologic antagonists. Presentation and treatment of patients who overdose with the various narcotic drugs are similar, with differences relating mostly to the time course of toxicity and of the required treatment.

One large study of heroin overdose (149 patients) provides a good source of clinical data.[55] Toxicity was related primarily to neurologic depression. Patients were asleep or comatose and respirations were depressed. Pupils were characteristically pinpoint, although severe hypoxia or the presence of other drugs sometimes produced dilation. Bradycardia and hypotension were typically present. Arrhythmias were not common (4 per cent); atrial fibrillation was the most frequently reported arrhythmia. Atrial fibrillation with slow ventricular response has also been described; nalorphine has been reported to effect coarse fibrillation with a faster ventricular response rate and then sinus rhythm.[115]

The most important cardiopulmonary toxic effect of opiate overdosage is pulmonary edema.[65] This is common and a universal finding in fatalities. It may occur after intravenous, oral, or intranasal administration of any narcotic. Although pulmonary edema usually arises shortly after injection of heroin, its onset may be delayed one to two hours, may become evident after administration of an antagonist, or may develop as long as six hours after ingestion of methadone. Most likely, sudden reversal of narcotic-induced venodilation and venous pooling, combined with pulmonary capillary injury so that fluid enters the lungs at relatively low cardiac filling pressures, accounts for naloxone-induced pulmonary edema. The clinical manifestations are pulmonary rales, severe hypoxemia, and a radiologic picture of either a bilateral butterfly or patchy infiltrate. The condition is usually transient, but there are unusual cases of recurrent hypotension and pulmonary edema, possibly resulting from coexistent cardiomyopathy and left ventricular failure.[2, 143]

Narcotics generally have little effect on the myocardium, although norpropoxyphene, a major metabolite of propoxyphene, may be cardiotoxic.[140] Central nervous system effects of narcotics result in increased vagal activity. Narcotics dilate peripheral veins and arterioles, presumably through a CNS-mediated effect on sympathetic tone. Consequently, hypotension and relative bradycardia are common.

Prolongation of the Q-T interval and conduction disturbances have been described in heroin users,[121, 143] but the role of the narcotic per se in causing these disturbances has not been proved. Quinine and procaine as well as other local anesthetics commonly adulterate heroin sold on the streets, and may themselves contribute to myocardial depression or even cardiac arrest.

Blood concentrations of narcotics are not usually helpful in evaluating narcotic overdose because of extensive tissue distribution. Heroin is rapidly metabolized to morphine and is detected as such in the urine. Determinations of narcotic as well as quinine levels in the urine are useful in diagnosis.

The first step in treatment of suspected narcotic drug overdose is the use of a narcotic antagonist. Naloxone (Narcan) is a pure antagonist without agonist activity. It is administered intravenously in doses of 0.4 to 2.0 mg until a response is observed, which is usually immediate. The effects of heroin, morphine, and other short-acting narcotics may outlast the effects of naloxone, so multiple doses may be necessary. Because the effects of methadone may last beyond 12 hours, it has been proposed that a dilute solution of naloxone (0.04 mg/ml) be infused to titrate the antagonist effect. However, naloxone dose-related narcotic abstinence syndrome can be precipitated in addicts; a balance between persistent narcotic effect and severity of abstinence is desirable. If respiration does not increase after administration of naloxone, intubation and ventilatory support are required. Propoxyphene overdose differs from most other narcotic overdoses in the frequency of convulsions and the extremely high mortality. Doses of naloxone needed to reverse signs of narcotic intoxication are greater after propoxyphene than those required for other narcotic overdoses. Ventilation with positive pressure is usually sufficient treatment for pulmonary edema. Steroids have been proposed for heroin-induced pulmonary edema, but since their benefit is unproved and other measures are usually effective, they do not seem to be indicated. Usually, no specific therapy for arrhythmias is necessary. Naloxone has been reported to convert coarse atrial fibrillation to fine atrial fibrillation with a faster ventricular response rate, and then to normal sinus rhythm.[115] If atrial fibrillation with a rapid ventricular response rate persists, digitalis, verapamil, or propranolol is indicated to slow the rate.

Membrane-Depressant Drugs*

Quinidine and Other Type I Antiarrhythmic Drugs

Quinidine is the prototype membrane-depressant drug. Quinidine and other type I antiarrhythmic drugs (including procainamide and disopyramide) impede the fast sodium current across cardiac cell membranes and slow conduction, particularly in the His-Purkinje system.[88] In toxic doses, slowed conduction is demonstrated by progressively marked Q-T prolongation, QRS widening, or AV block, with loss of atrial activity and slow ventricular rhythm.[62] Ventricular tachycardia and fibrillation may occur after therapeutic doses ("quinidine syncope") as well as overdose.[152] Ventricular tachycardia in the presence of long Q-T interval is characteristically of the polymorphous (torsades de pointes) type characterized by undulation of the QRS polarity about an isoelectric point.[172] The prolonged Q-T interval is believed to be caused by asynchronous repolarization of His-Purkinje fibers, which predisposes to ventricular arrhythmias. In addition to its electrophysiologic effects, quinidine in large doses depresses myocardial contractility and relaxes blood vessels, resulting in hypotension. In cases of massive overdose, this may produce shock. Disopyramide, and quinidine to a lesser extent, also have anticholinergic effects that may result in sinus tachycardia after a mild overdose.

Therapeutic options for ventricular tachycardia due to quinidine or quinidine-like drugs include lidocaine, phenytoin, isoproterenol, bretylium, and cardiac pacing.[6, 48, 106, 111, 141, 188] Isoproterenol, which increases the heart rate and shortens the Q-T interval, is recommended by some as the drug of choice, although the prospect of treating ventricular tachycardia with catecholamines is believed too hazardous by other clinicians. Treatment of conduction disturbances and hypotension are discussed below under tricyclic antidepressant toxicity. For a more detailed discussion of the pathogenesis and management of poisoning with quinidine and type I antiarrhythmic drugs, the reader is referred to a recent review.[22]

Tricyclic Antidepressant and Antipsychotic Drugs

Tricyclic antidepressants (TCAs) and antipsychotic drugs are in wide clinical use. Significant cardiovascular toxicity during therapeutic use and after overdosage is well documented. Although the severity of cardiovascular complications and the resultant fatalities are much greater with TCAs than with phenothiazine or other antipsychotic drugs, the pharmacologic effects of TCAs

*See Table 16–5.

Table 16–5. MANIFESTATIONS, MECHANISMS, AND TREATMENT OF COMPLICATIONS OF MEMBRANE-DEPRESSANT DRUG OVERDOSE

Drug	Manifestations	Mechanisms	Treatment
Membrane-depressant drugs (quinidine, tricyclic antidepressants, phenothiazines)	a. Arrhythmias		
	1. Sinus tachycardia (often with wide QRS complex)	Anticholinergic effects, inhibition of neuronal catecholamine uptake	None, propranolol, physostigmine (cautiously, see text)
	2. Atrial tachycardia or fibrillation	Anticholinergic effects, inhibition of neuronal catecholamine uptake	Same as above plus verapamil, cardioversion
	3. Conduction defects (↑ QRS, ↑ Q-T, AVB, BBB)	Depressed sodium conductance across myocardial cell membranes	Sodium bicarbonate or lactate, intracardiac pacing
	4. Ventricular premature beats and tachycardia (often polymorphous)	Depression of cardiac conduction (as above), with temporal dispersion of action potential duration and reentrant excitation	Sodium bicarbonate or lactate, lidocaine, phenytoin, overdrive pacing, isoproterenol, bretylium
	5. Bradyarrhythmias (usually junctional or ventricular)	Myocardial depression as described above	Atropine, isoproterenol, pacemaker*
	b. Hypotension	Blockade of peripheral alpha-adrenergic receptors, quinidine-like depression of myocardial function, inhibition of CNS sympathetic tone, arrhythmias (see above)	Fluids (hemodynamic monitoring advised if evidence of cardiac failure or myocardial depression), treat bradyarrhythmias, dopamine, norepinephrine (if low systemic vascular resistance), dobutamine, isoproterenol (if low cardiac output), intra-aortic balloon pump or cardiopulmonary bypass (if intractable cardiogenic shock)
	c. Convulsions, coma	?CNS antihistaminic and/or anticholinergic effects	Diazepam, phenytoin, phenobarbital, halothane, or barbiturate
	d. Hyperthermia	Muscular hyperactivity, anticholinergic inhibition of sweating as route of heat dissipation	Stop seizures, pancuronium if seizures are uncontrollable, external cooling; oxygen

*May require higher than usual pacing voltage.
AVB = atrioventricular block, BBB = bundle branch block.

and phenothiazines are similar. For this reason we discuss them together and point out important differences. There are several classes of antipsychotic drugs. The phenothiazines, such as chlorpromazine (Thorazine), have been most prescribed and studied best. In this chapter we refer to the phenothiazines as representative of the entire group of antipsychotic drugs except when specific differences among drugs are discussed.

A common cardiovascular effect of therapeutic doses of TCAs and phenothiazines is postural hypotension.[64, 102] Hypotension is most pronounced at the initiation of therapy, but tolerance develops after several weeks. Syncope and myocardial infarction, probably due to postural hypotension, have been reported to arise shortly after initiation of treatment with TCAs in the elderly and in patients with pre-existing cardiovascular disease. Electrocardiographic changes are quite common with both TCAs and phenothiazines,[28, 94] and occur in as many as 50 per cent of patients receiving thioridazine (Mellaril).[94] Abnormalities include prolongation of the P-R and Q-T intervals, U-wave and T-wave abnormalities such as broadening and notching, and T-wave inversion. With high doses, prolongation of the QRS interval and varying degrees and types of AV block have been observed. Prolongation of the QRS interval is believed to be a sign of therapeutic overdosage and is an indication to decrease the dose. The clinical significance of T-wave changes is unknown; they can be reversed in some cases by an overnight fast or by potassium loading.[5] Most clinicians do not believe that T-wave changes are a contraindication to continued treatment. Arrhythmias, including ventricular tachycardia, ventricular fibrillation, and AV block, followed by sudden death have been reported in patients (some otherwise healthy) receiving both TCAs and phenothiazines in therapeutic doses.[4, 28, 118] Although there is always concern in treating patients with heart disease, a recent report indicates that patients with chronic atherosclerotic or hypertensive heart disease, even with impaired myocardial function, can be treated safely with therapeutic doses of imipramine or doxepin.[190]

The mortality rate for cases of TCA overdose is substantial, the cause of death being primarily cardiovascular. Death from phenothiazine overdose does occur[54] but is relatively uncommon in adults. Arrhythmias and hypotension are the major cardiovascular complications. Hypertension has also been reported in less severe cases of overdose with TCAs.

The mechanisms of cardiotoxicity of TCA and phenothiazine drugs are similar. Differences in overall effect probably reflect different potencies with respect to various actions and different concentrations in cardiac tissue. The TCAs and their potentially toxic metabolites are concentrated in myocardial tissue to a greater extent than are the phenothiazines.[154] The major pharmacologic effects that contribute to cardiotoxicity are listed below. (1) Anticholinergic effects are particularly prominent with TCAs and sedative phenothiazines, and probably explain the commonly observed sinus tachycardia. Anticholinergic effects also delay gastric emptying and lead to erratic and delayed absorption, which may account for the sudden or late deterioration of patients overdosed with TCAs. (2) Neuronal catecholamine uptake is inhibited significantly by TCAs in therapeutic doses and by phenothiazines in large doses. This effect accounts for the hypertension that occurs when exogenous sympathomimetic drugs are administered to patients receiving TCAs.[50] The combination of the anticholinergic effect and the excessive effects of circulating catecholamines, resulting from inhibition of neuronal uptake, explains the high cardiac output with normal or increased blood pressure that is present after mild-to-moderate TCA overdose.[183] (3) Quinidine-like effects on the myocardium occur with both TCAs and phenothiazines.[12, 195] In therapeutic doses, TCAs and phenothiazines may have antiarrhythmic effects.[27] Depression of myocardial contractility and impaired intracardiac conduction can occur in overdosed patients.[192] (4) Peripheral alpha-adrenergic receptor blockade occurs with both classes of drugs and probably explains early postural hypotension. Hypotension in patients after TCA overdose may result in part from alpha-adrenergic blockade. (5) Phenothiazines and possibly also TCAs act on the cardiovascular control area of the central nervous system to inhibit sympathetic reflexes.[193]

Thus, in mild and moderate cases of TCA overdose, anticholinergic effects and increased circulating catecholamines result in supraventricular tachycardia, increased cardiac output, and normal or increased blood pressure.[184] In severe cases, impaired intracardiac conduction and depressed myocardial contractility predominate and hypotension occurs. Prolongation of the QRS interval is nearly universal in cases of serious TCA toxicity.[147] Bundle branch block, AV block, and slow ventricular rhythm and asystole occur in the most severe poisonings. Responsiveness to electrical stimulation is decreased so that pacing thresholds are often higher than normal, and in extreme cases the heart does not respond at all to pacing. Hypotension usually results from depressed cardiac output. Cardiac output may be reduced owing to venous pooling with inadequate cardiac filling (associated with low PCW pressure),[116] or in more severe poisoning to myocardial depression alone (with normal or high wedge pressure).

The cardiovascular complications of phenothiazine overdose are similar, but the arrhythmias tend not to be malignant and profound circulatory shock is uncommon. Clinically, it appears that mixed TCA and phenothiazine overdose poses a particular risk of high-degree AV block, severe bradyarrhythmias, and asystole.

In view of the substantial risk of cardiotoxicity with TCAs, there has been some concern about choosing the least cardiotoxic of them. Tertiary TCAs (amitriptyline [Elavil] and imipramine [Tofranil]) may be more toxic because of their greater anticholinergic effects and because the major metabolites are also cardioactive.[99, 154] Doxepin (Sinequan) is alleged to be less cardiotoxic and is a less potent inhibitor of catecholamine uptake than amitriptyline.[89] The claim of less cardiotoxicity is supported by one study that shows less depression of infranodal conduction during His bundle electrocardiography in patients overdosed with doxepin than in those overdosed with other TCAs;[192] although the clinical condition was reported to be comparable, the authors did not report blood levels of drug with which one might estimate myocardial tissue exposure. At similar concentrations, the electrophysiologic effects of imipramine and doxepin in vitro are similar.[34] Several new antidepressant drugs of different pharmacologic classes, including amoxapine, maprotiline, and trazodone, appear to have substantially less cardiac toxicity. There are reports of severe intoxication with amoxapine resulting in convulsions and even death, but without evidence of cardiac depression.[73, 114] Clinical experience with poisonings from maprotiline or trazodone is still scanty.

With respect to the relative cardiotoxicity of different phenothiazines, adverse electrophysiologic effects are reported most frequently with the piperidyl antipsychotics (thioridazine [Mellaril] and mesoridazine [Serentil]), less frequently with chlorpromazine, and infrequently with the butyrophenones (haloperidol [Haldol]). An inverse relationship between autonomic-cardiovascular and antipsychotic potency has been proposed.[33] Since adverse cardiovascular effects are relatively uncommon with haloperidol, it has been recommended for use in high-risk patients, despite reports of cardiotoxicity even with this drug.[161]

The relationship between blood levels of TCAs and effects in overdosed patients has received considerable attention. The best clinical correlate to a plasma level of 1000 ng per ml, signifying a severe overdose, is a QRS duration of 100 msec.[147] Conversely, an awake patient with no evidence of anticholinergic effects and a QRS interval of less than 100 msec, assuming absorption is complete, is unlikely to be seriously intoxicated. In a small series, TCAs were found to have a half-life ranging from 25 to 81 hours, with a mean of 45 hours in overdosed patients.[174]

Toxicologic analysis in cases of phenothiazine overdose consists of qualitative screening of blood and urine. Because of the large number of active metabolites, it is impossible to use blood levels to predict outcome or as a guide to therapy.

Management of cardiovascular complications of TCA and phenothiazine overdoses primarily involves treatment of arrhythmias and hypotension. In view of the frequency and unpredictability of arrhythmias, cardiac monitoring should be provided for patients in coma or with a wide QRS interval until they are free of arrhythmias and have normal ECG results for 24 hours.

Whether patients recovering from TCA overdose remain at risk of cardiac arrhythmias and sudden death for days or weeks has been a topic of considerable debate. Analysis of large series of poisoned patients indicates that late cardiac complications are indeed rare, and that nearly all "late" complications occur within 24 hours of resolution of manifestations of poisoning.[78] Intensive monitoring for 24 hours therefore appears reasonable.

Specific therapy for TCA overdose should be tailored to the particular cardiovascular disturbance. Sinus tachycardia and supraventricular arrhythmias, if associated with hemodynamic disturbances (either excessive hypertension or hypotension), can be controlled with physostigmine or propranolol. As discussed previously, these drugs can depress cardiac conduction and should be avoided, if possible, when membrane-depressant effects, manifested by the presence of a wide QRS interval, AV block, or bradyarrhythmias, are present, unless a temporary cardiac pacemaker is in place. Severe bradyarrhythmias and asystole have occurred after treatment with physostigmine.[145]

Administration of either sodium bicarbonate or lactate or hyperventilation to correct acidemia and induce alkalemia has a dramatic effect in reducing arrhythmias in animals and (anecdotally) humans.[35, 36] The use of bicarbonate may be safer than hyperventilation because the hypocapnia due to the latter may lower the seizure threshold, and seizures are a common and serious complication of TCA overdose. The mechanism of beneficial effects of sodium bicarbonate therapy is not proved, but most likely results from reducing extracellular potassium or increasing extracellular sodium concentrations, which improve membrane responsiveness and increase conduction velocity in fast-response (His-Purkinje) cells.

Administration of lidocaine or phenytoin is the treatment of choice for ventricular arrhythmias. Phenytoin therapy has been reported in an uncontrolled study to improve intraventricular conduction,[81] but its superior antiarrhythmic efficacy as compared with lidocaine or a more favorable outcome in patients treated with phenytoin is unproved. Type I antiarrhythmic drugs (quinidine, procainamide, disopyramide), which have additive membrane-depressant effects, should be avoided. Because of the possible role of excess catecholamine stimulation in causing ventricular arrhythmias, propranolol has also been recommended[66] but, as discussed earlier, may be hazardous in patients with bradycardia or AV block. Overdrive pacing has been used successfully to treat ventricular tachycardia due to quinidine[6] or phenothiazines,[123] and would be expected to be useful in treating TCA overdose also. Bretylium should be considered for refractory ventricular tachycardia or fibrillation, although it might worsen the hypotension.

Intracardiac pacing is indicated in patients with high-grade AV block. If intraventricular conduction is worsening (i.e., if the QRS complex is widening) early in the clinical course when the extent of ultimate myocardial depression is not yet known, prophylactic pacing is advised because of the chance of sudden deterioration. The presence of sinus or ventricular bradycardia, rather than the usual supraventricular tachycardia, indicates severe toxicity and warrants pacing also. Bradyarrhythmias associated with reduced cardiac output and hypotension can be treated with isoproterenol until intracardiac pacing can be accomplished.

In addition to the usual supportive methods, a number of specific treatments have been suggested for complicated TCA or phenothiazine overdose. Physostigmine (Antilirium) has been recommended because it is an inhibitor of acetylcholinesterase and reverses the atropine-like effect of TCAs.[139, 157] Physostigmine can awaken a comatose patient after TCA overdose[10] and has been alleged to stop seizures in some cases. It may also be effective in slowing sinus and supraventricular tachyarrhythmias, presumably by its vagotonic effect. Successful treatment of ventricular tachycardia with physostigmine has been described, but reports do not differentiate supraventricular tachycardia with rate-related aberrant conduction from ventricular tachycardia. In the presence of a wide QRS interval or other manifestations of heart block, physostigmine may produce sinus bradycardia or complete heart block, with a slow idioventricular rhythm or even asystole.[145] Physostigmine may also aggravate hypotension, unless it is secondary to rapid heart rate. Because of the potential for serious toxicity, we recommend physostigmine for only the following indications: (1) supraventricular tachyarrhythmias that are contributing to hypertension, hypotension, or myocardial ischemia; and (2) severe or prolonged coma in patients with underlying medical disease in whom coma, if untreated, would contribute to substantial morbidity or mortality. Physostigmine is administered by intravenous infusion slowly over 30 to 60 seconds. Recommended doses for adults are 0.5 to 2 mg, repeated at 10- to 20-minute intervals until a maximal dose of 4 mg has been given. The duration of action of physostigmine is 30 to 60 minutes, so it may be necessary to repeat the doses at those intervals. Patients receiving physostigmine should be monitored electrocardiographically, and atropine sulfate in a dose one half of the physostigmine dose should be ready to be administered, if necessary, to reverse any undesirable cardiovascular effects of physostigmine.

Hypotension is common after a TCA overdose. In many patients hypotension can be managed successfully with fluids. If pressors are required, alpha-adrenergic agonists such as norepinephrine or dopamine are preferred. In the presence of selective alpha-blockade due to TCAs, the predominant effects of mixed alpha- and beta-agonists, such as epinephrine, may be beta-mediated vasodilation and worsening of hypotension. Dobutamine may be useful in managing myocardial depression with normal or increased vascular resistance. Profound cardiogenic shock resulting from TCA overdose is often unresponsive to medical treatment and has a poor prognosis. In these cases, extracorporeal circulatory aids such as cardiopulmonary bypass or intra-aortic balloon pumping may be the only means of sustaining life until the body can eliminate the drug. The successful use of intra-aortic balloon pumping has been reported for quinidine intoxication associated with intractable shock.[163]

In view of extensive tissue distribution and a high degree of protein binding in the plasma, hemodialysis is not useful in patients with TCA or phenothiazine overdose. Although the percentage of total body TCA removed by hemoperfusion is small, some temporary clinical benefit has been attributed to this procedure.[187] In extremely severe cases of overdose in which a few extra hours might improve the chance of survival, hemoperfusion might be attempted.

Digitalis*

Mortality and major morbidity from digitalis overdose result from arrhythmias, heart block, and hyperkalemia.[171] Digitalis inhibits the sodium-potassium ATPase-dependent pump located on the cell membrane. In the therapeutic situation this results in greater calcium movement into the cell, which is believed to account for increased myocardial contractility. After an overdose, disruption of sodium and potassium movement across membranes results in depressed conduction velocity, as described for membrane-depressant drugs. In addition, automaticity of previously nonautomatic tissue is enhanced, which is related to an increased rate of diastolic depolarization and possibly to spontaneous after-depolarizations ("triggered" rhythms).[47] Digitalis may also increase sympathetic and parasympathetic neural activity.[173] Sympathetic stimulation enhances automaticity and excitability, whereas parasympathetic stimulation further decreases conduction velocity. Thus, an overdose with digitalis is characterized by arrhythmias demonstrating both increased automaticity and depressed intracardiac conduction.

Tachyarrhythmias from digitalis intoxication typically include ectopic atrial tachycardia with AV block, AV junctional tachycardia, and ventricular tachycardia or fibrillation. Ventricular arrhythmias are reported to occur more commonly in persons with underlying heart disease. Bradyarrhythmias include sinus bradycardia, sinoatrial block, second-degree and complete AV block, atrial fibrillation or flutter with slow ventricular response, idioventricular rhythm, and asystole. Severe hyperkalemia due to inhibition of sodium-potassium exchange in skeletal muscle can contribute to AV block and depressed myocardial excitability.

Therapy for digitalis-induced arrhythmias is directed at the specific arrhythmia and normalization of serum potassium. Supraventricular arrhythmias often do not require specific treatment because the ventricular response is usually moderate. If necessary, propranolol may be used to treat atrial tachycardia. Patients who have been taking diuretics chronically may be depleted of potassium,

*See Table 16–6.

Table 16–6. MANIFESTATIONS, MECHANISMS, AND TREATMENT OF COMPLICATIONS OF DIGITALIS OVERDOSE

Manifestations	Mechanisms	Treatment
a. Tachyarrhythmias		
1. Supraventricular: Atrial tachycardia with AV block, junctional tachycardia	Inhibition of sodium-potassium ATPase pump with increased automaticity, after-depolarizations, decreased AV conduction velocity, increased vagal and sympathetic activity	None, propranolol, potassium (only if serum potassium is low)
2. Ventricular		Phenytoin, lidocaine, propranolol, potassium (if serum level is low), digoxin antibodies
b. Bradyarrhythmias:		
1. Sinus bradycardia, sinoatrial block, high-grade AV block, atrial fibrillation with slow ventricular response, idioventricular rhythm	Increased refractory period of AV node, increased parasympathetic (vagal) activity, hyperkalemia	Correct hyperkalemia (resins, glucose and insulin), atropine, isoproterenol, intracardiac pacing, digoxin antibodies

Table 16–7. MANIFESTATIONS, MECHANISMS, AND TREATMENT OF COMPLICATIONS OF SYMPATHETIC-INHIBITORY DRUG OVERDOSE

Drug	Manifestations	Mechanisms	Treatment
Propranolol and other beta-blockers, methyldopa, clonidine, other antihypertensive drugs	a. Bradyarrhythmias: Sinus bradycardia, AV block, junctional or ventricular bradycardia	Beta- or central sympathetic blockade, membrane depression (propranolol)	None, atropine, isoproterenol, glucagon, cardiac pacing
	b. Ventricular arrhythmias	Escape during bradyarrhythmias, membrane depression (long Q-T)	Treat bradyarrhythmias, lidocaine, phenytoin, overdrive pacing
	c. Hypotension, cardiogenic shock	Beta- or central sympathetic blockade, membrane depression (propranolol)	Treat bradyarrhythmias as above, fluids, glucagon, dobutamine, dopamine
	d. Hypertension (clonidine and occasionally methyldopa, or guanethidine)	Direct alpha-agonist, catecholamine release	Phentolamine, nitroprusside

and supraventricular tachyarrhythmias may respond to potassium supplementation. However, potassium may depress AV conduction and, as described earlier, life-threatening hyperkalemia may be present. Quinidine-like membrane depressants should be avoided in treating digitalis-intoxicated patients. Phenytoin has been reported to be particularly effective in treating arrhythmias as it may enhance AV conduction while depressing automaticity.[158] Lidocaine and propranolol have likewise been used to treat ventricular arrhythmias; the latter may also worsen conduction disturbances.

Sinus bradycardia and AV conduction block, in light of the vagal actions of digitalis, may respond to atropine. Isoproterenol is usually effective in treating bradyarrhythmias refractory to atropine, but can result in increased ventricular excitability; intracardiac pacing is preferred in patients with complete AV or second-degree heart block, or when bradyarrhythmias result in hemodynamic compromise. Correction of hyperkalemia may in itself revert AV block.

Since the course of toxicity after ingestion of most digitalis preparations lasts for several days, an attempt to accelerate removal of digitalis from the body should be considered. Techniques include repeated doses of cholestyramine or activated charcoal to interrupt enterohepatic recycling[39, 148] and/or hemoperfusion for digitoxin, and digoxin-specific antibodies for digoxin or digitoxin.[170]

Sympathetic-Inhibiting Drugs*

Beta-Adrenergic Receptor Blockers

Cardiac disturbances due to beta-adrenergic receptor blockers result from both receptor blockade, which all drugs in this class demonstrate, and other actions such as membrane-depressant or sympathomimetic effects, which differ among drugs within the class.[47A, 68] Beta-adrenergic blockade itself is associated with sinus bradycardia, AV block (usually first-degree), and sometimes the emergence of ectopic escape pacemakers in healthy hearts. In persons with underlying cardiac conduction disease, advanced AV block with slow ventricular rhythms can occur. In the presence of underlying myocardial disease such that contractility is dependent on sympathetic activity, beta-adrenergic receptor blockade can result in hypotension or cardiac failure, including shock or acute pulmonary edema and death.

Large doses of beta-blockers such as propranolol with membrane-depressant effects can directly depress myocardial function and result in hypotension due to reduced cardiac output in previously healthy persons.[68] Drugs such as pindolol with intrinsic sympathomimetic activity can cause tachycardia and hypertension despite concurrent beta-blockade after an overdose.

*See Table 16–7.

Sinus bradycardia is usually well tolerated and requires no specific therapy. If it results in hemodynamic compromise, atropine, isoproterenol, glucagon, or intracardiac pacing should be considered. Owing to the competitive nature of drug-induced beta-blockade, extraordinary doses of isoproterenol may be required to increase the heart rate. The dose may be limited by peripheral vasodilation and a fall in blood pressure. Advanced AV block is an indication for intracardiac pacing.

Hypotension can usually be managed with fluids and correction of bradyarrhythmias. In the presence of myocardial depression, glucagon, which activates adenylate cyclase by a nonadrenergic mechanism, may enhance myocardial contractility and increase cardiac output.[96, 160] Dobutamine and epinephrine are potentially useful inotropic agents, although the doses may need to be higher than usual because of beta-blockade.

Sympatholytic Antihypertensive Drugs

Most patients who have ingested excessive doses of sympatholytic antihypertensive drugs have sinus bradycardia and hypotension when first seen. Drugs such as methyldopa, clonidine, and reserpine, which are active in the central nervous system, commonly cause sedation or coma. In addition, after an overdose of clonidine, miosis and respiratory depression resembling narcotic overdose can also be present.[45] However, after clonidine poisoning, hypotension and bradycardia are more prominent than respiratory depression. The reverse is true for narcotics. Clonidine (by direct alpha-adrenergic receptor agonist activity) and methyldopa, reserpine, and guanethidine (through systemic release of catecholamines) have also been associated with transient and sometimes severe hypertension.

In most cases, hypotension resulting from antihypertensive drug overdose is not severe and can be managed by placing the patient in the Trendelenburg position and by intravenous administration of fluids. When hypotension is severe in the presence of bradycardia, atropine, isoproterenol, or cardiac pacing will increase heart rate and cardiac output and may increase blood pressure. Although not often necessary, modest doses of dopamine or norepinephrine are usually effective. Hypertension resulting from clonidine or other sympatholytic drugs is best treated with the short-acting alpha-adrenergic receptor antagonist phentolamine, and if necessary by vasodilators such as nitroprusside. It should be recognized that the hypertensive phase is relatively brief, and treatment should be tapered before the subsequent hypotensive effects manifest.

Since clonidine exerts its hypotensive and sedating effects by actions on alpha-receptors in the brain, the use of centrally active alpha-blockers such as tolazoline has been recommended for treating clonidine overdose. Although tolazoline can reverse the effects of therapeutic doses of clonidine,[133] no benefit has been proved for its use in the treatment of clonidine overdose. Most clonidine-intoxicated patients respond to supportive care, and so we do not use tolazoline. Clonidine has been shown to reduce symptoms of narcotic withdrawal and is used as an adjunct in treating such symptoms.[71] (This explains recent epidemics of clonidine overdose in heroin addicts.) Conversely, high doses of naloxone in animals reverse the hypotension and bradycardia due to clonidine,[59] and might be expected to be of benefit in overdose cases in humans. Our experience and that of others[17] has not confirmed its usefulness in moderate doses (up to 0.1 mg/kg).

Salicylates*

Aspirin is the most widely used medication in the world. Salicylate intoxication is relatively common and occurs both in single, large, accidental or suicidal overdose situations and during the course of salicylate therapy. The latter occurs most commonly in young children, in the elderly, and in patients being treated for rheumatologic disorders. In a recent series of 73 cases, young suicidal patients were usually diagnosed early and responded well to treatment.[8] Mortality in this group was 2 per cent (one death), and there were a few complications. Older patients more often became intoxicated while taking salicylate for medical problems; diagnosis and treatment were often delayed and mortality was high (25 per cent), with frequent complications.

The ingestion of slow-release salicylate preparations may result in a misleading clinical picture of a patient who looks well six

*See Table 16–8.

Table 16–8. MANIFESTATIONS, MECHANISMS, AND TREATMENT OF COMPLICATIONS OF SALICYLATE OVERDOSE

Manifestations	Mechanisms	Treatment
a. Hyperventilation, respiratory alkalosis (with potassium loss)	Direct stimulation of CNS (medullary) respiratory center	Fluids, potassium
b. Metabolic acidosis	Uncoupling of oxidative phosphorylation, disruption of enzymes of secondary metabolism	Bicarbonate, hemodialysis (if unable to give bicarbonate owing to pulmonary edema or in presence of renal insufficiency)
c. Hyperthermia	Increase in metabolic rate secondary to above	Fluids, cooling
d. Pulmonary edema	Increased pulmonary vascular permeability	Positive end-expiratory pressure, assisted ventilation if necessary
e. Encephalopathy, seizures, coma, cardiopulmonary collapse	Cerebral hypoglycemia, cerebral edema	Glucose, bicarbonate to correct metabolic acidosis
		All: facilitate drug removal: alkalinization of urine (potassium, bicarbonate), active drug removal (hemodialysis, hemoperfusion)

hours after overdose, but who becomes severely intoxicated with rapid deterioration at home after discharge from the emergency room. Patients who ingest slow-release preparations should be monitored in the hospital with frequent measurement of blood salicylate concentrations, at least until concentrations are clearly declining.

Patients with salicylism can have significant cardiopulmonary manifestations on admission to the hospital.[180] Even at therapeutic blood levels of salicylate, uncoupling of oxidative phosphorylation occurs, resulting in increased oxygen consumption and production of carbon dioxide and consequent increased ventilation. At toxic blood levels of salicylate, the medullary respiratory center is stimulated directly, causing tachypnea, respiratory alkalosis, and dyspnea. Hypokalemia may occur owing to increased renal bicarbonate and potassium excretion or vomiting. Enzymes of secondary metabolism are disrupted, resulting in accumulation of organic acids and ketone bodies, and subsequently in metabolic acidosis. These enzymes are more easily disrupted in young children, so that metabolic acidosis and coma occur with lower blood levels of salicylate, and therefore after relatively smaller overdoses than in adults. The adult when first evaluated most commonly has respiratory alkalosis, but late in the course of the overdose this frequently develops into metabolic acidosis. A mixed stage may intervene in which blood pH is within normal limits owing to the balanced effects of metabolic acidosis and respiratory alkalosis. Fever is common throughout the course and contributes to hypovolemia.

Pulmonary edema is a common cause of salicylate morbidity.[8, 31, 85] In one report, pulmonary edema was present on admission to the hospital in 10 per cent of cases and developed in an additional 4 per cent during the course of aggressive fluid therapy. In another report, pulmonary edema was present at the time of admission in eight (22%) of 36 consecutive patients with blood levels of salicylate > 30 mg/dl.[85] Patients with pulmonary edema were more likely to be older cigarette smokers who ingested aspirin chronically, and frequently were lethargic or confused on admission. In four patients the pulmonary edema was mild and cleared rapidly, but in another four individuals severe pulmonary edema required intubation and ventilation with high concentrations of oxygen and positive end-expiratory pressures. Pulmonary capillary wedge pressures are reported to be normal or low after salicylate overdose, which is consistent with a defect in pulmonary vascular permeability, as discussed previously.[31, 91]

Other manifestations of salicylate poisoning, in approximate order of appearance and with increasing severity of intoxication, include tinnitus, decreased auditory acuity, confusion, agitation, and dysarthria. Generalized seizures and coma occur late and indicate a poor prognosis. Abnormal bleeding occasionally occurs as a result of salicylate-induced impairment of clotting factor synthesis and platelet function. Rarely, renal failure and hepatic toxicity occur.

Death from salicylate poisoning is usually due to cardiopulmonary arrest, which is believed to be an effect of salicylates on the central nervous system, or to medical complications during the course of prolonged coma. In either case, the emphasis in treatment is on prevention of toxicity to the central nervous system. In animals, the severity of intoxication has been correlated with brain salicylate levels and cerebral hypoglycemia.[37, 86, 185]

Blood levels of salicylate, when corrected for time of ingestion, have been found to be roughly predictive of severity of intoxication.[53] Salicylate is primarily metabolized by the liver at low doses, but with the high doses that occur in poisoned patients the metabolizing enzymes are saturated.[119] Thus, at high doses, renal excretion is the major route of elimination.

Therapy for cardiopulmonary complications is supportive. Particular therapeutic measures include replacement of potassium and fluid deficits, correction of acidosis, and treatment of hyperthermia with cooling. Since cerebral hypoglycemia can occur even with normal blood concentrations of glucose, glucose should be administered intravenously unless the blood level is already high. In experimental animals, glucose infusion has been shown to prevent hypoglycemic brain damage and death during the course of salicylate poisoning.[185] Correction of acidosis is also especially important because salicylate is a weak acid that preferentially partitions into the brain, thereby increasing toxicity to the central nervous system, during systemic acidosis.[37, 86] This explains the rapid clinical deterioration that can occur as salicylate-intoxicated patients pass from the stage of respiratory alkalosis to that of metabolic acidosis. Alkalinization of blood and urine minimizes passage of salicylate into the brain and enhances renal excretion. Realistic therapeutic goals are a normal or slightly alkaline blood pH and a urine pH of 7 or greater. Although forced diuresis increases renal excretion of salicylate,[117, 134] it is hazardous because of the risk of pulmonary edema. Urine alkalinization is usually accomplished with potassium repletion and bicarbonate supplementation. Bicarbonate therapy can be difficult to administer in the presence of fluid overload. Acetazolamide (Diamox) has been used to alkalinize the urine, but is best avoided because it produces systemic acidosis and thus increases salicylate toxicity.

With intact renal function, the elimination of salicylate can be accelerated by alkalinization of the urine, from a half-life of 20 hours to one as low as four hours.[152, 184] The latter is comparable to results with hemodialysis. However, with impaired renal function, in a situation in which bicarbonate cannot be administered because of pulmonary edema, or with acidosis refractory to bicarbonate therapy, peritoneal dialysis or hemodialysis is indicated to correct systemic acidosis.

Organophosphate and Related Insecticides*

Accidental and suicidal poisoning with organophosphate and carbamate insecticides seem to be occurring with increasing frequency, and may have serious cardiopulmonary effects.

Organophosphates inhibit acetylcholinesterase, resulting in excess acetylcholine in cholinergic synapses and myoneural junctions. The cardiovascular effects of organophosphates are unpredictable and often change over the time course of the poisoning.[136] Early in the course, acetylcholine stimulates nicotinic receptors at sympathetic ganglia, and causes tachycardia and mild hypertension. Later, the overabundant acetylcholine stimulates muscarinic receptors or blocks ganglionic transmission by hyperpolarization, resulting in bradycardia and hypotension. In severe poisoning, advanced AV block, bradyarrhythmias with hypotension, asystole, or ventricular fibrillation may occur.

Two recent reports describe Q-T interval prolongation, ventricular arrhythmias including polymorphous ventricular tachycardia (torsades de pointes), and sudden death after exposure to organophosphates.[110, 122] It is of particular interest that ventricular arrhythmias presented several days after ex-

*See Table 16–9.

Table 16–9. MANIFESTATIONS, MECHANISMS, AND TREATMENT OF COMPLICATIONS OF ORGANOPHOSPHATE AND CARBAMATE POISONING

Manifestations	Mechanisms	Treatment
a. Pulmonary secretions and/ or edema	Excess acetylcholine effects on bronchial tree	Atropine (high doses required), pralidoxime, positive end-expiratory pressure, assisted ventilation
b. Respiratory failure	Muscle paralysis (hyperpolarization blockade of neuromuscular transmission), CNS depression	Assisted ventilation, pralidoxime
c. Sinus tachycardia, hypertension	Autonomic ganglionic stimulation (early phase of poisoning)	None
d. Sinus, atrial, junctional, or ventricular bradycardia; AV block	Excess acetylcholine effects on postganglionic autonomic receptor	Atropine, pralidoxime, isoproterenol, cardiac pacing
e. Hypotension	Same as above	Treat bradyarrhythmias, fluids (central monitoring), pressors
f. Ventricular arrhythmias (may see long Q-T, polymorphous ventricular tachycardia)	Unknown	Lidocaine, phenytoin, isoproterenol, overdrive pacing
g. Other common manifestations: miosis, diaphoresis, lacrimation, salivation, urinary incontinence, abdominal cramps, diarrhea, coma	Cholinergic excess, muscarinic effects	Supportive, atropine (high doses required), pralidoxime
h. Fasciculations, muscle weakness and paralysis	Nicotinic excess, stimulation/ hyperpolarization blockade of neuromuscular transmission	Pralidoxime

posure at a time when patients seemingly had recovered from the manifestations of the poisoning. In some cases a transient electrocardiographic picture of myocardial infarction was seen. One patient died suddenly on the fifth day after exposure.[122] The mechanism of the long Q-T interval syndrome is presumably due to autonomic disturbances resulting in asynchronous ventricular repolarization.

Bradyarrhythmias, if hemodynamically significant, can usually be successfully treated by atropine administration. Atropine must compete with excess acetylcholine at the receptor site, and thus extremely large doses may be required. Doses should be increased until cholinergic signs such as salivation, diaphoresis, and bronchorrhea are reversed. Pralidoxime (2-PAM) regenerates cholinesterase and may also be effective in reducing manifestations of cholinergic excess. When atropine and 2-PAM are not effective, cardiac pacing is indicated. Sinus or atrial tachycardia causing hemodynamic compromise is a greater problem to treat, because drugs such as propranolol that might slow the rate might also worsen bronchoconstriction or aggravate conduction disturbances later in the course of the overdose. As discussed for quinidine, ventricular arrhythmias associated with a long Q-T interval respond best to isoproterenol or overdrive pacing, although lidocaine, phenytoin, or bretylium may also be effective.

Pulmonary secretions (sometimes presenting as acute pulmonary edema)[29] or respiratory failure may also result in hypoxia and acidosis, which aggravate arrhythmias and hypotension. Atropine is the treatment of choice for the bronchorrhea; 2-PAM may also be useful. Pralidoxime, but not atropine, is often effective in reversing the neuromuscular-blocking effects of organophosphates.

References

1. Abboud, R. T., Freedman, M. T., Rogers, R. M., et al.: Methaqualone poisoning with muscular hyperactivity necessitating the use of curare. Chest 65:204, 1974.
2. Addington, W. W., Cugell, D. W., Bazley, E. S., et al.: The pulmonary edema of heroin toxicity—an example of the stiff lung syndrome. Chest 62:199, 1972.
3. Afifi, A. A., Sacks, S. T., Liu, V. Y., et al.: Cumulative prognostic index for patients with barbiturate, glutethimide and meprobamate intoxication. N. Engl. J. Med. 285:1497, 1971.
4. Alexander, C. S., and Nino, A.: Cardiovascular complications in young patients taking psychotropic drugs. Am. Heart J. 78:757, 1969.
5. Alvarez-Mena, S. C., and Frank, M. J.: Phenothiazine-induced T-wave abnormalities. J.A.M.A. 224:1730, 1973.
6. Anderson, J. L., and Mason, J. W.: Successful treatment by overdrive pacing of recurrent quinidine syncope due to ventricular tachycardia. Am. J. Med. 64:715, 1978.
7. Anderson, R. J., Garza, H. R., Garriott, J. C., et al.: Intravenous propylhexedrine (Benzedrex) abuse and sudden death. Am. J. Med. 67:15, 1979.
8. Anderson, R. J., Potts, D. E., Gabow, P. A., et al.: Unrecognized adult salicylate intoxication. Ann. Intern. Med. 85:745, 1976.
9. Anonymous: Glutethimide—an unsafe alternative to barbiturate hypnotics. Br. Med. J. 1:1424, 1976.
10. Aquilonius, S.-M., and Hedstrand, U.: The use of physostigmine as an antidote in tricyclic anti-depressant intoxication. Acta Anaesthesiol. Scand. 22:40, 1978.
11. Arieff, A. I., and Friedman, E. A.: Coma following non-narcotic drug overdosage: management of 208 adult patients. Am. J. Med. Sci. 266:405, 1973.
12. Arita, M., and Surawicz, B.: Electrophysiologic effects of phenothiazine on canine cardiac fibers. J. Pharmacol. Exp. Ther. 184:619, 1973.
13. Avant, G. R., Speeg, K. V., Jr., Freemon, F. R., et al.: Physostigmine reversal of diazepam-induced hypnosis. Ann. Intern. Med. 91:53, 1979.
14. Axelson, J. A., and Hagaman, J. F.: Meprobamate poisoning and pulmonary edema. N. Engl. J. Med. 296:1481, 1977.
15. Bailey, D. N.: Methaqualone ingestion: evaluation of present status. J. Anal. Toxicol. 5:279, 1981.
16. Bailey, D. N.: Phencyclidine abuse. Clinical findings and concentrations in biological fluids after nonfatal intoxication. Am. J. Clin. Pathol. 72:795, 1979.
17. Banner, W., and Clawson, L.: Failure of Narcan to reverse clonidine toxicity. Vet. Hum. Toxicol. 23:361, 1981.
18. Banner, W., Jr., and Czajka, P. A.: Acute caffeine overdose in the neonate. Am. J. Dis. Child. 134:495, 1980.
19. Bayer, M. J., and Rumack, B. H. (eds.): Poisonings and overdose. *In* Topics in Emergency Medicine, Vol. 1, No. 3. Germantown, Aspen Publications, 1979.
20. Bell, E. F.: The use of naloxone in the treatment of diazepam poisoning. J. Pediatr. 87:803, 1975.
21. Benchimol, A., Bartall, H., and Desser, K. B.: Accelerated ventricular rhythm and cocaine abuse. Ann. Intern. Med. 88:519, 1978.
22. Benowitz, N. L.: Quinidine, procainamide, and disopyramide poisoning. *In* Haddad, L. M., and Winchester, J. F. (eds.): Clinical Management of Poisoning and Drug Overdose. Philadelphia, W. B. Saunders Co., 1983, pp. 853–862.
23. Benowitz, N. L., and Goldschlager, N.: Cardiac disturbances in the toxicologic patient. *In* Haddad, L. M., and Winchester, J. F. (eds.): Clinical Management of Poisoning and Drug Overdose. Philadelphia, W. B. Saunders Co., 1983, pp. 65–99.
24. Benowitz, N. L., Osterloh, J., Goldschlager, N., et al.: Massive catecholamine release due to caffeine poisoning. J.A.M.A. 248:1097, 1982.
25. Berger, R., Green, G., and Melnick, A.: Cardiac arrest caused by oral diazepam intoxication. Clin. Pediatr. 14:842, 1975.
26. Bernstein, E., and Diskant, B. M.: Phenylpropanolamine: a potentially hazardous drug. Ann. Emerg. Med. 11:311, 1982.
27. Bigger, J. T., Giardina, E. G. V., Perel, J. M., et al.: Cardiac antiarrhythmic effect of imipramine hydrochloride. N. Engl. J. Med. 296:206, 1977.
28. Bigger, J. T., Jr., Kantor, S. J., Glassman, A. H., et al.: Cardiovascular effects of tricyclic antidepressant drugs. *In* Lipton, M. A., DiMascio, A., and Killam, A. F. (eds.): Psychopharmacology: A Generation of Progress. New York, Raven Press, 1978, pp. 1033–1046.
29. Bledsoe, F. H., and Seymour, E. Q.: Acute pulmonary edema associated with parathion poisoning. Radiology 103:53, 1972.
30. Boakes, A. J., Laurence, D. R., Teoh, P. C., et al.: Interactions between sympathomimetic amines and antidepressant agents in man. Br. Med. J. 1:311, 1973.
31. Bowers, R. E., Brigham, K. L., and Owen, P. J.: Salicylate pulmonary edema: the mechanism in sheep and review of the clinical literature. Am. Rev. Respir. Dis. 115:261, 1977.
32. Bowyer, K., and Glasser, S. P.: Chloral hydrate overdose and cardiac arrhythmias. Chest 77:232, 1980.
33. Branchey, M. H., Lee, J. H., Amin, R., et al.: High- and low-potency neuroleptics in elderly psychiatric patients. J.A.M.A. 239:1860, 1978.
34. Brennan, F. J.: Electrophysiologic effects of imipramine and doxepin on normal and depressed cardiac Purkinje fibers. Am. J. Cardiol. 46:599, 1980.
35. Brown, T. C. K.: Sodium bicarbonate treatment for tricyclic antidepressant arrhythmias in children. Med. J. Aust. 2:380, 1976.
36. Brown, T. C. K.: Tricyclic antidepressant overdosage: experimental studies on the management of circulatory complications. Clin. Toxicol. 9:255, 1976.
37. Buchanan, N., Kundig, H., and Eyberg, C.: Experimental salicylate intoxication in young baboons. J. Pediatr. 86:225, 1975.
38. Burns, R. S., Lerner, S. E., Corrado, R., et al.: Phencyclidine—states of acute intoxication and fatalities. West. J. Med. 123:345, 1975.
39. Cady, W. J., Rehder, T. L., and Campbell, J.: Use of cholestyramine resin in the treatment of digitoxin toxicity. Am. J. Hosp. Pharm. 36:92, 1979.
40. Camarata, S. J., Weill, M. H., Hanashiro, P. K., et al.: Cardiac arrest in the critically ill. I. A study of predisposing causes in 132 patients. Circulation 44:688, 1971.

41. Catravas, J. D., and Waters, I. W.: Acute cocaine intoxication in the conscious dog: studies on the mechanism of lethality. J. Pharmacol. Exp. Ther. 217:350, 1981.
42. Chezan, J. A., and Garella, S.: Glutethimide intoxication: a prospective study of 70 patients treated conservatively without hemodialysis. Arch. Intern. Med. 128:215, 1971.
43. Chynn, K. Y.: Acute subarachnoid hemorrhage. J.A.M.A. 233:55, 1975.
44. Coleman, D. L., Ross, T. F., and Naughton, J. L.: Myocardial ischemia and infarction related to recreational cocaine use. West. J. Med. 136:444, 1982.
45. Conner, C. S., and Watanabe, A. S.: Clonidine overdose: a review. Am. J. Hosp. Pharm. 36:906, 1979.
46. Cook, C. E., Brine, D. R., Jeffcoat, A. R., et al.: Phencyclidine disposition after intravenous and oral doses. Clin. Pharmacol. Ther. 31:625, 1982.
47. Cranefield, P. F.: Action potentials, afterpotentials, and arrhythmias. Circ. Res. 41:415, 1977.
47A. Cruickshank, J. M.: The clinical importance of cardioselectivity and lipophilicity in beta blockers. Am. Heart. J. 100:160, 1980.
48. de Azevedo, I. M., Watanabe, Y., and Dreifus, L. S.: Electrophysiologic antagonism of quinidine and bretylium tosylate. Am. J. Cardiol. 33:633, 1974.
49. Dice, W. H., Ward, G., Kelley, J., and Kilpatrick, W. R.: Pulmonary toxicity following gastrointestinal ingestion of kerosene. Ann. Emerg. Med. 11:138, 1982.
50. DiLiberti, J., O'Brien, M. L., and Turner, T.: The use of physostigmine as an antidote in accidental diazepam intoxication. J. Pediatr. 86:106, 1975.
51. Domino, E. F.: Neurobiology of phencyclidine (Sernyl), a drug with an unusual spectrum of pharmacological activity. Int. Rev. Neurobiol. 6:303, 1964.
52. Domino, E. F., and Wilson, A. E.: Effects of urine acidification on plasma and urine phencyclidine levels in overdosage. Clin. Pharmacol. Ther. 22:421, 1977.
53. Done, A. K.: Salicylate intoxication: significance of measurements of salicylate in blood in cases of acute ingestion. Pediatrics 26:800, 1960.
54. Donlon, P. T., and Tupin, J. P.: Successful suicides with thioridazine and mesoridazine. Arch. Gen. Psychiatry 34:955, 1977.
55. Duberstein, J. L., and Kaufman, D. M.: A clinical study of an epidemic of heroin intoxication and heroin-induced pulmonary edema. Am. J. Med. 51:704, 1971.
56. Eastman, J. W., and Cohen, S. N.: Hypertensive crisis and death associated with phencyclidine poisoning. J.A.M.A. 231:1270, 1975.
57. Ehlers, S. M., Zaske, D. E., and Sawchuk, R. J.: Massive theophylline overdose. Rapid elimination by charcoal hemoperfusion. J.A.M.A. 240:474, 1978.
58. Espelin, D. E., and Done, A. K.: Amphetamine poisoning. N. Engl. J. Med. 278:1361, 1968.
59. Farsang, C., Ramirez-Gonzalez, M. D., Mucci, L., et al.: Possible role of an endogenous opiate in the cardiovascular effects of central alpha adrenoceptor stimulation in spontaneously hypertensive rats. J. Pharmacol. Exp. Ther. 214:203, 1980.
60. Fein, A., Grossman, R. F., Jones, J. G., et al.: The value of edema fluid protein measurement in patients with pulmonary edema. Am. J. Med. 67:32, 1979.
61. Ferguson, M. J., Germanos, S., and Grace, W. J.: Meprobamate overdosage: a report on the management of five cases. Arch. Intern. Med. 106:238, 1960.
62. Finnegan, T. R. L., and Trounce, J. R.: Depression of the heart by quinidine and its treatment. Br. Heart J. 16:341, 1954.
63. Fischer, V. W., and Barner, H.: Cardiomyopathic findings associated with methylphenidate. J.A.M.A. 238:1497, 1977.
64. Fowler, N. O., McCall, D., Chou, T., et al.: Electrocardiographic changes and cardiac arrhythmias in patients receiving psychotropic drugs. Am. J. Cardiol. 37:223, 1976.
65. Frand, U. I., Shim, C. S., and Williams, M. H.: Heroin-induced pulmonary edema: sequential studies of pulmonary function. Ann. Intern. Med. 77:29, 1972.
66. Freeman, J. W., and Loughhead, M. G.: Beta blockade in the treatment of tricyclic antidepressant overdosage. Med. J. Aust. 1:1233, 1973.
67. Frishman, W., Jacob, H., Eisenberg, E., et al.: Clinical pharmacology of the new beta-adrenergic blocking drugs. Part 8. Self-poisoning with beta-adrenoceptor blocking agents: recognition and management. Am. Heart J. 98:798, 1979.
68. Frishman, W., Silverman, R., Strom, J., et al.: Clinical pharmacology of the new beta-adrenergic blocking drugs. Part 4. Adverse effects. Choosing a beta-adrenoreceptor blocker. Am. Heart. J. 98:256, 1979.
69. Ginsberg, M. D., Hertzman, M., and Schmidt-Nowara, W. W.: Amphetamine intoxication with coagulopathy hyperthermia and reversible renal failure. A syndrome resembling heatstroke. Ann. Intern. Med. 73:81, 1970.
70. Glauser, F. L., Smith, W. R., Caldwell, A., et al.: Ethchlorvynol (Placidyl)-induced pulmonary edema. Ann. Intern. Med. 84:46, 1976.
71. Gold, M. S., Pottash, A. L. C., Sweeney, D. R., et al.: Efficacy of clonidine in opiate withdrawal: a study of thirty patients. Drug Alcohol Depend. 6:201, 1980.
72. Goldberg, M. J., and Berlinger, W. G.: Treatment of phenobarbital overdose with activated charcoal. J.A.M.A. 247:2400, 1982.
73. Goldberg, M. J., and Spector, R.: Amoxapine overdose: report of two patients with severe neurologic damage. Ann. Intern. Med. 96:463, 1982.
74. Goldfrank, L. R. (ed.): Toxicologic Emergencies, 2nd ed. New York, Appleton-Century-Crofts, 1982, pp. 1–29.
75. Goodman, J. M., Bischel, M. D., Wagers, P. W., et al.: Barbiturate intoxication, morbidity and mortality. West. J. Med. 124:179, 1976.
76. Greenblatt, D. J., Allen, M. D., Noel, B. J., et al.: Acute overdosage with benzodiazepine derivatives. Clin. Pharmacol. Ther. 21:497, 1977.
77. Greenblatt, D. J., and Koch-Weser, J.: Adverse reactions to intravenous diazepam: a report from the Boston Collaborative Drug Surveillance Program. Am. J. Med. Sci. 266:261, 1973.
78. Greenland, P., and Howe, T. A.: Cardiac monitoring in tricyclic antidepressant overdose. Heart Lung 10:856, 1981.
79. Gunne, L. M., and Anggard, E.: Pharmacokinetic studies with amphetamines—relationship to neuropsychiatric disorders. J. Pharmacokinet. Biopharm. 1:481, 1973.
80. Gustafson, A., Svensson, S.-E., and Ugander, L.:

Cardiac arrhythmias in chloral hydrate poisoning. Acta Med. Scand. 201:227, 1977.

81. Hagerman, G. A., and Hanashiro, P. K.: Reversal of tricyclic antidepressant-induced cardiac conduction abnormalities by phenytoin. Ann. Emerg. Med. 10:82, 1981.
82. Haider, I., Matthew, H., and Oswald, I.: Electroencephalographic changes in acute drug poisoning. Electroenceph. Clin. Neurophysiol. 30:23, 1971.
83. Hall, J. G., Morris, B., and Woolley, G.: Intrinsic rhythmic propulsion of lymph in the unanaesthetized sheep. J. Physiol. (Lond.) 180:336, 1965.
84. Hansen, A. R., Kennedy, F. A., Ambre, J. J., et al.: Glutethimide poisoning: a metabolite contributes to morbidity and mortality. N. Engl. J. Med. 292:250, 1975.
85. Heffner, J. E., and Sahn, S. A.: Salicylate-induced pulmonary edema. Ann. Intern. Med. 95:405, 1981.
86. Hill, J. B.: Current concepts—salicylate intoxication. N. Engl. J. Med. 288:1110, 1973.
87. Hitner, H., and DiGregoria, G. J.: Preliminary investigation of the peripheral sympathomimetic effects of phencyclidine. Arch. Int. Pharmacodyn. Ther. 212:36, 1974.
88. Hoffman, B. F., Rosen, M. R., and Wit, A. L.: Electrophysiology and pharmacology of cardiac arrhythmias. VII. Cardiac effects of quinidine and procaine amide. Am. Heart J. 90:117, 1975.
89. Hollister, L. E.: Doxepin hydrochloride. Ann. Intern. Med. 81:360, 1974.
90. Hooper, R. G., Conner, C. S., and Rumack, B. H.: Acute poisoning from over-the-counter sleep preparations. J.A.C.E.P. 8:98, 1979.
91. Hormaechea, E., Carlson, R. W., Rogove, H., et al.: Hypovolemia, pulmonary edema and protein changes in severe salicylate poisoning. Am. J. Med. 66:1046, 1979.
92. Horowitz, J. D., Lang, W. J., Howes, L. G., et al.: Hypertensive response induced by phenylpropranolamine in anorectic and decongestant preparations. Lancet 1:60, 1980.
93. Hulting, J., and Thorstrand, C.: Hemodynamic effects of norepinephrine in severe hypnotic drug poisoning with arterial hypotension. Acta Med. Scand. 192:447, 1972.
94. Huston, J. R., and Bell, G. E.: The effect of thioridazine hydrochloride and chlorpromazine on the electrocardiogram. J.A.M.A. 198:16, 1966.
95. Ilett, K. F., Jarrott, B., O'Donnell, S. R., et al.: Mechanism of cardiovascular actions of 1-(Cl-phenylcyclohexyl) piperidine hydrochloride (phencyclidine). Br. J. Pharmacol. Chemother. 28:73, 1966.
96. Illingworth, R. N.: Glucagon for beta-blocker poisoning. Practitioner 223:683, 1979.
97. Jacob, H. S., Craddock, P. R., Hammerschmidt, D. E., et al.: Complement-induced granulocyte aggregation: an unsuspected mechanism of disease. N. Engl. J. Med. 302:789, 1980.
98. Jacobs, M. H., Senior, R. M., and Kessler, G.: Clinical experience with theophylline: relationships between dosage, serum concentration, and toxicity. J.A.M.A. 235:1983, 1976.
99. Jandhyala, B. S., Steenberg, M. L., Perel, J. M., et al.: Effects of several tricyclic antidepressants on the hemodynamics and myocardial contractility of the anesthetized dogs. Eur. J. Pharmacol. 42:403, 1977.
100. Janson, P. A., Watt, J. B., and Hermos, J. A.: Doxepin overdose. Success with physostigmine and failure with neostigmine in reversing toxicity. J.A.M.A. 237:2632, 1977.
101. Jay, S. J., Johanson, W. G., and Pierce, A. K.: Respiratory complications of overdose with sedative drugs. Am. Rev. Respir. Dis. 112:591, 1975.
102. Jefferson, J. W.: A review of the cardiovascular effects and toxicity of tricyclic antidepressants. Psychosom. Med. 37:160, 1975.
103. Jorgensen, E. O.: EEG without detectable cortical activity and cranial nerve areflexia as parameters of brain death. Electroenceph. Clin. Neurophysiol. 36:70, 1974.
104. Josephson, G. W., and Stine, R. J.: Caffeine intoxication: a case of paroxysmal atrial tachycardia. J.A.C.E.P. 5:776, 1976.
105. Kalant, A., and Kalant, O. J.: Death in amphetamine users: causes and rates. Can. Med. Assoc. J. 112:299, 1975.
106. Kaplinsky, E., Yahini, J. H., Brazilai, J., et al.: Quinidine syncope; report of a case successfully treated with lidocaine. Chest 62:764, 1972.
107. Karp, H. N., Kaufman, N. D., and Anand, S. K.: Phencyclidine poisoning in young children. J. Pediatr. 97:1006, 1980.
108. Katz, M., Robertson, P. A., and Creasy, R. K.: Cardiovascular complications associated with terbutaline treatment for preterm labor. Am. J. Obstet. Gynecol. 139:605, 1981.
109. Kendrick, W. C., Hull, A. R., and Knochel, J. P.: Rhabdomyolysis and shock after intravenous amphetamine administration. Ann. Intern. Med. 86:381, 1977.
110. Kiss, Z., and Fazekas, T.: Arrhythmias in organophosphate poisonings. Acta Cardiol. (Tokyo) 34:323, 1979.
111. Koster, R. W., and Wellens, H. J. J.: Quinidine-induced ventricular flutter and fibrillation without digitalis therapy. Am. J. Cardiol. 38:519, 1976.
112. Kramer, J. C., Fischman, V. S., and Littlefield, D. C.: Amphetamine abuse pattern and effects of high doses taken intravenously. J.A.M.A. 201:305, 1967.
113. Krenzelok, E. P., Anderson, G. M., and Mirick, M.: Massive diphenhydramine overdose resulting in death. Ann. Emerg. Med. 11:212, 1982.
114. Kulig, K., Rumack, B. H., Sullivan, J. B., Jr., et al.: Amoxapine overdose. Coma and seizures without cardiotoxic effects. J.A.M.A. 248:1092, 1982.
115. Labi, M.: Paroxysmal atrial fibrillation of heroin intoxication. Ann. Intern. Med. 71:951, 1969.
116. Langou, R. A., Van Dyke, C., Tahan, S. R., et al.: Cardiovascular manifestations of tricyclic antidepressant overdose. Am. Heart J. 100:458, 1980.
117. Lawson, A. A. H., Proudfoot, A. T., Brown, S. S., et al.: Forced diuresis in the treatment of acute salicylate poisoning in adults. Q. J. Med. 38:31, 1969.
118. Leestma, J. E., and Koenig, K. L.: Sudden death and phenothiazines. Arch. Gen. Psychiatry 18:137, 1968.
119. Levy, G., and Tsuchiya, T.: Salicylate accumulation kinetics in man. N. Engl. J. Med. 287:430, 1972.
120. Lhoste, F., Lemaire, F., and Rapin, M.: Treatment of hypotension in meprobamate poisoning. N. Engl. J. Med. 296:1004, 1977.
121. Lipski, J., Stimmel, B., and Donoso, E.: The effect of heroin and multiple drug abuse on the electrocardiogram. Am. Heart J. 86:663, 1973.

122. Ludomirsky, A., Klein, H. O., Sarelli, P., et al.: Q-T prolongation and polymorphous ("torsade de pointes") ventricular arrhythmias associated with organophosphorus insecticide poisoning. Am. J. Cardiol. 49:1654, 1982.
123. Lumpkin, J., Watanabe, A. S., Rumack, B. H., et al.: Phenothiazine-induced ventricular tachycardia following acute overdose. J.A.C.E.P. 8:476, 1979.
124. Maddock, R. K., Jr., and Bloomer, H. A.: Meprobamate overdosage: evaluation of its severity and methods of treatment. J.A.M.A. 201:999, 1967.
125. Maher, J. F., Schreiner, G. E., and Westervelt, F. B., Jr.: Acute glutethimide intoxication. I. Clinical experience (twenty-two patients) compared to acute barbiturate intoxication (sixty-three patients). Am. J. Med. 33:70, 1962.
126. Mandelbaum, J. M., and Simon, N. M.: Severe methyprylon intoxication treated by hemodialysis. J.A.M.A. 216:139, 1971.
127. Marshall, A. J.: Cardiac arrhythmias caused by chloral hydrate. Br. Med. J. 2:994, 1977.
128. Massey, S. R.: Fake "speed" causes almost as much fear as the real thing. Wall Street J., Sept. 8, 1981.
129. Massumi, R. A., Mason, D. T., Amsterdam, E. A., et al.: Ventricular fibrillation and tachycardia after intravenous atropine for treatment of bradycardias. N. Engl. J. Med. 287:336, 1972.
130. Matthew, H., Proudfoot, A. T., Brown, S. S., et al.: Mandrax poisoning: conservative management of 116 patients. Br. Med. J. 1:101, 1968.
131. Mawer, G. E., and Lee, H. A.: Value of forced diuresis in acute barbiturate poisoning. Br. Med. J. 2:790, 1968.
132. Meldrum, B. S., Vigouroux, R. A., and Brierley, J. B.: Systemic factors and epileptic brain damage. Arch. Neurol. 29:82, 1973.
133. Merguet, P., Heimsoth, V., Murata, T., et al.: Experimental study on the circulatory effect of 2-(2,6-dichlorophenylamino)-2-imidazoline-hydrochloride in man. Pharmacol. Clin. 1:30, 1968.
134. Morgan, A. G., and Polak, A.: The excretion of salicylate in salicylate poisoning. Clin. Sci. 41:475, 1971.
135. Namba, T., Greenfield, M., and Grob, D.: Malathion poisoning: a fatal case with cardiac manifestations. Arch. Environ. Health 21:533, 1970.
136. Namba, T., Nolte, C. T., Jackrel, J., et al.: Poisoning due to organophosphate insecticides: acute and chronic manifestations. Am. J. Med. 50:475, 1971.
137. Neuvonen, P. J., and Elonen, E.: Effect of activated charcoal on absorption and elimination of phenobarbitone, carbamazepine and phenylbutazone in man. Eur. J. Clin. Pharmacol. 17:51, 1980.
138. Neuvonen, P. J., Elonen, E., and Mattila, M. J.: Oral activated charcoal and dapsone elimination. Clin. Pharmacol. Ther. 27:823, 1980.
139. Newton, R. W.: Physostigmine salicylate in the treatment of tricyclic antidepressant overdosage. J.A.M.A. 231:941, 1975.
140. Nickander, R., and Smits, S.: Some effects of *d*-propoxyphene (Darvon). Pharmacologist 15:203, 1973.
141. Nickel, S. N., and Thibaudeau, Y.: Quinidine intoxication treated by isoproterenol (Isuprel). Can. Med. Assoc. J. 85:81, 1961.
142. Ober, K. F., and Wang, R. I. H.: Drug interactions with guanethidine. Clin. Pharmacol. Ther. 14:190, 1973.
143. Parathaman, S. K., and Khan, F.: Acute cardiomyopathy with recurrent pulmonary edema and hypotension following heroin overdosage. Chest 69:117, 1976.
144. Pentel, P. R., Mikell, F. L., and Zavoral, J. H.: Myocardial injury after phenylpropanolamine ingestion. Br. Heart J. 47:51, 1982.
145. Pentel, P. R., and Peterson, C. D.: Asystole complicating physostigmine treatment of tricyclic antidepressant overdose. Ann. Emerg. Med. 9:11, 1980.
146. Peterson, R. B., and Vasquez, L. A.: Phenylpropanolamine-induced arrhythmias. J.A.M.A. 223:324, 1973.
147. Petit, J. M., Spiker, D. G., Ruwitch, J. F., et al.: Tricyclic antidepressant plasma levels and adverse effects after overdose. Clin. Pharmacol. Ther. 21:47, 1976.
148. Pond, S., Jacobs, M., Marks, J., et al.: Treatment of digitoxin overdose with oral activated charcoal. Lancet 2:1177, 1981.
149. Pond, S., Rosenberg, J., Benowitz, N. L., et al.: Pharmacokinetics of haemoperfusion for drug overdose. Clin. Pharmacokinet. 4:329, 1979.
150. Prewitt, R. M., McCarthy, J., and Wood, L. D. H.: Treatment of acute low pressure pulmonary edema in dogs. Relative effects of hydrostatic and oncotic pressure, nitroprusside, and positive end-expiratory pressure. J. Clin. Invest. 67:409, 1981.
151. Reidt, W. U.: Fatal poisoning with methyprylon (Noludar), a nonbarbiturate sedative. N. Engl. J. Med. 255:231, 1956.
152. Reynolds, E. W., and Vander Ark, C. R.: Quinidine syncope and the delayed repolarization syndromes. Mod. Concepts Cardiovasc. Dis. 45:117, 1976.
153. Richman, S., and Harris, R. D.: Acute pulmonary edema associated with Librium abuse. A case report. Radiology 103:57, 1972.
154. Robinson, D. S., and Barker, E.: Tricyclic antidepressant cardiotoxicity. J.A.M.A. 236:2089, 1976.
155. Rosa, R. M., Silva, P., Young, J. B., et al.: Adrenergic modulation of extrarenal potassium disposal. N. Engl. J. Med. 302:431, 1980.
156. Rosenberg, J., Benowitz, N. L., and Pond, S.: Pharmacokinetics of drug overdose. Clin. Pharmacokinet. 6:161, 1981.
157. Rumack, B. H.: Pharmacology for the pediatrician. Anticholinergic poisoning: treatment with physostigmine. Pediatrics 52:449, 1973.
158. Rumack, B. H., Wolfe, R. R., and Gilfrich, H.: Phenytoin (diphenylhydantoin) treatment of massive digoxin overdose. Br. Heart J. 36:405, 1974.
159. Russo, M. E.: Management of theophylline intoxication with charcoal-column hemoperfusion. N. Engl. J. Med. 300:24, 1979.
160. Salzberg, M. R., and Gallagher, E. J.: Propranolol overdose. Ann. Emerg. Med. 9:26, 1980.
161. Scialli, J. V. K., and Thornton, W. E.: Toxic reactions from a haloperidol overdose in two children. Thermal and cardiac manifestations. J.A.M.A. 239:48, 1978.
162. Setter, J. G., Maher, J. F., and Schreiner, G. E.: Barbiturate intoxication: evaluation of therapy including dialysis in a large series selectively referred because of severity. Arch. Intern. Med. 117:224, 1966.
163. Shub, C., Gau, G. T., Sidell, P. M., et al.: The management of acute quinidine intoxication. Chest 73:173, 1978.
164. Shubin, H., and Weil, M. H.: Shock associated with barbiturate intoxication. J.A.M.A. 215:263, 1971.
165. Shubin, H., and Weil, M. H.: The mechanism of

shock following suicidal doses of barbiturate, narcotics and tranquilizer drugs, with observations on the effects of treatment. Am. J. Med. 38:853, 1965.
166. Siegel, J. H.: The myocardial contractile state and its role in the response to anesthesia and surgery. Anesthesiology 30:519, 1969.
167. Simpson, D. L., and Rumack, B. H.: Methylenedioxyamphetamine: clinical description of overdose, death, and review of pharmacology. Arch. Intern. Med. 141:1507, 1981.
168. Smith, H. J., Roche, A. H. G., Jagusch, M. F., et al.: Cardiomyopathy associated with amphetamine administration. Am. Heart J. 91:792, 1976.
169. Smith, L. L., Wright, A., Wyatt, I., et al.: Effective treatment for paraquat poisoning in rats and its relevance to treatment of paraquat poisoning in man. Br. Med. J. 4:569, 1974.
170. Smith, T. W., Haber, E., Yeatman, L., et al.: Reversal of advanced digoxin intoxication with Fab fragments of digoxin-specific antibodies. N. Engl. J. Med. 294:797, 1976.
171. Smith, T. W., and Willerson, J. T.: Suicidal and accidental digoxin ingestion. Circulation 44:29, 1971.
172. Smith, W. M., and Gallagher, J. J.: "Les torsades de pointes": an unusual ventricular arrhythmia. Ann. Intern. Med. 93:578, 1980.
173. Somberg, J. C., and Smith, T. W.: Localization of the neurally mediated arrhythmogenic properties of digitalis. Science 204:321, 1979.
174. Spiker, D. G., and Biggs, J. T.: Tricyclic antidepressants. Prolonged plasma levels after overdose. J.A.M.A. 236:1711, 1976.
175. Staub, N. C.: The pathogenesis of pulmonary edema. Prog. Cardiovasc. Dis. 23:53, 1980.
176. Strubelt, O., Hoffman, A., Siegers, C.-P., et al.: On the pathogenesis of cardiac necrosis induced by theophylline and caffeine. Acta Pharmacol. Toxicol. 39:383, 1976.
177. Suarez, C. A., Arango, A., and Lester, J. L., III: Cocaine—condom ingestion. Surgical treatment. J.A.M.A. 238:1391, 1977.
178. Takki, S., Gambertoglio, J. G., Honda, D. H., et al.: Pharmacokinetic evaluation of hemodialysis in acute drug overdose. J. Pharmacokinet. Biopharm. 6:427, 1978.
179. Teeham, B. P., Maher, J. F., Carey, J. J., et al.: Acute ethchlorvynol (Placidyl) intoxication. Ann. Intern. Med. 72:875, 1970.
180. Temple, A. R.: Pathophysiology of aspirin overdosage toxicity, with implications for management. Pediatrics 62:873, 1978.
181. Theodore, J., and Robin, E. D.: Pathogenesis of neurogenic pulmonary oedema. Lancet 2:749, 1975.
182. Thorstrand, C.: Cardiovascular effects of poisoning by hypnotic and tricyclic antidepressants. Acta Med. Scand. 198:583, 1975.
183. Thorstrand, C.: Cardiovascular effects of poisoning with tricyclic antidepressants. Acta Med. Scand. 195:505, 1974.
184. Thorstrand, C.: Clinical features in poisonings by tricyclic antidepressants with special reference to the ECG. Acta Med. Scand. 199:337, 1976.
185. Thurston, J. H., Pollock, P. G., Warren, S. K., et al.: Reduced brain glucose with normal glucose in salicylate poisoning. J. Clin. Invest. 49:2139, 1970.
186. Tong, T. G., Benowitz, N. L., Becker, C. E., et al.: Phencyclidine poisoning. J.A.M.A. 234:512, 1975.
187. Trafford, J. A. P., Jones, R. H., Evans, R., et al.: Haemoperfusion with R-004 amberlite resin for treatment of acute poisoning. Br. Med. J. 2:1453, 1977.
188. Vander Ark, C. R., Reynolds, E. W., Kahn, D. R., et al.: Quinidine syncope. A report of successful treatment with bretylium tosylate. J. Thorac. Cardiovasc. Surg. 72:464, 1976.
189. van Swearingen, P.: Placidyl and pulmonary edema. Ann. Intern. Med. 84:614, 1976.
190. Veith, R. C., Raskind, M. A., Caldwell, J. H., et al.: Cardiovascular effects of tricyclic antidepressants in depressed patients with chronic heart disease. N. Engl. J. Med. 306:954, 1982.
191. Vellar, I. D. A., Richardson, J. P., Doyle, J. C., et al.: Gastric necrosis: a rare complication of chloral hydrate intoxication. Br. J. Surg. 59:317, 1972.
192. Vohra, J., Burrows, G., Hunt, D., et al.: The effect of toxic and therapeutic doses of tricyclic antidepressant drugs on intracardiac conduction. Eur. J. Cardiol. 3:219, 1975.
193. Wang, H.-H., Kanai, T., Markee, S., et al.: Effects of reserpine and chlorpromazine on the vasomotor center in the medulla oblongata of the dog. J. Pharmacol. Exp. Ther. 144:186, 1964.
194. Weisdorff, D., Kramer, J., Goldbarg, A., et al.: Physostigmine for cardiac and neurologic manifestations of phenothiazine poisoning. Clin. Pharmacol. Ther. 24:663, 1978.
195. Weld, F. M., and Bigger, J. T., Jr.; Electrophysiological effects of imipramine on ovine cardiac Purkinje and ventricular muscle fibers. Circ. Res. 46:167, 1980.
196. Wetli, C. V., and Wright, R. K.: Death caused by recreational cocaine use. J.A.M.A. 241:2519, 1979.
197. Wright, N., and Roscoe, P.: Acute glutethimide poisoning: conservative management of 31 patients. J.A.M.A. 214:1704, 1970.
198. Yudis, M., Swartz, C., Onesti, G., et al.: Hemodialysis for methyprylon (Noludar) poisoning. Ann. Intern. Med. 68:1301, 1968.
199. Zwillich, C. W., Sutton, F. D., Neff, T. A., et al.: Theophylline-induced seizures in adults: correlation with serum concentrations. Ann. Intern. Med. 82:784, 1975.

17

Diagnosis and Treatment of Pulmonary Embolism

G. V. R. K. SHARMA,
M. SCHOOLMAN,
and A. A. SASAHARA

Pulmonary thromboembolism is a common disease occurring most often as a complication in hospitalized patients. The exact incidence is not known but, on the basis of our own and other studies, fatal pulmonary embolism can be estimated to occur in about 150,000 patients per year and nonfatal pulmonary embolism in about 600,000 patients per year.[5, 13] Untreated pulmonary embolism carries a high (18–38%) mortality rate, but once it is recognized and treated a substantial reduction in mortality (8.3%) occurs.[2] This observation underscores the importance of early diagnosis and prompt treatment.

The diagnosis of pulmonary embolism usually rests on clinical suspicion in the proper setting and confirmation by appropriate laboratory tests. Major diagnostic problems that the physician faces are: (1) pulmonary embolism can and does occur with few or minimal symptoms and signs, and may be mistaken for other cardiopulmonary disorders such as congestive heart failure, pneumonia, and atelectasis; (2) common laboratory tests usually yield nonspecific results; and (3) the more specific studies such as ventilation-perfusion lung scanning and selective pulmonary angiography are not always readily available. Therapeutic considerations include the mode of heparinization, the duration of anticoagulant treatment, and the role of thrombolytic agents and surgery. This chapter represents an attempt to evaluate the features of history and physical findings that are of diagnostic aid, to assess the specificity and sensitivity of laboratory tests, and to discuss the therapeutic approach with emphasis on recent advances.

HISTORY

When the presentation is typical, pulmonary embolism is readily suspected. The classical presentation, however, occurs infrequently. It is, therefore, helpful to consider the clinical setting in which the disease occurs, since most patients suffer pulmonary embolism in a hospital during confinement for another illness. Conditions recognized as placing the patient at high risk for pulmonary embolism include heart disease (especially with congestive heart failure), trauma (especially fractures of the hip), the postoperative state, chronic obstructive pulmonary disease, previous pulmonary embolism, and malignant disease. Other predisposing conditions include advanced age, obesity, pregnancy, and ingestion of oral contraceptive drugs. Any of these factors, in the presence of appropriate cardiopulmonary symptoms, should alert the physician to the possibility of pulmonary embolism. A history of previous thrombophlebitis is a helpful pointer, but often is not forthcoming. It is useful from a therapeutic standpoint to classify the predisposing factors into those that result from acute processes and those that represent continuing sources of thromboembolism. Acute self-limited conditions include immobilization after injuries, especially trauma to the legs, and the postoperative and postpartum periods. Once the patient returns to normal activity, the risk of embolism usually ceases. The threat of thromboembolism continues when the predisposing factors are chronic, e.g., chronic congestive heart failure and chronic venous insufficiency of the lower extremities.

	PREVALENCE %		
	ALL	MASSIVE	SUBMASSIVE
DYSPNEA	81	79	83
PLEURAL PAIN	72	62	84*
APPREHENSION	59	61	56
COUGH	54	50	60
HEMOPTYSIS	34	27	44
SWEATS	26	27	24
SYNCOPE	14	22*	4

Figure 17–1. An analysis of the presenting symptoms of pulmonary embolism from the Urokinase–Pulmonary Embolism Trial. Asterisks indicate significant correlation with submassive and massive pulmonary embolism.

SYMPTOMS AND SIGNS

Symptoms and signs depend on the mode of presentation of pulmonary embolism, which could be one of the following three clinical syndromes: (1) pulmonary infarction, with acute onset of pleuritic pain, dyspnea, hemoptysis, and pleural friction rub; (2) acute cor pulmonale, with sudden development of dyspnea, cyanosis, right ventricular failure, and hypotension; and (3) unexplained dyspnea. Two factors play important roles in the genesis of these clinical syndromes: pre-embolic cardiopulmonary status and "massivity" of embolism. Whereas most patients without previous cardiopulmonary disease exhibit some clinical clue suggestive of pulmonary embolism, patients with a background of chronic obstructive pulmonary disease or congestive heart failure have only nonspecific symptoms and signs.[20] It is indeed unusual for patients with pulmonary embolism to present with the complete clinical picture of apprehension, dyspnea, pleuritic pain, hemoptysis, pleural friction rub, and phlebitis. Often, tachypnea may be the only clinical finding. When symptoms and signs occur in patients without previous cardiopulmonary disease, they constitute clues to the diagnosis, whereas when they arise in patients with previous heart or lung disease, they may be mistaken for manifestations of the underlying disease state. The following analysis of symptoms and signs was made from data obtained from the National Institutes of Health–sponsored Urokinase–Pulmonary Embolism Trial (UPET) (Fig. 17–1).[15]

Dyspnea was the most common symptom, occurring in 81 per cent of patients with proved pulmonary embolism. Characteristically, this respiratory complaint by the patient appears to be out of proportion to the degree and extent of objective abnormal findings.

Chest pain, frequently pleuritic in nature, occurred in 72 per cent of patients. Usually it is not associated with hemoptysis and is noted more often with submassive than with massive embolism (massive defined as the obstruction of at least two or more lobar arteries or equivalent obstruction of 40 per cent of the pulmonary vasculature).

Apprehension, although very nonspecific, was noted in 59 per cent of patients. In minor embolism, varying degrees of anxiety occur and appear to be more than apparently warranted by the physical findings noted.

Cough occurred in 54 per cent of patients. It is usually nonproductive, unless the patient has underlying chronic obstructive pulmonary disease.

Hemoptysis, at one time considered necessary before pulmonary embolism/infarction would be considered in the differential diagnosis, was seen in only 34 per cent of patients. The hemoptysis is characteristically blood-streaking, in contrast to diseases such as mitral stenosis in which blood alone is expectorated. In addition, serious blood loss is uncommon.

Syncope, usually associated with massive pulmonary embolism, occurred in 14 per cent of patients.

The physical examination, also tabulated from the UPET study, showed relatively nonspecific findings that could be associated with other cardiopulmonary disorders (Fig. 17–2).

Tachypnea (respiratory rate greater than 20/min) was most frequently encountered, having occurred in 87 per cent of patients. It is

	ALL	PREVALENCE % MASSIVE	SUBMASSIVE
RALES	53	50	57
↑ P_2	53	60*	44
PHLEBITIS	33	42	21
S_3, S_4	34	47*	17
SWEATING	34	41	24
CYANOSIS	18	28*	6
↑ RESP (>16)	87		
↑ PULSE (>100)	44		
FEVER (≥ 37.8)	42		

Figure 17–2. An analysis of the physical findings of pulmonary embolism from the Urokinase–Pulmonary Embolism Trial. Asterisks indicate significant correlation with massive pulmonary embolism.

generally characterized as "fast and shallow" respiration.

Tachycardia (heart rate greater than 100 beats/min) occurred in 44 per cent of patients. In general, there tends to be a direct relationship between the size of the embolus and the heart rate. However, when tachycardia ceases suddenly in a patient with massive embolism, it is an ominous sign that may herald a cardiac arrest.

Rales were noted in 53 per cent of patients and were a manifestation of congestive heart failure, which generally occurs in patients with underlying cardiopulmonary disease.

Fever was found in 42 per cent of patients. It was generally of modest elevation (100°–102°F) and lacked the "spiking" nature of systemic infectious processes.

Sweating occurred in 34 per cent of patients. It results from the sympathetic discharge that takes place in patients with anxiety and cardiopulmonary distress; hence, it is more a sign of massive pulmonary embolism.

Thrombophlebitis was an uncommon finding in these patients, although asymptomatic deep vein thrombosis was not. This latter observation is of clinical importance since most pulmonary emboli arise from thrombi in the deep venous system of the legs. Only by application of objective diagnostic studies can deep vein thrombi be detected with any degree of sensitivity.

Accentuation of the pulmonary closure sound (S2P) occurred in 53 per cent of patients. Since it is usually a manifestation of large pulmonary emboli and the development of sudden pulmonary hypertension, its detection generally denotes significant embolic obstruction. The occurrence of S3 and S4 gallop heart sounds was detected in 35 per cent of patients, but mostly in those with extensive embolic obstruction. Their occurrence pathophysiologically is related to the abnormal right ventricular hemodynamics that result from sudden significant elevation of the pulmonary arterial pressure. At the bedside, their right ventricular origin can occasionally be confirmed by their variation with phasic respiration.

Cyanosis, a finding noted in 18 per cent of patients, represented a more severe degree of the very frequent hypoxemia that occurs in patients with pulmonary embolism; hence, it is a finding of massive pulmonary embolism.

It is clear from this analysis that most patients with pulmonary embolism have signs and symptoms that could be part of other heart and lung disorders. The physician must be prepared to accept a clinical presentation short of the classical hemoptysis, pleural pain, and thrombophlebitis, and intitiate as expeditiously as possible a diagnostic evaluation to make or to exclude the diagnosis.

DIAGNOSTIC EVALUATION

The fact that potentially fatal recurrent embolism can occur rules against a standard, routine algorithmic approach to diagnosis, in contrast to many other major diseases that do not have serious consequences if diagnosis is delayed for a few days. Hence, the diagnostic evaluation should be tailored to the clinical urgency and the facilities readily available to the physician.

Laboratory Tests

Although a number of biochemical and coagulation tests have been described in the past as being useful in the diagnostic evaluation, none have been sensitive or specific enough. The tests generally performed in this clinical setting, however, may help in differentiating pulmonary embolism from the two conditions that figure prominently in the differential diagnosis, namely, pneumonia and acute myocardial infarction.

The white blood cell count rarely exceeds 15,000 per cu mm in pulmonary embolism and in many instances is less than 10,000 with little or no shift to the left on the differential count. Pneumonia, on the other hand, usually is associated with white cell counts greater than 10,000, frequently greater than 15,000, with a distinct shift to the left. Initial reports[26] stressing the value of the serum enzymes, glutamic oxaloacetic transaminase (SGOT) and lactic dehydrogenase (LDH), with the serum bilirubin in establishing the diagnosis of pulmonary embolism have not been borne out by subsequent studies.[22] Changes in the levels of SGOT have been inconsistent. Elevation of bilirubin appears to be related more to the presence of congestive heart failure and hepatic congestion than pulmonary embolism. The triad of elevated LDH, normal SGOT, and increased bilirubin occurs infrequently. An elevated LDH alone is common, but a normal LDH does not exclude pulmonary embolism. In addition, elevated LDH may occur in pneumonia, acute myocardial infarction, and congestive heart failure, disease states that may mimic or accompany pulmonary embolism.

Other biochemical tests considered useful in the past include degradation products of fibrin(ogen) (FDPs). Because of lack of specificity, these tests are no longer ordered as part of the routine work-up. When pleural effusion is present, a study of pleural fluid may be helpful. A hemorrhagic or serosanguineous effusion raises the suspicion of pulmonary infarction, but many embolic effusions can be serous. In general, unless the pleural effusion poses a major mechanical hindrance to respiration, pleural taps are discouraged.

Although active investigations are currently being carried out in determining the usefulness of the specific products of thrombosis or fibrinolysis in diagnosis, none, as yet, have sufficient data supporting their use in clinical pulmonary embolism.

Chest Radiograph

Most of the radiographic changes in pulmonary embolism are subtle and nonspecific and therefore need careful scrutiny. The x-ray findings described by Fleischner consist of high position and diminished excursion of the diaphragm, plate-atelectases, pleural effusion, diminished vasculature, dilatation of hilar arteries, and right ventricular enlargement.[6] The complete picture, however, is the exception. A useful combination of findings was described by the panel of experts who reviewed the chest films for the NIH-sponsored clinical trials of thrombolytic agents in pulmonary embolism: the combination of a pulmonary infiltrate and an elevated hemidiaphragm on the same side was found in 41 per cent of the patients. The pulmonary infiltrate represents a pulmonary infarct, although most of these infiltrates were originally considered to represent pneumonia. The elevated hemidiaphragm on the involved side represents the decreased lung volume that results from the frequent atelectasis occurring in pulmonary embolism. The combination, therefore, of a pulmonary infiltrate and an elevated diaphragm on the affected side should suggest pulmonary embolism/infarction rather than penumonia.

Electrocardiogram

Although a number of electrocardiographic findings have been described in pulmonary embolism, few are specific enough to raise suspicion of the disease. Aside from the well-known pattern of acute cor pulmonale, or the S1-Q3-T3 pattern (Fig. 17–3), the other findings are nonspecific and can be encountered in many other cardiopulmonary disease states: arrhythmias, QRS abnormalities, and ST-segment and T-wave changes.[21]

The most frequently encountered arrhythmias are ventricular and atrial ectopics; the most common sustained arrhythmia is paroxysmal atrial fibrillation. Although paroxysmal atrial flutter may occur in pulmonary embolism with a high degree of specificity, its occurrence is not common. QRS abnormalities are frequently observed, having been noted in 65 per cent of patients in the NIH trials. A number of other abnormalities were observed, including right axis and left axis deviation, right bundle branch blocks, incomplete and complete, and the S1-Q3-T3 pattern. Nonspecific ST-segment and T-wave changes were common, being found in 40 to 44 per cent of patients in the trials. Aside from the S1-Q3-T3 pattern and the T-wave inversions over the right precordial leads, which generally occur only with significant pulmonary embolism, the other described findings were observed without any apparent relationship to the size of the embolic event. In essence, the ECG may be quite sensitive in patients with pulmonary embolism although many of the changes are nonspecific.

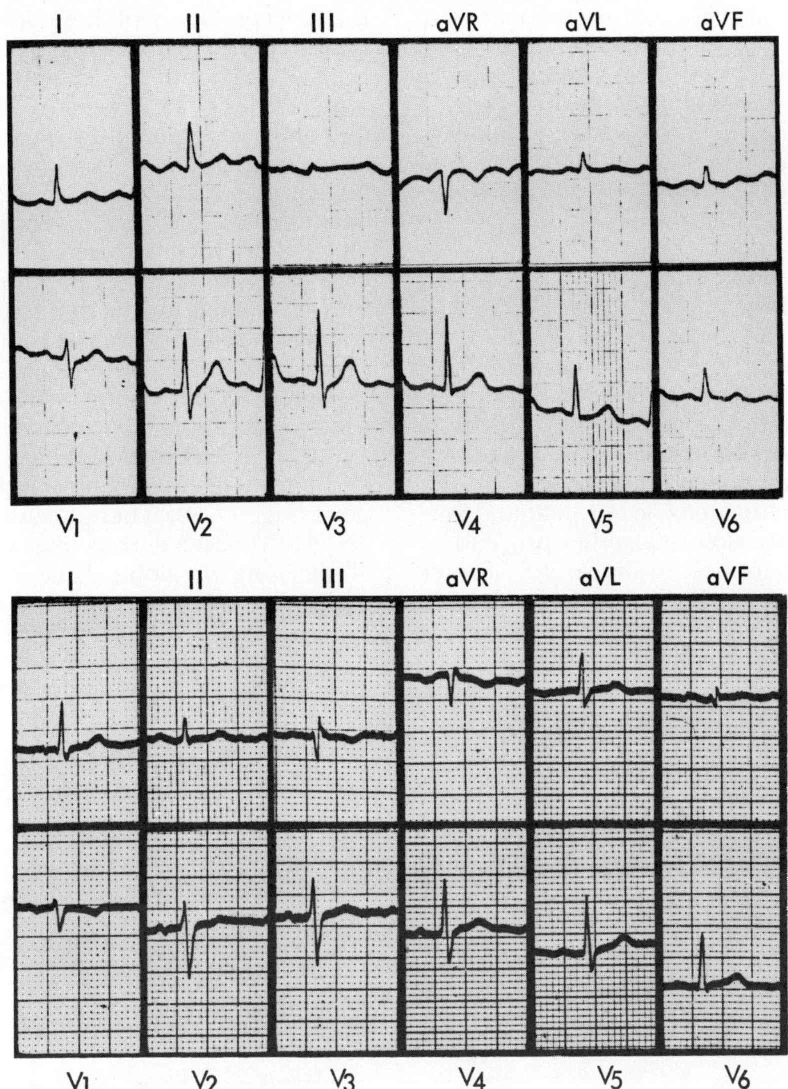

Figure 17–3. *Bottom panel,* Twelve-lead ECG from a patient with massive pulmonary embolism showing the S1, Q3, T3 pattern and right precordial ST- and T-wave changes. Compare this tracing with the normal ECG in the same patient prior to the embolic episode *(top panel).*

Nonetheless, it remains an important part of a work-up for cardiopulmonary disease and should be obtained. It is particularly useful in patients who suffer syncope or have extensive chest discomfort in which one must consider acute myocardial infarction in the differential diagnosis.

Arterial Oxygen Tension

One of the more commonly used laboratory tests for the evaluation of patients suspected of having pulmonary embolism is the measurement of arterial oxygen tension. Its usefulness derives from the fact that the vast majority of patients who suffer pulmonary embolism have some degree of hypoxemia. It is now known that, in patients without previous cardiopulmonary disease, there is an inverse relationship between the size of the embolic process and the level of the arterial Po_2: large emboli result in low Po_2 while smaller emboli show a lesser degree of hypoxemia.[9] Approximately 6 per cent of patients have a value of 90 mm Hg or more, despite the size of the embolic process. As a general rule, therefore, it can be stated that if the Po_2 is 90 mm Hg or more in patients suspected of having sustained pulmonary embolism, the likelihood that pulmonary embolism is present is only about 6 per cent. The test is most useful in patients without previous heart or lung disease in whom a normal P_{O_2} may help to exclude pulmonary embolism with a reasonably high degree of probability. Nevertheless, no diagnostic decision should be based on P_{O_2} alone.

Lung Scanning

The perfusion lung scan is an extremely useful aid in confirming the clinical impression or in excluding the diagnosis. If multiple-view scans are normal, clinical pulmonary embolism is extremely unlikely and the diagnostic evaluation may be terminated. However, if these are abnormal, other procedures should be performed to arrive at a firmer basis for diagnosis. The modern approach to the interpretation of lung scans is a more realistic approach that considers the limitations of scanning. It recognizes the fact that lung scanning is a procedure that characterizes only the regional distribution of pulmonary arterial blood flow. Since it is now known that a number of abnormalities may alter the distribution of pulmonary arterial blood flow, the interpretation of abnormal lung scaans as it relates to pulmonary embolism must take into account the probability of pulmonary embolism as the causative disease.[2]

High-probability lung scans are those in which the lesions or scan defects (1) are multiple (in one or both lungs) and (2) have configuration(s) compatible with vascular lesions (Fig. 17–4). These include lesions that occur as concave defects on the lateral edges of the lung or along a pleural surface, or wedge-shaped or segmental lesions that con-

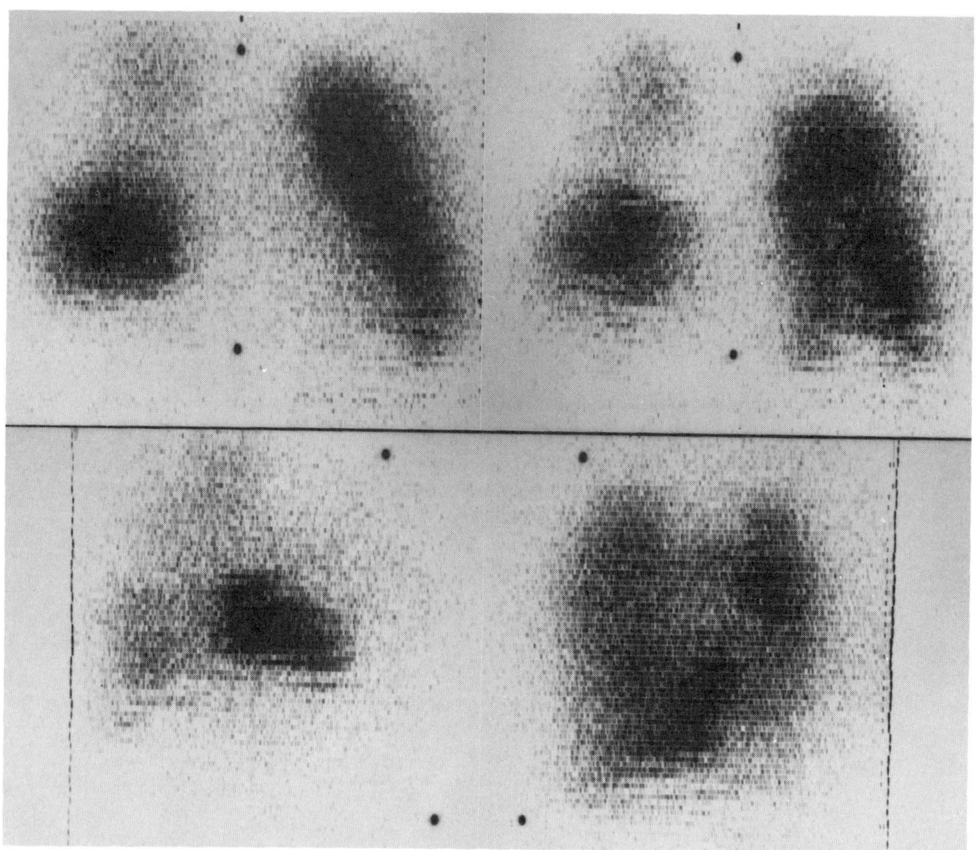

Figure 17–4. Multiple-view perfusion lung scans in a patient with massive pulmonary embolism. The top scans represent the anterior *(left)* and posterior *(right)* views. Note the marked perfusion defect in the upper two thirds of the right lung on both the anterior and posterior views. The lower panel represents the right lateral *(left)* and left lateral *(right)* views. In addition to the obvious perfusion defect on the right lateral view, the perfusion defects in the upper apical and lower posterior segments of the left lung are well visualized. The dots represent markers over the suprasternal notch and xiphoid.

form to a vascular pattern. Low-medium–probability lung scans are those in which the lesions may be either single or multiple, generally corresponding with some other abnormality on the plain chest film. The lesions are not clearly definable as segmental or vascular in origin. They tend to be round or elongated, crossing lung segments—commonly noted in those with chronic obstructive airway disease. It should be noted, however, that patients with obstructive airway disease may also show segmental or other types of lesions that have a vascular configuration. The only difference is that these vascular lesions occur much more frequently in patients with pulmonary embolism.

The simultaneous performance of ventilation (before or shortly after perfusion scanning) will add specificity to lung scanning.[10] Characteristically, a normal ventilation scan over an area that shows a perfusion defect or defects is said to be highly specific for pulmonary embolism. Such mismatched defects are generally seen only in patients with pulmonary embolism. Lesions that are matched (poor ventilation and perfusion) are indicative of other disease states such as chronic obstructive airway disease. However, it is in this category of patients that the specificity of combined ventilation and perfusion scanning is less secure. If pulmonary embolism occurred in an area of lung that already had poor perfusion and ventilation, the lung scan would not change significantly and the resulting "matched" lesions would be interpreted as consistent with chronic lung disease. Hence, in these clinical situations, other diagnostic aids such as pulmonary angiography should be performed. If the latter is not available, objective assessment of the deep venous system of the legs may be helpful. In general, however, a compatible history for pulmonary embolism in a young patient without underlying heart or lung disease plus an abnormal lung scan with V/Q mismatched lesion(s) may be adequate documentation to begin therapy.

Selective Pulmonary Angiography

Selective pulmonary angiography was popularized in 1964 and used routinely since then, becoming the standard by which pulmonary embolism can be diagnosed with assurance during life.[16] All other tests are indirect and at best may suggest a level of probability high enough to warrant therapy without adding the risks and costs of angiography. Although there is considerable current research on new diagnostic techniques to provide simple tests or a combination of tests that will yield sufficient diagnostic specificity to replace pulmonary angiography, the potential seriousness of the disease and the significant risks of treatment justify the use of angiography whenever the diagnosis is in reasonable doubt. Injection of contrast media into a peripheral vein or right atrium results in inadequate definition of the pulmonary vasculature. Selective angiography, therefore, is the desirable approach. Performance of selective views is helpful in reducing the number of equivocal results. The two accepted angiographic criteria for the diagnosis of pulmonary embolism are: vessel cut-off and intravascular filling defect (Fig. 17–5). Others, such as flow retardation, pruning, and alteration in vessel caliber, are nonspecific.

Pulmonary angiography is most helpful in demonstrating thromboembolism in patients with underlying heart or lung disease, in whom the clinical presentation may be nonspecific and compatible with an exacerbation

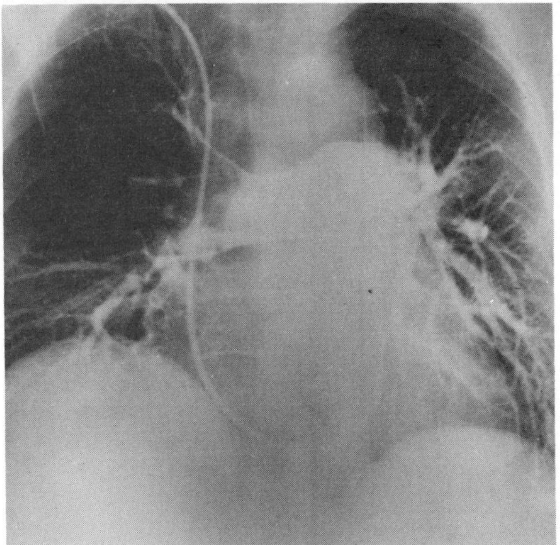

Figure 17–5. Selective pulmonary angiogram from the same patient with massive pulmonary embolism as in Figure 17–4. There is a large saddle embolus straddling the right upper and right intermediate lobar arteries, as well as an extension into the right lower lobar artery. The left upper lobar artery with its markedly compromised segmental artery perfusion is also evident, in addition to several intravascular filling defects in the left lingular and lower lobe arteries.

of the underlying disease and in whom the V/Q scan may be less specific. Visualization of the offending emboli secures the diagnosis and obviates the need for other studies.

Pulmonary angiography is also very useful in other patients without previous heart or lung disease who are suspected of having pulmonary embolism. In addition to confirming the diagnosis, the measurement of pressures in the pulmonary circulation and right heart provides an index of the degree of competency of the heart in coping with the embolic process. Since there is a direct relationship between the size of the embolic process and right heart pressures, these measurements can provide valuable diagnostic and therapeutic information.

Recurrence of pulmonary embolism is also best confirmed by pulmonary angiography. At the bedside, it is virtually impossible to differentiate true recurrence from fragmentation of the original emboli with distal migration. The performance of a repeat pulmonary angiogram may be the only reliable method in making this distinction. If a repeat angiogram shows the disappearance of a previous proximal embolus with poor or no visualization of the distal vessels subserved by the larger, originally occluded vessel, one can conclude that the original embolus fragmented, resulting in distal migration or embolization of the smaller fragments. Such a process is important to characterize because, in contrast to true recurrence, fragmentation and migration is not considered a failure of treatment that requires a change in therapy.

Pulmonary angiography, however, is an invasive procedure that has some morbidity and mortality, albeit very small. It is one of the more difficult angiographic procedures to perform well and requires expensive equipment and a trained team to perform it safely and expertly. Because of its invasive nature, it does not lend itself to serial performance, and thus other diagnostic measures have been sought. One such test is impedance plethysmography.

Electrical Impedance Plethysmography

The assessment of the deep venous system of the legs as a diagnostic aid stems from the observations made by Sevitt and Gallagher in 1961 that the great majority of their patients who died of massive pulmonary embolism had their source of emboli in the deep venous system of the legs, as demonstrated on postmortem examination.[17] Some years later, Kakkar noted a similar correlation from his radioactive fibrinogen leg scan survey of patients undergoing elective abdominal or thoracic surgery.[7] Since radioactive fibrinogen was not available for leg scans in the United States until recently, we chose to assess impedance plethysmography as the noninvasive diagnostic aid in pulmonary embolism, a technique originally described by Mullick and colleagues.[11]

This technique is practiced by elevating the foot of the bed 15°, which empties the normal venous system. The knee is bent at 30° to 35° and the hip is rotated externally, which is usually facilitated by having the patient shift his weight onto the hip of the side being tested.

Four circumferential electrodes are placed around the calf with the inner two electrodes approximately 10 cm apart. A 7-inch wide pneumatic cuff is wrapped around the lower thigh. The thigh cuff is inflated to a pressure of 45 cm of water for 45 seconds, after which it is quickly released. The initial increase in venous volume following inflation of the cuff is recorded as well as a fall in the venous volume within 3 seconds after release of the tourniquet. These two variables, reflecting venous capacitance and maximal rate of venous outflow, are then plotted as functions of each other.

If the test appears normal, the procedure is concluded. If it appears abnormal, technical factors must be excluded as the cause. The most common cause for a technical false-positive is the position of the leg. Other factors may be the tightness of the electrodes, the pneumatic cuff, the patient's clothing, or bandages. A test should not be considered positive unless repositioning of the leg has been performed several times and the other factors listed above have been checked.

The procedure is a physiologic test that detects and measures venous outflow obstruction in the deep veins, as well as the capability of the venous system to expand and constrict, as it would do in the normal state. It does this task very effectively and has a sensitivity reported to average 97 per cent and a specificity of 93 per cent.[29] It does not, however, detect thrombi in the calf veins as efficiently as it does in the deep system. Nonetheless, because of the noninvasive nature of the procedure, serial observations can be made in a patient who is in a high-risk clinical situation for developing thromboembolism.

In our validating study, 95 per cent of patients who had confirmed pulmonary embolism by angiography showed an abnormal impedance tracing indicative of deep venous obstruction. None of these patients had a history or evidence of major pelvic disease, pelvic surgery, or major pelvic manipulation that might predispose them to thrombosis of the pelvic veins. In a subsequent study, it was shown that if an assessment of the deep venous system is positive in patients with suspected pulmonary embolism, the probability of pulmonary angiographic confirmation is 90 per cent whereas, if the impedance assessment is normal bilaterally, the probability of pulmonary angiographic *exclusion* is 90 per cent.[19]

These results were very encouraging and prompted the routine clinical use of electrical impedance plethysmography in our institution, because it established the same strong relationship between pulmonary embolism and the deep veins of the legs as the source of the emboli. This procedure can now be a valuable noninvasive diagnostic aid that can lend weight to the diagnostic process in patients with suspected pulmonary embolism.

An Approach to Diagnosis

One of the most important and controversial clinical problems in pulmonary embolic disease is to decide how many and which studies are necessary for diagnosis before therapy can be instituted (Fig. 17–6). It is unrealistic to insist that all patients with suspected pulmonary embolic disease be studied in an identical manner.

In approaching this problem, several factors should be considered: (1) suspicion of pulmonary embolism, (2) urgency of diagnosis, and (3) availability of diagnostic tests or procedures. For all patients, an awareness of the possibility of pulmonary embolism, together with thorough history-taking and physical examination, is fundamental to early diagnosis. The secondary consideration concerns the urgency of diagnosis, which is determined by the clinical picture of the patient suspected of embolism.

Pulmonary Embolism (Usually Submassive) Without Significant Cardiopulmonary Decompensation or Shock. If the patient has only minimal symptoms and signs, there is adequate time for a complete laboratory work-up, which is helpful in differentiating among the various diagnostic possibilities. In addition to the routine evaluation, which includes plain chest radiography and the ECG, V/Q lung scanning with multiple views is an

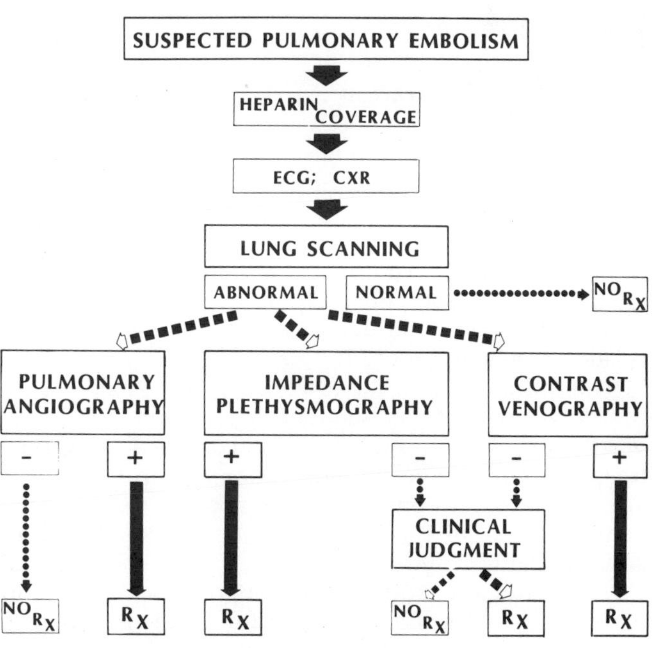

Figure 17–6. Recommended diagnostic pathways for the diagnosis of pulmonary embolism. Optimal is the use of both perfusion lung scanning and pulmonary angiography. When pulmonary angiography is not available, either scanning and impedance plethysmography or scanning and contrast venography can be employed.

important diagnostic screen. When facilities are available for performing impedance phlebography, detection of deep venous thrombosis of the legs greatly strengthens the suspicion of coexistent pulmonary embolism.

If the patient is markedly symptomatic with characteristic presentation for pulmonary embolism, an immediate V/Q lung scan is helpful to confirm the clinical suspicion and to quantify the degree of embolic occlusion. In either event—whether the clinical features are minor or major—if the subject is without previous cardiopulmonary disease and the lung scan reveals characteristic V/Q defects, treatment with heparin may be started without pulmonary angiography. If, on the other hand, preexisting cardiopulmonary disease underlies the clinical picture and the diagnosis is less certain, selective pulmonary angiography should be performed.

Pulmonary Embolism (Usually Massive) With Significant Cardiopulmonary Decompensation or Shock. In the clinical setting of marked dyspnea, air hunger, anxiety, severe right-sided failure with distended neck veins, and shock, emergency angiography is indicated, without recourse to lung scanning and to other less definitive investigative procedures, provided a thoracic surgical team capable of performing pulmonary embolectomy is available. Among other tests, only an ECG may be important.

TREATMENT

Heparin Administration

Heparin administration has been the mainstay of therapy for venous thromboembolism for over 30 years. Despite the long history of effective use, there has not been, until recently, a consensus concerning the mode of administration and the requirements for monitoring. Following demonstration of the relationship between the frequency of bleeding complications and the level of heparin in the blood,[28] and the subsequent clinical demonstration of reduced bleeding complications, the intravenous administration of heparin by continuous pump infusion appears to be the optimal method of administering the anticoagulant.[12]

Heparinization should be instituted by administering a loading dose of 3000 to 5000 units intravenously, followed immediately by a continuous pump infusion regulated to deliver 1200 units per hour. After several hours, any of several clotting tests (activated partial thromboplastin time or thrombin time) should be obtained to maintain the level of anticoagulation at approximately two to three times the control value. Following each adjustment, several hours should elapse for stabilization before another blood monitoring sample is obtained. Generally, most patients require between 1200 and 1800 units per hour to maintain the blood clotting test values in the recommended therapeutic range.

When heparin was administered in this fashion, Salzman and colleagues observed only a 1 per cent major bleeding complication, in contrast to the 8 to 10 per cent complication when heparin was given intravenously on an intermittent basis every four hours.[12] Our experience, as well as that of others, confirms these findings.

The duration of heparin administration depends on the subsidence of the acute process, which is assessed by clinical improvement. However, it has been shown in the experimental animal that seven to 12 days are required before a thrombus stabilizes, becomes firmly crosslinked, shows cellular infiltration, and becomes more firmly attached to the vein wall.[27] The process of vein wall attachment is particularly important in preventing recurrence of pulmonary embolism. Thus, it seems reasonable to maintain the most effective anticoagulant for the period of seven days or so that the patient is confined to bed.

Although the subcutaneous route of administration has been popular for many years, particularly because an intravenous line was not required, the inability to maintain smooth control of the anticoagulant levels makes this method suboptimal in achieving effective antithrombotic therapy. The intramuscular route, on the other hand, is not recommended as a safe means of drug administration.

Oral Anticoagulation

Oral anticoagulants are necessary to maintain the antithrombotic state on a more chronic basis, depending on the duration of the high-risk state for recurrent thromboembolism. The oral anticoagulant drugs have no direct effect on blood coagulation. The action is based on their antagonism with vitamin K so that the activity of vitamin K–dependent clotting factors (II, VII, IX, and X) is reduced. Sodium warfarin is the most widely used agent.

In critically ill patients who have complicating congestive heart failure, hypotension, or other morbid conditions, it is recommended that only heparin be administered during this period of complete bed rest when venous blood stasis is maximal. When clinical improvement is sufficient to project ambulation, warfarin should be begun concurrently with heparin, bearing in mind that three to four days are necessary before all the vitamin K–dependent clotting factors are sufficiently depleted to achieve an effective anticoagulated state. Because of the short half-life of six hours for Factor VII, which most influences the prothrombin time, it is possible to prolong the prothrombin time within 36 to 48 hours to therapeutic levels without achieving an antithrombotic state. Since Factor II has a half-life of 60 hours, a minimum of three or more days is required to achieve an antithrombotic state. At this point, heparin can be discontinued.

When the patient is not critically ill, oral drugs may be initiated simultaneously with heparin, providing a longer time in which to achieve the desired therapeutic range. When heparin is discontinued, only minor adjustments of dosage are generally required.

There is no unanimity concerning the optimal duration of chronic oral anticoagulant therapy. Coon and Willis, on the basis of their clinical studies,[3] showed that after four to six months of outpatient therapy there was no significant difference in the recurrence rate of thromboembolism when the anticoagulated group was compared with nonanticoagulated patients. Up to that time, however, the frequency of recurrences was strikingly higher in the nonanticoagulated group. On this empiric basis, then, it can be recommended that patients be anticoagulated for a period of at least six months. After this time, if the patient is well and fully ambulatory, without leg swelling or other abnormalities, the oral agent can be discontinued. Those with chronic venous insufficiency of the postphlebitic leg syndrome should be continued on oral anticoagulants for longer periods.

On an objective basis, impedance plethysmography and perfusion lung scanning can be carried out at monthly intervals following discharge from the hospital. When the lung scan normalizes or stabilizes on two successive monthly visits, and particularly when the impedance measurement returns to normal, indicating that no venous outflow block exists, oral anticoagulants can be terminated. In patients who have received heparin, followed by oral drugs, this status is achieved in approximately three to four months; in those who have received thrombolytic agents it takes much less time. If the impedance does not return to normal after six months, it is recommended that contrast venography be performed to assess the deep venous system. Usually, an abnormal system with occlusions and collateral vessel formation are found, which may require long-term oral anticoagulation therapy.

Thrombolytic Therapy

The investigational use of thrombolytic agents has had a long history of use in venous thromboembolism, although it was not until several years ago that the two major activators of the fibrinolytic system, streptokinase and urokinase, became available to the professional community. Streptokinase is a bacterial catabolite with a single chain that indirectly activates plasminogen through a streptokinase-plasminogen complex, whereas urokinase, produced by the parenchymal cells of the kidney, directly converts plasminogen to plasmin (Fig. 17–7).

The efficacy of these agents was established in the United States by the two major cooperative clinical trials sponsored by the National Heart, Lung, and Blood Institute: the Phase I Urokinase–Pulmonary Embolism Trial (UPET)[15] and the Phase II Urokinase-Streptokinase–Pulmonary Embolism Trial (USPET).[25] The Phase I UPET was designed to compare therapeutic efficacy of heparin therapy and of urokinase followed by heparin therapy. The Phase II USPET was designed to compare therapeutic efficacy among three thrombolytic regimens: 12-hour urokinase, 24-hour urokinase, and 24-hour streptokinase infusions, all followed by heparin and oral anticoagulant therapy. In the Phase I UPET, it was demonstrated that the 12-hour urokinase infusion regimen was superior to heparin alone when clot resolution was estimated by pre- and postinfusion pulmonary angiography, when the extent of

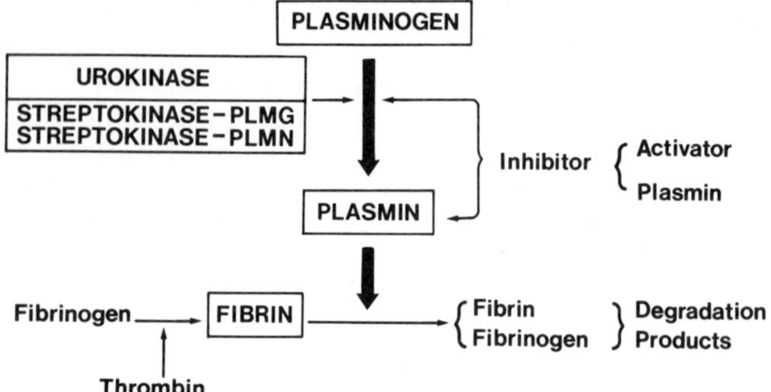

Figure 17–7. Schematic illustration of natural fibrinolysis. Streptokinase may activate this system by combining with plasminogen, whereas urokinase may activate it directly. Plasmin is the active enzyme that dissolves fresh fibrin clots.

improved perfusion was estimated by serial lung scans, and when the extent of improved hemodynamic measurements was assessed by pre- and postinfusion measurements of right atrial, right ventricular systolic and diastolic, and pulmonary arterial mean pressures, pulmonary vascular resistance, and arterial oxygen tensions. In the Phase II USPET, it was demonstrated that therapeutic efficacy was comparable among the three thrombolytic regimens and that all three were superior to heparin. The most striking changes in improvement were noted in patients with massive pulmonary embolism, and it is for this group that thrombolytic therapy is now being recommended.

Although the trials were not designed to test mortality differences because of the huge number of patients that would have been required, there are other studies showing patient benefits with thrombolytic therapy that were not associated with conventional heparin therapy. These included the much higher frequency of preservation of venous valve cusps and valve function, which may have long-term implications in preventing chronic venous hypertension and venous insufficiency.[1, 8] In addition, it has been shown that thrombolytic therapy may prevent permanent damage to the pulmonary vasculature by lysing thromboemboli and restoring the pulmonary circulation to normal,[18] as judged by our studies on pulmonary capillary blood volume and diffusing capacity. In contrast, residual emboli are usually present in patients treated with heparin alone. Such residual emboli, particularly significant in those who suffer recurrent thromboembolism, may result in persistent pulmonary hypertension. These benefits have been emphasized in a Consensus Development Conference on Thrombolytic Therapy in Thrombosis sponsored by the National Institutes of Health, and the results of this Conference have been published in a Consensus Statement.[23]

Clinical Use of Thrombolytic Therapy

Urokinase has been released for use in acute pulmonary embolism and occluded access shunts and intravascualr lines, whereas streptokinase currently has broader applications in deep vein thrombosis, pulmonary embolism, occluded access shunts and intravascular lines, and arterial thrombosis, and most recently in acute myocardial infarction. On the basis of the two NIH-sponsored trials UPET and USPET, in which the most striking clot resolutions were noted in individuals with significant embolic occlusions (more than 30 per cent obstruction of the pulmonary vasculature), it has been recommended that thrombolytic agents be used primarily in patients with the more extensive embolic obstructions in whom symptoms have been present for less than seven days. However, in view of the evidence that lytic therapy tends to preserve the anatomy of the venous valve cusps and that thromboemboli from the pulmonary vasculature are removed much more completely than with conventional heparin therapy, it seems reasonable that thrombolytic therapy be used in all patients with clinical pulmonary embolism and in those with deep vein thrombosis extending above the knee.

Selection of Patients

Patients selected for thrombolytic therapy should have had an adequate diagnostic confirmation of venous thromboembolism, preferably with pulmonary angiography or venography. It is important that the duration of symptoms be less than seven days, otherwise thromboemboli may have aged and passed the point at which reasonable lysis can be expected.

Although a number of relative contraindications are noted in the official package inserts of these two agents, the decision to treat must be made by the clinician who is in the best position to assess questions of risk and benefit.

The two absolute contraindications are an active internal bleeding state and a history of any cerebrovascular disease or procedure within the previous two months. Since it is not really known when a "safe" period begins in patients with cerebrovascular disease or following a neurosurgical procedure, lytic therapy should not be considered unless two months have elapsed. Even after this period, there should be a strong relative contraindication. Other relative contraindications include recent (less than 10 days) surgery or organ biopsy, recent serious internal trauma, pregnancy, and CPR with rib fractures. However, if a patient with a relative contraindication suffers massive, life-threatening pulmonary embolism, the clinician may decide to proceed with lytic therapy. Procedures or punctures of femoral, subclavian, or jugular vessels also constitute a relative contraindication because adequate pressure hemostasis cannot be achieved, and serious bleeding in these areas may take place before it is recognized and appropriate hemostatic measures can be instituted.

Overall, the guiding principle should be the clinician's assessment of the risk-benefit ratio, upon considering the severity of the embolic process, the projected benefits of lytic therapy, and the risk of bleeding.

Drug Administration

The initiation of thrombolytic therapy with either urokinase or streptokinase should begin with a loading dose, administered intravenously by continuous pump infusion: for urokinase, 4400 U/kg over 10 minutes; for streptokinase, 250,000 U over 30 minutes.

Since some patients may have had occult streptococcal infections before therapy, a small percentage of patients may require more than 250,000 U of streptokinase to overcome the high titers of antibodies that may be present. More than 90 per cent of patients, however, respond to this loading dose. Urokinase is a human protein and therefore does not stimulate antibody production. A predictable response can be anticipated from the loading dose.

The maintenance dose, again by continuous pump infusion, should be: for urokinase, 4400 U/kg/hr for 12 to 24 hours; for streptokinase, 100,000 U/hr for 24 to 72 hours.

The minimal duration of 12 hours for urokinase infusion was based on the observations in the USPET and UPET, concerned only with acute pulmonary embolism. However, since the vast majority of patients also have deep vein thrombosis, which responds more completely to a longer infusion, it is recommended that infusion of drug be continued for 24 hours or longer when possible.

During the administration of streptokinase for deep vein thrombosis, daily noninvasive assessments using impedance plethysmography or Doppler ultrasound should be carried out to obtain an estimate of the degree of improvement. As long as improvement continues, drug infusion should be maintained.

Monitoring of Drug Infusion

Since the loading and maintenance dosages are fixed for thrombolytic therapy, laboratory monitoring is obtained to ensure that some degree of systemic fibrinolysis has been established. As long as some degree of lysis is obtained and the fibrin clots are fresh (less than seven days), vigorous clot dissolution can be expected. When streptokinase is administered, it is particularly important to monitor lysis because of the occasional patient with very high titers of streptococcal antibodies from a previous infection, and in whom the streptokinase infusion is thus ineffective. Moreover, without the lytic and anticoagulant effects, the patient is at risk of recurrent thromboembolism.

Since most clinical laboratories do not routinely perform the thrombin time test, arrangements should be made to have it available. It is very sensitive to the depletion of fibrinogen and the generation of fibrin(ogen) degradation products. As measurable amounts of these products are generated, the thrombin time becomes prolonged, reflecting an active fibrinolytic state.

Alternatively, the partial thromboplastin (PTT) and prothrombin (PT) times can be substituted, although they do not reflect the fibrinolytic state as sensitively as the thrombin time. However, when degradation products of thrombolysis are generated, functioning as circulating anticoagulants, the PTT and PT become prolonged, indicating a fibrinolytic state.

The performance of laboratory monitoring tests is less important when urokinase is employed since it is a human protein, evoking no antigenic response. Nevertheless, it is reassuring to know that systemic fibrinolysis has been achieved that reflects the functional integrity of the pump infusion system. Thus, after the infusion is begun, one of the tests, thrombin time, whole blood euglobulin lysis time, or PT and PTT, should be obtained three to four hours later. If systemic fibrinolysis has been established, no further tests are necessary. If no changes from the control value are obtained, the urokinase infusion system should be checked. With streptokinase, another loading dose should be administered and the infusion continued. The monitoring test should be rechecked in three to four hours and, if the test value persists unchanged, streptokinase should be discontinued and urokinase instituted. Alternatively, lytic therapy should be abandoned and heparin therapy begun.

Upon completion of lytic therapy, heparin administration should be begun to prevent rethrombosis and re-embolization. To effect a smooth transition, a PTT should be obtained after discontinuing thrombolytic therapy. When the value is twice that of a normal control, a continuous infusion of heparin should be instituted without a loading dose. Adjustments of dosage are based on the PTT as is conventionally done and maintained for the usual five to ten days, overlapping with oral anticoagulants.

Adjunctive Therapy

Since most patients with clinically detectable pulmonary embolism have some degree of hypoxemia, oxygen therapy is an important adjunct. Administration of oxygen relieves or diminishes the symptoms of hypoxemia in many patients. Since hypoventilation is rarely a cause of hypoxemia in pulmonary embolism, oxygen may be given comfortably by nasal catheter without fear of suppressing ventilation.

In patients who sustain major to massive pulmonary edema, cardiac failure frequently is observed, particularly when there is preexisting cardiopulmonary disease. The cardiac index may fall below 2.0 liters/min/meter^2. In such circumstances, the administration of an isoproterenol hydrochloride drip (2–4 mg/500 ml 5% dextrose in water) is helpful as a cardiotonic agent; it increases cardiac output and decreases pulmonary arterial pressure. Occasionally, when central venous pressure is low, administration of intravenous fluids may be helpful in restoring near-normal hemodynamics. Digitalis glycosides, intravenously administered diuretics, and various antiarrhythmic agents should be used in the appropriate clinical situation in the usual dosages.

Surgical Therapy

The role of surgery in pulmonary embolism is twofold: (1) prevention by interruption of venous flow and (2) reversal of the lethal effects of massive pulmonary embolism by embolectomy.

Prevention of Pulmonary Embolism

Since more than 90 per cent of emboli originate in thrombi in the lower extremities, surgical maneuvers have been directed toward interruption of the venous system from this region of the body. Most emboli from the lower extremities originate from thrombosis of the deep venous system rather than from the superficial system; ligation of the saphenous vein(s) at the groin therefore has long been recognized as a futile maneuver and has been discarded. However, it is indicated in the rare instance (1%) when superficial venous thrombosis propagates above the midthigh.

Similarly, single or bilateral superficial femoral vein or deep femoral vein ligations in the groin, which were in vogue some 20 years ago, are rarely used today. Interruption of the superficial femoral vein offers no protection from the more common embolization from the deep femoral venous system. Thrombi were often present above the ligation. Analysis of considerable data has demonstrated that femoral vein ligation is not as effective as anticoagulation alone in preventing subsequent pulmonary embolism. Furthermore, leg morbidity from venous stasis following deep femoral vein ligation was unacceptably high.

1. CONTRAINDICATIONS TO ANTICOAGULATION
2. RECURRENCE DURING *ADEQUATE* ANTICOAGULATION
3. SEPTIC PELVIC THROMBOPHLEBITIS WITH EMBOLI
4. RECURRENT PULMONARY EMBOLI
5. NEAR-FATAL PULMONARY EMBOLI
6. PULMONARY EMBOLECTOMY

Figure 17–8. Indications for inferior vena caval interruption.

Currently, the inferior vena cava is considered the most effective site for venous interruption and has replaced more distal ligational sites.

There is still controversy regarding the indications for inferior vena caval interruption. Some physicians use this technique quite frequently after an episode of pulmonary embolism, regardless of its severity. However, since the morbidity of vena caval interruption is significant and since the procedure carries a mortality of over 5 per cent,[4] conservatism is warranted. Before caval interruption is decided upon, there should be reasonable assurance that the source of embolism is in the venous system below the proposed site of interruption.

Our indications for inferior vena caval interruption are listed in Figure 17– 8, and are discussed below.

(1) Significant pulmonary embolism with contraindications to anticoagulation. This is the most common indication for caval interruption. One contraindication to anticoagulants may be actual or potential bleeding from mucosal lesions. Recent surgery (one to seven days) on the brain, spinal cord, or retroperitoneum is a relative contraindication, depending on the magnitude of the procedure and the degree of hemostasis in the preceding 48 hours. Discontinuation of anticoagulants, usually due to the development of complications, is a variant of the above. Recurrent emboli during *adequate* anticoagulant (heparin) therapy represent a failure of anticoagulants. As mentioned before, it is imporant to distinguish between a true recurrence of pulmonary embolism from a fragmentation and distal migration of the original emboli. The former represents treatment failure that usually calls for a change in therapy; the latter does not. It is also important to know that "recurrence" arose during adequate heparinization in which the clotting tests were maintained at therapeutic levels for at least several days. Pulmonary embolism has recurred during the early stage of heparinization in which the clotting test values were near, but not in, therapeutic range. It seems reasonable in this situation to continue with heparin therapy.

(2) Multiple episodes of PE over a period of weeks or months. This is a situation in which the risk of very prolonged anticoagulation must be weighed against the risk of caval interruption.

(3) Uncontrolled septic pelvic thrombophlebitis with multiple septic pulmonary emboli. "Uncontrolled" means lack of a rapid response to heparin-antibiotic administration. This condition is potentially lethal and represents an urgent indication for caval and left ovarian vein *ligation.* Partial interruption should not be performed in this clinical setting.

(4) Concurrently with pulmonary embolectomy.

(5) Occurrence of paradoxical embolism into the systemic circulation through an atrial septal defect or patent foramen ovale, or through a ventricular septal defect. As mentioned previously, the development of pulmonary hypertension as a result of massive pulmonary embolism increases the likelihood of paradoxical embolism. This demands total rather than partial interruption of the cava.

(6) Massive pulmonary embolism, not requiring embolectomy, but when recurrent embolization could be lethal. This is a controversial indication, and considerable thought should be given in each case before the decision to interrupt the cava is made. For example, when the source of emboli is from nonocclusive iliofemoral vein thrombosis, caval interruption may be desirable. Because of the length and diameter of these veins, emboli tend to be massive and poorly tolerated. In general, however, the severity in compromise of the baseline cardiopulmonary status should be the determinant factor in the decision to perform caval interruption.

(7) Prophylactic. In patients undergoing major abdominal surgery (gastric, colonic, uterine, ovarian, pancreatic, or aortic aneu-

rysm resection) with a previous history of venous thromboembolism, some surgeons would interrupt the cava as a prophylactic measure. This is, however, a controversial indication and must be considered on an individual basis. The additional presence of obesity, malignancy, or compromise in cardiac function might also favor caval interruption. Many surgeons, in contrast, would employ low-dose heparin or other effective means of prophylaxis for venous thrombosis.

To avoid using general anesthesia and to reduce the mortality and morbidity of the plication procedures, a number of vena caval filter devices have been introduced during the past ten years. The earliest of these is the Mobinuddin umbrella filter, which can be introduced under local anesthesia through an incision in the internal jugular vein. Thousands of these filters have so far been employed, the only major complication being dislodgement of the filter (1%). The Kim-Ray-Greenfield filter has been introduced recently; it can be inserted through the femoral vein and positioned in the inferior vena cava more easily than the umbrella filter.

Pulmonary Embolectomy

As mentioned above, there is now an increased awareness of the natural history of pulmonary embolism, with its predominant tendency for spontaneous lysis during anticoagulant therapy and accelerated lysis with thrombolytic agents. This awareness has considerably limited the indications for pulmonary embolectomy. Barring recurrent embolism, if the circulation can be supported to sustain perfusion to the vital organs, the patient will improve over a period of hours and days. On the whole, patients with massive pulmonary embolism who re-establish circulatory compensation respond rapidly and impressively with thrombolytic therapy.[15] If thrombolytic agents are not available, heparin therapy is satisfactory.

The indications for pulmonary embolectomy have not changed from those stated in an editorial in 1973:[14] "If maximal medical treatment (oxygen, isoproterenol, heparin or lytic therapy) does not succeed within an hour in re-establishing and maintaining an adequate circulation (systolic blood pressure greater than 90 mm Hg, urine output greater than 20 ml/hour, arterial oxygen tension greater than 60 mm Hg and absence of peripheral vasomotor collapse), then the decision for embolectomy should be made." Massive pulmonary embolism must be confirmed by pulmonary angiography before embolectomy is attempted. If it is evident that renal, cerebral, and pulmonary functions are well maintained, embolectomy may be deferred. Although some authors have advocated an aggressive approach, recommending embolectomy before the onset of circulatory failure, it is strongly recommended that embolectomy not be done "on the unwarranted assumption that a patient would deteriorate at some future time without an operation. On the other hand, it would be equally wrong to persist in medical treatment until the patient is moribund before an embolectomy is attempted."[14] If these indications are closely observed, the survival rate can be expected to be between 35 and 50 per cent. We believe, therefore, that pulmonary embolectomy is not indicated in the great majority of patients who suffer massive pulmonary embolism. In those few individuals who have persistent and refractory circulatory failure, however, it may be lifesaving.

References

1. Arnesen, H., Heilo, A., Jakobsen, E., et al.: A prospective study of streptokinase and heparin in the treatment of deep vein thrombosis. Acta Med. Scand. 203:457, 1978.
2. Barritt, D. W., and Jordan, S. C.: Anticoagulant drugs in the treatment of pulmonary embolism. Lancet 1:1309, 1960.
3. Coon, W. W., and Willis, P. W.: Deep venous thrombosis and pulmonary embolism. Prediction, prevention and treatment. Am. J. Cardiol. 4:611, 1959.
4. Crane, C.: Femoral vs. caval interruption for venous thromboembolism. N. Engl. J. Med. 270:819, 1964.
5. Dalen, J. E., and Alpert, J. S.: Natural history of pulmonary embolism. Prog. Cardiovasc. Dis. 17:259, 1975.
6. Fleischner, F. G.: Observations on the radiologic changes in pulmonary embolism. *In* Sasahara, A. A., and Stein, M. (eds.): Pulmonary Embolic Disease. New York, Grune & Stratton, 1965, p. 312.
7. Kakkar, V. V., Howe, C. T., Flanc, C., and Clark, M. B.: Natural history of postoperative deep vein thrombosis. Lancet 2:230, 1969.
8. Kakkar, V. V., Howe, C. T., Laws, J. W., and Flanc, C.: Late result of treatment of deep vein thrombosis. Br. Med. J. 1:810, 1969.
9. McIntyre, K. M., and Sasahara, A. A.: The hemodynamic response to pulmonary embolism in patients without prior cardiopulmonary disease. Am. J. Cardiol. 28:288, 1971.
10. McNeil, B. J.: A diagnostic strategy using ventilation perfusion studies in patients suspect for pulmonary embolism. J. Nucl. Med. 17:613, 1976.

11. Mullick, S. C., Wheeler, H. B., and Songster, G. F.: Diagnosis of deep vein thrombosis by measurement of electrical impedance. Am. J. Surg. 119:417, 1970.
12. Salzman, E. W., Deykin, D., Shapiro, R. M., and Rosenberg, R.: Management of heparin therapy: controlled prospective trial. N. Engl. J. Med. 292:1046, 1975.
13. Sasahara, A. A.: Current problems in pulmonary embolism: introduction. *In* Sasahara, A. A., Sonnenblick, E. H., and Lesch, M. (eds.): Pulmonary Emboli. New York, Grune & Stratton, 1975. p. 1.
14. Sasahara, A. A., and Barsamian, E. M.: Another look at pulmonary embolectomy. Ann. Thorac. Surg. 16:317, 1973.
15. Sasahara, A. A., Hyers, T. M., Cole, C. M., et al.: The Urokinase–Pulmonary Embolism Trial: a national cooperative study. Circulation 47(Suppl. II):66, 1973.
16. Sasahara, A. A., Stein, M., Simon, M., and Littmann, D.: Pulmonary angiography in the diagnosis of thromboembolic disease. N. Engl. J. Med. 270:1075, 1964.
17. Sevitt, S., and Gallagher, N. G.: Venous thrombosis and pulmonary embolism: a clinicopathological study in injured and burned patients. Br. J. Surg. 48:475, 1961.
18. Sharma, G. V. R. K., Burleson, V. A., and Sasahara, A. A.: Effect of thrombolytic therapy on pulmonary capillary blood volume in patients with pulmonary embolism. N. Engl. J. Med. 303:842, 1980.
19. Sharma, G. V. R. K., Greenfield, D. H., McIntyre, K. M., and Sasahara, A. A.: Venous thrombosis and pulmonary embolism. *In* Parisi, A. F., and Tow, D. E. (eds.): Noninvasive Approaches to Cardiovascular Diagnosis. New York, Appleton-Century-Crofts, 1979, pp. 181–198.
20. Sharma, G. V. R. K., and Sasahara, A. A.: Diagnosis of pulmonary embolism in patients with chronic obstructive pulmonary disease. J. Chronic Dis. 28:255, 1975.
21. Stein, P. D., Dalen, J. E., McIntyre, K. M., et al.: The electrocardiogram in pulmonary embolism. *In* Sasahara, A. A., Sonnenblick, E. H., and Lesch, M. (eds.): Pulmonary Emboli. New York, Grune & Stratton, 1975, pp. 65–75.
22. Szucs, M. M., Brooks, H. L., Grossman, W., et al.: Diagnostic sensitivity of laboratory findings in acute pulmonary embolism. Ann. Intern. Med. 74:161, 1971.
23. Thrombolytic Therapy in Thrombosis: NIH Consensus Development Conference Summary. Vol. 3, No. 1, 1980.
24. Tow, D. E., and Simon, A. L.: Comparison of lung scanning and pulmonary angiography in the detection and follow-up of pulmonary embolism: The Urokinase–Pulmonary Embolism Trial experience. Prog. Cardiovasc. Dis. 17:239, 1975.
25. Urokinase-Streptokinase–Pulmonary Embolism Trial: Phase II results. J.A.M.A. 229:1606, 1974.
26. Wacker, W. E. C., Rosenthal, M., Snodgrass, P. J., and Amador, E.: A triad for the diagnosis of pulmonary embolism and infarction. J.A.M.A. 178:8, 1961.
27. Wessler, S., Freiman, D. G., Ballon, J. D., et al.: Experimental pulmonary embolism with serum-induced thrombi. Am. J. Pathol. 38:89, 1961.
28. Wessler, S., and Gitel, S. N.: Control of heparin therapy. Prog. Hemost. Thromb. 3:311, 1976.
29. Wheeler, H. B., O'Donnell, J. A., Anderson, F. A., and Benedick, K.: Occlusive impedance phlebography: a diagnostic procedure for deep vein thrombosis and pulmonary embolism. Prog. Cardiovasc. Dis. 17:199, 1974.

18

Diagnosis and Treatment of Acute Respiratory Failure

JEANINE P. WIENER-KRONISH

and MICHAEL A. MATTHAY

In this chapter, we focus on the diagnosis and treatment of the two most frequent causes of acute respiratory failure: (1) acute pulmonary edema, both cardiogenic and noncardiogenic; and (2) decompensated chronic obstructive lung disease. These two types are discussed separately, since their pathophysiology and clinical features are quite different. In respiratory failure from acute pulmonary edema, severe hypoxemia is the main physiologic disturbance, whereas in respiratory failure from decompensated chronic obstructive lung disease, both hypercapnia and hypoxemia are the major abnormalities.

PULMONARY EDEMA

In order to administer the appropriate treatment to patients in respiratory failure from acute pulmonary edema, it is important to understand why they are so hypoxic. Severe hypoxemia occurs when there is markedly decreased or absent ventilation to many lung units that still receive blood flow. These lung units are called shunt units, because the blood flowing by these units is not oxygenated. Most of the alveoli are filled with edema fluid, so that these lung units have a ventilation-perfusion ratio of zero (Fig. 18–1). Therefore, giving the patient with pulmonary edema high concentrations of oxygen to breathe does not relieve the severe hypoxemia, as very little oxygen can reach the perfusing blood.

Less severe hypoxemia is seen when the majority of lung units receive some ventilation or have ventilation-perfusion ratios less than one, but greater than zero. In patients with asthma and chronic obstructive pulmonary disease (COPD), ventilation-perfusion mismatch is the major cause of hypoxemia. In contrast to those with shunts, patients with ventilation-perfusion mismatch can experience a marked increase in their oxygenation with relatively low concentrations of inspired oxygen. Improved oxygenation occurs in the latter because their lung units can receive some of the oxygen that is inspired, and the perfusing blood absorbs this oxygen.*

Patients with shunting and ventilation-perfusion mismatch can also have other abnormalities that make their hypoxemia more severe. If these patients develop decreased

*In order to determine the severity of a patient's hypoxemia, arterial PaO_2 should be compared with alveolar oxygen tension. This can be done by simply calculating the difference between alveolar oxygen tension and arterial oxygen tension; normally, the difference is small. Since direct measurements of alveolar gas tension are difficult, alveolar oxygen tension (PAO_2) is estimated by using the alveolar gas equation:

$PAO_2 = P_IO_2 \times \frac{PACO_2}{R}$ where P_IO_2 is the Po_2 of the inspired gas (760 mm Hg − 47 mm Hg (water pressure) × % FIO_2) (FIO_2 = fraction inspired oxygen concentration.) $PACO_2$ is the alveolar Pco_2 (assumed to be equal to the arterial Pco_2) and R is the respiratory exchange ratio (normally 0.8). Once alveolar oxygen tension is calculated, the measured arterial oxygen tension is subtracted from it to obtain the alveolar-arterial oxygen difference (A-aO_2). While breathing room air, the normal value for the A-aO_2 difference is less than 30 mm Hg. A larger difference indicates lung disease. Measuring the A-aO_2 on an FIO_2 greater than 70% oxygen will give an estimate of the hypoxemia caused by shunt units in the lungs (Fig. 18–2).[40]

Figure 18–1. Alveoli filled with edema fluid, protein, and cellular debris cannot be penetrated by oxygen flowing into the lungs. Gas transfer does not occur, so that the blood perfusing these alveoli remains unoxygenated. The ventilation-perfusion ratio is thus zero.

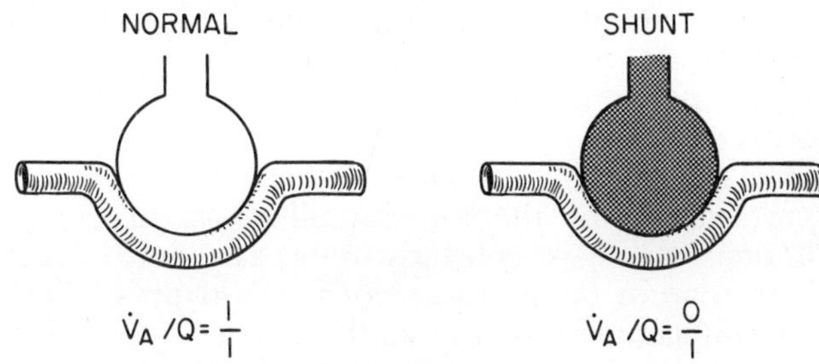

cardiac output, their lung units with low ventilation-perfusion ratios will be perfused by blood with lower oxygen tensions owing to the long circulation time.[23, 25] The end result is more severe hypoxemia (Fig. 18–3).

Some critically ill patients with pulmonary edema and severe hypoxemia may develop hypercapnia ($PaCO_2 > 40$ mm Hg) because of muscle weakness, concomitant airway disease, or a decreased central ventilatory drive from sedatives or analgesics (such as morphine). The hypercapnia worsens the arterial hypoxemia because alveolar oxygen tension falls as arterial and alveolar CO_2 rises. As the alveolar O_2 tension falls, arterial oxygen tension declines also.

Cardiogenic Pulmonary Edema

In this section, we first discuss approaches to determine the etiology of the cardiogenic pulmonary edema. Secondly, we reveiw the principles of diagnosis and treatment of the respiratory failure that occurs with cardiogenic pulmonary edema.

Many patients require measurement of pulmonary arterial wedge pressure, which reflects left atrial pressure, to determine whether elevated pulmonary capillary wedge (PCW) pressure is the cause of the pulmonary edema.

The type of pulmonary edema can sometimes be discerned by analyses of the protein concentration of airway edema fluid. In patients with cardiogenic pulmonary edema, a low ratio of the protein in edema fluid to the

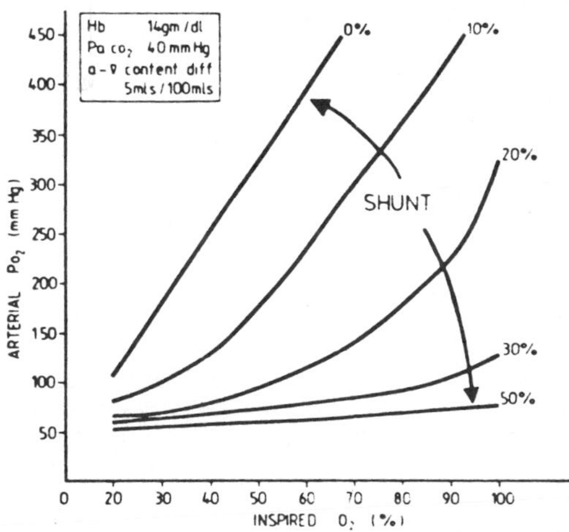

Figure 18–2. The relationship among the inspired oxygen concentration (FIO_2, %), the arterial PaO_2, and the shunt fraction is shown. The patient is assumed to have a normal hemoglobin concentration, a normal $PaCO_2$, and a normal cardiac output. (From Flenly, D. C.: Blood gas and acid base interpretations. Basics of Respiratory Disease, ATS News, Fall, 1981. Reproduced with permission.)

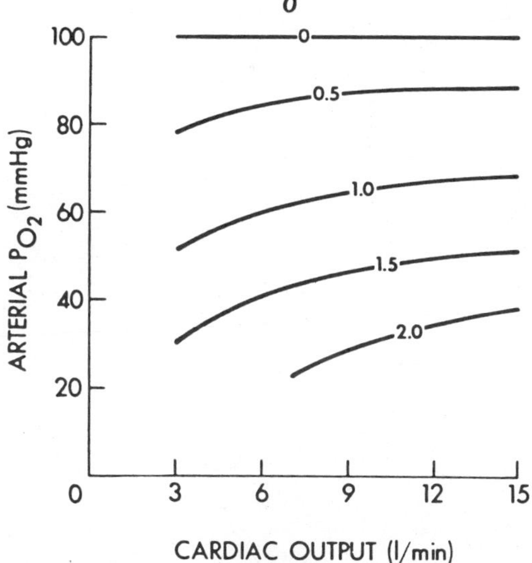

Figure 18–3. The relationship between arterial PO_2 and cardiac output is shown, when there are varying amounts of ventilation-perfusion inequality (V/Q). When there is no ventilation-perfusion inequality (Q = 0), changing the cardiac output has no effect on PaO_2. However, as the ventilation-perfusion inequality worsens (Q = 0.5–2), a decrease in cardiac output decreases the PaO_2 and an increase in cardiac output increases the PaO_2. (From West, J. B., and Wagner, P. D.: Bioengineering Aspects of the Lungs. New York, Marcel Dekker, Inc., 1977. Reprinted by courtesy of Marcel Dekker, Inc.)

protein in plasma protein concentration ($\leq 55\%$) is found. In contrast, noncardiogenic pulmonary edema has a high protein concentration in the edema fluid close to that of plasma ($\leq 80\%$) because of the increased permeability of the alveolocapillary membrane.[29, 48, 108] A recent study found that there is overlap in these airway edema fluid protein-to-plasma ratios, so that there may be an intermediate form of pulmonary edema with both increased hydrostatic pressures and increased permeability.[97]

As described in Chapter 2, patients with acute cardiogenic pulmonary edema should be categorized into hemodynamic subsets according to their stroke work index and left ventricular filling pressure.[57] In general, the principal goals of therapy are to reduce the left ventricular filling pressures and to reduce myocardial oxygen consumption. These goals can usually be accomplished by bed rest, morphine, and diuretics. In patients whose systemic vascular resistance is markedly elevated, sodium nitroprusside can be used to reduce arterial pressures and also to further decrease left ventricular pressures.[57]

In addition to decreasing pressures and oxygen consumption of the heart, attempts should be made to increase myocardial oxygen supply. Patients with cardiogenic pulmonary edema often respond resonably well to supplemental oxygen and diuretics and, if necessary, vasodilator therapy.

In some patients with cardiogenic pulmonary edema, the acute respiratory distress is not satisfactorily relieved by the above measures. Arterial oxygen tension remains below 60 mm Hg and the work of breathing is high (Fig. 18–4). These patients will benefit from nasotracheal intubation and positive-pressure ventilation. Tracheal intubation can usually be accomplished by the nasotracheal route without the need for sedation or paralyzing agents.[24]

There are several reasons why positive-pressure ventilation treats both the cardiac and respiratory problems. First, it reduces preload by decreasing venous return to the heart. Second, it may decrease afterload on the left heart by abolishing wide swings in pleural pressure produced by the dyspneic, spontaneously breathing patient. Also, it almost invariably improves arterial oxygenation because of better ventilation of lung units that previously were poorly ventilated. Finally, positive-pressure ventilation takes over the work of breathing so that myocardial oxygen demand is reduced and the patient can rest.

Noncardiogenic Pulmonary Edema

The adult respiratory distress syndrome (ARDS) is a clinical syndrome of patients who have developed acute respiratory failure pri-

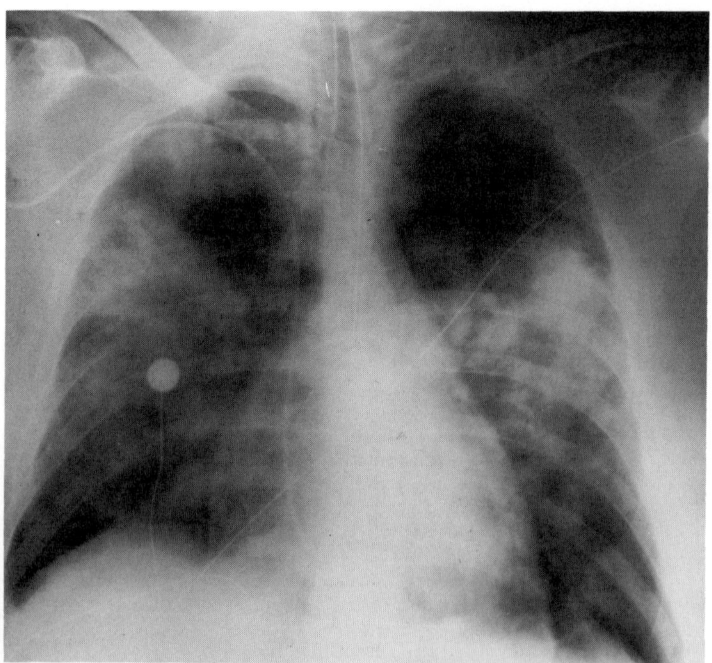

Figure 18–4. An anteroposterior chest roentgenogram showing the butterfly pattern of cardiogenic pulmonary edema. Note that the patient is intubated and has a Swan-Ganz pulmonary arterial catheter in place.

marily from noncardiogenic pulmonary edema. There are three classic hallmarks: severe hypoxemia refractory to high inspired oxygen fractions, diffuse bilateral infiltrates on the chest radiograph, and reduced lung compliance.[42, 74] The causes of ARDS are numerous (Table 18–1); the important ones to remember are those that are treatable, particularly sepsis and primary lung infections.

Table 18–1. ETIOLOGIES OF THE ADULT RESPIRATORY DISTRESS SYNDROME*

Sepsis
Trauma
Fat emboli
Lung contusion
Nonthoracic trauma
Shock of any etiology
Aspiration of liquid
Gastric contents
Fresh and salt water (drowning)
Hydrocarbon fluids
Associated with drugs
Heroin
Methadone
Propoxyphene
Barbiturates
Colchicine
Ethchlorvynol
Aspirin
Hydrochlorothiazide
Inhaled toxins
Smoke
Oxygen (high concentration)
Corrosive chemicals (NO_2, Cl_2, NH_3, phosgene)
Hematologic disorders
Massive blood transfusion
Thrombotic thrombocytopenic purpura
Disseminated intravascular coagulation
Metabolic disorders
Acute pancreatitis
Uremia
Miscellaneous
Lymphangiography
Lymphangitic carcinomatosis
Increased intracranial pressure
Postcardiopulmonary bypass
Eclampsia
Radiation pneumonitis
Air emboli
Amniotic fluid embolism
Ascent to high altitude
Primary pneumonias
Viruses
Bacteria (including legionnaires' disease)
Mycobacterium tuberculosis
Fungi
Pneumocystis carinii
Mycoplasma pneumoniae

*From Matthay, M. A., and Hopewell, P. C.: The adult respiratory distress syndrome: pathogenesis and treatment. *In* Simmons, D. H. (ed.): Current Pulmonology, Vol. 3. New York, John Wiley & Sons, 1981. Reprinted by permission of John Wiley & Sons, Inc.

Pathophysiology

The common abnormality in patients with ARDS, regardless of the associated clinical disorder, is increased permeability of the alveolocapillary membrane so that protein-rich fluid collects in the interstitium and airspaces of the lung. A review of the mechanism of this increased permeability edema is beyond the scope of this chapter but has appeared in various articles.[58, 98, 99] The abnormalities of pulmonary function in patients with noncardiogenic pulmonary edema are similar even though the causes initiating the syndrome are varied. Hypoxemia is always present, mainly because right-to-left shunts are created by alveolar flooding and atelectasis.*[22, 105]

The diffuse bilateral infiltrates seen on the chest roentgenograms of these patients are also caused by the alveolar flooding and atelectasis (Fig. 18–5). The fluid in the alveoli displaces air, so that the density is increased on the radiograph. Measurements of the lung volume are decreased because of the fluid in the alveoli;[99] air cannot penetrate the fluid-filled alveoli, so the measured vital capacity and functional residual capacity are reduced.[28, 64] There is also a decrease in lung compliance that is due to the fluid in the alveoli and interstitium, and perhaps to a reaction between the protein and surfactant in the alveoli, causing increased surface tension and alveolar instability.[99]

The reduced compliance means that for any distending pressure the lung volume is smaller than normal. Therefore, high pressures are required to ventilate these patients at normal tidal volumes. Indeed, serial measurements of the static compliance of the chest wall and lung, utilizing the plateau airway pressure at end-inspiration and the expired tidal volume, can be useful to follow the course of ARDS patients.[12, 100]

Patients with noncardiogenic pulmonary edema can also have abnormal cardiac function. Studies evaluating right ventricular function have shown that some patients with severe noncardiogenic pulmonary edema have markedly decreased right ventricular

*Although carbon dioxide elimination is not usually a problem, it can become one later in the syndrome when interstitial fibrosis and capillary obliteration occur. This morphologic change means that instead of having mostly lung units with low ventilation-perfusion ratios, there are areas of high ventilation-perfusion ratios. This means that physiologic dead space is increased and carbon dioxide elimination may be impaired.

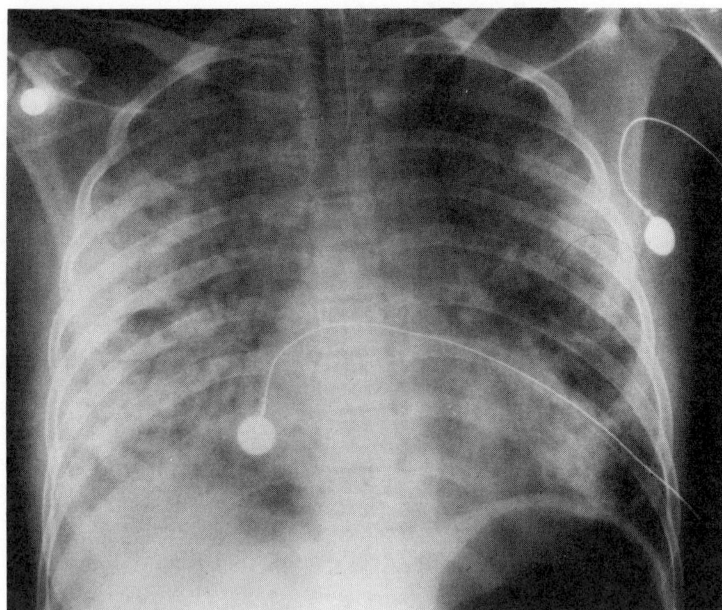

Figure 18–5. An anteroposterior chest roentgenogram showing diffuse bilateral infiltrates that obscure the heart borders. Note that the patient is intubated. A Swan-Ganz catheter was passed into the pulmonary artery and the wedge pressure measured 2 mm Hg. This low-pressure pulmonary edema was due to increased vascular permeability from gram-negative sepsis.

performance.[10, 52] As the lung injury progresses, the right ventricular ejection fraction decreases, suggesting that the ventricular dysfunction is caused by increased afterload from acute pulmonary hypertension.[52, 95] This increase in pulmonary arterial pressure is caused in part by vascular obstruction.[35, 112] The pulmonary arterial hypertension may also be caused by hypoxic pulmonary vasoconstriction, since vasodilators can reduce pulmonary arterial pressures modestly.[110]

Finally, abnormal muscle performance can be seen in noncardiogenic pulmonary edema and can even make the respiratory failure worse. Respiratory muscle fatigue may occur as the work of breathing rises to ventilate the "stiff" lungs. This muscle fatigue is worsened by arterial hypoxemia and a decrease in cardiac output[8, 56, 84]

Treatment

Mechanical Ventilation and Positive End-Expiratory Airway Pressure. Patients with noncardiogenic pulmonary edema usually require mechanical ventilation for four reasons: (1) to assume the high work of breathing, (2) to ventilate mechanically with large tidal volumes, (3) to deliver high concentrations of inspired oxygen, and (4) to deliver positive end-expiratory airway pressure (PEEP) (see Fig. 18–5). These patients often have muscle fatigue so that they need mechanical ventilation to take over the work of their breathing. They also have decreased functional residual capacities so that they need mechanical ventilation to increase their lung volume with larger tidal volumes and PEEP.

The ventilator has the important role of supplying high concentrations of oxygen to

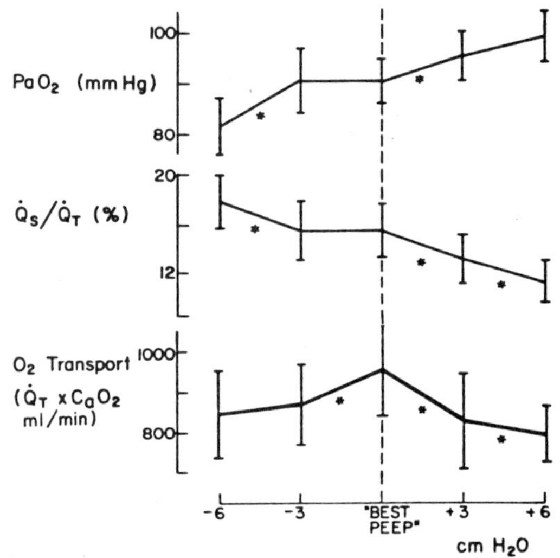

Figure 18–6. The figure shows that at the "best PEEP" level the PaO_2 is high, the shunt ($\dot{Q}_S/\dot{Q}_T$) has decreased, and the oxygen transport has increased. Levels of PEEP above the "best PEEP" increase the PaO_2 and the shunt also decreases further, but the oxygen transport decreases. (From Suter et al.: Optimum end-expiratory airway pressure in patients with acute pulmonary failure. N. Engl. J. Med. 292:286, 1975. Reprinted by permission of the New England Journal of Medicine.)

these hypoxemic patients. However, inspired oxygen concentrations above 40 per cent are associated with an increased risk of oxygen toxicity.[109] Thus, one of the goals of supportive therapy is to achieve adequate oxygenation at the lowest possible fraction of inspired oxygen (FIO_2). PEEP is the proved adjunct to mechanical ventilation that usually results in improved arterial oxygenation and a lower FIO_2. Levels of PEEP in the range of 5 to 15 cm H_2O usually improve PaO_2 markedly. PEEP primarily increases PaO_2 by increasing functional residual capacity and thereby increasing ventilation to previously underventilated lung units.[26, 28, 70, 103] Sometimes, however, this beneficial effect is offset by a decrease in cardiac output that results in a net decrease in oxygen transport, even though PaO_2 is higher (Fig. 18–6). Therefore, it is not sufficient to follow a patient's PaO_2; cardiac output and calculated oxygen transport should also be monitored.[23, 100]

In fact, it has been shown that the clinical improvement in arterial oxygenation seen with PEEP is in part due to a decrease in cardiac output.[23, 55] The reason for improved arterial oxygenation may be a reduction in blood flow to poorly ventilated lung units because of the fall in cardiac output, and thus less intrapulmonary shunting and less return of unoxygenated blood to the systemic circulation.

The reason for the decrease in cardiac output with PEEP has ben extensively investigated. Wood and Prewitt[21, 106, 110] and Fewell et al.[31] looked at the effects of PEEP on left ventricular mechanics in dogs and in patients with noncardiogenic pulmonary edema, and concluded that cardiac output decreased because of decreased venous return. Decreased left ventricular compliance secondary to septal shift from the right to the left ventricular cavity may also decrease cardiac output in patients with severe pulmonary arterial hypertension and high right ventricular pressures and ARDS.[46]

Although PEEP improves PaO_2, it does not decrease extravascular lung water.[25, 41, 78] Thus, PEEP treats the hypoxemic manifestations of ARDS without altering the formation or clearance of edema. It is also important to remember that a PEEP-induced decrease in cardiac output decreases the amount of calculated shunt, so shunt fraction should not be followed as the sole indicator of disease progression (Fig. 18–7).[55]

Fluids. Increased permeability of the alveolocapillary membrane means that pulmonary edema occurs in the presence of normal or even low capillary pressures.[98, 99] Experiments have shown that the amount of edema fluid can be decreased experimentally by lowering left atrial pressure to below normal values (Fig. 18–8).[78, 98] This means that pulmonary arterial wedge pressures should be monitored closely, and normal to below-normal pressure should be maintained to ensure that the amount of edema fluid is minimized. Measured cardiac output must also be adequate, which can be confirmed by following clinical indicators of tissue oxygenation such as urine flow, mental status, and arterial pH.

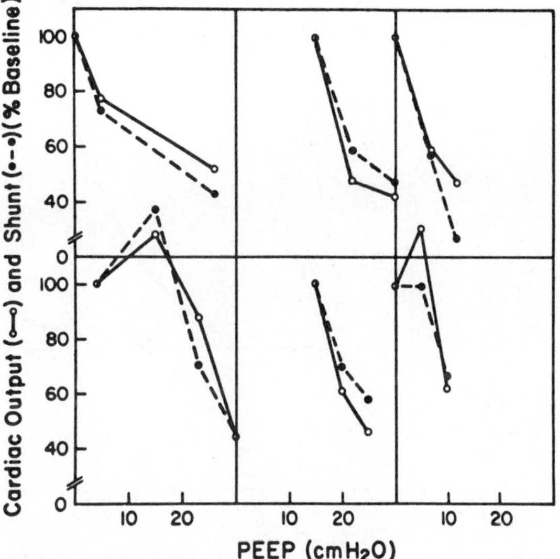

Figure 18–7. The relationship between changes in cardiac output and shunt is shown in six patients with adult respiratory distress syndrome. Note that as PEEP is increased, the cardiac output and shunt decrease in each patient. (From Dantzker et al.: Depression of cardiac output is a mechanism of shunt reduction in the therapy of acute respiratory failure. Chest 77:638, 1980. Reproduced with permission.)

Experimental and clinical studies to evaluate the role of albumin administration have not shown a beneficial effect from this therapy. In fact, albumin administration can increase edema in the presence of increased vascular permeability by raising vascular filling pressures.[78, 102]

Pharmacologic Agents. Antibiotics should be given promptly in any patient with ARDS who is suspected of having sepsis. If there is a possibility of a treatable, primary lung infection, diagnosis can be undertaken by open lung biopsy if the usual noninvasive methods prove diagnostically ineffective. If the patient

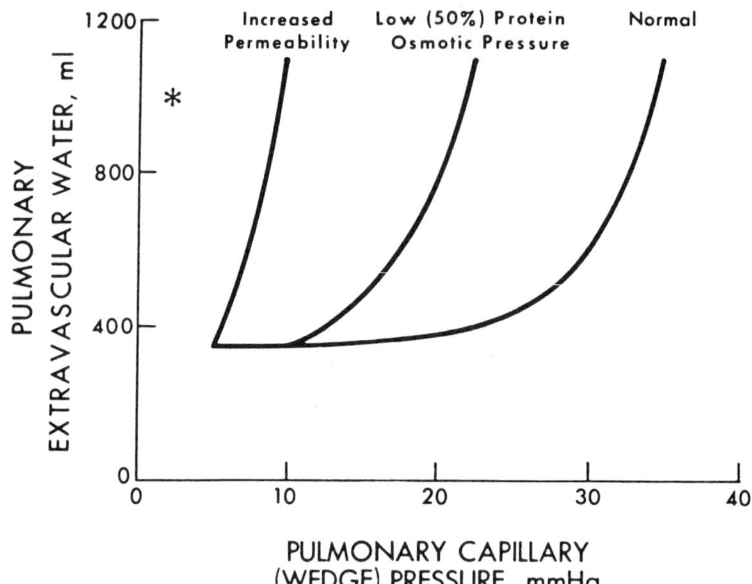

Figure 18–8. Schematic design showing the effect of wedge pressure on the amount of extravascular lung water (pulmonary edema). Note that when there is increased permeability and the wedge pressure increases, the amount of pulmonary edema increases exponentially. (From Hinshaw, H. C., and Murray, J. F. (eds.): Diseases of the Chest, 4th ed. Philadelphia, W. B. Saunders Co., 1980. Reproduced with permission.)

is too ill to tolerate a surgical procedure, broad-spectrum antibiotic coverage against likely pathogens should be administered.

Vasodepressors and vasodilators are useful because they can help maintain an adequate cardiac output and perhaps reduce overall fluid requirement. Nitroprusside, a vasodilator, can increase stroke volume and cardiac output and decrease PCW pressure in experimental models of ARDS.[77, 79, 80] However, nitroprusside also increases intrapulmonary shunting and thus often necessitates an increase in the F_{IO_2} or level of PEEP.[77, 80] Dopamine and dobutamine, vasopressors, increase stroke volume and cardiac output, and can also increase intrapulmonary shunting.[86] Since all these drugs increase cardiac output, this may be part of the explanation for their increasing the shunt. There may also be a direct effect from their action in vasodilating constricted pulmonary vessels.[55, 110] In some ARDS patients, these vasoactive drugs can be used to decrease fluid requirements and maintain cardiac output at a lower ventricular filling pressure.[110] Eventually, as more is known about the pathophysiology of the acute long injury, this class of drugs may be used for more specific therapy.

A recent report of pulmonary vascular obstruction in severe ARDS once again raises the issue of the possible role of anticoagulation therapy.[35] Although some pathologic studies of patients dying with ARDS demonstrate fibrin thrombi in small vessels of the lung, experimental studies of acute lung injury, in general, have shown minimal to no benefit from heparin.[35] In fact, in the national study to evaluate the role of extracorporeal membrane oxygenation (ECMO), the mortality rate in the ECMO-treated group was as high as the control group, and all the ECMO patients were heparinized.[50]

High-dose corticosteroids (30 mg/kg/day of methylprednisolone) may be useful in ameliorating the acute lung injury in endotoxin-induced ARDS, if the steroids are given very early.[90] A recent study of ARDS in septic patients documented a mild reduction in transvascular protein flux in some individuals treated with corticosteroids.[69, 89, 90, 91] The beneficial effect of the drugs may relate to the inhibition of complement activation and granulocyte aggregation.[15] No beneficial effect has been demonstrated in other cases of ARDS (e.g., aspiration, primary lung infection, acute pancreatitis).

Thus, the best available treatment for patients with noncardiogenic pulmonary edema is supportive. There is no specific therapy to restore normal vascular permeability once the lung is injured. Research is in progress on the role of superoxide dismutase and antiprostaglandin therapy, two specific treatments for lung injury.

Supportive therapy in patients with ARDS can result in survival rates of approximately

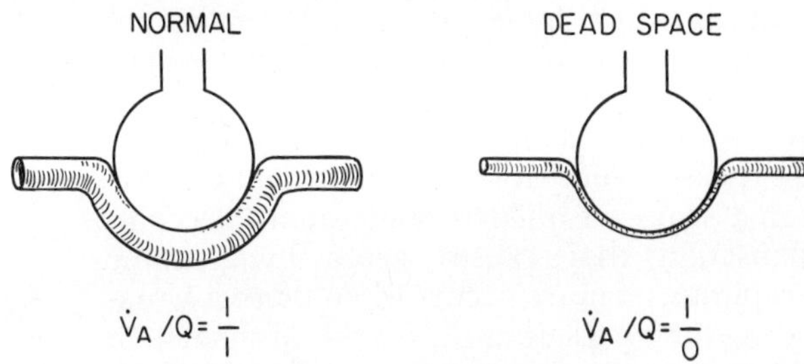

Figure 18–9. Alveoli that still receive oxygen flowing into the lungs, but have little or no blood perfusing them, cause dead-space ventilation. Gas transfer does not occur because there is no blood flowing by the airspace, and the ventilation-perfusion ratio is infinity (one part ventilation divided by zero part perfusion).

50 per cent.[42, 44] Those who survive acute respiratory failure usually recover normal lung function.[27, 51, 82]

DECOMPENSATED CHRONIC OBSTRUCTIVE PULMONARY DISEASE

In order to properly treat patients in respiratory failure from decompensated COPD, it is important to recall how normal arterial carbon dioxide tension is maintained by the balance between production ($\dot{V}CO_2$) and excretion or alveolar ventilation ($\dot{V}A$). These two factors determine the PCO_2 in arterial blood, as shown in this equation: $PaCO_2 = \frac{\dot{V}CO_2}{\dot{V}A}$. Thus, hypercapnia or an increased arterial PCO_2 can result from an increase in production of CO_2, a decrease in alveolar ventilation ($\dot{V}A$), or a combination of both.

Alveolar ventilation is that portion of minute ventilation (70–75%) that results in alveolar gas exchange. Minute ventilation ($\dot{V}E$), which is the tidal volume multiplied by the respiratory rate, is equal to the sum of alveolar ventilation ($\dot{V}A$) and dead-space ventilation ($\dot{V}D$): $\dot{V}E = \dot{V}A + \dot{V}D$. Dead-space ventilation is that fraction of the minute ventilation (usually 20–25%) that does not exchange gas, but remains in the conducting airways.

A decrease in alveolar ventilation can occur in one of two ways: (1) An absolute decrease in minute ventilation ($\dot{V}E$), which results in a decrease in alveolar ventilation ($\dot{V}A$), without a change in dead space: $\downarrow \dot{V}E = \downarrow \dot{V}A + \dot{V}D$. Clinically, a decrease in minute ventilation can occur either from a decrease in central respiratory drive (as in drug overdose) or from a neuromuscular disorder (as in myasthenia gravis or Guillain-Barré syndrome). (2) Alveolar ventilation may be decreased by ventilation-perfusion mismatch in the lung with a normal or elevated minute ventilation: $\dot{V}E$ (normal or $\uparrow$) $= \downarrow \dot{V}A$ plus $\uparrow \dot{V}D$. In this case, there is an increase in the measured dead space because alveoli that are ventilated are not perfused, as in emphysema with capillary obliteration (Fig. 18–9). A decrease in alveolar ventilation and an increase in dead-space ventilation occurs in many lung diseases, although COPD from emphysema is the classic example. Table 18–2 summarizes the different categories of dis-

Table 18–2. CAUSES OF HYPERCAPNIC RESPIRATORY FAILURE*

1. Central nervous system depression
   - A. Overdose of sedatives, narcotics, tranquilizers, anesthetics
   - B. CNS trauma, tumors, vascular accident
   - C. Primary hypoventilation ("Ondine's curse")
   - D. Obesity-hypoventilation (pickwickian) syndrome
   - E. Myxedema
2. Neuromuscular disorders
   - A. Infections—poliomyelitis, tetanus, botulism
   - B. Drug-induced—curare and cogeners, acetylcholinesterase inhibitors, antibiotics (colistin, polymyxin B, aminoglycosides)
   - C. Spinal cord tumors, trauma
   - D. Weakness or trauma of diaphragms or phrenic nerves
   - E. Guillain-Barré syndrome
   - F. Amyotrophic lateral sclerosis
   - G. Multiple sclerosis
   - H. Myasthenia gravis
   - I. Muscular dystrophy
3. Ventilation-perfusion mismatch
   - A. Foreign bodies in airway
   - B. Airway obstruction by tumors
   - C. Asthma
   - D. Infection and secretions
   - E. Emphysema
   - F. Chronic bronchitis
   - G. Bronchiolitis
   - H. Bronchiectasis

*Modified from Shibel, E. M., and Moser, K. M.: Respiratory Emergencies. St. Louis, C.V. Mosby Co., 1977.

eases in which hypercapnia is the major abnormality. In all patients with COPD, there is some contribution of chronic ventilation-perfusion imbalance, because the airway disease makes ventilation abnormal and emphysema causes capillary obliteration. Decompensation that causes acute hypercapnic respiratory failure occurs when there is worsening of ventilation-perfusion mismatch, a decrease in neuromuscular ventilatory effort, or a decrease in central ventilatory drive. In some patients, one, two, or all three of these factors may contribute to the acute hypercapnia.

Diagnosis

The diagnosis of decompensated chronic obstructive lung disease may be difficult because of the varied clinical presentations. The patient with decompensated COPD may be agitated and dyspneic and appear in acute distress with tachypnea, cyanosis, and marked use of the accessory muscles to breathe. On the other hand, such a patient may exhibit signs of carbon dioxide narcosis with somnolence, confusion, and even a normal respiratory rate. On physical examination, there may be increased blood pressure and tachycardia and marked pulsus paradoxus. On chest examination, the patient will have decreased breath sounds, a decreased inspiratory expiratory ratio, and a variable degree of wheezing. There may be signs of right-sided heart failure including prominent neck veins, hepatomegaly, peripheral edema, and a right-sided gallop.

Arterial blood gases must be measured to assess the severity of hypoxemia, hypercapnia, and acidosis.[67] Arterial blood gases usually show an acute respiratory acidosis with hypercapnia and hypoxemia. Since many patients may have elevated serum bicarbonate because they are chronically hypercapnic, the best way to determine whether there is a superimposed acute respiratory acidosis is to look at the nomograms defining the pH and bicarbonate limits associated with respiratory acidosis. These nomograms can reveal other metabolic disturbances such as new metabolic alkalosis with chronically abnormal arterial blood gases (Fig. 18–10).

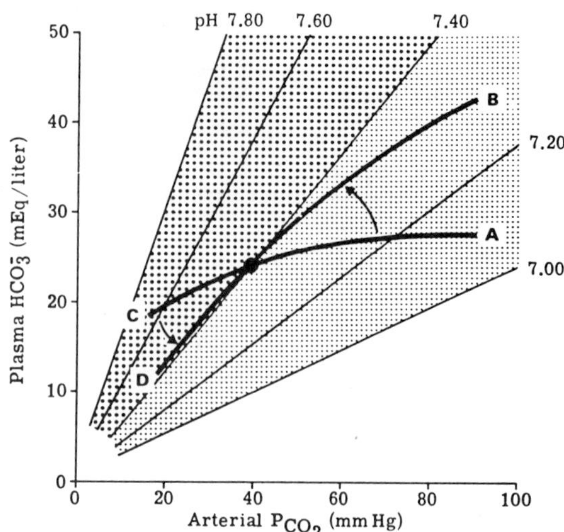

Figure 18–10. Pooled results from several studies of the effects of acute and chronic variations in arterial P_{CO_2} on plasma HCO_3^- and pH. When P_{CO_2} is raised acutely (acute respiratory acidosis), HCO_3^- and pH values lie along line *A*. After compensation by retention of HCO_3^- is complete (chronic respiratory acidosis), values lie along line *B*. When P_{CO_2} is lowered acutely (acute respiratory alkalosis), resulting HCO_3^- and pH values lie along line *C*. After compensation by rejection of HCO_3^- is complete (chronic respiratory alkalosis), values lie along line *D*. (From Murray, J. F.: The Normal Lung. Philadelphia, W. B. Saunders Co., 1976. Reproduced with permission.)

Causes of Decompensation in COPD

Patients with COPD decompensate and develop acute respiratory failure because of the following clinical problems: (1) worsening airway obstruction, (2) a new parenchymal pulmonary process, (3) muscle fatigue, and/or (4) decreased central ventilatory drive.

More severe airway obstruction often develops when patients develop a superimposed acute viral or bacterial bronchitis. Clinically, this is usually manifest by increased sputum production, change in sputum color, and fever without other objective evidence of a bacterial infection.[38, 101] There may also be more dyspnea, and the pulmonary function tests of airflow (forced expiratory volume in one second and forced vital capacity) will tend to be decreased. In a recent study of acute exacerbations of airway obstruction in patients with COPD, only 20 per cent of these episodes were proved to be associated with viral infections, and the latter seemed to predispose to subsequent bacterial infections.[94] The cause for most of these exacerbations of airway obstruction is unknown, although some patients seem to develop more obstruction because of changes in the weather, exposure to a seasonal allergen, or failure to comply with their prescribed medical therapy.

Pneumonia can lead to respiratory failure in COPD patients. The most common organisms found are *Streptococcus pneumoniae* and *Hemophilus influenzae*, although sputum cultures and blood cultures should always be obtained to discover the pathogen.[38]

Another clinical cause of a parenchymal process and decompensation in COPD patients is pulmonary thromboembolism. Postmortem studies of patients with COPD report that 28 to 51 per cent have thromboemboli.[9, 53, 76] However, in a recent prospective study looking at deep vein thrombosis as a source of emboli in patients with COPD in acute respiratory failure, only four of 45 patients were found to have deep vein thrombosis, and two of the four developed the thrombosis during hospitalization.[76] Lippmann and Fein[53] described three patients with COPD who had pulmonary thromboembolism, and these represented 18 per cent of their emphysema patients hospitalized for acute exacerbations. Several studies in the past have found an incidence of pulmonary emboli of up to 30 per cent in COPD patients.[9, 88] Thus, the exact incidence of pulmonary thromboemboli as a cause of acute respiratory failure in COPD is still unclear.

Cardiogenic pulmonary edema causes a pulmonary parenchymal process and can occur in patients with COPD, causing pulmonary decompensation.[39] Various studies have found fairly normal left ventricular function in COPD patients when there is no history of valvular or ischemic heart disease.[11, 17, 19, 93] There is still controversy over whether right heart dysfunction also makes this population more prone to left ventricular failure. In any case, some patients with acute respiratory failure and COPD do have coexistent left heart failure. Diagnosis usually depends on measurement of pulmonary arterial wedge pressures, although interpretation of these pressures can be difficult because of large pleural pressure variations in the spontaneously breathing dyspneic patients in acute respiratory distress. Recent reports also demonstrate that noncardiogenic pulmonary edema may cause respiratory failure in COPD patients.[39, 97]

Acute muscle fatigue may contribute to respiratory failure. Hyperinflated lungs, a common finding in COPD, increase the elastic work of breathing because the inspiratory muscles have to contract throughout the whole breathing cycle.[6, 56, 83] Hypoxia also decreases the endurance of the muscles. Clinically, muscle fatigue can be detected by the development of rapid, shallow breathing; abdominal paradoxical motion; and alterations between predominantly rib-cage and predominantly abdominal displacements during inspiration (Fig. 18–11).[13, 56]

It has often been suggested that an acute decrease in ventilatory drive causes patients with COPD to develop hypercapnic respiratory failure.[49] This is partly based on evidence that many COPD patients have blunted ventilatory drives chronically.[66] However, when COPD patients develop acute hypercapnic respiratory failure, the latest evidence indicates that an acute decrease in ventilatory drive is not usually present. The rise in $PaCO_2$ that occurs with supplemental oxygen therapy is mostly related to increasing ventilation-perfusion mismatch that occurs with oxygen therapy.[7, 37, 71] Nevertheless, it is still true that some patients with COPD do have decreased ventilatory drive chronically, and use of sedative or tranquilizing drugs can further decrease ventilatory drive and precipitate acute hypercapnic respiratory failure.

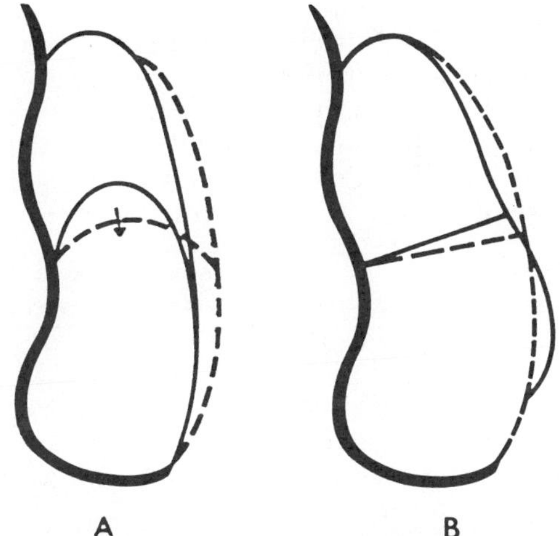

Figure 18–11. During normal inspiration, the diaphragm descends *(A)*. The thorax and abdomen move outward synchronously. On expiration, the chest and abdomen move inward synchronously. With asynchronous breathing *(B)*, an outward movement of the abdomen occurs during expiration. Asynchronous breathing probably results from inefficient position of the diaphragm plus maximal use of accessory muscles of respiration. (From Bone, R. C.: Treatment of respiratory failure due to advanced chronic obstructive lung disease. Arch. Intern. Med. 140:1019, 1980. Reproduced with permission. Copyright 1980, American Medical Association.)

Cardiac Effects of Acute Respiratory Failure in Patients with COPD

The major hemodynamic abnormality in COPD patients is pulmonary arterial hypertension.[10, 11, 45] Matthay and co-workers[62] evaluated chest radiographs of 61 patients with COPD and found an enlarged pulmonary artery (either a right descending artery greater than 16 mm or a left descending artery greater than 18 mm) in 45 of 46 patients with elevated pulmonary arterial pressures (Fig. 18–12). The chest roentgenogram is therefore a reasonably sensitive detector of pulmonary arterial hypertension in COPD patients.[59]

Overall, decompensated cor pulmonale or right ventricular dysfunction secondary to lung disease constitutes 30 to 40 per cent of clinical heart failure.[32] Detection of right heart failure by electrocardiographic criteria (Table 18–3) is possible only when severe cardiomegaly is present. There may be moderate increases in right ventricular mass that cannot be detected by the ECG because of the increase in total lung capacity or rotation of the heart.[36] More subtle signs of right ventricular hypertrophy or dilatation may be observed with echocardiography.

Patients with mild obstructive disease and mild hypoxemia usually have normal cardiac function at rest, with normal to slightly increased pulmonary arterial pressures.[11, 17] However, even in these mildly affected patients, exercise causes pulmonary arterial hypertension and right ventricular dysfunction.[11, 17, 93] In fact, about 50 per cent of patients with chronic bronchitis who had abnormal right ventricular ejection fractions with exercise but no clinical evidence of cor pulmonale at rest eventually developed acute respiratory failure and right heart failure.[11, 59] Thus, exercise may be a useful prognostic stress test to show which of these mildly affected patients are at risk of developing acute cor pulmonale with increases in hypoxemia or airway obstruction.

Patients with more severe obstructive lung disease, those with chronic hypercapnia and hypoxemia, have pulmonary hypertension at rest. Although their cardiac output remains normal at rest, it cannot increase during exercise.[63] Exercise again shows that these patients have abnormal cardiac function and that they are clearly at a higher risk of developing acute cor pulmonale with even slight increases in hypoxemia or airway obstruction.

Treatment

Oxygen. The most important therapy is to administer oxygen in order to relieve the hypoxemia and thereby decrease pulmonary arterial pressure. A decrease in pulmonary arterial pressure will decrease right ventricular afterload and thus increase cardiac output. The risk of fatal arrhythmias will also be reduced as the hypoxemia is relieved.[43]

As already discussed, oxygen therapy was believed to decrease the COPD patient's hy-

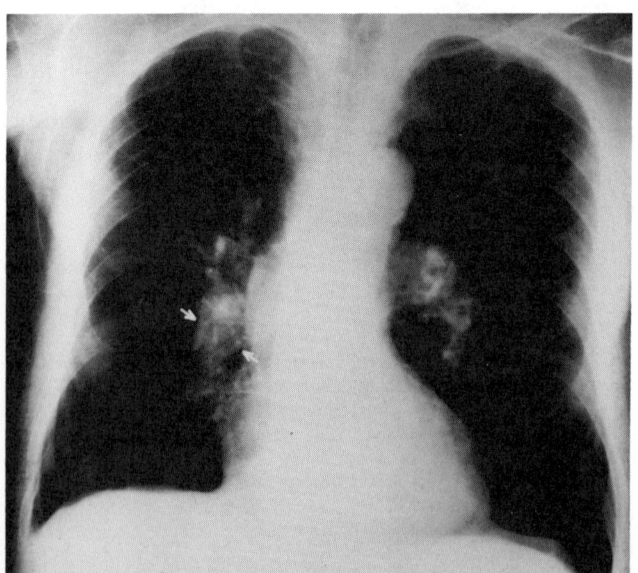

Figure 18–12. Arrows outline an enlarged right descending pulmonary artery, 22 mm in its widest diameter (a normal artery is ≤16 mm in width). Note also the enlarged left main pulmonary artery. (From Matthay, R. A., and Berger, H. J.: Cardiovascular performance in chronic obstructive pulmonary disease. Med. Clin. North Am. 65:496, 1977. Reproduced with permission.

Table 18–3. ELECTROCARDIOGRAPHIC CHANGES CHARACTERISTIC OF RIGHT VENTRICULAR ENLARGEMENT IN CHRONIC COR PULMONALE WITH OBSTRUCTIVE DISEASE OF THE AIRWAYS*

1. Isoelectric P waves in lead I or right axis deviation of the P vector
2. P-pulmonale pattern (an increase in P-wave amplitude in II, III, and aV_1)
3. Tendency for right axis deviation of the QRS
4. R/S amplitude ratio in $V_6<1$
5. Low-voltage QRS
6. S1-Q3 or S1-S2-S3 pattern
7. Incomplete (and rarely complete) right bundle branch block
8. R/S amplitude ratio in $V_4>1$
9. Marked clockwise rotation of the electrical axis
10. Occasional large Q wave or QS in the inferior or mid-precordial leads, suggesting healed myocardial infarction

*From Holford, F. D. *In* Fishman, A. P. (ed.): Pulmonary Diseases and Disorders. New York, McGraw-Hill Book Co., 1980. Copyright © 1980 by McGraw-Hill, Inc. Used by permission of McGraw-Hill Book Company.

poxic stimulus to breathe, resulting in carbon dioxide retention as PaO_2 rises with oxygen therapy.[49,65] It now appears that the respiratory drive is not reduced in most patients with acute respiratory failure. The $PaCO_2$ rises with oxygen therapy because there is a shift of ventilation to high ventilation-perfusion zones, or an increase in dead-space ventilation. Oxygen might have this effect by vasodilating vessels near alveoli that were receiving inadequate ventilation.[7,37] Nevertheless, whatever the exact mechanism, oxygen therapy can cause hypercapnia, which can lead to more respiratory acidosis and CO_2 narcosis.[65] Therefore, controlled, low-flow oxygen therapy, 1 to 4 liters per minute, should be instituted and arterial blood gases closely monitored.

Low-flow oxygen therapy usually results in a substantial rise in oxygen saturation (Fig. 18–13).[13,14] For example, with an increase in PaO_2 from 40 to 60 mm Hg, there will be a large increase in oxygen saturation because of the shape of the oxyhemoglobin dissociation curve. Small increases in PaO_2 on the steep portion of this curve result in larger increases in saturation. Patients who become more severely hypercapnic on low-flow oxygen therapy, and therefore manifest worsening respiratory acidosis, are candidates for intubation and mechanical ventilation if the overall prognosis warrants such aggressive treatment.[92] The oxygen therapy must not be withdrawn in an effort to decrease the hypercapnia, because the risk of hypoxemia is more dangerous than the hypercapnia.

Bronchodilators. Aerosolized bronchodilators, the beta-2-agonists (terbutaline, albuterol and fenoterol), have rapid onset of action, are potent bronchodilators, have minimal cardiovascular effects, and have more prolonged durations of action than aerosols such as isoproterenol.[107] These agents can be delivered via metered-dose inhalers, compressed-air–driven nebulizers, or intermittent positive-pressure devices. The last-named have come into disfavor because they are no more effective than other delivery systems, are more expensive and may increase the risk of pneumothorax.[47,54] Terbutaline may be given subcutaneously to patients with the goal of dilating small airways that aerosols cannot reach.[72] However, with parenteral administration these agents lose much of their beta-2 selectivity. Parenteral (subcutaneous) terbutaline can improve right and left ventricular ejection fraction, and decrease pulmonary and systemic vascular resistances.[59]

Beta-2-agonists may also have an effect additive to the bronchodilating effect of theophylline.[111] Theoretically, these agents provide stimulation of mucociliary transport[107] and thus help patients clear secretions.

Intravenous theophylline has been used

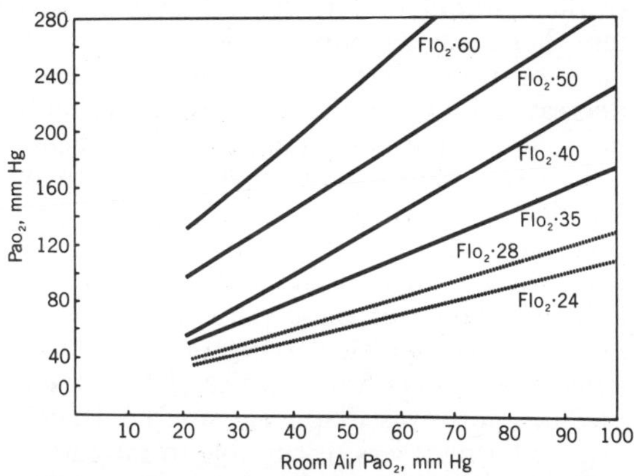

Figure 18–13. The relationship of PaO_2 to FIO_2 administered to patients with COPD. Each line gives the expected arterial oxygen tension for the FIO_2 administered. These lines were obtained in a study of patients with acute respiratory failure and stable patients with COPD. (From Bone, R. C.: Treatment of respiratory failure due to advanced chronic obstructive lung disease. Arch. Intern Med. 140:1020, 1980. Reproduced with permission. Copyright 1980, American Medical Association.)

for years in the treatment of acute and chronic bronchospasm. Much has been learned recently about the therapeutic-toxic dose range and about the mechanism by which it produces clinical improvement. Studies have shown that theophylline is metabolized more quickly by smokers than by nonsmokers, but patients with liver disease, congestive heart failure, severe hypoxia, or cor pulmonale require much smaller doses.[72, 75, 107] Generally, a maintenance dose of 0.4 mg per kg per hour is used in patients with severe COPD. Theophylline serum levels should be monitored closely to maintain a level of 10 to 20 μg per ml.[13, 107] Theophylline toxicity can be heralded by agitation, central nervous system symptoms, and gastrointestinal side effects. Grand mal seizures are the dreaded complication of theophylline toxicity and have a high mortality rate.[113] Minor symptoms of theophylline toxicity do not precede cardiac arrhythmias or seizures. Serum levels and not symptoms must be followed for protection from severe side effects.[13, 113]

Theophylline therapy has at least four mechanisms that may be beneficial to COPD patients with acute respiratory failure. First, theophylline produces bronchodilation by relaxing bronchial smooth muscle. How this effect is mediated, however, is unclear. Theophylline may inhibit phosphodiesterase (and thereby increase cyclic AMP) or it may act as a prostaglandin antagonist.[72] Second, theophylline stimulates the central nervous system, but most patients develop rapid tolerance of this effect.[81] Also, as mentioned, decreased CNS ventilatory drive is probably not so important in the pathogenesis of acute respiratory failure in COPD. Third, theophylline can improve right ventricular ejection fraction and decrease pulmonary arterial pressure in patients with COPD and cor pulmonale.[61] Some of these patients also show improved left ventricular performance.[60] Finally, preliminary work indicates that theophylline improves diaphragmatic contractility, rendering it less susceptible to fatigue.[6]

Corticosteroids. Studies have shown that treatment with methylprednisolone (0.5 mg/kg every 6 hr for 72 hr) results in a more rapid clinical recovery from acute respiratory failure in patients with decompensated COPD (without pneumonia, heart failure, or pulmonary embolism).[1] Corticosteroids increase the sensitivity of the airways to bronchodilation with beta-agonists[2] and can increase Po_2 in hypoxic patients.[107] Use for less than two weeks is probably free of serious toxicity.[96] Once a patient has stabilized, the corticosteroids can be decreased to a lower dose, or discontinued if objective assessment does not warrant their continued use.

Antibiotics. It is reasonable to administer antibiotics if there is clinical suspicion that bacterial infection has contributed to the events causing the acute respiratory failure.[9] Generally, *Streptococcus pneumoniae* and *Hemophilus influenzae* are the most common organisms found in the sputum of patients with COPD. Pathogenicity in these patients is unclear. Therefore, broad-spectrum antibiotics (ampicillin and tetracyline) are usually recommended.[13, 18] For *Hemophilus influenzae* resistant to ampicillin, trimethoprim sulfamethoxazole can be used. Sputum cultures, tracheal aspirates, and blood cultures are indicated to determine the infecting organisms in the presence of pneumonia or bronchitis unresponsive to empiric, broad-spectrum therapy.

Diuretics and Digitalis. Diuretics usually are not indicated for acute respiratory failure from decompensated COPD unless there is evidence of pulmonary congestion from left ventricular failure. Diuretics can be dangerous because they can decrease intravascular volume and thereby decrease cardiac output. Also, they can cause a hypokalemic metabolic alkalosis that may decrease ventilatory drive in some patients.

The use of digitalis for cor pulmonale usually is not recommended. Consensus favors its use only when the patient has left heart failure or arrhythmias that may be responsive to digitalis therapy.[34]

Treatment of Arrhythmias. Arrhythmias are frequent in COPD patients who are admitted for acute respiratory failure. In one report, 47 per cent of such patients had supraventricular arrhythmias; 70 per cent of those with ventricular arrhythmias died.[43] The conclusion of this study was to suggest continuous monitoring of all patients. Arrhythmias are usually caused by the respiratory failure, complicated by acid-base imbalances. Occasionally, the sympathomimetic drugs used to treat the airway obstruction aggravate or cause the arrhythmias. In general, treatment of the underlying respiratory failure should be continued. If the arrhythmias are potentially life threatening, the appropriate antiarrhythmic agents should be used (see Chapter 5).

Nutrition. Studies have shown that advanced COPD is associated with weight loss and that this has a negative effect on lung function. Patients with COPD who have lost weight have higher mortality rates and increased incidence of cor pulmonale.[44, 104] Most of the stable COPD patients lose weight not because of inadequate caloric intake but because of increased total energy requirements.[44] Patients in acute respiratory failure are often in worse nutritional condition, as they tend to be receiving only low caloric intravenous fluids. Individuals unable to eat should be given enteral alimentation if possible, and at least supplemental phosphorus if intravenous glucose alone is administered.[13] Hypophosphatemia is particularly detrimental to these patients, as it can impair oxygen delivery to tissues, and depresses the chemotaxis and phagocytosis of neutrophils.[20, 68]

Some reports indicate that over-vigorous nutritional supplement (more than 3000 calories per day), especially with high carbohydrate content, can result in a rise in CO_2 production.[4] This increase can cause persistent, severe hypercapnia in COPD patients, since they have a limited ability to increase their alveolar ventilation.[3] Some COPD patients have been successfully weaned from mechanical ventilators once their supplemental nutrition was adjusted into a more normal range.

Mechanical Ventilation. There are at least five indications for mechanical ventilation in patients with acute respiratory failure from

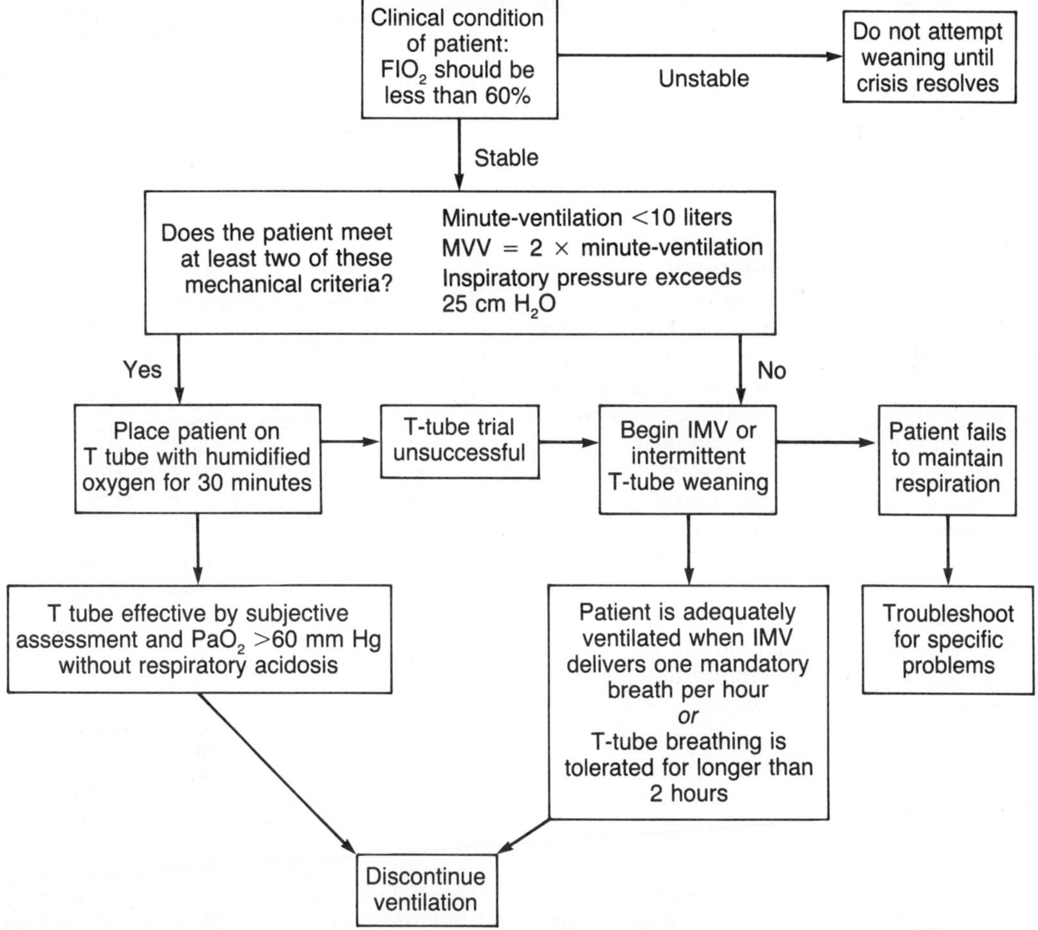

Figure 18–14. A flow chart on how to wean patients with COPD off mechanical ventilation. Note that only stable patients should be considered for weaning. (From Scoggin, C. H.: Weaning respiratory patients from mechanical support. J. Resp. Dis., 1:16, 1980. Reproduced with permission.)

COPD: (1) when low-flow oxygen does not raise the PaO_2 above 50 mm Hg, usually in patients with pneumonia or severe atelectasis; (2) a rising $PaCO_2$ that results in dangerous respiratory acidosis (pH <7.25); (3) somnolence from hypercapnia or some other process, such as a cerebrovascular accident with inability to protect the airway from aspiration; (4) an unmanageable quantity of secretions that the patient cannot adequately expectorate; (5) severe fatigue from the high work of breathing.

When COPD patients are being mechanically ventilated, it should be remembered that they are at increased risk of barotrauma because of their chronic lung disease, bullae, and nonhomogenous distribution of ventilation. In general, PEEP is contraindicated because the patients are already breathing at a high functional residual capacity. Flow rates should be adjusted to allow a longer period for expiration. Patients who are chronically hypercapnic should not be made eucapnic as this will cause a posthypercapnic metabolic alkalosis, and can depress ventilatory drive and cardiac output.

Patients can be gradually weaned from the ventilator once the acute pulmonary infection is clearing, the acute increase in airway resistance has returned toward baseline levels, the nutritional status is improved, and they are rested (Fig. 18–14).[85] They can be placed on a decreasing intermittent mandatory ventilation mode or can have increasingly longer T-piece trials during the weaning phase. When adequate arterial blood gases can be maintained with a minute ventilation of less than 10 to 12 liters for a few hours, most patients are ready for extubation.[85, 87]

Studies of acute exacerbations in patients with COPD show that the mortality rate ranges from 10 to 40 per cent.[5, 16, 73] Although a large majority of patients with decompensated COPD can recover from an episode of acute respiratory failure, many have a poor long-term prognosis.[5, 16, 110]

References

1. Albert, R. K., Martin, T. R., and Lewis, S. W.: Controlled clinical trial of methylprednisolone in patients with chronic bronchitis and acute respiratory insufficiency. Ann. Intern. Med. 92:753, 1980.
2. Arnaud, A., Vervloet, D., Dugue, P., et al.: Treatment of acute asthma: effect of intravenous corticosteroids and $beta_2$-adrenergic agonists. Lung 156:43, 1979.
3. Askanazi, J., Elwyn, D. H., and Silverberg, P. A.: Respiratory distress secondary to a high carbohydrate load: a case report. Surgery 87:596, 1980.
4. Askanazi, Rosenbaum, S. H., Hyman, A. J., et al.: Respiratory changes induced by the large glucose loads of total parenteral nutrition. J.A.M.A. 243:1444, 1980.
5. Asmundsson, T., and Kilburn, K. H.: Survival after acute respiratory failure. Ann. Intern. Med. 80:54, 1974.
6. Aubier, M., DeTroyer, A., Sampson, M., et al.: Aminophylline improves diaphragmatic contractility. N. Engl. J. Med. 305:249, 1981.
7. Aubier, M., Murciano, D., Fournier, M., et al.: Central respiratory drive in acute respiratory failure of patients with chronic obstructive pulmonary disease. Am. Rev. Respir. Dis. 122:191, 1980.
8. Aubier, M., Trippenbach, T., and Roussis, C.: Respiratory muscle fatigue during cardiogenic shock. J. Appl. Pnysiol. 51:499, 1981.
9. Baum, G., and Fisher, D.: Relationship of total pulmonary insufficiency with cor pulmonale and pulmonary emboli. Am. J. Med. Sci. 111:609, 1960.
10. Berger, H. J., and Matthay, R. A.: Noninvasive radiographic assessment of cardiovascular function in acute and chronic respiratory failure. Am. J. Cardiol. 47:950, 1981.
11. Berger, H. J., Matthay, R. A., Loke, J., et al.: Assessment of cardiac performance with quantitative radionuclide angiocardiography: right ventricular ejection fraction with refefence to findings in chronic obstructive pulmonary disease. Am. J. Cardiol. 41:897, 1978.
12. Bone, R. C.: Diagnosis of causes for acute respiratory distress by pressure-volume curves. Chest 70:740, 1976.
13. Bone, R. C.: Acute respiratory failure and chronic obstructive lung disease: recent advances. Symposium on chronic obstructive lung disease. Med. Clin. North Am. 65:563, 1981.
14. Bone, R. C., Pierce, A. K., and Johnson, R. L.: Controlled oxygen administration in acute respiratory failure in chronic obstructive pulmonary disease: a reappraisal. Am. J. Med. 65:896, 1978.
15. Brigham, K. L.: Mechanism of lung injury. Clin. Chest Med. 3:9, 1982.
16. Burk, R. H., and George, R. B.: Acute respiratory failure in chronic obstructive pulmonary disease. Arch. Intern. Med. 132:865, 1973.
17. Burrows, B., Kettel, L. J., Niden, A. H., et al.: Patterns of cardiovascular dysfunction in chronic obstructive lung disease. N. Engl. J. Med. 286:912, 1972.
18. Burrows, B., and Nevin, W.: Antibiotic management in patients with chronic bronchitis and emphysema. Ann. Intern. Med. 77:993, 1972.
19. Christianson, L. C., Shah, A., and Fisher, V. J.: Quantitative left ventricular cineangiography in patients with chronic obstructive pulmonary disease. Am. J. Med. 66:399, 1979.
20. Craddock, P. R., Yawata, Y., Van Santen, L., et al.: Acquired phagocyte dysfunction: a complication of the hypophosphatemia of parenteral hyperalimentation. N. Engl. J. Med. 290:1403, 1974.
21. Craven, K. D., Prewitt, R. M., and Wood, L. D. H.: Does the change in esophageal pressure (ΔPES) with PEEP accurately reflect the change in pressure

outside the pericardium (ΔPo). Fed. Proc. 39:1169, 1980 (abstr.).

22. Dantzker, D. R., Brook, C. J., Dehart, P., et al.: Ventilation-perfusion distributions in the adult respiratory distress syndrome. Am. Rev. Respir. Dis. 120:1039, 1979.
23. Dantzker, D. R., Lynch, J. P., and Weg, J. G.: Depression of cardiac output is a mechanism of shunt reduction in the therapy of acute respiratory failure. Chest 77:636, 1980.
24. Danzyl, D. F., and Thomas, D. M.: Nasotracheal intubations in the emergency department. Crit. Care Med. 8:677, 1980.
25. Demling, R. H., Staub, N. C., and Edmunds, L. H., Jr.: Effect of end-expiratory airway pressure on accumulation of extravascular lung water. J. Appl. Physiol. 38:907, 1975.
26. Dueck, R., Wagner, P. D., and West, J. B.: Effects of positive end-expiratory pressure on gas exchange in dogs with normal and edematous lungs. Anesthesiology 47:359, 1977.
27. Elliott, C. G., Morris, A. H., and Cengiz, M.: Pulmonary function and exercise gas exchange in survivors of adult respiratory distress syndrome. Am. Rev. Respir. Dis. 123:492, 1981.
28. Falke, K. J., Pontoppidan, H., Kumar, A., et al.: Ventilation with end-expiratory pressure in acute lung disease. J. Clin. Invest. 51:2315, 1972.
29. Fein, A., Grossman, R. F., Jones, J. G., et al.: The value of edema fluid protein measurement in patients with pulmonary edema. Am. J. Med. 67:32, 1979.
30. Ferrer, M. I.: Management of patients with cor pulmonale. Symposium on cardiac emergencies. Med. Clin. North Am. 63:251, 1979.
31. Fewell, J. E., Abendschein, D. R., Carlson, C. J., et al.: Continuous positive-pressure ventilation decreases right and left ventricular end-diastolic volumes in the dog. Circ. Res. 46:125, 1980.
32. Fishman, A. P.: Regulation of the pulmonary circulation. *In* Fishman, A. F. (ed.): Pulmonary Diseases and Disorders. New York, McGraw-Hill Book Co., 1980, pp. 397–409.
33. Flick, M. R., Hoeffel, J., and Staub, N. C.: Superoxide dismutase prevents increased lung vascular permeability after air emboli in unanesthetized sheep. Fed. Proc. 40:405, 1981 (abstr.).
34. Green, L. H., and Smith, T. W.: The use of digitalis in patients with pulmonary disease. Ann. Intern. Med. 87:459, 1977.
35. Greene, R., Zapol, W. M., Snider, M. T., et al.: Early bedside detection of pulmonary vascular occlusion during acute respiratory failure. Am. Rev. Respir. Dis. 124:593, 1981.
36. Gregoratos, G., Karliner, J. S., and Moser, K. M.: Mechanisms of disease and methods of assessment. *In* Moser, K. M. (ed): Pulmonary Vascular Diseases. New York, Marcel Dekker, 1979, pp. 279–340.
37. Guenard, H., Verhas, M., Todd-Prokopek, A., et al.: Effects of oxygen breathing on regional distribution of ventilation and perfusion in hypoxemic patients with chronic lung disease. Am. Rev. Respir. Dis. 125:12, 1982.
38. Gump, D. W., Phillips, C. A., Forsyth, B. R., et al.: Role of infection in chronic bronchitis. Am. Rev. Respir. Dis. 113:465, 1976.
39. Heffner, J. E., Silvers, G. W., and Petty, T. L.: Diagnosis of adult respiratory distress syndrome associated with underlying severe emphysema. Arch. Intern. Med. 141:1684, 1981.
40. Hinshaw, H. C., and Murray, J. F. (eds.): Respiratory failure. *In* Diseases of the Chest, 4th ed. Philadelphia, W. B. Saunders Co., 1980, pp. 955–1016.
41. Hopewell, P. C.: Failure of positive end-expiratory pressure to decrease lung water content in alloxan-induced pulmonary edema. Am. Rev. Respir. Dis. 120:813, 1979.
42. Hopewell, P. C., and Murray, J. F.: The adult respiratory distress syndrome. Annu. Rev. Med. 27:343, 1976.
43. Hudson, L. D., Kurt, T. L., Petty, T. L., et al.: Arrhythmias associated with acute respiratory failure in patients with chronic airway obstruction. Chest 63:661, 1973.
44. Hunter, A. M. B., Carey, M. A., and Larsh, H.: The nutritional status of patients with chronic obstructive pulmonary disease. Am. Rev. Respir. Dis. 124:376, 1981.
45. Inter-Society Commission for Heart Disease Resources: Primary prevention of pulmonary heart disease. Circulation 41:A17, 1970.
46. Jardin, F., Farcot, J. C., Boisante, L., et al.: Influence of positive end-expiratory pressure on left ventricular performance. N. Engl. J. Med. 304:387, 1981.
47. Karantzky, M. S.: Asthma mortality associated with pneumothorax and IPPB. Lancet 1:828, 1975.
48. Katz, S., Aberman, A., Frand, U. I., et al.: Heroin pulmonary edema: evidence for increased pulmonary capillary permeability. Am. Rev. Respir. Dis. 106:472, 1972.
49. Kepron, W., and Cherniack, R. M.: The ventilatory response to hypercapnia and to hypoxemia in chronic obstructive lung disease. Am. Rev. Respir. Dis. 108:843, 1973.
50. Kirby, R. R.: Membrane oxygenators: what role (if any) in acute ventilatory insufficiency? Crit. Care Med. 6:19, 1978.
51. Lakshminarayan, S., Stanford, R. E., and Petty, T. L.: Prognosis after recovery from adult respiratory distress syndrome. Am. Rev. Respir. Dis. 113:7, 1976.
52. Laver, M. B., Strauss, H. W., and Pohost, G. M.: Right and left ventricular geometry: adjustments during acute respiratory failure. Crit. Care Med. 7:509, 1979.
53. Lippmann, M., and Fein, A.: Pulmonary embolism in the patient with chronic obstructive pulmonary disease. Chest 79:39, 1981.
54. Loren, M., Chai, A., Miklich, D., et al.: Comparison between single nebulization and intermittent positive-pressure in asthmatic children with severe bronchospasm. Chest 72:145, 1977.
55. Lynch, J. P., Mhyre, J. G., and Dantzker, D. R.: Influence of cardiac output on intrapulmonary shunt. J. Appl. Physiol. 46:315, 1979.
56. Macklem, P. T.: Respiratory muscles: the vital pump. Chest 78:753, 1980.
57. Massie, B. M., and Chatterjee, K.: Vasodilator therapy of pump failure complicating acute myocardial infarction. Med. Clin. North Am. 63:25, 1979.
58. Matthay, M. A., and Hopewell, P. C.: The adult respiratory distress syndrome: pathogenesis and treatment. Curr. Pulmonol. 3:1, 1981.

59. Matthay, R. A., and Berger, H. J.: Cardiovascular performance in chronic obstructive pulmonary disease. Symposium on obstructive lung diseases. Med. Clin. North Am. 65:489, 1981.
60. Matthay, R. A., Berger, H. J., Davies, R., et al.: Prolonged improvement in cardiac performance by oral long-acting theophylline in chronic obstructive pulmonary disease. Circulation 60:107, 1979 (abstr.).
61. Matthay, R. A., Berger, H. J., Loke, J., et al.: Effects of aminophylline upon right and left ventricular performance in chronic obstructive pulmonary disease. Noninvasive assessment by radionuclide angiocardiography. Am. J. Med. 65:903, 1978.
62. Matthay, R. A., Schwartz, M. I., Ellis, J. H., Jr., et al.: Pulmonary artery hypertension in chronic obstructive pulmonary disease: chest radiographic assessment. Invest Radiol., 16:95, 1981.
63. McFadden, E. R., and Braunwald, E.: Cor pulmonale and pulmonary thromboembolism. *In* Braunwald, E. (ed.): Heart Disease. A Textbook of Cardiovascular Medicine. Philadelphia, W. B. Saunders Co., 1980, pp. 1643–1680.
64. McIntyre, R. W., Laws, A. K., and Ramachandran, P. R.: Positive expiratory pressure plateau: improved gas exchange during mechanical ventilation. Can. Anaesth. Soc. J. 16:477, 1969.
65. Mithoefer, J. C., Karetzky, M. S., and Mead, G. D.: Oxygen therapy in respiratory failure. N. Engl. J. Med. 277:947, 1967.
66. Mountain, R., Zwillich, C., and Weil, J.: Hypoventilation in obstructive lung disease. N. Engl. J. Med. 298:521, 1978.
67. Murray, J. F.: The Normal Lung: The Basis for Diagnosis and Treatment of Pulmonary Disease. Philadelphia, W. B. Saunders Co., 1976, pp. 199–222.
68. Newman, J. H., Neff, T. A., and Ziporin, P.: Acute respiratory failure associated with hypophosphatemia. N. Engl. J. Med. 296:1101, 1977.
69. Nicholson, D. P.: Glucocorticoids in the treatment of shock and the adult respiratory distress syndrome. Symposium on adult respiratory distress syndrome. Clin. Chest Med 3:121, 1982.
70. Noble, W. H., Kay, J. C., and Obdrzalek, J.: Lung mechanics in hypervolemic pulmonary edema. J. Appl. Physiol. 38:681, 1975.
71. Pardy, R. L., Rwington, R. N., Millic-Emili, J., et al.: Control of breathing in chronic obstructive pulmonary disease. The effect of histamine inhalation. Am. Rev. Respir. Dis. 125:6, 1982.
72. Patterson, J. W., Woolcock, A. J., and Shenfield, G. M.: Bronchodilator drugs. Am. Rev. Respir. Dis. 120:1149, 1979.
73. Petheram, I. S., and Branthwaite, M. A.: Mechanical ventilation for pulmonary disease, a six year survey. Anesthesiology 35:467, 1980.
74. Petty, T. L.: Adult respiratory distress syndrome: definition and historical perspective. Symposium on adult respiratory distress syndrome. Clin. Chest Med. 3:3, 1982.
75. Powell, J. R., Vozeh, S., Hopewell, P. C., et al.: Theophylline disposition in acutely ill hospitalized patients. Am. Rev. Respir. Dis. 118:229, 1978.
76. Prescott, S. M., Richards, K. L., Tikoff, G., et al.: Venous thromboembolism in decompensated chronic obstructive pulmonary disease. A prospective study. Am. Rev. Respir. Dis. 123:32, 1981.
77. Prewitt, R. M., Greenberg, D., Mackeen, B., et al.: Effects of nitroprusside on left ventricular mechanics in dogs with pulmonary capillary leak. Fed. Proc. 38:500, 1979 (abstr.).
78. Prewitt, R. M., McCarthy, J., and Wood, L. D. H.: Treatment of acute low pressure pulmonary edema in dogs. J. Clin. Invest. 67:409, 1981.
79. Prewitt, R. M., Oppenheimer, L., Sutherland, J. B., et al.: Acute effects of nitroprusside on hemodynamics and oxygen exchange in patients with hypoxemic respiratory failure. Am. Rev. Respir. Dis. 121:179, 1980 (abstr.).
80. Prewitt, R. M., and Wood, L. D. H.: Nitroprusside increases pulmonary shunt and improves left ventricular function in dogs with oleic acid pulmonary edema. Am. Rev. Respir. Dis. 117:382, 1978 (abstr.).
81. Ritchie, J. M.: The xanthines. *In* Goodman, L. S., and Gilman, A. (eds.): The Pharmacological Basis of Therapeutics, 5th ed. New York, Macmillan Publishing Co., 1975, pp. 367–378.
82. Rotman, H. H., Lavelle, T. F., Jr., Dimcheff, D. G., et al.: Long-term physiologic consequences of the adult respiratory distress syndrome. Chest 72:190, 1977.
83. Roussos, C., Fixley, M., Gross, D., et al.: J. Appl. Physiol. 46:897, 1979.
84. Roussos, C. S., and Macklem, P. T.: Diaphragmatic fatigue in man. J. Appl. Physiol. 43:189, 1977.
85. Sahn, S. A., and Lakshminarayan, S.: Bedside criteria for discontinuation of mechanical ventilation. Chest 63:1002, 1973.
86. Santman, F. W., Prewitt, R. M., Sutherland, J. B., et al.: Effect of dopamine on cardiac output and left ventricular mechanics in dogs. Fed. Proc. 39:708, 1980 (abstr.).
87. Scoggin, C. H.: Guidelines for discontinuing ventilation weaning respiratory patients from mechanical support. J. Resp. Dis., 1:13, 1980.
88. Scott, K. W. M.: A clinicopathological study of fatal chronic airway obstruction. Thorax 31:693, 1976.
89. Shine, K. I., Kuhn, M., Young, L. S., et al.: Aspects of the management of shock. Ann. Intern. Med. 93:723, 1980.
90. Sibbald, W., Holliday, R., and Driedger, A.: Corticosteroids in the prevention and reversal of microvascular injury. *In* Conference on Mechanisms of Lung Microvascular Injury. Ann. N.Y. Acad. Sci. 384:496, 1982.
91. Sladen, A.: Methylprednisolone. Pharmacologic doses in shock lung syndrome. J. Thorac. Cardiovasc. Surg. 71:800, 1976.
92. Sluiter, H. H., Blokziji, E. J., Van Dijl, W., et al.: Conservative and respirator treatment of acute respiratory insufficiency in patients with chronic obstructive lung disease. Am. Rev. Respir. Dis. 105:932, 1972.
93. Slutsky, R. A., Ackerman, W., Karliner, J. S., et al.: Right and left ventricular dysfunction in patients with chronic obstructive lung disease. Am. J. Med. 68:197, 1980.
94. Smith, C. B., Golden, C. A., Kanner, R. E., et al.: Association of viral and *Mycoplasma pneumoniae*

infections with acute respiratory illness in patients with chronic pulmonary diseases. Am. Rev. Respir. Dis. 121:225, 1980.
95. Snider, M. T., Rie, M. A., Bingham, J. B., et al.: Right ventricular performance in ARDS: radionuclide scintiscan and thermal dilution studies. Am. Rev. Respir. Dis. 121:192, 1980 (abstr.).
96. Spiegel, R. J., Oliff, A. I., Burton, J., et al.: Adrenal suppression after short-term corticosteroid therapy. Lancet 1:630, 1979.
97. Sprung, C. L., Rackow, E. C., Fein, I. A., et al.: The spectrum of pulmonary edema: differentiation of cardiogenic, intermediate and noncardiogenic forms of pulmonary edema. Am. Rev. Respir. Dis. 124:718, 1981.
98. Staub, N. C.: Pulmonary edema due to increased microvascular permeability to fluid and protein. Circ. Res. 43:143, 1978.
99. Staub, N. C.: Pulmonary edema. Physiol. Rev. 54:679, 1974.
100. Suter, P. M., Fairley, H. B., and Isenberg, M. D.: Optimum end-expiratory airway pressure in patients with acute pulmonary failure. N. Engl. J. Med. 292:284, 1975.
101. Tager, I., and Speizer, F. E.: Role of infection in chronic bronchitis. N. Engl. J. Med. 292:563, 1975.
102. Tranbaugh, R. F., Elings, V. B., Christensen, J., et al.: Pulmonary effects of massive crystalloid infusion and lowered colloid osmotic pressure in severely traumatized patients. Chest 80:372, 1981 (abstr.).
103. Uzawa, T., and Ashbaugh, D. G.: Continuous positive-pressure breathing in acute hemorrhagic pulmonary edema. J. Appl. Physiol. 26:427, 1969.
104. Vandenbergh, E., van de Woestijne, K. P., and Gyselen, A.: Weight changes in the terminal stages of chronic obstructive pulmonary disease. Am. Rev. Respir. Dis. 95:556, 1967.
105. Wagner, P. D., Laravuso, R. B., Uhl, R. R., et al.: Distributions of ventilation-perfusion ratios in acute respiratory failure. Chest 65:325, 1974.
106. Wally, K., Prewitt, R. M., and Wood, L. D. H.: Reduced end-systolic volume (ESV) during reduced resistive afterload is not due to increased contractility. Fed. Proc. 39:814, 1980 (abstr.).
107. Weinberger, M., Hendeles, L., and Ahrens, R.: Pharmacologic management of reversible obstructive airways disease. Symposium on chronic obstructive lung disease. Med. Clin. North Am. 65:579, 1980.
108. Wilen, S., Rubin, J., and Lyons, H.: Vascular leakage of protein in noncardiac and cardiac pulmonary edema. Circulation 52:11, 1975.
109. Witschi, H. R., Haschek, W. M., Klein-Szanto, A. J. P., et al.: Potentiation of diffuse lung damage by oxygen: determining variables. Am. Rev. Respir. Dis. 23:98, 1981.
110. Wood, L. D. H., and Prewitt, R. M.: Cardiovascular management in acute hypoxemic respiratory failure. Am. J. Cardiol. 47:963, 1981.
111. Wyatt, R., Weinberger, M., and Hendeles, L.: Oral theophylline dosages for the management of chronic asthma. J. Pediatr. 92:125, 1978.
112. Zapol, W. M., Kobayashi, K., and Snider, M. T.: Vascular obstruction causes pulmonary hypertension in severe acute respiratory failure. Chest 71:306, 1977.
113. Zwillich, C. W., Sutton, F. D., Jr., Neff, T. A., et al.: Theophylline-induced seizures in adults—correlation with serum concentrations. Ann. Intern. Med. 82:784, 1975.

INDEX

Note: Page numbers in *italics* indicate illustrations; page numbers followed by t indicate tables.